Clinical Radiology in the Tropics

Peter Cockshott
Professor of Radiology, McMaster University

Howard Middlemiss
Professor of Radiology, University of Bristol

CHURCHILL LIVINGSTONE
EDINBURGH LONDON AND NEW YORK 1979

CHURCHILL LIVINGSTONE
Medical Division of Longman Group Limited

Distributed in the United States of America by Churchill Livingstone Inc., 19 West 44th Street, New York, N.Y. 10036 and by associated companies, branches and representatives throughout the world.

First published 1979

ISBN 0 443 01676 3 (cased)
ISBN 0 443 01987 8 (ELBS)

British Library Cataloguing in Publication Data

Clinical radiology in the tropics.
1. Diagnosis, Radioscopic—Addresses, essays, lectures 2. X-rays—Addresses, essays, lectures 3. Tropical medicine—Addresses, essays, lectures
I. Cockshott, Peter II. Middlemiss, Howard
616.07'572'0913 RC78 79-40190

Printed in Great Britain by Butler & Tanner Ltd, Frome and London

Preface

This book is written primarily for those working in the tropical world, though we expect that the contents will be useful to radiologists in other climes who have patients who come from, or have lived in the tropics.

We recognise that medical and radiological facilities are limited in many tropical areas and that for many years to come there will be a shortage of radiologists there. Therefore we have attempted to provide information in a manner that will be helpful to both radiologists and to those clinicians who have perforce to conduct their own radiological studies and interpretations. It is for this reason that we have chosen to organise the contents by body systems since this is the usual way that a clinical problem declares itself—symptoms and signs referrable to an organ or system. For those preferring an aetiological approach we believe that the index will cater for their needs. To avoid repetition on the geographic prevalence or life cycles of parasites, such information is covered under the main body system affected in clinical practice.

The primary reference sources on tropical disorders are dispersed in many journals printed in several languages and for these reasons inevitably difficult to obtain in most places. Accordingly we have not been comprehensive in our coverage but have quoted mainly helpful references.

What to include in the contents posed difficulties. Obviously a disorder had to have radiological features. If a disease was ubiquitous, well known, and posed similar clinical and radiographical changes everywhere we have omitted it since standard texts already contain excellent descriptions of the radiological management. We have, however, not confined ourselves to the maladies that make up what was traditional 'tropical medicine', but have also considered entities that are seen in the tropics because of genetic, environmental and unexplained factors.

Both authors have experience of work in tropical countries; both have previously written relatively extensively on the radiological features of conditions occurring in the tropics, and have previously collaborated over a book with similar objectives (*Tropical Radiology* (1961) Ed. Middlemiss, H. London: Heinemann). But obviously no two authors can hope to have a comprehensive global grasp of all the clinical problems seen in the tropics in which radiology has a useful role. There are obvious omissions and some conditions are too briefly discussed. Personal idiosyncrasies and experience have doubtless influenced our selection of topics. Our choice has also been affected by financial constraints. A larger book would be expensive and defeat our objective of being helpful at the x-ray department level.

Many of our friends in the tropics have been our guides and informants over the years and their experience has remedied some of our deficiencies of experience. We have been lucky to have illustrative material provided by many colleagues who are acknowledged in the text. We count ourselves fortunate in having contributions from several radiologists working in the tropics who have made certain fields particularly their own.

1979

P.C.
H.M.

We dedicate this book to Colina and Mary who have endured our many absences abroad over the years and yet have at all times given us encouragement and advice.

Acknowledgements

We wish to express our thanks to the many individuals and organisations that have provided assistance to make this work possible.

The World Health Organisation, through Professor Thomas Lambo (Deputy Director) and Dr. W. Seelentag (Chief Officer, Radiation Medicine) have given us encouragement and provided facilities that have broadened our experience of tropical disorders.

One of us (W.P.C.), who recently spent a sabbatical year in Africa, the South Pacific and the Far East, gratefully acknowledges the support from the Picker Foundation and McMaster University and McMaster University Medical Center that made this possible.

A grant from the Commonwealth Fund of New York helped to defray production, photographic and secretarial expenses.

Finally, as stated in the preface, this work would have been impossible without the kind help of colleagues all over the world who have educated us and provided us with radiographs over many years.

Contributing authors

Professor *Stanley Bohrer*, MD, MPH, FMCR, Rochester, New York
Formerly Professor of Radiology, University of Ibadan

Professor *D. Cabrera*, MD, MPH, TM, Manila, Philippines
Dean, Institute of Public Health, University of the Philippines

Professor *S. Chawla*, MB, BS, DMRD, New Delhi, India
Professor of Radiology, Lady Hardinge Medical College

Professor *T. M. Kolawole*, MB, BS, DMRD, FRCR, Ibadan, Nigeria
Professor of Radiology, University of Ibadan

Professor *S. B. Lagundoye*, MB, BS, DMRD, FMCR, Ibadan, Nigeria
Professor of Radiology, University of Ibadan

Dr. *James Lambeth*, MD, FACR, Papaikou, Hawaii
Formerly Faculty at University of Saigon and University of Malaya

Dr. *James S. Macdonald*, MB, ChB, MRCPE, FRCR, London
Director of Radiology, The Royal Marsden Hospital
Honorary Senior Lecturer to the Institute of Cancer Research

Professor *Joginder Singh*, MB, BS, DMRD, Kuala Lumpur, Malaysia
Professor Madya of Radiology, University of Malaya

Dr *T. M. Walker*, MB, BS, DMRD, FRCR,
Lately Senior Lecturer in Radiology, University of the West Indies

Professor *Leslie R. Whittaker*, MB, FRCR, Nairobi, Kenya
Professor of Radiology, University of Nairobi

Contents

Introduction xi

Chapter 1
Soft tissues

Calcification in the soft tissues 1
- Injection site calcification 1
- Tumoral calcinosis 1
- Myositis ossificans 3
- Guinea worm 5
- Loiasis 6
- Onchocerciasis 7
- Wuchereria and Brugia filariasis 7
- Sarcocystis 7
- Sparganosis 8
- Cysticercosis 9
- Porocephalosis—Pentastomiasis 10
- Unknown calcifications 12

Pyomyositis 12
Subcutaneous lesions 14
Lymphoedema 15
- Filarial lymphoedema 16

Kaposi's sarcoma 17

Chapter 2
Bone diseases

growth and maturation — Professor *S. P. Bohrer* 22
Determining population norms
Effects of malnutrition — Professor *S. P. Bohrer* 23
Deficiency rickets 24
Endemic fluorosis 24
Bone infections 26
- Haematogenous osteomyelitis 27
- Bone and joint tuberculosis 27
- Tropical ulcer 34
- Brucellosis 36
- Melioidosis 38
- Klebsiella osteomyelitis 39
- Granuloma inguinale osteomyelitis 40
- Salmonella vertebral osteomyelitis 41
- Treponematosis 42
- Leprosy 46
- Fungal osteitis due to yeasts 50
- Mycetoma 56
- Sporotrichosis 59
- Aspergillus bone infections 60
- Rhinophycomycosis 61
- Rhinoscleroma 62
- Viral bone infections 63
- Parasitic bone infection 65
- Hydatid disease 66

Tetanus—fractures 67
Ainhum 69
Miscellaneous skeletal topics 69
- Anatomic anomalies 69
- Carpal fusions 70
- Congenital dislocation of the hip 70
- Hallux valgus 71
- Blount's disease 71
- Ectopic nasal dentition 72
- Pregnancy pubic changes 72
- Frontal mucocele 72

Haemoglobin diseases 73
- Sickle cell anaemia 74
- Hb SC disease 76
- Thalassaemia 77
- Hb E/Thalassaemia 79
- Hb S/Thalassaemia 79

Bone tumours 81
Arthritis in the tropics 85
- Septic arthritis — Professor *S. P. Bohrer* 85
- Guinea worm arthritis 85
- Rheumatoid arthritis — Professor *S. P. Bohrer* 86
- Acute tropical polyarthritis — Professor *S. P. Bohrer* 87

Chapter 3
Alimentary system

Cancrum oris 88
Chagasic mega-oesophagus 88
Corrosive oesophageal strictures 89
Peptic ulceration 90
Infective and inflammatory lesions 92
- Anisakiasis 92
- Hookworm 94
- Strongyloidiasis 95
- Ascariasis 97
- Giardiasis 98
- Intestinal capillariasis — Professor *D. Cabrera* 101
- Taenia saginata 101
- Taenia solium 103
- Other cestodes 103
- Typhoid 103
- Intestinal tuberculosis — Professor *S. Chawla* 105
- Intestinal schistosomiasis 110
- Helminthoma 112
- Amoebiasis 113
- Lymphogranuloma venereum 117
- Chagasic megacolon 119
- Fungal inflammatory bowel disease 119
- Trichuris trichiuria 119
- Crohn's disease and ulcerative colitis 120
- Non-specific colitis 120

Acute intestinal obstruction 122
- Obstructed hernia 122
- Intussusception 122
- Sigmoid volvulus 122
- Volvulus of the small bowel 124

Idiopathic tropical sprue 125
Disaccharide deficiency 126
Diverticular disease 126
Malignancy of the gastro-intestinal tract 127
Mediterranean lymphoma — Dr. *J. S. Macdonald* 129
Biliary calculi 130

Amoebic liver abscess 130
Hydatid liver disease 133
Biliary infections 136
Biliary ascariasis 136
Clonorchiasis—Opisthorchiasis 137
Liver flukes 139
Portal hypertension 140
Pyogenic cholangitis 142
Hepatic malignancy 142
Hepatoma — Professor *S. B. Lagundoye* 142
Pancreatic lithiasis 142
The spleen 145
Tropical splenomegaly syndrome 148

Chapter 4 Respiratory system

Eosinophilia and the lung 149
Filarial disease 149
Larval ascariasis 150
Pulmonary capillariasis 152
Strongyloides stercoralis 153
Gnathostomiasis 153
Pneumonias 154
Measles pneumonia 154
Plague 154
Leptospirosis — Dr. *T. M. Walker* 156
Melioidosis — Dr. *James Lambeth* 158
Nocardiosis 159
Pulmonary mycoses 160
Tuberculosis — Professor *T. M. Kolawole* 160
Paragonimiasis 162
Hydatid disease 165
Amoebic involvement 167
Malaria–'shock lung' 169
Parasitic lung infarction 169
Respiratory distress syndrome 170
Black fat lipid pneumonia 170
Pulmanary neoplasia 170
Malignant trophoblastic disease 171
Rib and extrapleural lesions 173

Chapter 5 Cardiovascular system

Malnutrition, kwashiorkor and the heart 175
Anaemia and the heart 175
Sickle cell anaemia 177
Hypertension 177
Annular subvalvar ventricular aneurysms 178
Idiopathic cardiomegaly 182
Endomyocardial fibrosis 184
Chagas' cardiomyopathy 188
African trypanosomiasis 190
Pulmonary hypertension in the tropics 190
Altitude pulmonary hypertension 191
Domestic air pollution 191
Schistosomal pulmonary hypertension 191
'Filarial' pulmonary hypertension 193
Trophoblastic pulmonary hypertension 193
Pulmonary embolism 193
Cardiac hydatid disease 194
Cardiac Burkitt's lymphoma 195
Pericardial diseases 196
Aortic pan arteritis 197
Tuberculous aortitis and aneurysms 201
Idiopathic peripheral gangrene 201
Buerger's disease — Professor *J. Singh* 202
Venous thrombosis and varicose veins 204

Chapter 6 Genito-urinary system

Renal outlines 205
Calculi 205
Schistosomiasis 206
Filarial chyluria 210
Renal hydatid disease 211
Papillary Necrosis 212
Urethral strictures 213
Obstetrics 213
Advanced extra-uterine gestation 215
Vesico vaginal fistulae 215
Malignant trophoblast disease 216

Chapter 7 Central nervous system

Pineal calcification 219
Cerebral parasitism 219
Echinococcus 219
Paragonimiasis 220
Cysticercosis 222
Tuberculoma 223
African trypanosomiasis 224
Paraplegia 224
Tuberculosis 224
Yeast infections 225
Brucellosis myelopathy 225
Schistosomiasis 225
Guinea worm 226
Gnathostomiasis 226
Hydatid disease 226
Haematopoiesis paraplegia 226
Burkitt's 227

Introduction

At the present time shortage of trained manpower, x-ray equipment and other resources severely limit the practice of radiology in the tropics. The competing demands between the preventive and curative sector of health care on a small budget ensure that radiology facilities are often scanty and that radiologists are confined to large urban centres and teaching hospitals.

A few charts will indicate the degree of difference between various countries in and out of the tropics.

The relative number of radiologists is shown (Fig. 1) on a logarithmic scale as the population to be served per radiologist. It will be noticed that the country best endowed with radiologists, Sweden, has about 180 times more per capita than the country least well off. It would have been possible to name areas without a single radiologist but these could not be accommodated on such a graph! In some societies about 4 per cent of all doctors are radiologists whereas in most countries in the tropics the figure is around 1 per cent, perhaps expressing the economic realities and priorities of those countries. Where it is higher it is due to the artificial beneficial effects of aid programmes and military presence. In the case of Tahiti, which has the highest number of radiologists relative to other doctors in the world, to the two factors mentioned above must be added the many undoubted attractions which has ensured the presence of radiologists in the private sector!

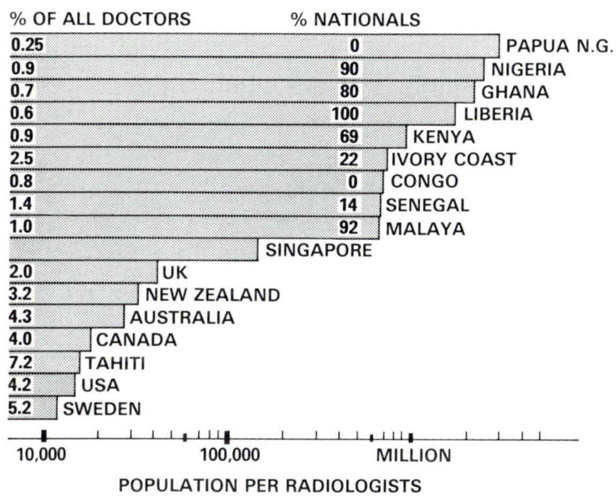

Fig. 1

The proportion of nationals practising radiology is growing compared to a decade ago. As training programmes grow and develop in the tropics, often in collaboration with an overseas centre, the numbers of expatriates will dwindle further. Unfortunately to offset this progress are the forces of the international marketplace competing for trained radiologists. The higher remuneration and better facilities in more affluent societies have inevitably had some adverse effects on the manpower situation in the tropics.

In radiography the provision of trained personnel is analogous to that of radiologists—a comparative shortage in many countries (Fig. 2). In the English-speaking areas good training schools have produced an excellent and growing cadre of radiographers. But the demands are such that, for the provision of radiographical services outside the largest cities, it may be more realistic to provide a less highly trained individual to supplement the radiographers. It will be noted in Figure 2 that in Senegal the number of radiographers is low but if the 'technicians' (locally briefly trained x-ray operators) are included, the level of service to the public is much improved. Lest we be accused of restricting and cheapening the role of the radiographer, we hasten to add a proviso. Since better radiological service to the public is the aim we feel that there is room for experimentation in developing an expanded task for some radiographers. In areas where there are few radiologists, selected radiographers should be trained to do contrast procedures. Not to diagnose but to carry out and record examinations on films. This would provide a valuable service in certain settings. Such changes in practice require adjustments in thinking of the

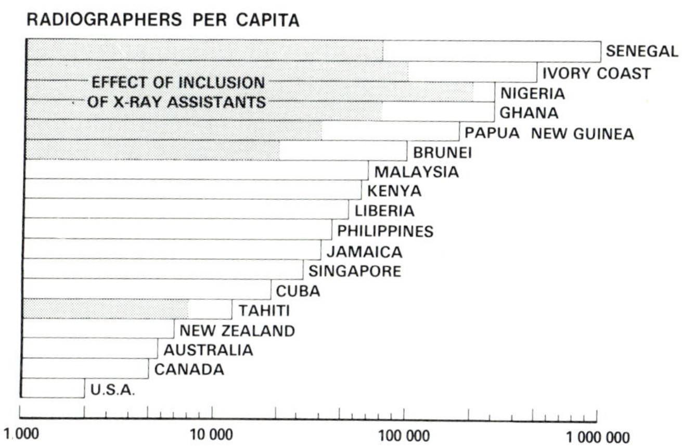

Fig. 2

stereotypes of their professions by both radiologists and radiographers. There is no reason to perpetuate everywhere what has evolved historically in temperate climates.

The provision of radiographical units (Fig. 3) parallels that of the medical and radiographical staff. The shortage

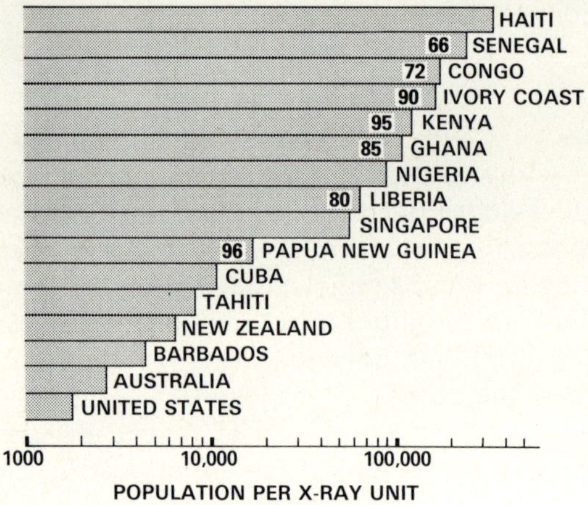

Fig. 3

of equipment is often accentuated by poor maintenance. We make a plea that in the selection of equipment simplicity be emphasised. The likelihood of a breakdown is determined not by the sum of the parts but by a multiplication of the number of the parts. The more complex, the considerably greater frequency of breakdowns. Where simple equipment will do the task it should be chosen. In a recent survey over two-thirds of remote-controlled T.V. fluoroscopy units in Africa were not fully functional due to breakdowns in the imaging system. In areas far removed from factories and stores we believe that fluoroscopy units should have stand-by mirror optics available. The new type of thin actual size image intensifiers are ideal for the tropics as they not only avoid the use of television and ceiling suspension but are also considerably cheaper than T.V. fluoroscopy chains.

Another weak link is the automatic processor. Before purchase it is essential to determine whether the water supply is suitable. It is equally important to obtain an ample set of spare rollers, chains, cogs, etc. Needless to say automatic processors are only warranted in large centres with skilled staff able to monitor performance. Hand processing is much more economical and reliable.

RADIOLOGY UTILISATION

The amount of radiology carried out is shown in the histogram displaying the number of radiographic examinations

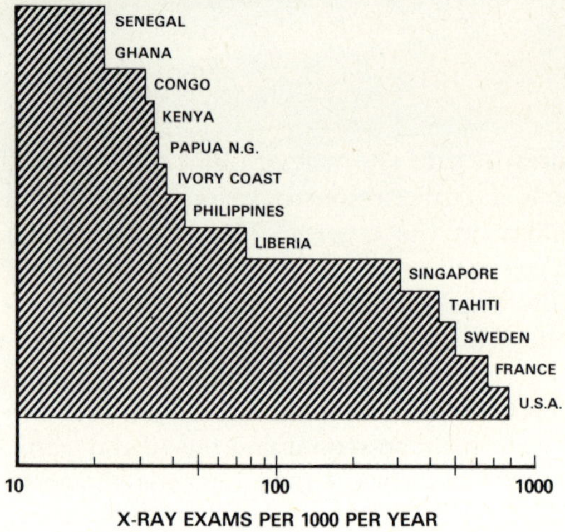

Fig. 4

per 1000 population per year (Fig. 4). This indicates that there is a disparity of usage of the order of 30 times between nations.

We do not suggest that there is an absolute optimal level of use but that perhaps a desirable level lies between the two extremes. The cost of radiological examinations is difficult to express in terms of population dosage or even in monetary terms. Radiology has a necessary role in health care but it can be abused. Radiology uses high technology and is one of the more expensive sectors of modern health care. It is ultimately the users who are aware of the benefits and can equate these with other competing local claims to determine the appropriate priorities. The simpler radiographical techniques are generally the cheapest and most reliable and quantitatively provide the greatest impact on health care. The complex procedures with their high demands on staff resources need to be reserved initially for the referral specialized hospitals. In many countries radiology is not available to the public outside the capital due to maldistribution of facilities and trained staff. Provision of basic simple units at the periphery recognises these realities and will increase the availability of radiology where the majority of people live.

1. Soft Tissues

CALCIFICATION IN THE SOFT TISSUES

Standard works of radiology describe most of the calcifications and ossifications that may develop in soft tissues. These include congenital disorders such as the Ehlers Danlos syndrome and myositis ossificans progressiva; inflammatory lesions such as sarcoid and scleroderma; metabolic diseases attendant upon renal dialysis, etc. Such conditions and many others are ubiquitous. In the tropics various other entities must also be considered that are infective (parasitic) and of idiopathic origin. This section will discuss these briefly to emphasise their diagnostic features. Interpretation is often aided by knowledge of the endemicity of a particular lesion, since the appearance is not always pathognomic. Furthermore, one should be aware that calcification is indicative of a chronic process which may have little to do with a patient's present complaint.

Cultural artefacts may also produce densities in radiographs. Superficial applications to the skin may be visible if the material is radio-opaque and is viewed tangentially. Metallic materials may be used for tattooing. Kohl, antimony, may be applied around the eyelashes.

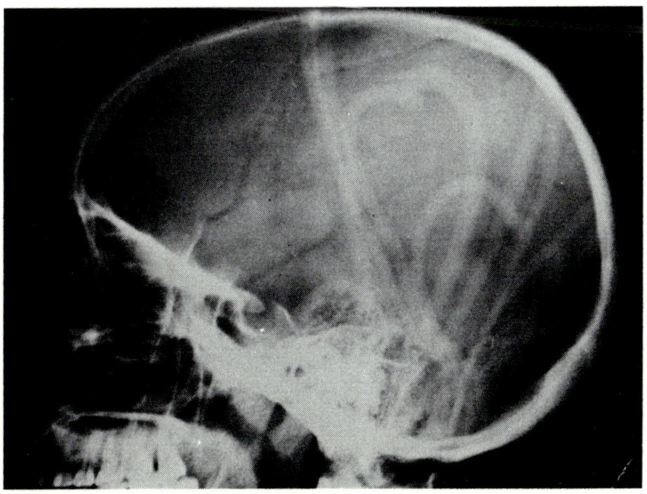

Fig. 1.1 Lateral skull of Yoruba lady who had plaited hair bound by black cotton.

Binding of hair may produce symmetrically disposed densities of varying patterns over the calvarium extending beyond the scalp (Fig. 1.1).

INJECTION SITE CALCIFICATION

It is not unusual to detect rounded calcified opacities in the gluteal region which are often multiple and bilateral. Their size is variable, extending from 4 mm to over 2 cm, as is their density which may be homogeneous or show a denser periphery. Borders are well defined (Fig. 1.2).

These areas of dystrophic calcification follow injections of various substances that result in local tissue necrosis. Quinine and emetine are notorious in this respect, but many other drugs can produce the same results. Heavy metal or radio-opaque densities may also be injected, but these interstitial deposits appear denser and may track somewhat in the line of muscle fibres rather than being rounded and confined.

Other materials may be introduced by unqualified healers leading to septic abscesses which also occasionally later develop calcification within them.

TUMORAL CALCINOSIS

This condition, in which there are multiple, often symmetrical, swellings around joints, particularly the thighs, buttocks, shoulder girdle, elbows and feet, is often diagnosed from radiographs.

The lesions are superficial, usually on the extensor side of a bony prominence, painless and the overlying skin is generally freely mobile. The swellings may ulcerate and discharge some of their contents. Local recurrence can follow incomplete excision. The condition is benign and of unknown cause.

Though the lesion has been recorded in caucasians in North America, Europe and Iran, it has a much higher incidence in those of African ancestry. It is seen through-

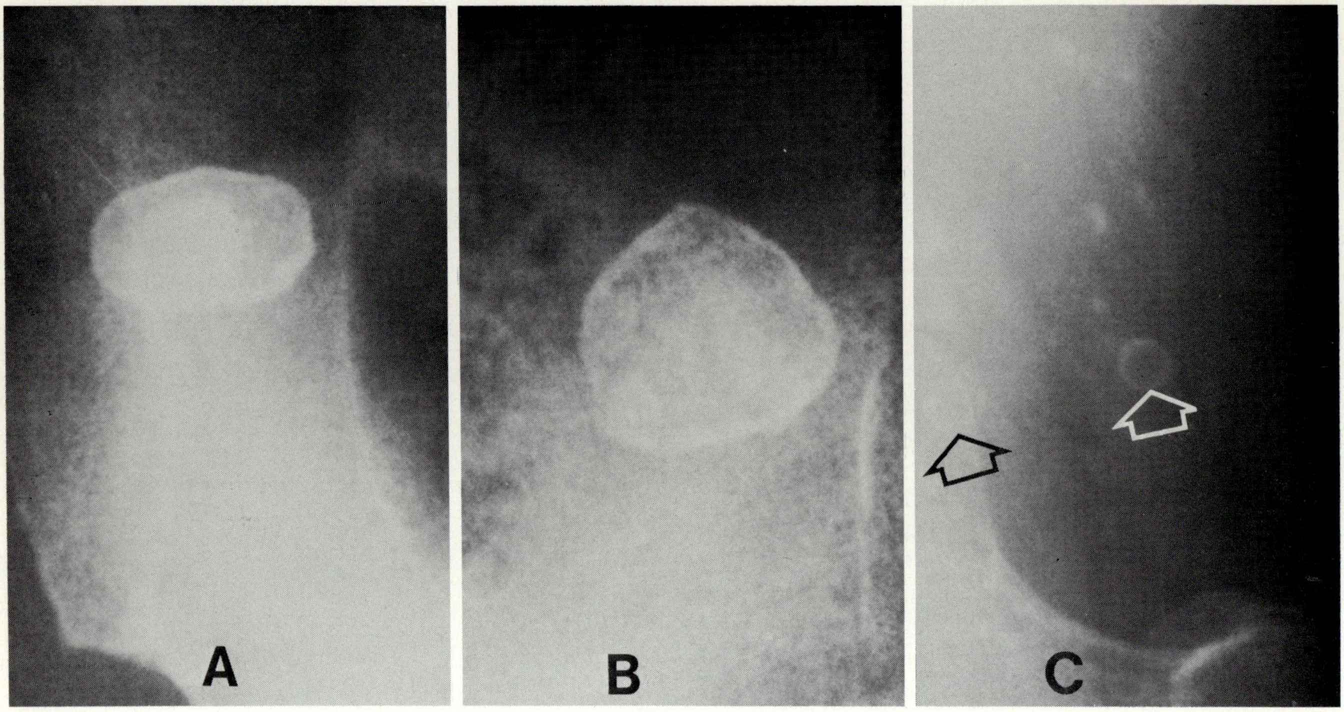

Fig. 1.2 Three forms of gluteal injection site calcifications. **A.** Dense nucleus and amorphous periphery. **B.** Diffuse amorphous calcification. **C.** Multiple calcified foci with 2 ring forms (arrowed).

out sub-saharan Africa including the Sudan (Palmer, 1966; Veress *et al.*, 1976). It is also prevalent in the Melanesians of Papua New Guinea (Cooke, 1969; Onuigbo, 1977). In the Eastern and Central Highlands it has been termed locally hip stone. We have also seen the condition in the Malay. The patients are well and show no obvious metabolic disorder though biochemically a high serum phosphorus may be evident (Kolawole & Bohrer, 1974). Calcinosis has been observed in four siblings with hyperphosphatemia, but this was an isolated observation. Palmer considers that the location fits with pressure from sleeping on the ground or hard mats. Chronic trauma from carrying loads on the backs by females has been implicated as the cause of the lumbar and iliac crest calcified bursae found in the Kikuyu (Maathuis, 1972; Owor, 1972) (Figs. 1.3 and 1.4). Tumoral calcinosis can occur in the first decade or may be present in the seventies, but it is most common in the twenties.

In radiographs the calcific densities are well defined and may show a lobular formation due to septa separating the amorphous cloudy collections of calcium carbonate and phosphate (Fig. 1.5). Soft tissue views indicate that the shape of the deposits is moulded by adjacent bone and by fascial planes that confine the directions of expansion (Fig. 1.6).

In the early stages of the lesion the calcareous material may be milky and can be aspirated, but later it becomes more gritty, thicker and fixed. On incising into a deposit the material exudes from multiple cyst-like cavities.

In erect films some layering of calcium is sometimes

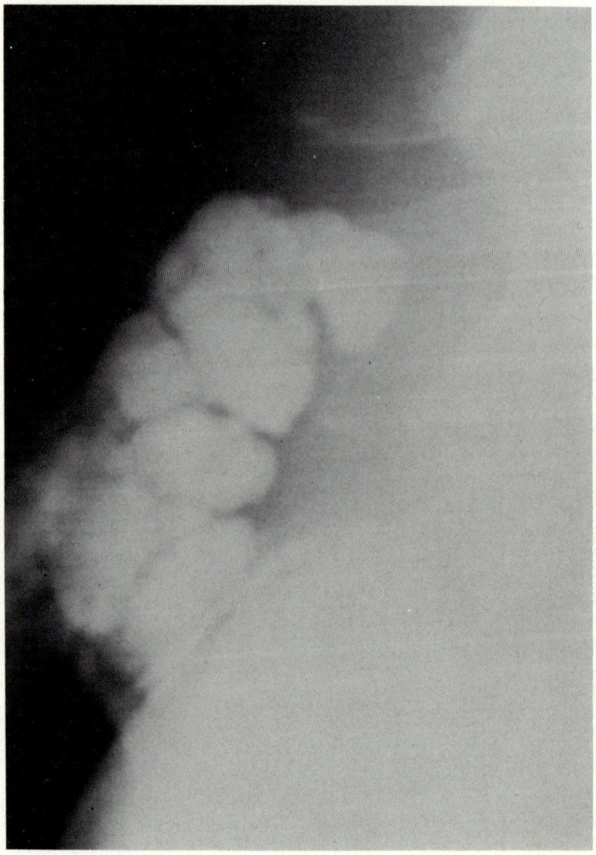

Fig. 1.3 Multinodular calcification present in posterior lumbar area in a Kikuyu bursa. (Courtesy of Prof. L. Whittaker, Nairobi.)

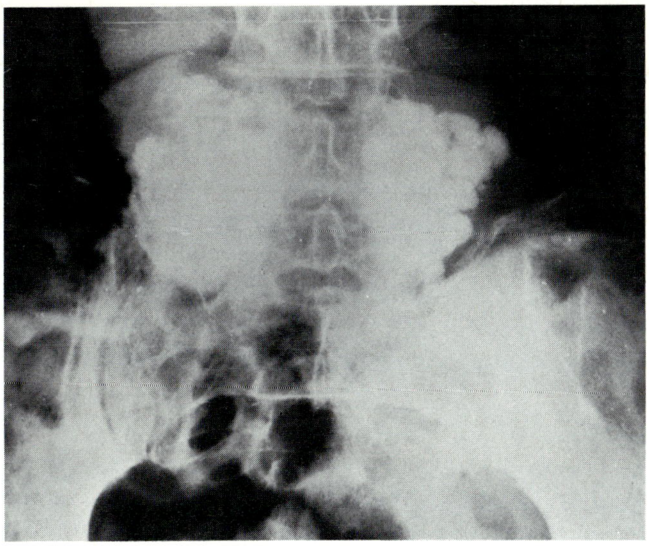

Fig. 1.4 Paired lumbar 'Kikuyu bursa' at typical site where heavy loads rest. (Courtesy of Dr. S. Malik.)

seen with the formation of levels (Kolawole & Bohrer, 1974; Hug & Guncaga, 1974).

Though the clinical differential diagnosis of nodules is large, the presence of calcium, the typical location and symmetry usually makes the designation clear. Calcium deposits in patients being dialysed can superficially resemble this lesion. A calcified abscess such as a tuberculous bursa or dystrophic parasitic calcifications are unlikely to be confused with tumoral calcinosis.

REFERENCES
Cooke, R. A. (1969) Tumoral calcinosis, *British Medical Journal*, **1**, 644.
Hug, I. & Guncaga, J. (1974) Tumoral calcinosis with sedimentation sign, *British Journal of Radiology*, **47**, 734–736.
Kolawole, T. M. & Bohrer, S. P. (1973) Tumoral calcinosis, *Tropical and Geographical Medicine*, **25**, 18–22.
Kolawole, T. M. & Bohrer, S. P. (1974) Tumoral calcinosis with 'fluid levels' in the tumoral masses, *American Journal of Roentgenology*, **120**, 461–465.
Maathuis, J. B. (1972) Kikuyu bursa in Kenya, *Tropical and Geographical Medicine*, **24**, 130–133.
Onuigbo, W. I. B. (1977) Tumoural Calcinosis in Nigeria and Papua New Guinea. *Papua New Guinea Medical Journal*, **20**, 78–79.
Ower, R. (1972) Tumoral calcinosis in Uganda, *Tropical and Geographical Medicine*, **24**, 39–43.
Palmer, P. E. S. (1966) Tumoral calcinosis, *British Journal of Radiology*, **39**, 518–525.
Veress, B., Malik, M. O. A. & El Hassan, A. M. (1975) Tumoral lipocalcinosis: a clinicopathological study of 20 cases, *Journal of Pathology*, **119**, 113–117.

MYOSITIS OSSIFICANS
TRAUMA, TETANUS AND TRYPANOSOMIASIS

Bone tissue developing from metaplasia in the reparative process around a haematoma or a fracture is a well-recognised complication of trauma to muscle tissues (Fig. 1.7).

In under-doctored areas there may be early activity after a dislocation that can result in massive exuberant myositis ossificans. Bone in muscle tissue is also seen in paraplegics and in patients with poliomyelitis, but here physiotherapy may sometimes be responsible.

In tetanus strong muscular contractions occur that can fracture bones, particularly the dorsal vertebrae and less commonly the ulna and the sternum. Such forces can equally damage muscle with later myositis ossificans. Lesions develop around joints in either flexors or extensors and can involve ligamentous structures. The process is associated with joint rigidity and by the third week a faint flocculent type of calcium density can be seen in the affected muscle or ligaments (Gunn & Young, 1959;

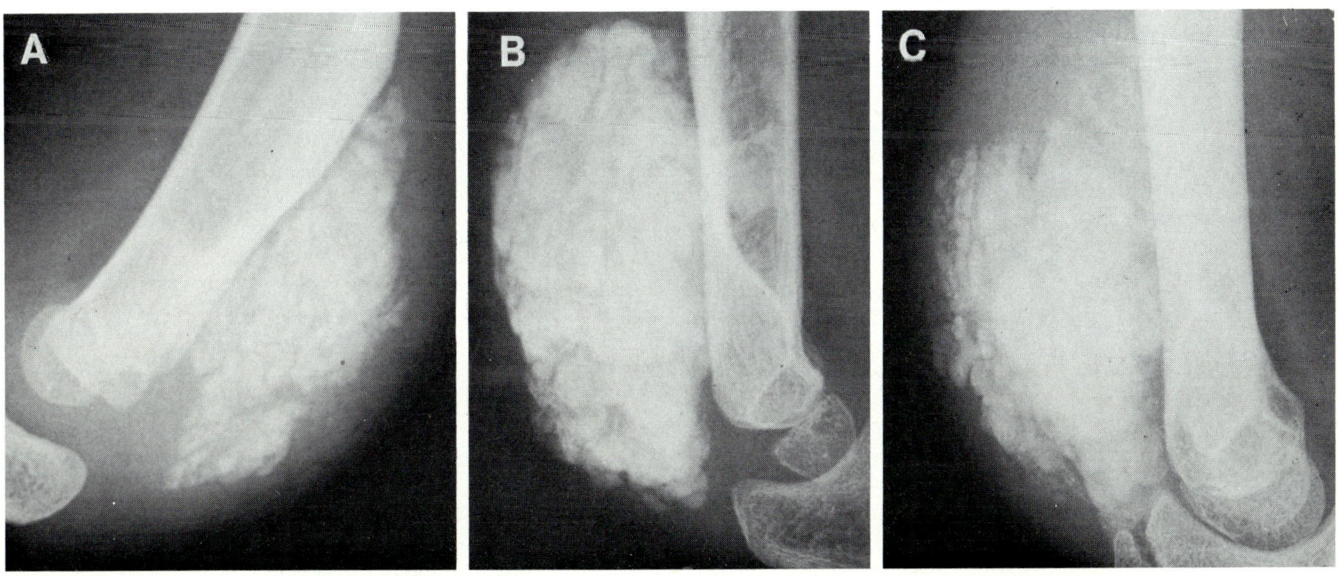

Fig. 1.5 Large deposits of tumoural calcinosis around the elbow. **A.** The calcified mass has eroded the posterior humerus and also provoked new bone formation. **B.** Well encapsulated multinodular form. **C.** Large nodular mass. (Courtesy of Prof. Philip Palmer, Sacramento.)

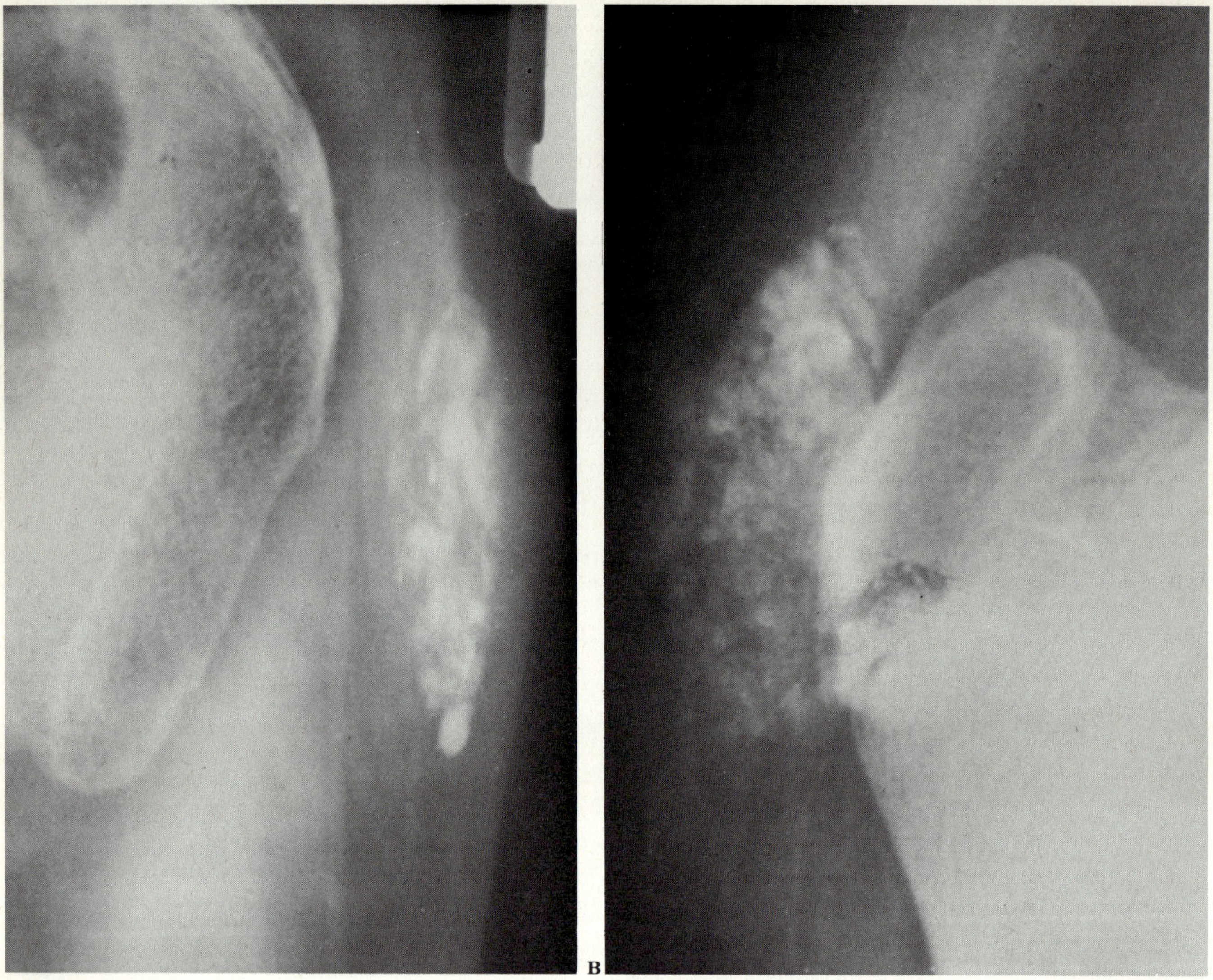

A B

Fig. 1.6 A, B. Soft tissue views of early tumoural calcinosis related to iliac crest and trochanteric area to show moulding effects of fascial planes.

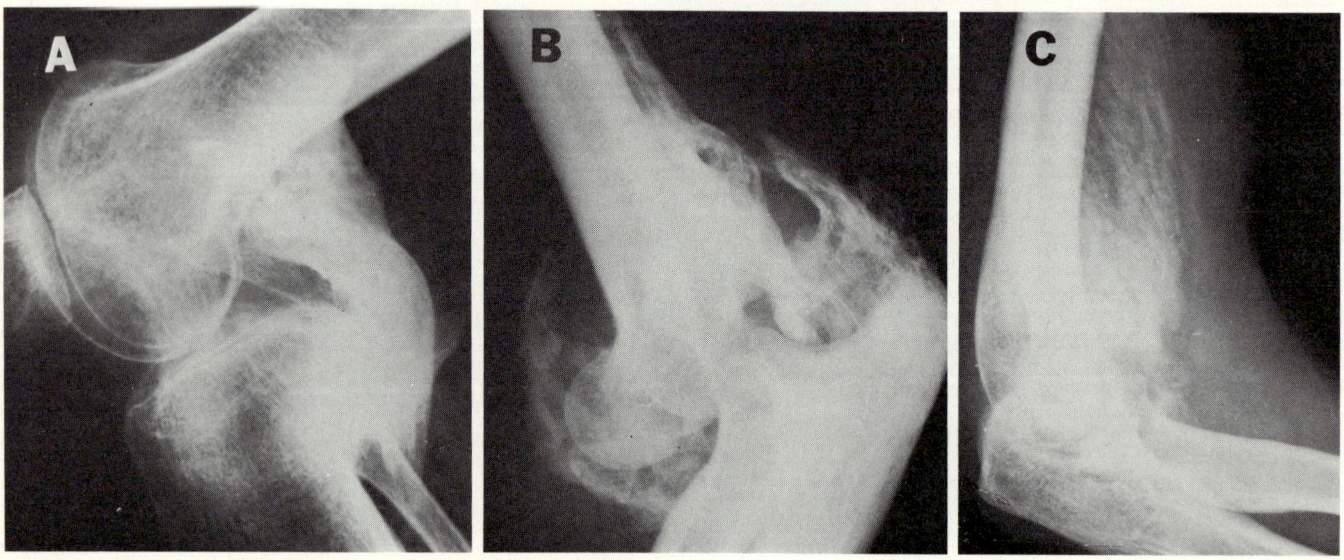

Fig. 1.7 A & B. Post-traumatic myositis ossificans demonstrating typical bone formation in line of muscle fibres after trauma. **C.** Bone formation in brachialis following tetanus. (Courtesy of Prof. Bohrer.)

Femi-Pearse & Olowu, 1971; Diop Mar & Sow, 1973). The calcification and ossification though in the shape of the muscle affected does not display the linear muscle fibre bundle trajectories seen in the more common post-dislocation myositis, perhaps because there is less haemorrhagic infiltration and dissection. Later, with remodelling, the two forms of myositis cannot be differentiated by radiography.

A further cause of myositis ossificans has been noted in patients with sleeping sickness due to T. gambiense. Some weeks following the encephalitic stage of the disease stiffness and pain may be noted around the joints and eventually limitation of movement is evident (Norredam & Kandelhart, 1971). Radiographically cloudy para-articular calcification can be detected which, within three months, matures from an amorphous structure to well defined trabecular bone. This new bone formation never actually merges with the normal cortex as there is always a thin plane of lucent connective tissue separating normal and new bone. The new bone can totally invest the tissues around a joint, particularly the hips. The shoulders, elbows, knees and hips can all be affected usually in a symmetrical fashion.

REFERENCES

Diop Mar, I. & Sow, A. (1973) Les osteopathies para-articulaires du tetanos, *Abstracts Ninth International Congress of Tropical Medicine and Malaria*, Athens, 195.

Femi-Pearse, D. & Olowu, A. D. (1971) Myositis ossificans—a complication of tetanus, *Clinical Radiology*, **22**, 89–92.

Gunn, D. R. & Young, W. B. (1959) Myositis ossificans as a complication of tetanus, *Journal of Bone and Joint Surgery*, **41B**, 535–540.

Norredam, K. & Kandelhart, E. (1971) Para-articular ossification: a complication of African trypanosomiasis, *Annales de la Société Belge de Médecine Tropicale*, **57**, 325–334.

GUINEA WORM
DRACONTIASIS, DRACUNCULOSIS

Dracontiasis is a disease well known in antiquity and still presenting problems in Arabia, Iran, India, parts of West Africa, the Sudan and the Congo. It is now rare in South America and has disappeared from the West Indies.

The disease is associated with polluted water supplies and disappears with the provision of protected wells and a piped water supply. In some rural areas the disability from the disease has serious socio-economic implications. In rural communities with a 13·5 per cent incidence each episode averaged 100 days off productive work (Kale, 1977).

The clinical manifestations are due to the female worm which can vary from 30 cm to 1 metre in length. The shorter male of approximately 3 cm in length does not appear to cause any direct disability. The female worms lie in subcutaneous tissues, predominantly in the lower limbs, and actively seek the skin surface. The head and the gravid uterus which contains ova and first stage larvae are extruded through a skin ulcer. On contact with water the uterus discharges larvae until eventually after several weeks it empties. These larvae are taken up by various cyclops (water fleas) where they maturate and moult. If man swallows an infected cyclops, the larvae are released by digestion in the stomach. These then migrate into subcutaneous tissues, or between muscle planes.

The exact route of migration in man is unknown, but in the dog immature worms appear first to gather in the axillae and groin (Onabamiro, 1956). The gravid females eventually move to the limbs in order to reach the exterior and repeat the cycle, the whole process taking about one year. At the time of the initial infection there may be systemic hypersensitivity urticarial reactions. However, it is the later reactions to a dead worm in the tissues that is the chief cause of disability.

In the acute phase a localised aseptic inflammatory reaction may take place or a cellulitis and abscess which lies between tissue planes. The localisation is a useful differential point between this process and pyomyositis (Cockshott & Evans, 1964).

Soft tissue radiographs and angiography show distinctive features, but are rarely necessary (see section on pyomyositis).

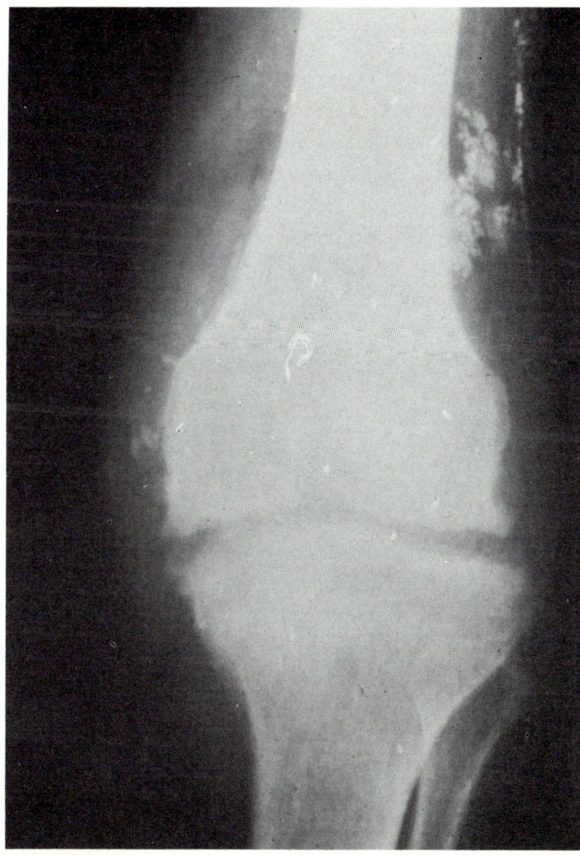

Fig. 1.8 Severely arthritic knee—a sequel to previous septic arthritis from guinea worm. Numerous calcified worms in soft tissues.

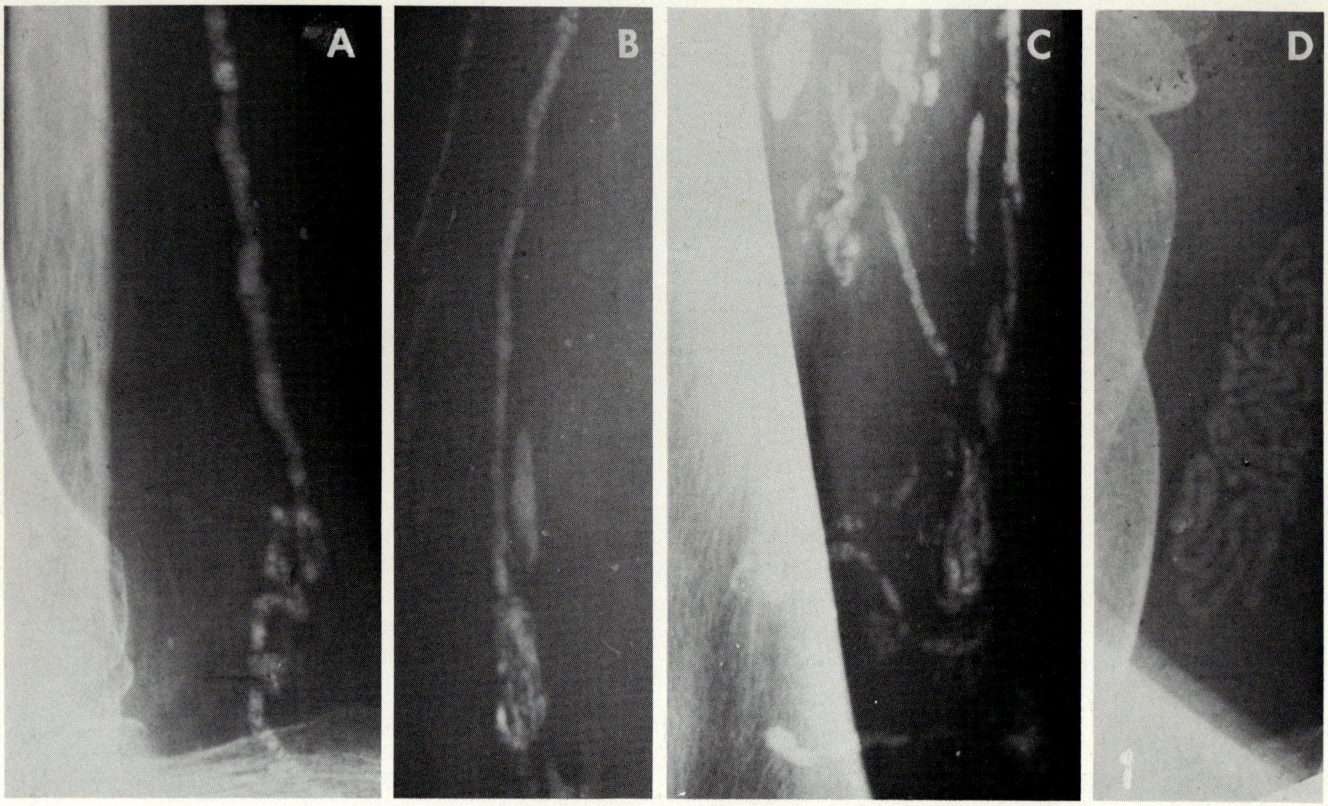

Fig. 1.9 Calcified guinea worms. **A & B**. Extended forms showing typical slight nodularity. **C.** Linear segments and amorphous forms. **D.** Convoluted forms.

Calcification around a guinea worm represents the sarcophagus around a long departed parasite. In itself the finding is of little significance except in perhaps explaining the aetiology of disease in an adjacent joint that shows evidence of long standing septic arthritis (Fig. 1.8).

Calcified worms tend to lie along tissue planes in the limbs but elsewhere they are often coiled and convoluted. The width is around 2 mm (Fig. 1.9). When reaction is marked the individual loops of a coiled worm may not be recognised as the calcium is laid down as an amorphous mass.

REFERENCES

Cockshott, W. P. & Evans, K. T. (1964) The place of soft tissue arteriography, *British Journal of Radiology*, **37,** 367–375.

Kale, O. O. (1977) The clinico-epidemiological profile of guinea worm in the Ibadan district of Nigeria, *American Journal of Tropical Medicine and Hygiene*, **24,** 208–214.

Onabamiro, S. D. (1956) The early stages of the development of Dracunculus medinensis (Linnaeus) in the mammalian host, *Annals of Tropical Medicine and Parasitology*, **50,** 157–166.

LOIASIS
LOA LOA INFECTION

This form of filariasis has a relatively limited geographical distribution encompassing southern and eastern Nigeria and Cameroons, and extending in an easterly fashion towards central Africa and Angola.

Human infection is acquired through the bite of tabanid flies of various Chrysops species which implant larvae. These mature and worms of both sexes appear in the subcutaneous tissue up to a year after the initial episode. The fertilised female worm releases microfilariae into the circulation, particularly at night—the period when chrysops flies bite man, acquire the microfilariae and maintain the cycle. Diagnosis is most readily made from blood film examinations.

The adult female worms that lie in the subcutaneous tissues measure approximately 65 mm by 5 mm and the males are approximately half this size. When alive these worms are mobile and wander in subcutaneous tissues where their passage can be detected in loose skin areas such as the conjunctival sac. At times the worms liberate antigenic material and produce local swellings classically called 'Calabar swellings' after the town in Nigeria. These subcutaneous lesions may develop anywhere. On the death of a worm a more violent granulomatous foreign body reaction takes place and dystrophic calcification may occur later. Polyarthritis can be associated with Loa Loa infection (Bouvet *et al.*, 1977).

Radiologically the calcified worms may be extended or coiled and show a continuous linear or a beaded calcified density (Fig. 1.10). The thickness of the calcification is usually under 3 mm and the length, because of coiling, is difficult to assess. For technical reasons the worms are most readily detected in hand and foot radiographs (Williams, 1955). This apparent prevalence probably does not represent the real distribution as worms are recognised incidentally at surgery and necropsy at many sites.

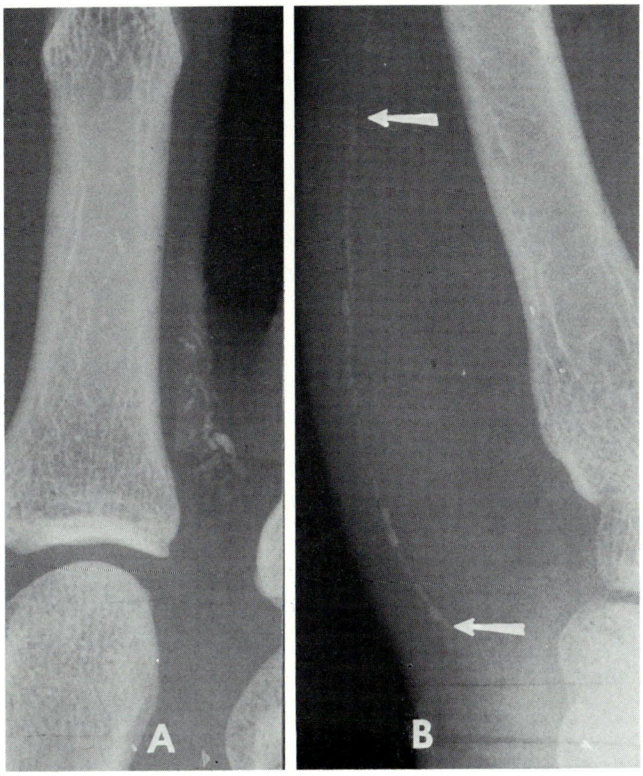

Fig. 1.10 Calcified Loa loa. **A.** convoluted. **B.** Extended form.

REFERENCES

Bouvet, J. P., Therizol, M. & Auquier, L. (1977) Microfilarial polyarthritis in a massive Loa Loa infestation, *Acta Tropica*, **34,** 281–284.

Williams, I. (1955) Calcification in loiasis, *Journal of the Faculty of Radiologists*, **6,** 142–144.

ONCHOCERCIASIS
RIVER BLINDNESS

This form of filariasis which occurs in sub-saharan Africa, Central America, the northern parts of South America and in south-west Arabia has negligible radiological manifestations. The worms, of which the male adult is 4 cm and the female 50 mm, have not been reported as calcifying radiologically though O. volvulus does calcify histologically in subcutaneous nodules. The liberated microfilariae causes skin thickening and later atrophy and local lymphoedema from lymphatic obstruction. This can cause pendulous bulging lesions such as the 'hanging groin'. Material excised from such lesions during hernia repairs contains calcified areas that can be seen in specimen radiographs but not in the *in situ* films. Further radiologico-pathological correlations are needed in this field. Clinical diagnosis depends on identification of adult worms in biopsies or of microfilariae from skin snips.

REFERENCES

Chartres, J. C. (1955) Onchocerciasis, *The West African Medical Journal*, **4,** 130–135.

Foy, H. & Konda, A. (1958) Symposium on Onchocerciasis, *Transactions of the Royal Society of Tropical Medicine and Hygiene*, **52,** 59–134.

WUCHERERIA BANCROFTI FILARIASIS
BRUGIA MALAYI. FILARIASIS

Remarks on these filariae will be confined to calcification, as other aspects are considered under lymphoedema, chyluria, and eosinophilic lung. In an excellent radiological, pathological and clinical study O'Connor and his colleagues (1930) convincingly demonstrated that W. bancrofti worms calcify. Calcified worms can be seen, but very infrequently, in subcutaneous lymph channels of the legs, thighs, and scrotum as well as in lymph glands in the groin. The calcified structures are 3 to 4 mm by under 1 mm and can be straight or slightly coiled. They are thus smaller than Loa loa in length and larger than onchocercal histologic calcification. Nevertheless precise identification unless there is additional epidemiological data or evidence of lymphoedema is probably not possible. B. malayi worms calcify histologically but do not appear to be detected radiologically.

REFERENCE

O'Connor, F. W., Golden, R. & Auchingloss, H. (1930) The roentgen demonstration of calcified filaria bancrofti in human tissue, *American Journal of Roentgenology*, **23,** 494–502.

SARCOCYSTIS
SARCOSPORIDIAL INFECTION

Sarcocystis infections exist throughout the world, but the recorded instances in man are rare. This is attributed to the negligible scrutiny of muscular tissue in routine autopsies. Establishment of the diagnosis is by muscle biopsy.

The organism responsible, Sarcocystis lindemanni, has an uncertain life cycle. Consumption of infected muscle is considered to be the method of infection with the protoplasts passing through the intestine and carried by the blood stream to voluntary and cardiac muscles. There the

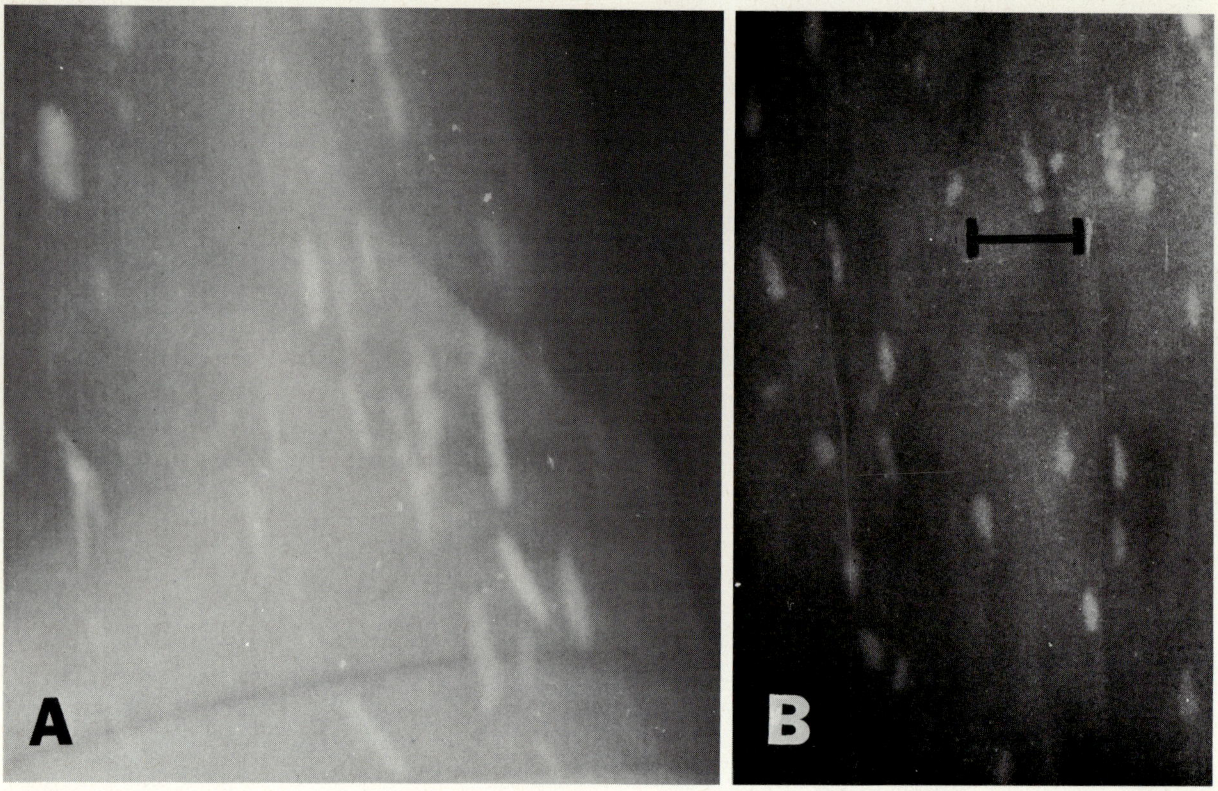

Fig. 1.11 Calcified thigh lesions. **A.** Kenyan with linear calcification in line of muscle fibres—sarcosporidiosis. (Courtesy Prof. L. Whittaker, Nairobi.) **B.** Small calcifications in line of muscle fibres in a Nigerian. Black bar indicates 1 cm. Identical features were seen in a Rhodesian and attributed to sparganosis (see text). No definite diagnosis in this case.

organism gives rise to urticarial or granulomatous reactions. The parasite in the muscle cell initially excites little reaction as it replaces the sarcoplasm of the cell with a cyst containing spores formed by binary fission. Ultimately the cyst bursts and a reparative scarring process takes place.

Radiological changes have been described in this disease. Scars and granulomatous nodules around dead cysts (the cysts themselves are microscopic) may cast densities different from the muscle (Mandour, 1965), but eventual multiple calcification in granulomata are readily seen (Fig. 1.11). In a case from Greece multiple densities were seen in the muscles and subcutaneous tissue of the arms and legs (Kremmydas *et al.*, 1964). The opacities were amorphously calcified with no particular orientation.

There is still considerable ignorance of this area as few fully proven cases with calcification are known. By that stage proof of diagnosis may be impossible.

REFERENCES

Kremmydas, B. N., Papadakis, A. M., Theodosin, A. & Antonopoulos, G. (1964) A case of sarcosporidial infection in a woman, *Radiology*, **83,** 1064–1067.

Mandour, A. M. (1965) Pathology and symptomatology of Sarcocystis infection in man, *Transactions of the Royal Society of Tropical Medicine and Hygiene*, **59,** 432–435.

SPARGANOSIS

Sparganum is the term applied to the larval form of diphyllobothriid (pleocercoid) tapeworms. Man acquires the infection by ingesting water containing cyclops (water fleas) infected with procercoid larvae; by eating or handling inadequately cooked infected chicken, frogs or snakes harbouring the pleocercoid larvae; or by applying, as in Indo China, the flesh of live frogs to wounds or ulcers.

The distribution of the organism is worldwide, albeit cases are scanty. Reports have come from China, Indonesia, Korea, Australia, sub-saharan Africa, Madagascar, Central and South America, the United States and Canada (Huang & Kirk, 1962).

The pleocercoid larvae migrate and give rise to localised granulomata and nodules retroperitoneally, around the bowel to cause helminthoma (vide section on colon), nodules in subcutaneous tissues, and typically in the orbital tissues. The nodule contains a live or dead white coiled ribbon-like larva termed a spargana. Involvement of lymph channels and glands can result in lymphoedema.

Rhodesian workers describe a patient who showed multiple scattered oval calcified opacities of varying size aligned in the direction of muscle fibres and measuring apparently under 1 cm long. These were thinner than cysterci and showed a somewhat different structure. Biopsy revealed a sparganum (Alves *et al.*, 1954). Thus it would seem that subcutaneous and possibly muscular calcified foci may be attributed to sparganosis, but this is the only recorded case with these features. We have encountered patients from southern Nigeria with similar features (Fig. 1.11) but have no histologic or parasitic information on the nature of the infestation that does appear to differ from cysticercosis. The alignment of the calcified parasites in muscle is also unusual for sparganum foci. Sarosporidiosis calcification would also have to be excluded. Much remains unknown in this field.

REFERENCES

Alves, W. D., Gelfand, M. & Weinberg, R. (1954) A case of sparganosis in an African from Portuguese East Africa, *Transactions of the Royal Society of Tropical Medicine and Hygiene*, **48,** 87–88.

Huang, C. T. & Kirk, R. (1962) Human sparganosis in Hong Kong, *Journal of Tropical Medicine and Hygiene*, **65,** 133–138.

CYSTICERCOSIS

Cysticercosis represents infection with the larval stage of the tapeworm taenia solium which normally occurs in the pig. Man becomes infected with the tapeworm by eating inadequately cooked pork harbouring cysticerci. (Discussed in alimentary section.) Humans may acquire cysticercosis by ingesting food contaminated with the ova of the tapeworm and so become an intermediate host. Food becomes infected through faecal contamination, but it has been postulated that reverse peristalsis in a person with a tapeworm could lead to cysticercosis. Even if theoretically possible this must be a rare event (Brailsford, 1941).

The condition is seen extensively in Mexico, Central and South America; to a lesser extent in Eastern Europe, the Middle East, India, the Far East and Africa. It is rare in Moslem areas.

Following gastric digestion the eggs, derived from the mature tapeworm proglottid, liberate active oncosphores which penetrate the gut wall, enter the circulation and are carried to various tissues, particularly the central nervous system, cerebrospinal fluid pathways and muscle and subcutaneous tissues.

The location of the embryo that encyst (cysticercus cellulosae) in the body is controversial. Some authors emphasise a considerable predominance in the brain (Arseni & Samitca, 1957; Sautin & Vargas, 1966), but this is vigorously contested by others (Brailsford, 1941). Radiological evidence of muscle involvement is higher than pathology records which suggest only 3·5 per cent of cases have muscle cysticerci, whereas Brailsford believed this to be more frequent than in the brain. Probably a third to a half of cases have muscle or subcutaneous deposits.

The distribution in muscle is probably according to its volume and so the bulky thighs are the most rewarding area to study radiographically. The encysted cysticerci live in muscle for some years and only become calcified after five years or so. The calcium deposit forms initially in the fluid around the parasite, then in the body apart from the scolex and only later in the cyst wall. The cysts measure 10 mm by 6 mm but shrink slightly over a few years through desiccation, fibrosis and absorption of contents. Characteristically these lie according to the orientation of the muscle fibre bundles (Fig. 1.12).

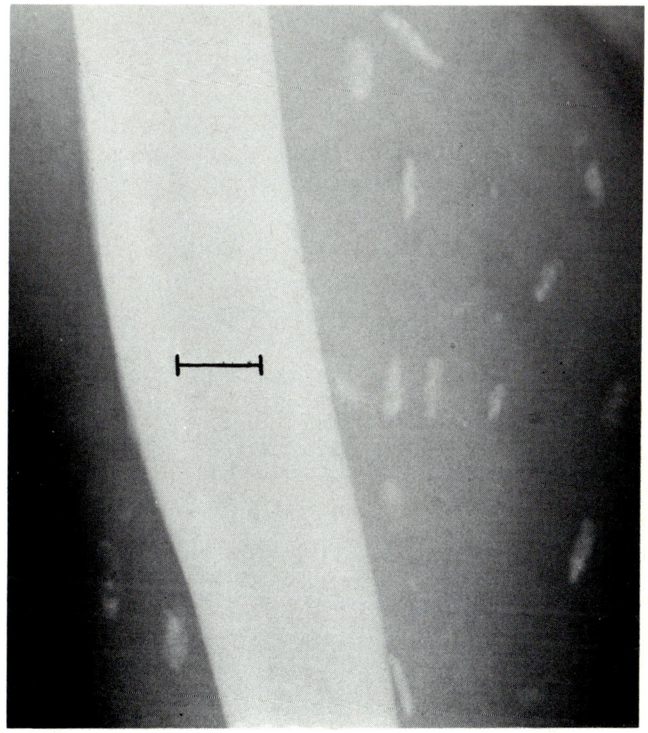

Fig. 1.12 Typical calcified cysticerci lying in plane of muscle fibres and showing internal structure. Bar is 1 cm.

When the typical features are seen the appearance is characteristic enough for a presumptive diagnosis. Complement fixation and antigen precipitation test exist with varying degrees of specificity, but these are rarely available or required.

The brain cysticerci, when they calcify, are considerably smaller, about 2 mm in size and are difficult to detect.

REFERENCES

Arseni, C. & Samitca, D. C. (1957) Cysticercosis of the brain, *British Medical Journal*, **2,** 494–497.

Brailsford, J. F. (1941) Cysticercus cellulosae—its radiographic detection in the musculature and the central nervous system, *British Journal of Radiography*, **14,** 79–93.

Sautin, G. & Vargas, J. (1966) Roentgen study of cysticercosis of central nervous system, *Radiology*, **86,** 520–527.

POROCEPHALOSIS—PENTASTOMIASIS ARMILIFFER INFECTIONS

In certain parts of the tropics, particularly in West Africa, calcified nymphs of porocephalida are the most frequent cause of discrete rounded soft tissue calcifications seen in abdominal or chest radiographs. Their presence is pathognomic of porencephalosis.

The parasites are pentastomomida which have two orders: the porencephaloidea and the linguiatuloidea.

The former infect the lungs of snakes and exist in nymph forms in mammals on which the serpent feeds. Man acquires infection accidentally from eating inadequately cooked snake or food and drink contaminated by eggs from snakes' saliva—perhaps via well water or food 'wrapping leaves'.

The exact pathway of infected eggs in man, the emerging larvae, and the several moulting stages of nymphs is not well understood. The fully developed sixth moult is the stage usually recognised. By then the nymph assumes a crescentic shape in a fibrous capsule. These are usually situated subperitoneally in an organ such as the liver, bowel wall, or mesentery, subpleurally, or less frequently in other sites. Nymphs can exist more deeply embedded in tissues. Nymphs are seen within the liver parenchyma related to tributaries of the hepatic veins. Granulomatous reaction often develops. In Ibadan in western Nigeria, porocephalosis is the third commonest cause of hepatic fibrosis after tuberculosis and schistosomiasis (Smith *et al.*, 1975). More rarely nymphs can cause submucosal nodules in the stomach or jejunum or in the lung parenchyma. Even lymph glands can be affected (Pons & Noc, 1922). Symptoms are few if any in the majority of instances. The nymphs eventually die in their fibrous capsules and undergo dystrophic calcification to present radiologically as multiple calcified densities which appear crescent-shaped *en face* and oval in profile—4×8 mm in size (Fig. 1.13). They have no particular alignment as do cysticerci. They are more frequent in the upper abdomen than in the lower abdomen or the pleural cavities. Other ectopic sites do not feature radiologically. The calcified Malaysian forms are smaller than the West African nymphs.

The incidence of this infection may be as high at autopsy as 45 per cent in Malaysian Aborigines (Prathap *et al.*, 1969a, b) and 6 per cent in the Cameroons (Loehlein, 1912) but radiologically the incidence is much less, the highest figure being from Ibadan—2 per cent of adult males and 4 per cent in females (Lindner, 1965).

Porocephalosis by one of these species: P. crotali, P. sublifer, Armiliffer armillatus, A. grandis, A. monilformis, has been recorded from Liberia, Ivory Coast, Ghana, Nigeria, Cameroon, and the Congo. It is rare in Rhodesia and East Africa. Malaysia, Borneo and the Philippines have recorded cases. In the new world infection is virtually unknown.

In the foregoing emphasis has been placed on the calcified stigmata of previous infestation. Symptoms can be apparent early in the disease such as peritonism, 'acute abdomen', intestinal obstruction by bands (Manuwa, 1947). It is likely that these more acute features are the result of infection in an individual previously sensitised

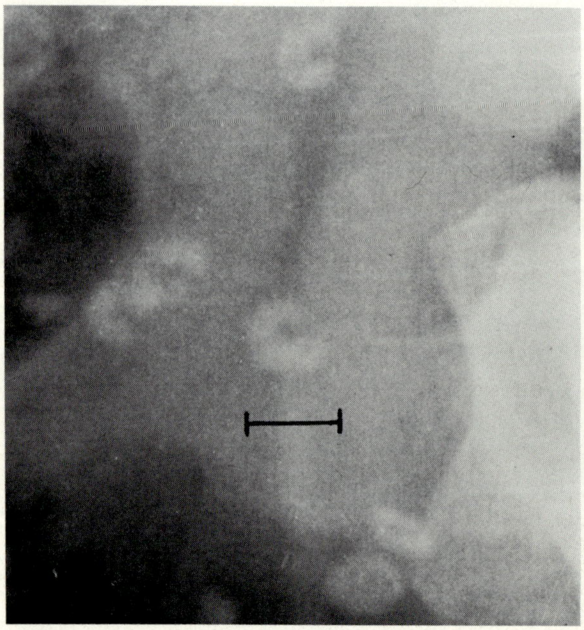

A

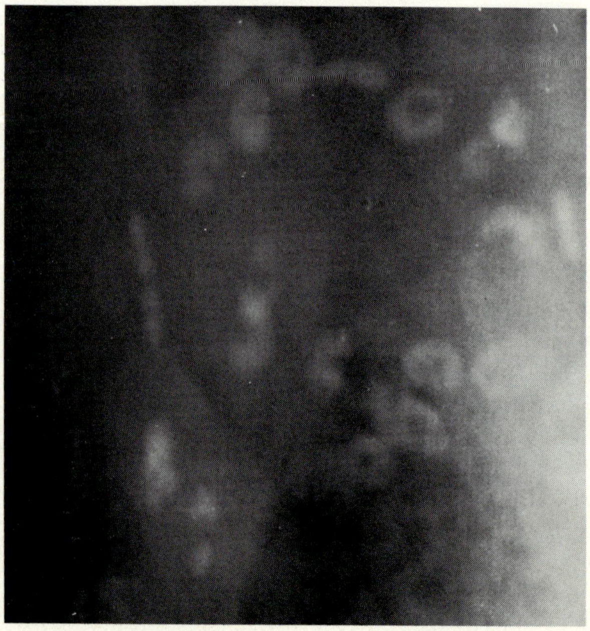

B

Fig. 1.13 A, B. Typical C-shape calcified Armiliffer armilatus when seen *en face*. The linear forms represent lateral views. Bar is 1 cm.

to pentastomal antigen by a previous infection, or release of material from recently deceased nymphs.

An excellent general review of this disorder is in the paper by Self *et al.*, 1975.

Recently, Smith and his colleagues noted in an autopsy survey that patients dying of malignancy had a 33 per cent rate of porocephalosis whereas in non-malignant conditions the rate was 16 per cent. This was based on 2,764 autopsies and seemed to be a statistically significant difference.

The linguatuloidea or tongue worm can also be acquired by man in a different stage of the life cycle after eating inadequately cooked meat of sheep, goats or wild cattle that has lymph glands harbouring third stage nymphs of L. serrata. These migrate from man's stomach to the nasopharynx where they cause local symptoms due to the presence of the tongue worm at that site. This form of disease, the Halzoun syndrome, is recorded from the Sudan, Greece and the Middle East. No radiographic changes have been described.

REFERENCES

Lindner, R. R. (1965) Retrospective x-ray survey of Porocephalosis, *Journal of Tropical Medicine and Hygiene*, **68,** 155–156.

Loehlein, M. (1912) Beitrage zur pathologie der bingeborenem in Kamerun. Summarised in *Tropical Diseases Bulletin*, **1,** 517.

Manuwa, S. L. A. (1946) Porocephalosis, *Transactions of the Royal Society of Tropical Medicine and Hygiene*, **40,** 507–508.

Pons, R. & Noc, F. (1922) Porocephaliose ganglionaire a lymphademie tuberculeuse a èvolution rapide chez un tirailleur sènegalais, *Bulletin Sociètè Pathologie Exotique*, **15,** 951–954.

Prathap, K., Lau, K. S. & Bolton, J. M. (1969a) Pentastomiasis: a common finding at autopsy in Malaysian aborigines, *American Journal of Tropical Medicine and Hygiene*, **18,** 20–27.

Prathap, K., Burns-Cox, C. J., Clark, E. & Gillman, R. (1969b) Porocephalosis in Western Malaysia, *Transactions of the Royal Society of Tropical Medicine and Hygiene*, **63,** 409–411.

Self, J. T., Hopps, H. C. & Olufemi Williams, A. (1975) Pentastomiasis in Africans, *Tropical and Geographical Medicine*, **27,** 1–13.

Smith, J. A., Oladiran, B., Lagundoye, S. B., Lawson, E. A. L. & Francis, T. T. (1975) Pentastomiasis and Malignancy, *Annals of Tropical Medicine and Parasitology*, **69,** 503–512.

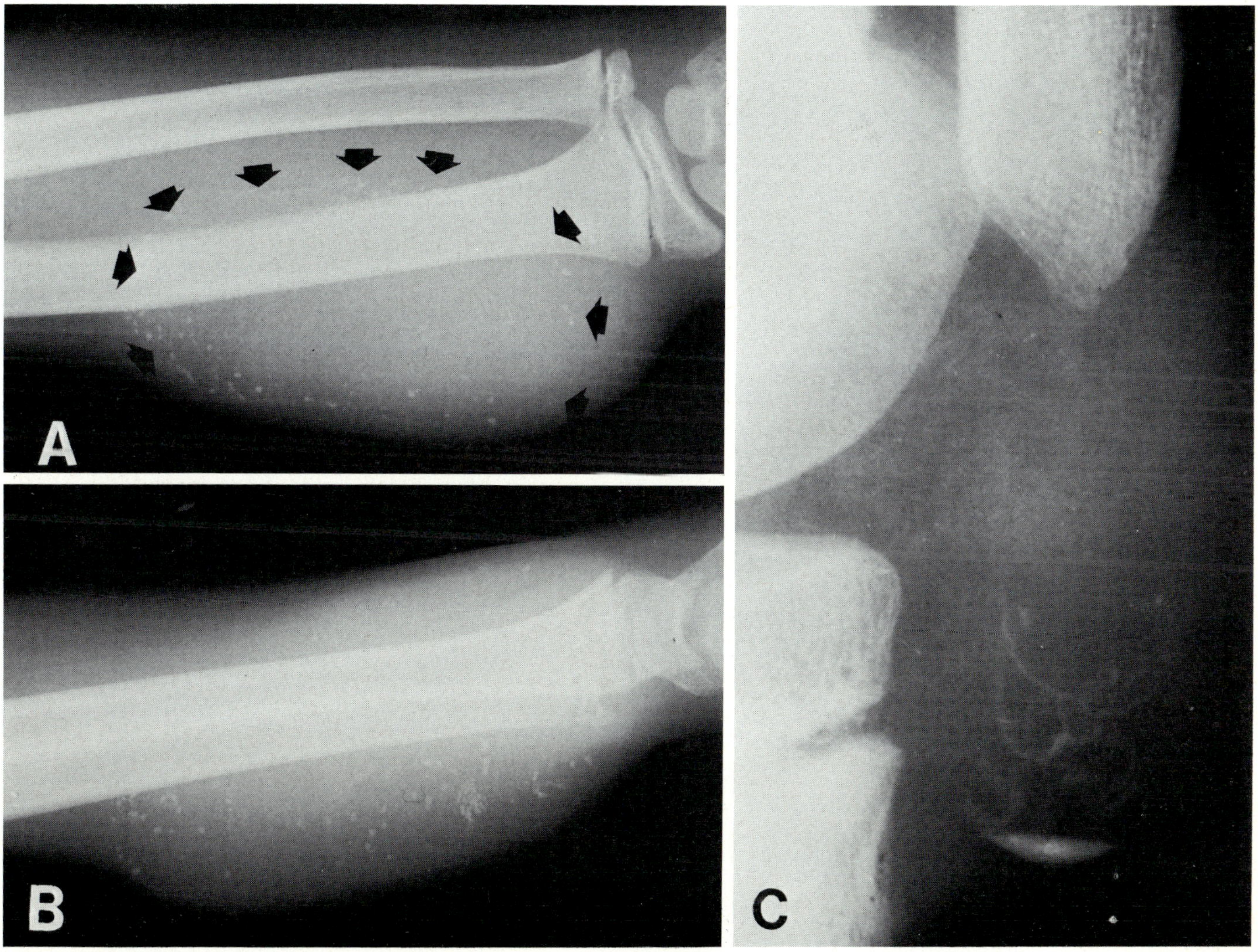

Fig. 1.14 A & B. Limb with fluctuant subcutaneous cyst in two positions showing some fixed mural calcific densities and some mobile fragmented linear 'parasitic' fragments. **C.** Infrapatellar cyst with curvilinear fragments and a settled deposit in this erect view. The identity of the parasite in these Nigerian patients is unknown.

UNKNOWN CALCIFICATIONS

In the preceding discussion on sparganosis, sarcosporidiosis and some filaria, it is obvious that some forms of calcification defy precise diagnosis radiologically and often histologically, since calcification destroys identifying morphologic features. We have seen on several occasions cystic lesions containing linear or particulate calcified fragments that appear to be parasitic in nature. Particles may be mobile, changing position in response to gravity as the area is moved or tilted (Fig. 1.14); we do not know the nature of the parasitism.

PYOMYOSITIS INTRAMUSCULAR AND INTERMUSCULAR ABSCESSES

Pyomyositis is a suppurative inflammatory process within muscle bellies due usually to Staphylococcus pyogenes. It is frequent in many tropical areas including sub-Saharan Africa, South America, Malaysia, Ceylon, the Pacific Islands and the West Indies. Though it develops in all ages its peak incidence is the second and third decades. There is a preponderance of male cases.

The etiology is unknown, but it seems likely that the lesion represents haematogenous infection of an injured muscle that may have a small tear or haematoma. Strong

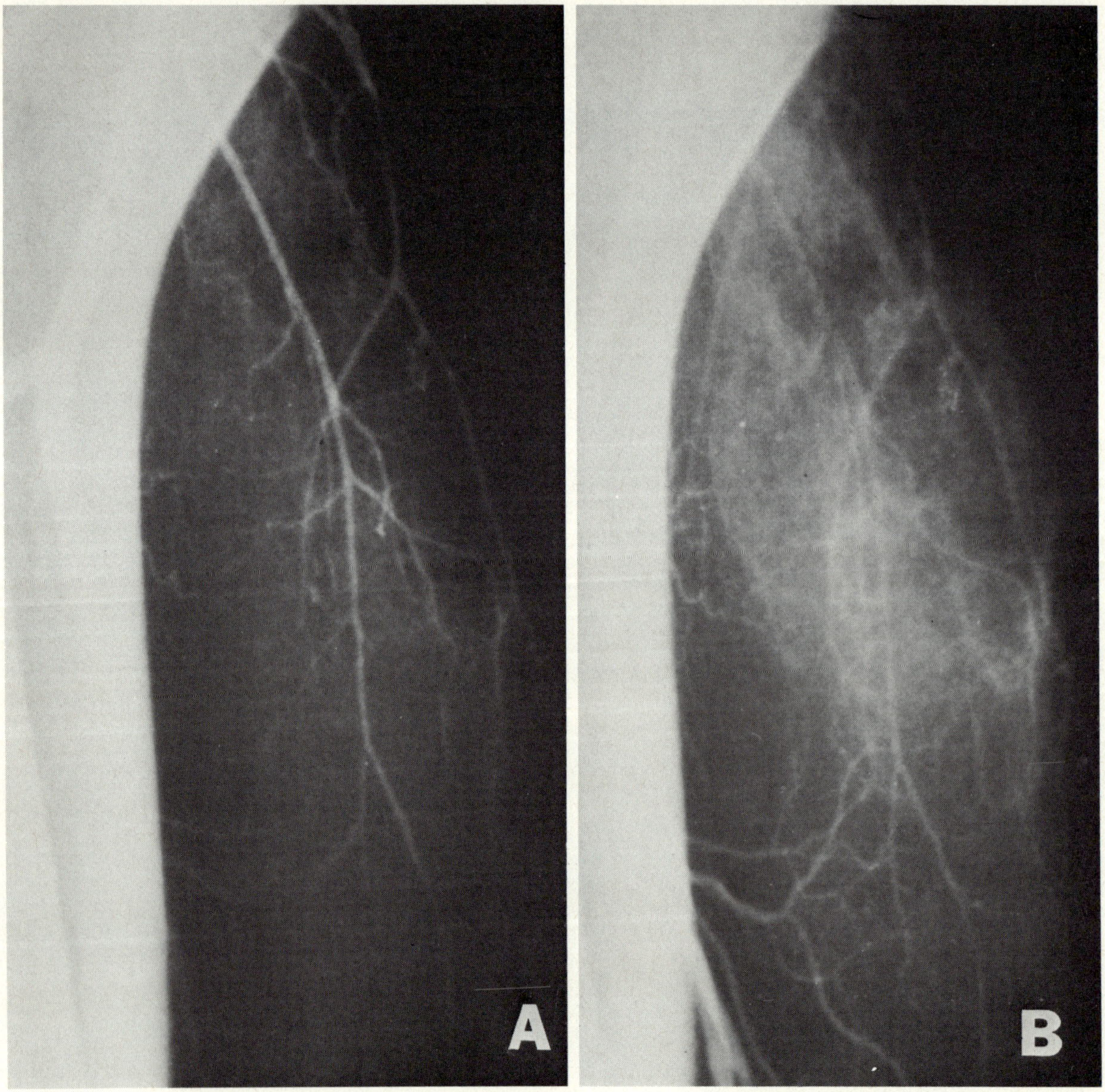

Fig. 1.15 Gastrocnemius pyomyositis showing early arterial **A** and later stage **B** of angiogram. Vessels are stretched and a capillary blush is evident but no macroscopic new vessels.

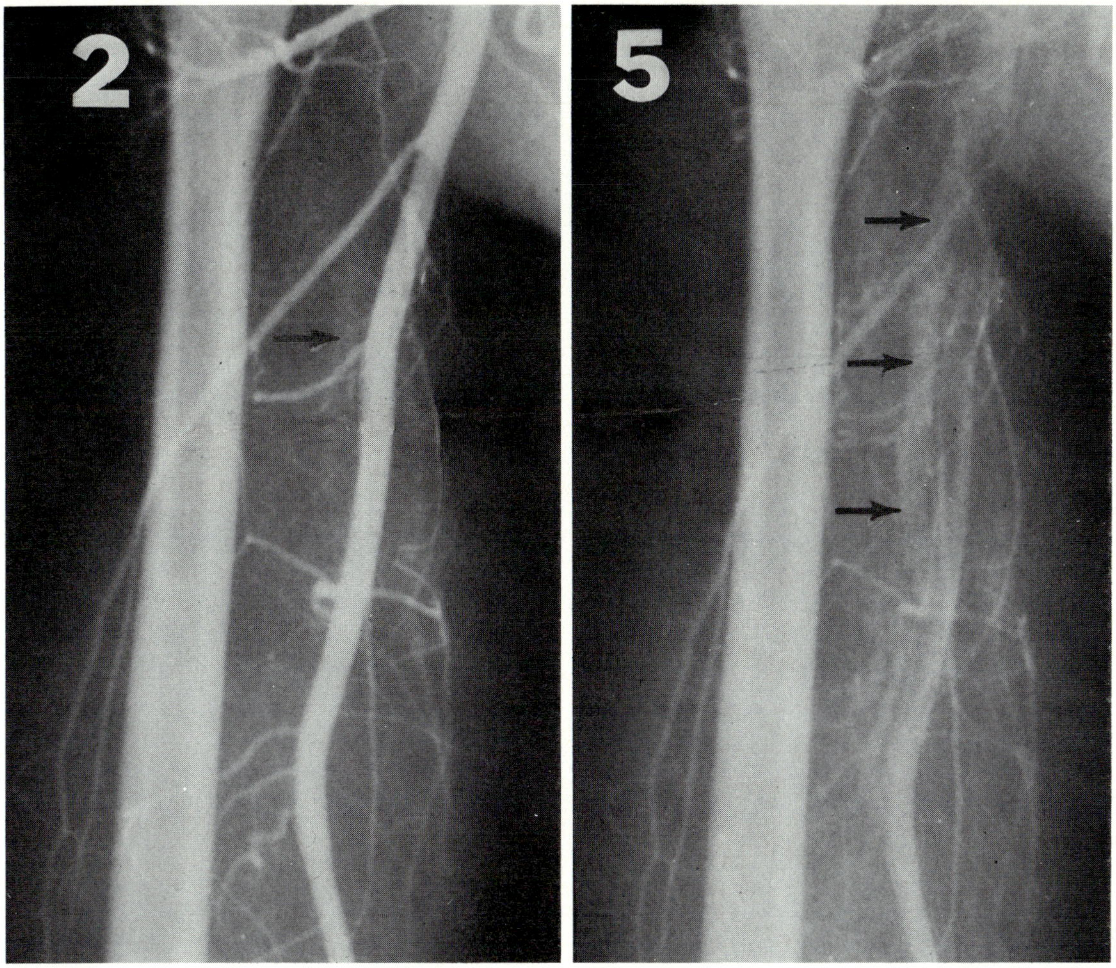

A B

Fig. 1.16 **A, B.** Biceps pyomyositis in early and late arterial phases at 2 and 5 seconds. Note early venous drainage and some opacification of hyperaemic wall. (Courtesy of *British Journal of Radiology*.)

large muscles are most often involved, particularly in the thigh on the right side (Coots & Gelfand, 1977). Patients present with pyrexia, toxicity and a tender swelling.

Plain film examination is not as a rule particularly informative though it may be possible in soft tissue films to relate the lesion to a particular muscle. Arteriography will show more specific features (Cockshott & Evans, 1964). The bulk of the inflammatory mass may displace the main arterial trunks. Dilated branches stretch around the affected area which shows diffuse vascularity due to the hyperaemia of the inflammatory cavity in the muscle. There is thus a capillary blush and early venous opacification (Figs. 1.15–1.16). We do not wish to suggest that angiography has a significant role to play in the diagnosis of what is often a clear clinical entity. Angiography can serve to identify indurated soft tissue sarcoma which at times can resemble this condition. A much more perplexing problem is the type of abscess that lies between muscle planes rather than within the muscle belly. As so clearly shown by Anand & Evans (1964), the intermuscular abscesses are due to reaction around dead guinea worms. Clinically these cause less toxicity and are less painful. The swelling may be more diffuse. The lesions contain pus and remnants of the worms. On arteriography they do not reveal a hyperaemic boundary and merely displace vessels (Fig. 1.17). Early venous filling is not a feature.

There are a large number of parasites that can invade muscle and cause a reaction. These often calcify and are discussed in sections on cysticerci, sparganum, sarcocystis, etc. During the more acute phase parasites exciting a strong reaction can simulate pyomyositis as has been recorded with oesophagostomum (Curan *et al.*, 1974).

REFERENCES

Anand, S. V. & Evans, K. T. (1964) Pyomyositis, *British Journal of Surgery*, **51**, 917–920.

Cockshott, W. P. & Evans, K. T. (1964) The place of soft tissue arteriography, *British Journal of Radiology*, **37**, 367–375.

Coots, D. & Gelfand, M. (1977) Tropical myositis in Rhodesian Africans. *Journal of Tropical Medicine and Hygiene*, **80**, 9–10.

Curan, D., Kassi, M., Essoh Nohel, P., Pothier, M.A., Badoual, J. & Doucet, J. (1974) Myosite provoquée par un oesophagostomum. *Annales de l'Université d'Abidjan*, **8**, 227.

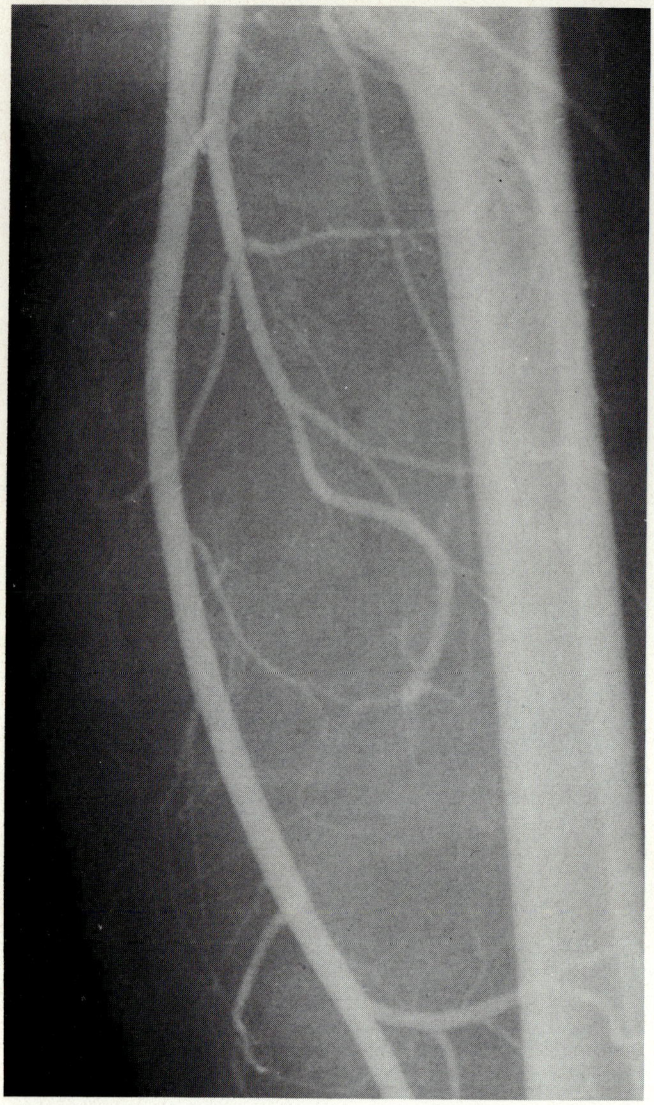

Fig. 1.17 Intermuscular abscess due to guinea worm displacing vessels. Hyperaemia of wall and early venous opacification were not seen in later films.

SUBCUTANEOUS LESIONS

Subcutaneous phycomycosis

Subcutaneous phycomycosis is an inflammatory lesion affecting the subcutaneous tissues leading to indurated thickened plaques fixed to the skin. Though these can occur anywhere, the limbs are most often involved. Most patients are children or adolescents who are otherwise healthy. The responsible organisms are various species of Basidiobolus, notably B. meristoporus and B. ranarum. The disease has been reported from equatorial Africa, Indonesia, New Guinea, Burma and the West Indies.

Since the radiographic density of the phycomycotic process is that of water and similar to muscle, a low kilovoltage technique is necessary not only to show the skin thickening and subcutaneous fat involvement but to reveal muscle invasion. This occurs in histologic studies, but can only be inferred radiographically if fat around a muscle belly is infiltrated. Even if this can be demonstrated the appearance in the radiograph does not permit differentiation from soft tissue sarcomata, and some forms of lymphoedema. Radiology can document the extent of the process, but diagnosis requires biopsy and cultural studies.

REFERENCE

Clark, B. M. (1968): Epidemiology of phycomycosis in systemic mycoses, *Ciba Foundation Symposium* pp. 179–192. London: Churchill.

Subcutaneous granulomata and Mycobacteria ulcerans

There are many parasites, fungi and other organisms that

A

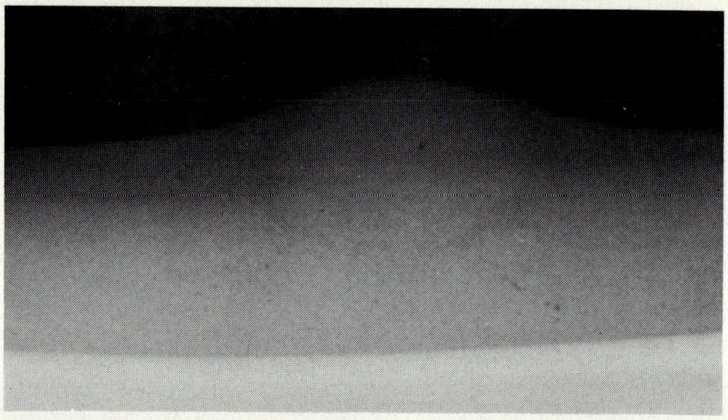

B

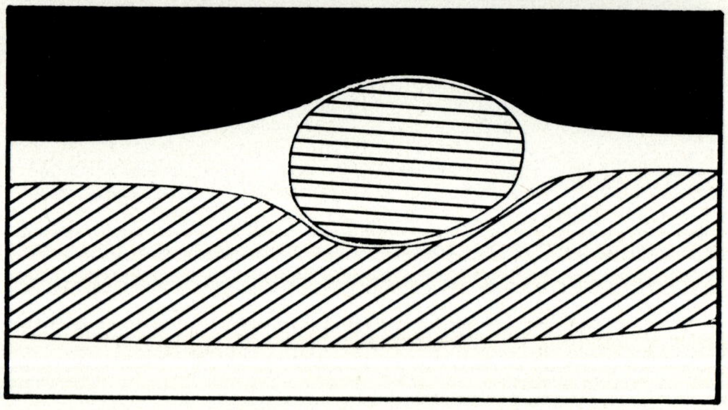

Fig. 1.18 A, B. Low kilovoltage soft tissue tangential view demonstrating Histoplasma duboisii subcutaneous granuloma.

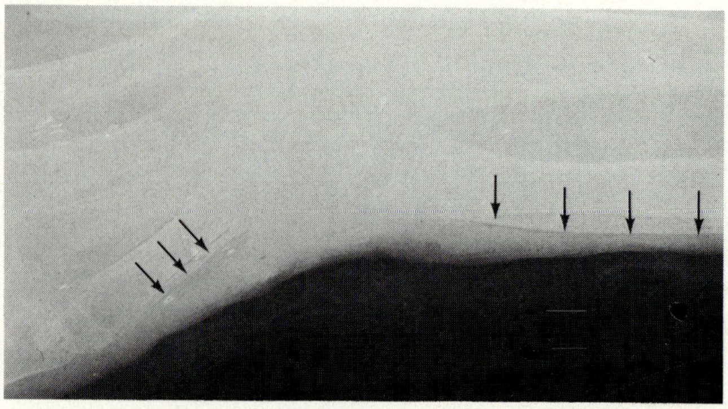

Fig. 1.19 Soft tissue view of wrist reveals periosteal reaction in bones adjacent to a Buruli ulcer. Note soft tissue deformities. (Courtesy of Prof. S. P. Bohrer.)

can cause subcutaneous nodules. These inflammatory lesions have a different density from adjacent subcutaneous fat and can be demonstrated by tangential low kilovoltage films (Fig. 1.18). Sometimes a cutaneous ulcer may produce reactionary periosteal reaction as with Mycobacteria ulcerans—Buruli ulcer (Figs. 1.19 and 1.20). This is seen in Africa and New Guinea with frequency and also occurs in Queensland.

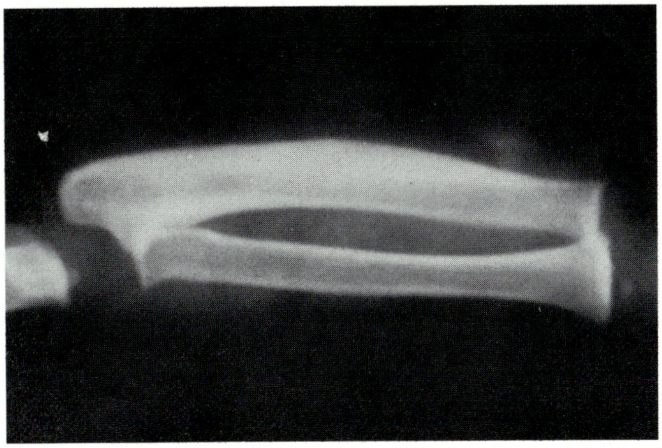

Fig. 1.20 Mycobacteria ulcerans subcutaneous granuloma has caused formation of dense ulnar periosteal new bone in this Queensland patient. (Courtesy of Mr Clive Felmingham, Cairns.)

REFERENCE

Radford, A. J. (1974) Mycobacteria ulcerans, *Papua and New Guinea Medical Journal*, 17, 129–149.

LYMPHOEDEMA

In the tropics lymphoedema of the lower limbs, scrotum and vulva can be caused by several conditions, additional to those seen in temperate climates rendering the differential diagnosis complex. Because a patient comes from an area where there is a high endemicity of a particular entity the assumption cannot be made that a local specific disease is responsible in an individual case.

In temperate zones venous circulatory stasis is an important factor, but in the tropics where phlebothrombosis and thrombo-embolic disease is rare, this aetiology is of low incidence.

Inflammatory lesions and filarial disease are important causes of lymphoedema. Certain clinical features help to differentiate the various possibilities (Ngu & Konstam, 1964), but laboratory tests and histologic methods are more definitive. Lymphangiography can be of occasional value in the investigation of these patients.

Tuberculous adenopathy

Tuberculous adenopathy may cause severe lymphoedema in the lower limbs, genitalia, breast and arm if the regional glands are involved. Caseation in glands leads to obstructive lymphatic phenomena. Later the glands may calcify. Lymphangiography has occasionally been carried out and reveals at first filling defects in glands and later, if obstruction becomes severe, dilated racemose channels bypassing the glands.

Lymphostatic verrucosis

Lymphostatic verrucosis from chronic sepsis often has distinguishing clinical features. The oedema is usually sharply limited to the lower limb below the knee as the obstructive element involves the vertical lower group of inguinal glands (Ngu, 1964). Presumably repeated wounds and abrasions in those walking bareshod contributes to this fibrosing adenopathy. Foot abrasions may permit certain irritants in the soil to enter that may have a lymphatic sclerosing effect. Surveys in Ethiopia, Guatemala and Rwanda Burundi in areas with no filariasis suggest that iron and trace elements in lava may be responsible (Price, 1976). Following on this process episodes of lymphangitis occur and result in a lymphatic obstructive process, marked lymphoedema and often hyperkeratosis of the skin of the foot. This can reach grotesque proportions with a markedly lobulated enlarged foot (Fig. 1.21).

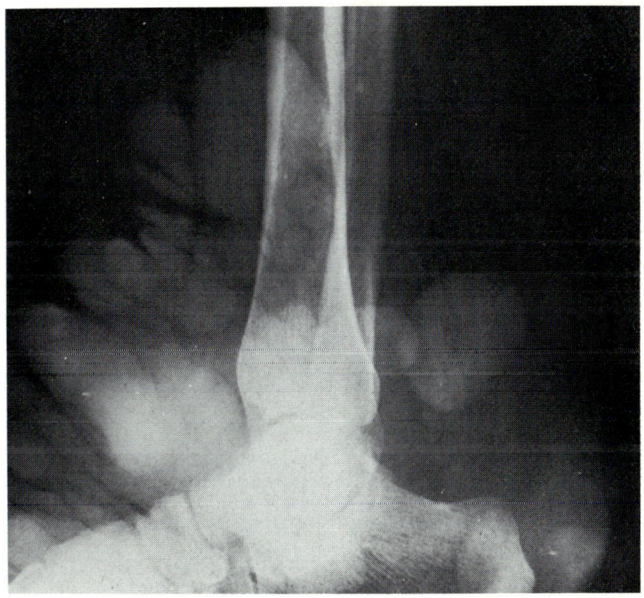

Fig. 1.21 Large soft tissue lobular deformities in lymphostatic verrucosis.

Lymphangiography in these patients can be difficult owing to the greatly thickened skin as well as the paucity of lymph trunks to inject, as many have been obliterated. The lymphatics are of small calibre and irregular, unlike those seen in filariasis.

Tropical phlebitis

Tropical phlebitis is a poorly understood syndrome

reported mainly from Central and East Africa (Manson-Bahr, 1955). This often occurs in small outbreaks in acute episodes and leads to a swollen leg and calf, often sparing the foot. Initially it is most painful and there is marked tenderness over the affected veins. Thrombo-embolism and recurrent episodes are not features of this entity. The lymphatics are apparently normal. We do not know of any documented venographic study of this syndrome.

Mossy foot

Mossy foot is a non-specific term to describe the greatly swollen hyperkeratotic foot seen in elephantiasis and lymphostatic verrucosis. In addition inflammatory lesions due to chromoblastomycosis from Phialaphora verrucosa, P. pedroisi and Cladosporium carrionni can simulate the condition if the foot and leg are involved. This is seen in Brazil, equatorial Africa, Malagasy, Indonesia, Polynesia, New Guinea, the Far East and in the West Indies. Protothecosis, a rare subcutaneous granuloma of the foot seen in Sierra Leone and in the southern United States due to an algae, can also simulate this condition (Davies *et al.*, 1964). In all these lesions the radiographic appearance of the soft tissues is distorted, but the appearances are not specific. Mycetoma, which may also cause great foot enlargement, is discussed in the section on bone diseases.

An exceptional cause of lymphatic obstruction has been recorded clinically and experimentally in sparganosis (Mueller, 1938).

REFERENCES

Davies, R. R., Spencer, H. & Wakelin, P. O. (1964) A case of human protothecosis, *Transactions of the Royal Society of Tropical Medicine and Hygiene*, **58**, 448–451.

Manson-Bahr, P. E. C. (1955) Tropical phlebitis, *East African Medical Journal*, **32**, 165–168.

Mueller, J. F. (1938) The life history of Diphyllobothrium mansonoides, Mueller 1935 and some considerations with sparganosis in the United States, *American Journal of Tropical Medicine*, **18**, 41–66.

Ngu, V. A. (1964) The lymphatic drainage of the leg and its implications. *Clinical Radiology*, **16**, 197–201.

Ngu, V. A. & Konstam, P. (1964) Chronic lymphoedema in Western Nigeria. *British Journal of Surgery*, **51**, 101–110.

Price, E. W. (1976) Endemic elephantiasis of the lower legs in Rwanda Burundi. *Tropical and Geographical Medicine*, **28**, 283–290.

FILARIAL LYMPHOEDEMA WUCHERERIA BANCROFTI FILARIASIS BRUGIA MALAYI FILARIASIS

These two parasites are considered jointly as their soft tissue features are similar and their life cycles have an affinity in that both require a vertebral host and an arthropod vector for completion of the cycle. Man is the only known host for bancroftian filariasis but man, other primates and dogs can harbour the malayan form. Transmission is by various species of mosquitoes. As this is a complex matter readers are referred to works of parasitology for details of the species and the development stages.

The bancroftian form is widespread, existing in Central and South America, some of the West Indian islands, India, Sri Lanka, Burma, Thailand, Malaysia, Indonesia and Melanesia, South Japan as well as in West, Central and East Africa. The malayan species is more restricted, affecting Burma, Eastern India, Indonesia and South China.

Man becomes infected through a bite of a mosquito when a larva from the insect enters the patient's lymphatics through the skin puncture. The larvae migrate within the lymphatic passages and mature over a period of approximately three months. After fertilisation they eventually shed, over several years, microfilariae into the blood stream in a periodic fashion, usually during sleep. Examination of blood films for microfilariae and noting the nuclear structure of the parasites provides specie determination. As in so many parasitic disorders the clinical course is determined by the immune state, the number of parasites, and the degree of reinfection. The immune aspect is important as the disease takes a different form in those coming from a non-endemic area and developing an infection for the first time and those with established residence in a filarial area.

Following the initial infection in an individual coming from a non-endemic area lymphadenopathy, particularly inguinal, develops, often associated in the male with funiculitis, hydrocele and focal lymphoedema. Pain and tenderness may be accurately localised to the glands that harbour the worms. Lymphangitis can also cause tenderness. In inhabitants of an endemic region the course is more insidious, though acute episodes from death of worms and release of its products may follow therapy. Progressive lymphoedema and elephantiasis may ensue as well as other complications such as chylous fistulae and chyluria. Microfilariae may not be readily recovered from patients with chronic infections. Eventually worms may die and calcify as described by O'Connor and his colleagues (1930).

Radiologically the lymphoedema shows itself as loss of differentiation between the fat and muscle densities consequent on accumulations of fluid and post-cellulitis scarring. The limb is thickened. Calcified worms 1×3 or 4 mm may be apparent in the subcutaneous tissues of legs or thighs, scrotum or epitrochlear regions.

Lymphangiography will show the degree of lymphatic involvement. Because of glandular obstruction tortuous dilated vessels develop and there may be a significant amount of dermal backflow (Fig. 1.22). Collateral pathways to bypass the obstruction develop peripherally within the limb and close to glands so that the number of lymphatic channels is increased. Gradually because of dilatation the valves are no longer evident and lymphatics can become as large as veins. In abdominal films more glands than normal or unusual glandular groups may

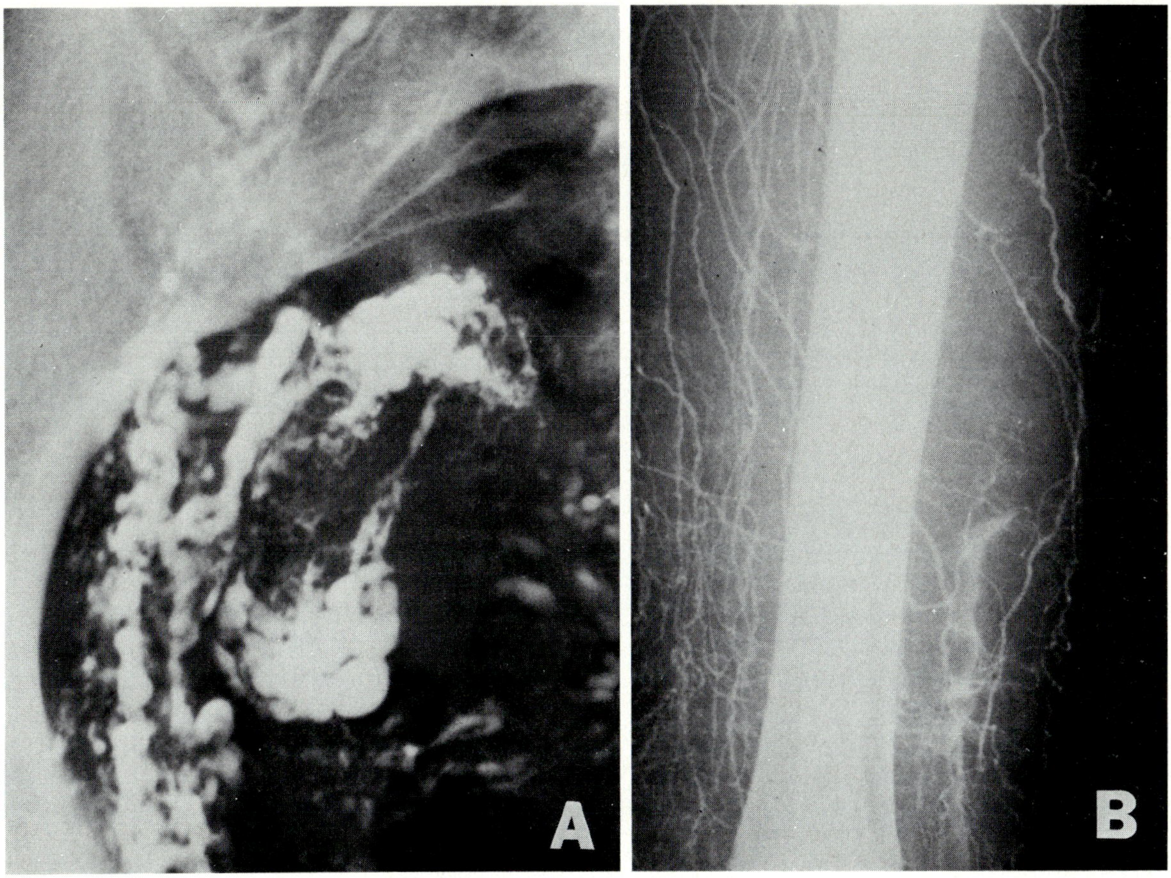

Fig. 1.22 Natural size—no reduction. Lymphangiogram. **A.** Large varicose redundant lymphatic channel from filarial obstruction. Patient also had chyluria. (Courtesy Dr. R. Tuttle, Hamilton.) **B.** Gross filarial leg oedema with increased and dilated channels and some dermal backflow.

become opacified as the normal pathways have become obliterated. The thoracic duct is usually shown (Akisada & Tani, 1968; Koehler *et al.*, 1968; Rajaram, 1970).

REFERENCES

Akisada, M. & Tani, S. (1968) Filarial chyluria in Japan, *Radiology*, **90,** 311–317.

Koehler, P. R., Chiang, T., Lin, C., Chen, K. & Chen, K. (1968) Lymphography in chyluria, *American Journal of Roentgenology*, **102,** 455–465.

O'Connor, F. W., Golden, R. & Auchingloss, H. (1930). The roentgen demonstration of calcified filaria bancrofti in human tissues, *American Journal of Roentgenology*, **23,** 494–502.

Rajaram, P. C. (1970) Lymphatic dynamics in filarial chyluria and prechyluric state—lymphographic analysis of 52 cases. *Lymphology*, **3,** 114–127.

KAPOSI'S SARCOMA

This tumour was once associated mainly with certain Eastern European ethnic groups but it is now realised that it is a frequent lesion in sub-saharan Africa (Basset & Payet, 1961; Palmer, 1962; Maclean, 1963). It is of interest that those of African descent living in the new world do not share in this high incidence. No aetiologic environmental factor has been implicated in this diffuse malignant vascular tumour of ambiguous cell derivation.

Several clinical forms of the disease are recognised, but these can overlap: a peripheral nodular cutaneous type initially involving the distal parts of the limbs; a rapidly progressive childhood form where adenopathy is the striking feature and visceral lesions may develop; and an infiltrative type with deep-seated muscle and bone deposits which may manifest exuberant ulcerative skin tumours (Cook, 1963).

In the rapidly progressive childhood form radiological study generally provides little specific diagnostic assistance beyond documenting the presence of such lesions as hilar and paratracheal adenopathy and perhaps nasopharyngeal or palatal masses.

By contrast, in the limb forms radiological study is of considerable value in indicating the initial extent of the disease and at follow-up to demonstrate regression or progression after therapy. In the presence of the typical tender, darkish purple skin nodules and lymphoedema the clinical diagnosis is readily confirmed by biopsy of an accessible lesion. The sites of tumour deposits can be established by soft tissue and standard radiographs supplemented by angiography (Fig. 1.23).

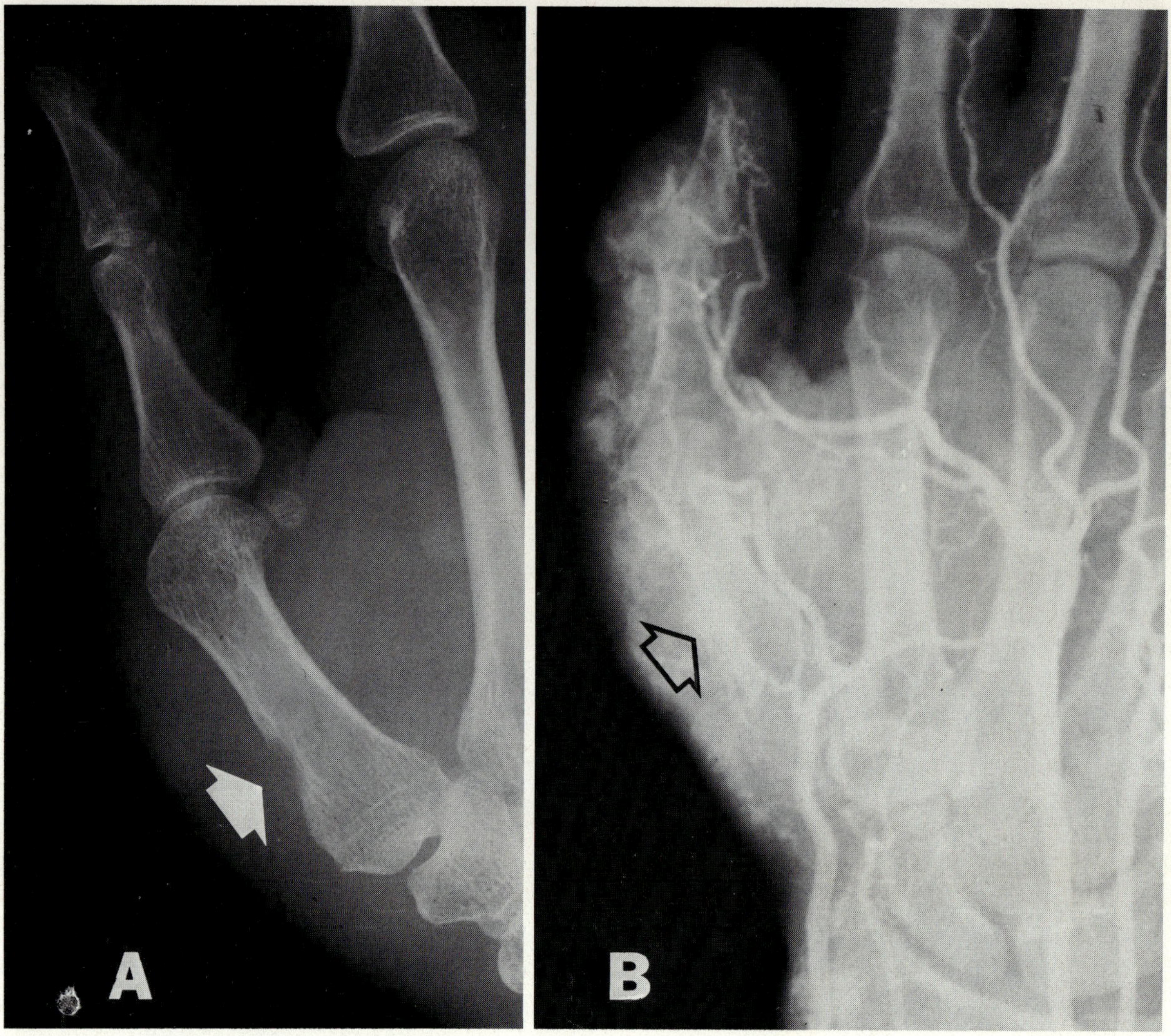

Fig. 1.23 **A.** Erosive marginal cortical bone destruction. **B.** Extensive vascular soft tissue deposits and a focus (open black arrow) occupies area of Kaposi bone erosion.

In soft tissue studies superficial Kaposi deposits and those in subcutaneous fat are readily evident in tangential projection.

The extensive lymphoedema that often accompanies this condition may cause difficulty in interpretation. Palmer (1962) in his experience of 200 cases, mentions the occasional presence of visible small calcium fleck-like deposits which may be in veins draining deposits.

Bony structures can be affected in several fashions as indicated by Davies (1957). Osteoporosis of the phalanges and juxta articular bone is common, particularly in patients with lymphoedema. Osseous destructive foci may arise apparently by erosion from an external deposit (Fig. 1.18). Other deposits appear to develop within the medullary space and destroy bone by expanding so that they form cyst-like lesions, often with fairly well-defined or invasive edges (Figs. 1.24, 1.25, 1.26).

Angiography demonstrates the site of most deposits (Palmer, 1962; Haylock, 1963). They are fed by a single vessel that fans out into the interwoven vessels that make up a nodular deposit. Contrast pools there and drains by single or often paired dilated venous channels. There is a degree of shunting through the deposits which may impair perfusion distally. Deep-seated nodules that are clinically not suspected can be opacified as may lymphatic deposits. The latter can also be shown in lymphangiograms as filling defects. Oedema is shown to be due to lymphatic obstruction. Nodules may communicate directly with lymphatics (Baddeley & Bhana, 1971).

Visceral deposits are often not clinically apparent but can exist almost anywhere within the thoracic or abdominal cavities. The gastro-intestinal lesions cause intramural masses that may obstruct, ulcerate and bleed. Such lesions can be demonstrated in barium studies and by angiography. Renal, pulmonary and cardiac deposits show evidence of mass lesions and their nature can be suspected when there are skin manifestations and adenopathy accessible to biopsy.

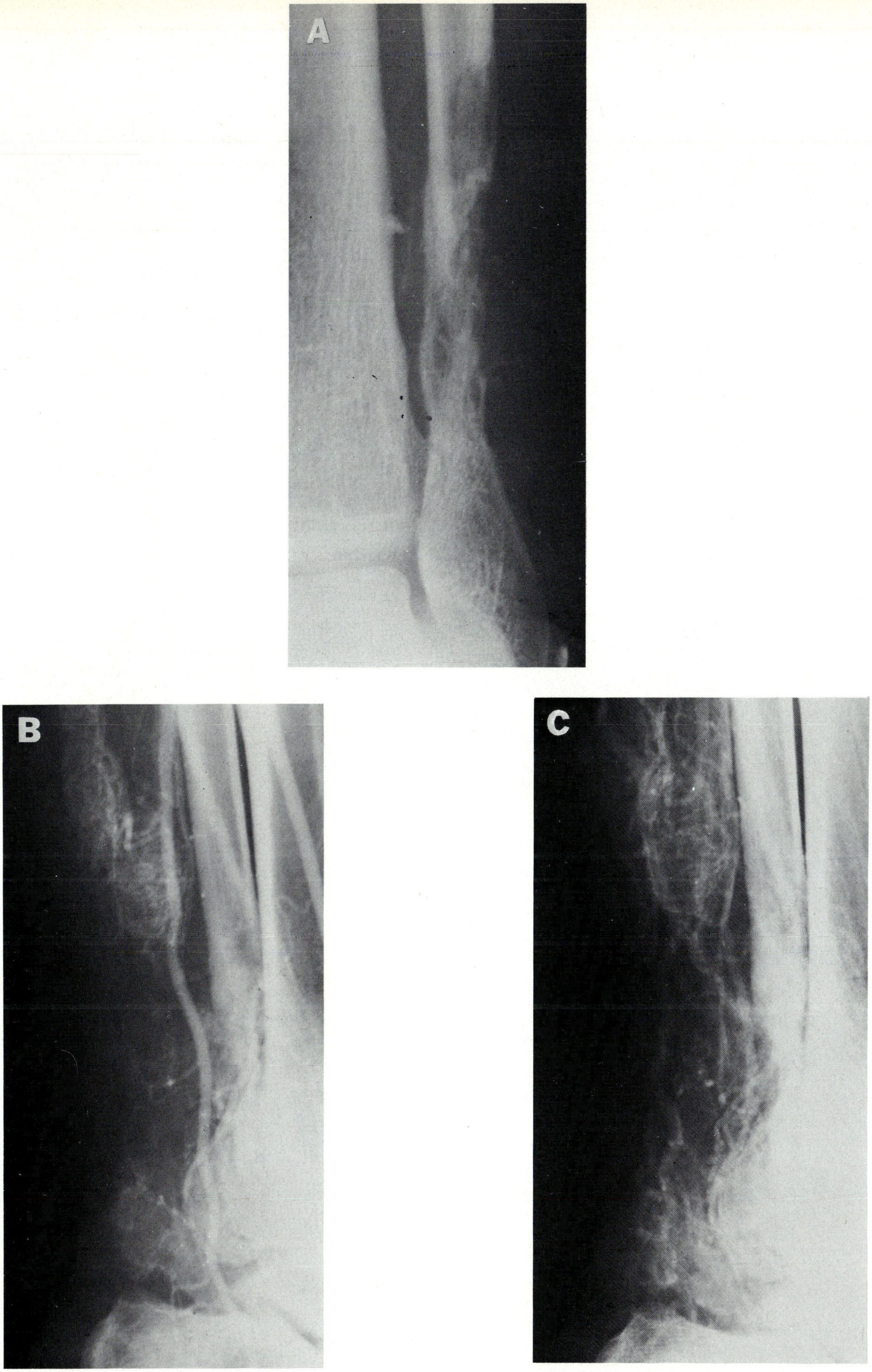

Fig. 1.24 **A.** Multiple rounded lytic defects in fibula. **B.** Early angiogram shows filling of muscle and subcutaneous nodules with a plexus of small vessels. **C.** Later phase reveals well opacified venous channels during arterial phase. (Courtesy of Dr. A. Haylock and *British Journal of Radiology*.)

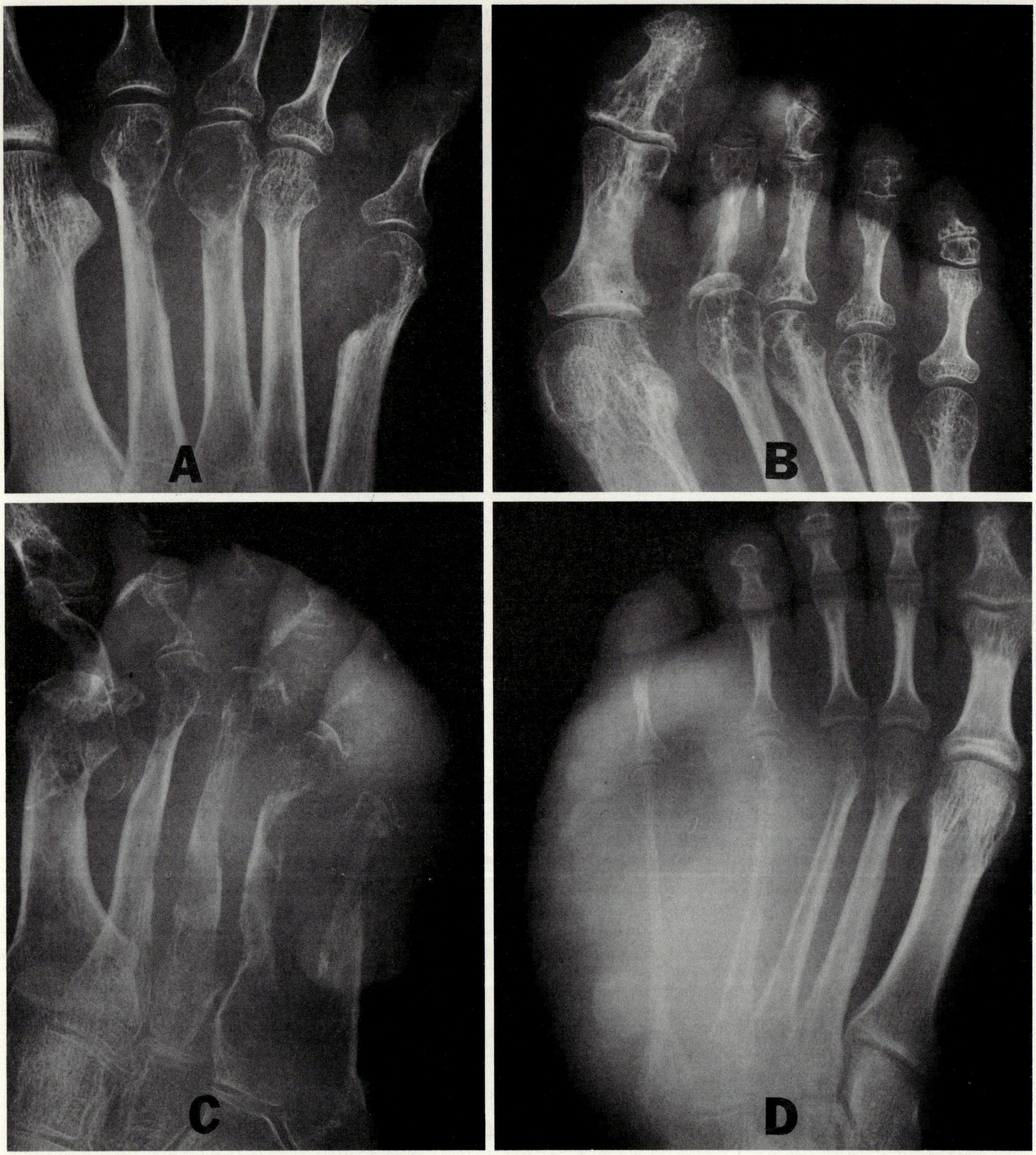

Fig. 1.25 Kaposi sarcoma. **A.** Multiple metatarsal defects and erosions. **B.** Many intramedullary foci. **C.** Extensive erosive bone destruction. **D.** Soft tissue mass with extrinsic bone attenuation.

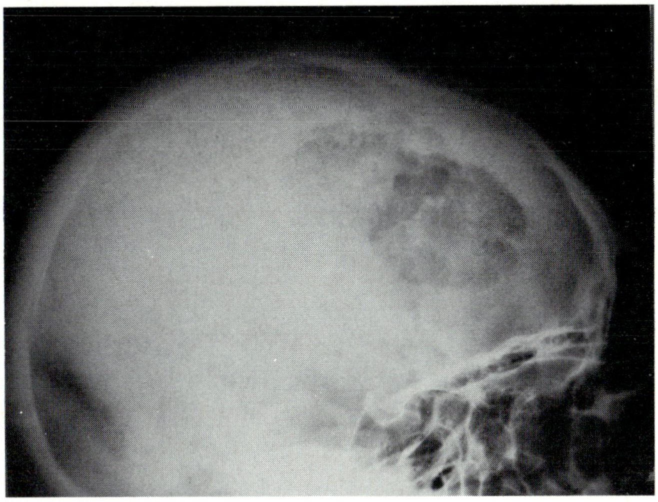

Fig. 1.26 Erosive skull defects due to Kaposi.

The differential diagnosis in the typical case is limited. The visceral forms are exceedingly perplexing as mentioned above. Mycetoma before the development of sinuses could be a problem in the pedal forms. Obviously the differential diagnosis of lymphoedema is large, but this feature is rare in isolation. In all doubtful cases the findings of a thorough clinical examination provide invaluable information to assist radiological interpretation.

REFERENCES

Baddeley, H. & Bhana, D. (1971) Lymphography in Kaposi's sarcoma, *Clinical Radiology*, **22,** 391–400.

Basset, A. & Payet, M. (1961) Caractères clinique de la maladie de Kaposi dans l'ouest African. Differences avec le Kaposi européen, *Bulletin et Mémoires de la Faculté de Médecine de Dakar*, **2,** 280–283.

Cook, J. (1963) *Symposium on Kaposi's Sarcoma.* pp. 75–85. Basel: S. Karger.

Davies, A. G. M. (1956) Bone changes in Kaposi sarcoma, *Journal of the Faculty of Radiologists*, **8,** 32–40.

Haylock, A. (1963) Angiography in Kaposi sarcoma, *Clinical Radiology*, **14,** 304–309.

Hutt, M. S. R. (1973) Kaposi sarcoma, *Tropical Pathology*. ed. Spencer, H., pp. 710–715. New York: Springer.

MacLean, C. M. U. (1963) Kaposi's sarcoma in Nigeria, *The British Journal of Cancer*, **17,** 195–205.

Palmer, P. E. S. (1962) The radiological changes of Kaposi's sarcoma, *Acta Union Internationale Contre le Cancer*, **18,** 400–412.

2. Bone Diseases

BONE GROWTH AND MATURATION

S. P. Bohrer

Bone growth and maturation are affected by both genetic and enviromental factors (Garn & Rohmann, 1966). Sex and race are the most important genetic factors. Parental height is also correlated with height of the offspring. Nutrition and disease are the most important environmental factors. Because of the genetic variation between races, it is not appropriate to measure one group's status by another group's standards. For example in the U.S.A. blacks have advanced skeletal maturation relative to the white population; they also have greater cortical thickness, skeletal mass, metacarpal length and height (at least to the age of 12) than comparable whites (Garn *et al.*, 1972; Garn *et al.*, 1973; Owen, 1973; Garn & Clark, 1975). Because protein calorie malnutrition causes slowed growth, delayed bone maturation and increased endosteal resorption, it is wrong to determine normative values for a population if the sample children evaluated contained any that were malnourished. It would then be a survey study rather than the establishment of the genetic norm for the group. Well-nourished children of the same racial make-up need to be studied to determine reference norms for the population—then the malnourished can be evaluated with a reference. Furthermore a standard once established is not immutable as substantial changes, in growth at least, have been recorded over decades in, for example, the average height of 18-year-old army recruits entering the forces of several countries. This probably expresses nutritional changes with alterations in economic circumstances.

Early bone age studies in Africa did not separate the genetic and environmental factors (Mackay, 1952). Africans were reported to have delayed skeletal maturation relative to American standards. Recent studies have shown that they are probably advanced in most areas if well-nourished children are studies. Poor nutrition may account for the observed retardation rather than genetic influences. An average maturation rate was determined for the group rather than a genetically determined ideal norm to be achieved with good nutrition.

DETERMINING POPULATION NORMS

The ideal study cohort should be composed of well-nourished healthy children aged from birth until growth plate closure. Longitudinal, cross section, or mixed longitudinal studies can be used to obtain sufficient data. The exact birthdate of each child should be known. The physical measurements studied, depending on the comprehensiveness desired (height, weight, circumferences and skin fold thickness), can be measured at an exact known age. Similarly hand radiographs obtained in a standardised fashion are taken to study bone maturation and to record cortical thickness, metacarpal length, etc. assigned to a specific chronological age.

Measurements such as growth, metacarpal length and cortical thickness have no predetermined value as the end point—as all children do not eventually grow to the same height. Accordingly these measurements can simply be plotted to show the norm and standard deviations for the group.

Bone maturation is however different. Everyone reaches an identical finite end point with closure of the growth plates and cessation of growth along with full maturation of the small bones of the wrist. A different approach is needed to 'plot' the findings.

One can make an atlas for the population under study similar to the established atlases in current use (Greulich & Pyle; Tanner–Whitehouse) or more simply one can relate maturation in the group studied to an existing atlas using a correction factor. For example if the mean bone age of all the male *chronologically* six-year-olds in the study population comes out to have a bone age of 5 years using the atlas, then an atlas correction factor of plus one year is needed for six-year-olds. Then the bone age equals chronological age with the reference atlas. It is also important to evaluate the standard deviation since bone age determinations show considerable biologic variations—as do other biomedical measurements. If this is done for each age group and for each sex, a correction chart can then be constructed (Fig. 2.1). It must be emphasised that the correction chart can only be applied to the specific atlas initially used. The two major atlases currently employed differ from each other by about one year for most ages,

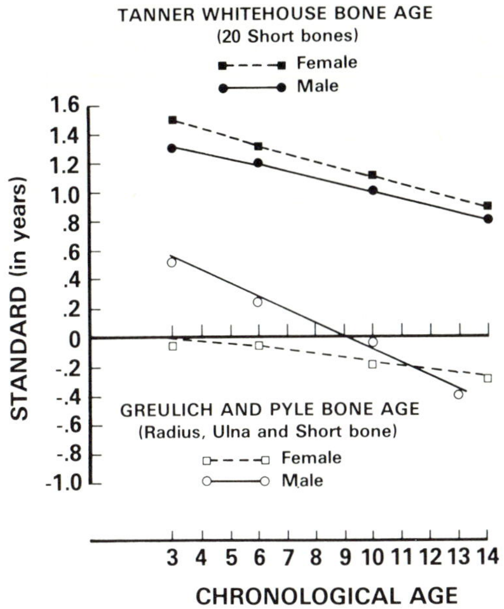

Fig. 2.1 Example of correction chart applied to maturation atlases.

as they were developed using different populations at different times.

For simplicity, and possibly greater consistency and accuracy, it is advisable to ignore the carpal bones when determining bone age. These show more developmental variability and asymmetry than epiphyses and are more prone to observer errors when evaluated (Acheson & Fowler, 1963, 1964, 1966; Levine, 1972).

EFFECTS OF MALNUTRITION

S. P. Bohrer

Bone formed by children with protein calorie undernutrition (malnutrition) is normal bone although it may be mechanically weak because of decreased quantity. Skeletal growth continues under conditions of even severe malnutrition, but it is slowed. Height and metacarpal length are decreased relative to the norms of well-nourished children. Periosteal appositional new bone continues to be laid down but there is endosteal resorption reducing the cortical thickness, cortical area and per cent cortical area (Garn & Rohmann, 1964; Garn, 1966; Garn *et al.*, 1969; Frisaucho *et al.*, 1970).

Bone maturation is also retarded permitting some 'catch-up' growth to take place as the growth plates remain open longer; but nevertheless the full growth potential is not reached. Chronic malnutrition results in smaller adults, both male and female, as bone maturation is less delayed than growth so that there is inadequate time to catch up before the epiphyses fuse. The degree of maturational retardation is greater during childhood than during adolescence (Frisaucho *et al.*, 1970). Thus the ossific centres appearing late are not as delayed as those appearing early. There is relative acceleration of maturation in the adolescent despite continued malnutrition, so that complete maturation (fusion) is only slightly delayed. The relative maturation spurt may be related to the onset of sexual maturation.

One study group has found that in malnutrition maturation of the metacarpal and phalangeal epiphyses are more affected than the development of the carpal bones (Masse & Hunt, 1963).

The appearance of transverse dense lines of arrested growth has an uncertain relationship with Kwashiorkor or subnutrition. Some process that allegedly interrupts growth of the cartilage leads to piling up and thickening of the zone of provisional ossification so that it extends laterally rather than longitudinally. The density is often emphasised by adjacent porosis. Certainly patients with kwashiorkor may show or develop transverse lines but these occur in children who have had an acute illness and may appear in premature baby units. Two studies indicate that protein calorie malnutrition *per se* is not responsible for the transverse linear bands, though they may be apparent in patients with subnutrition (Jones & Dean, 1956; Adams & Berridge, 1969).

REFERENCES

Acheson, R. M., Fowler, G., Fry, E. I., Koski, K., Urbano, P. & Van Der, J. J. (1963) Studies in the reliability of assessing skeletal maturity from x-rays. Part I. Greulich–Pyle Atlas, *Human Biology*, **35,** 317–349.

Acheson, R. M., Vicinus, J. H. & Fowler, G. B. (1964) Studies in the reliability of assessing skeletal maturity from x-rays. Part II. The bone specific approach, *Human Biology*, **36,** 211–228.

Acheson, R. M., Vicinus, J. H. & Fowler, G. B. (1966) Studies in the reliability of assessing skeletal maturity from x-rays. Part III. Greulich–Pyle Atlas and Tanner–Whitehouse method contrasted, *Human Biology*, **38,** 204–218.

Adams, P. & Berridge, F. R. (1969) Effects of kwashiorkor on cortical and trabecular bone, *Archive Diseases of Childhood*, **44,** 705–709.

Frisaucho, A. R., Garn, S. M. & Ascoli, W. (1970) Unequal influence of low dietary intakes on skeletal maturation during childhood and adolescence, *American Journal of Nutrition*, **23,** 1220–1227.

Garn, S. M. & Rohmann, B. A. (1964) Compact bone deficiency in protein calorie malnutrition, *Science*, **145,** 1444–1445.

Garn, S. M. & Rohmann, B. A. (1966) Interaction of nutrition and genetics in the timing of growth and development, *Pediatric Clinics of North America*, **13,** 353–379.

Garn, S. M. (1966) Malnutrition and skeletal development in the preschool child. In *Pre School Child Malnutrition*, pp. 43–62. Washington D.C.: National Academy of Sciences—National Research Council.

Garn, S. M., Guzman, M. A. & Wagner, B. (1969) Sub-periosteal gain and endosteal loss in protein calorie malnutrition, *American Journal of Physical Anthropology*, **30,** 153–155.

Garn, S. M., Sandusky, S. T., Nagy, J. M. & McCann, M. B. (1972) Advanced skeletal development in low income negro children, *The Journal of Pediatrics*, **80,** 965–969.

Garn, S. M., Clark, D. C. & Trowbridge, F. L. (1973) Tendency towards greater stature in American black children, *American Journal Diseases of Children*, **126,** 164–166.

Garn, S. M. & Clark, D. C. (1975) Nutrition, growth, development and maturation: Findings from the ten state nutrition survey of 1968–70, *Pediatrics*, **56,** 306–319.

Jones, P. R. M. & Dean, R. F. A. (1956) The effects of kwashiorkor on the development of bones of the hand, *Journal of Tropical Paediatrics*, **2,** 51–68.

Levine, E. (1972) The contributions of the carpal bones and the epiphyseal centers of the hand to the assessment of skeletal maturity, *Human Biology*, **44,** 317–327.

Mackay, D. M. (1952) Skeletal maturation in the hand: a study of development in East African children, *Transactions of the Royal Society of Tropical Medicine and Hygiene*, **46,** 136–150.

Masse, G. & Hunt, E. E., Jnr. (1963) Skeletal maturation of the hand and wrist in West African children, *Human Biology*, **35,** 3–25.

Owen, G. M. (1973) Anthropometric differences between black and white preschool children, *The Journal of Pediatrics*, **80,** 965–969.

DEFICIENCY RICKETS

Where the nutritional intake of vitamin D is low, rickets may develop in childhood, and osteomalacia in girls and women when custom deprives them of sunlight. This is seen classically in areas of adequate sunlight when there is strict observance of purdah. Asians and Africans emigrating to Europe may also develop the disease. There air pollution that filters out the ultraviolet light may be a factor in the aetiology.

The radiological features are well known. There is metaphyseal widening, with cupping and increase in depth of the growth plate translucent zone which is poorly and irregularly defined on its diaphyseal aspect (Fig. 2.2). In severe long-standing disease the skeleton is poorly mineralised, there may be bone plasticity with bowing or angular deformities of weight-bearing bones. The translucent bands of Looser's zones, which are of course not fractures, are the main radiological feature of the adult disease.

Treatment can give rise to temporary changes that may be confusing. The metaphysis becomes denser and more regular on the diaphyseal aspect. Calcium may appear around the shaft as osteoid previously laid down becomes mineralised. This is not inflammatory periosteal new bone. We have found that generalised loss of the lamina dura, particularly around the germinal follicle of unerupted teeth, is frequent in rickets (Fig. 2.3) (Braband *et al.*, 1965). Since part of a child's mandible is often shown in a chest radiograph this observation is useful to confirm a suspicion of rickets suggested by enlarged costochondral junctions.

REFERENCE

Braband, H., Cockshott, W. P. & Evans, K. T. (1965) Die röntgendiagnostische Bedeutung der Lamina dura des Zahnes, *Fortschritte Röntgenstrahlen*, **102,** 447–453.

ENDEMIC FLUOROSIS

Fluorine is a surprisingly prevalent substance and it has been estimated that one-thirteenth of the earth's crust contains compounds with this halogen (Eagers, 1969). Fortunately it is only deleterious to man when presented in excess in water-soluble form with ionic dissociation. In industrialised countries certain chemical and manufacturing processes release inorganic fluorides that can prove very toxic to workers through inhalation or by ingestion of contaminated materials.

Here we are concerned with endemic fluorosis where increased chronic uptake of fluorine occurs through the water supply or from foods grown in soils with high fluorine content: notably volcanic or those close to outcrops of rocks of high phosphate content. Wells, usually of the deep variety, may contain water with increased fluorine content. Some years ago when communities began to add fluorides to water supplies to inhibit dental caries, studies showed that 1 part per million protected

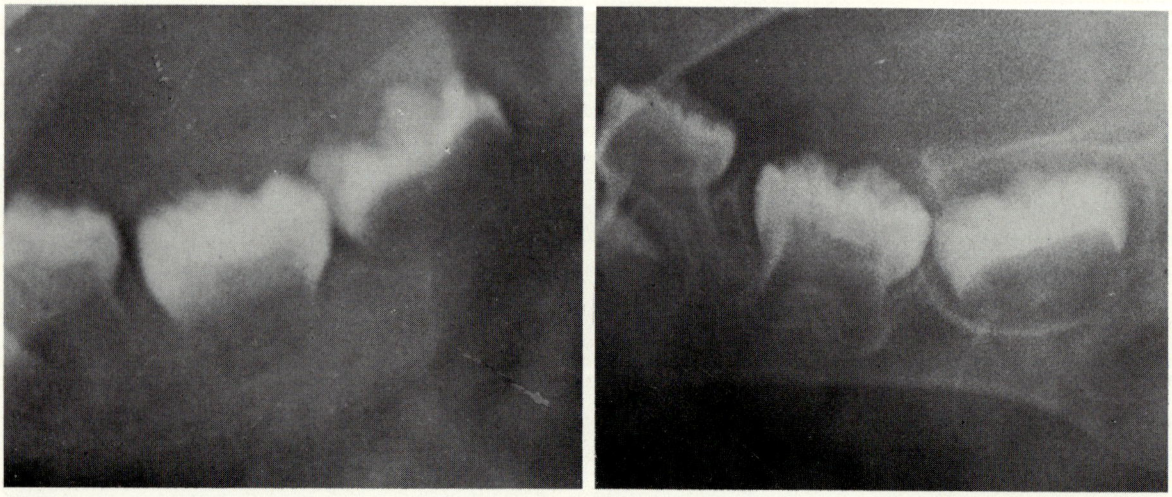

A B

Fig. 2.2 A, B. Young child with rickets on left. At time of diagnosis there is no trace of lamina dura investing the teeth. After six months therapy (right) the lamina dura of tooth sockets and of germinal follicles has returned.

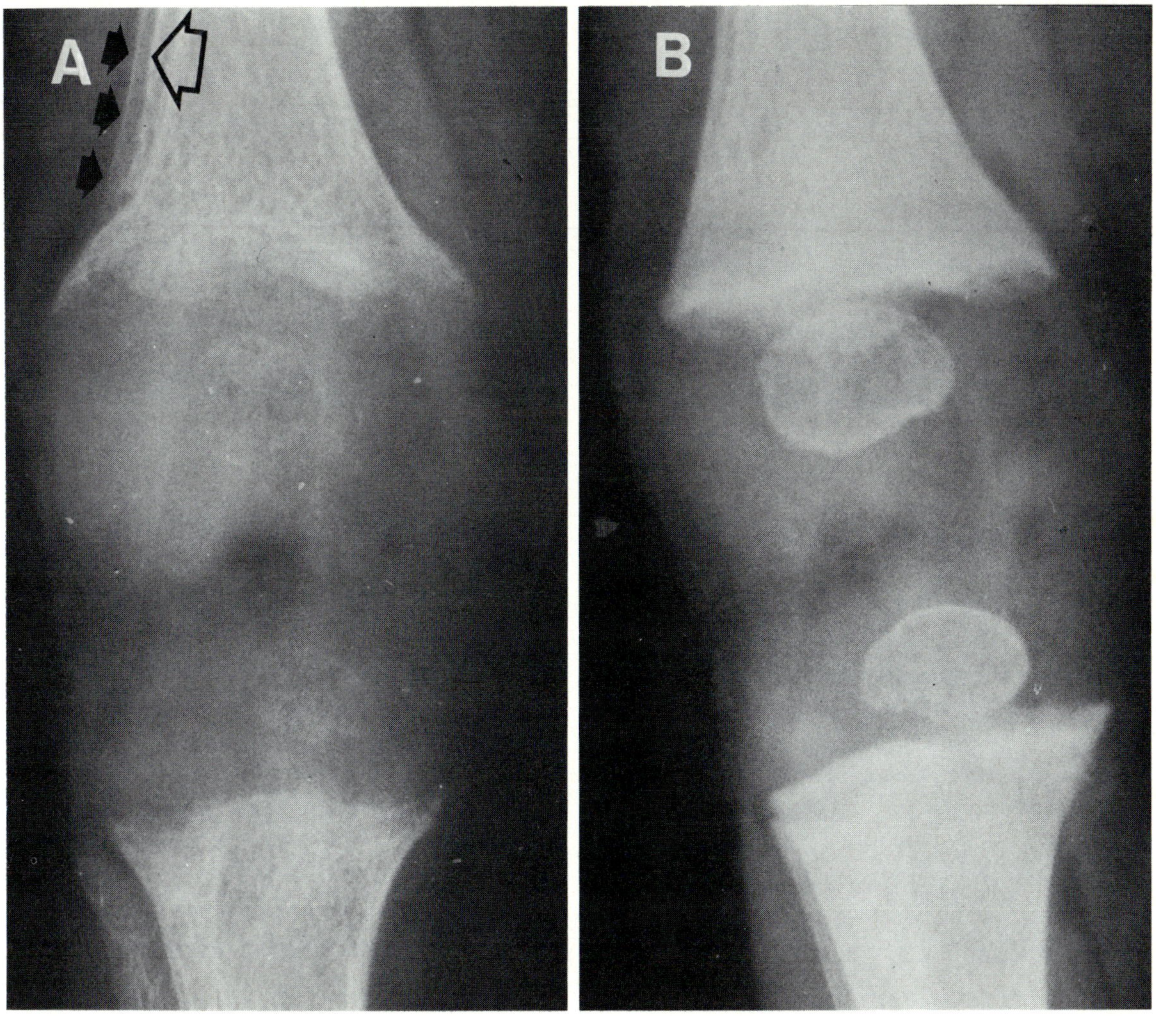

Fig. 2.3 **A.** Acute rickets two weeks following start of treatment. Note the lamellated lines due to mineralisation of pre-existing osteoid around the shaft. **B.** Three months later note the nearly normal metaphysis, the reappearance of the epiphyseal ossification centres and the general increase in mineralisation.

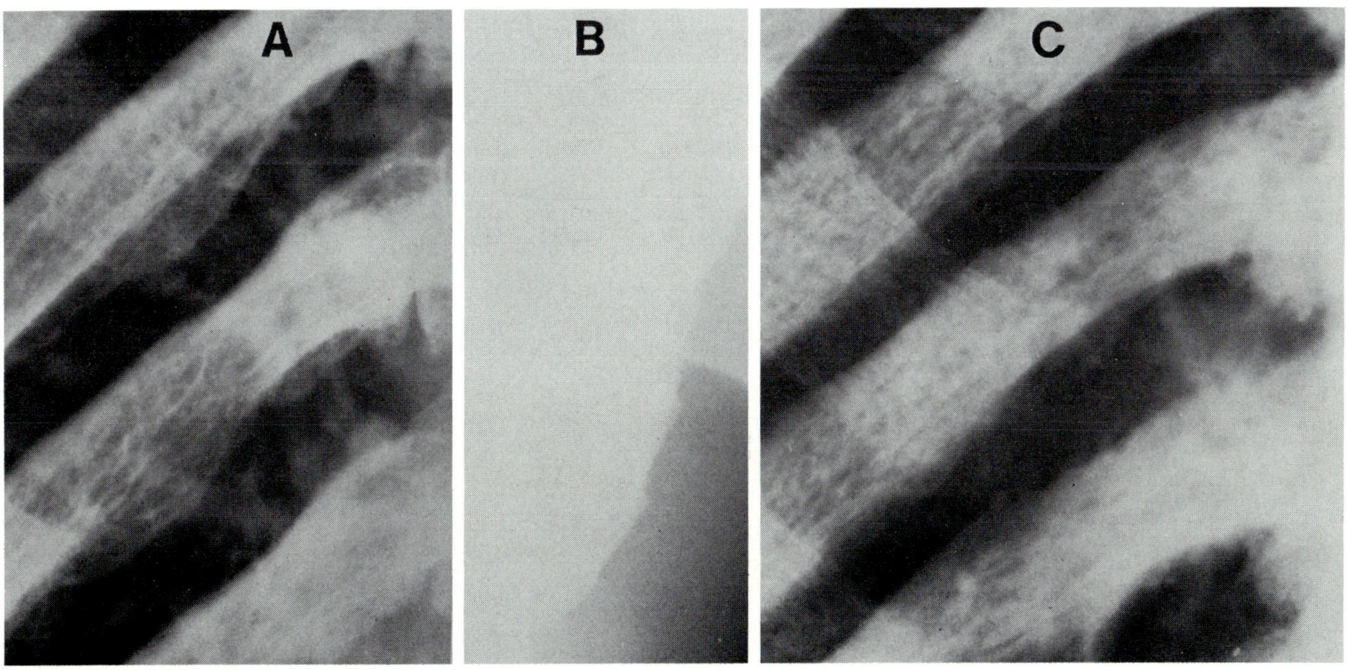

Fig. 2.4 Fluorosis from Kuwait. **A.** Note coarse rib structure and new bone on inferior aspect of rib. **B.** Axillary border of scapula to show density and irregular marginal new bone proliferation. **C.** Typical coarse rib trabecular structure and areas of homogeneous density.

dental health and that 2 parts per million might lead to dental mottling, but that consumption of water containing up to 8 parts per million over many years need not produce deleterious signs or symptoms (Stevenson & Watson, 1957). However, severe bony changes have been described from drinking well water with 6 parts per million (Kumar & Kemp Harper, 1963). Nevertheless, in a survey of 170 000 radiographs of the spine and pelvis of Texans and Oklahomans (Stevenson & Watson, 1957) living in areas with a high fluorine content in the water, only 23 patients with skeletal fluorosis were found. None developed in communities with less than 4 parts per million of fluoride in their water supply. The relationship of skeletal fluorosis to a given fluorine water content is not purely dose related since in India and elsewhere it has been clearly shown that the state of overall nutrition is also relevant.

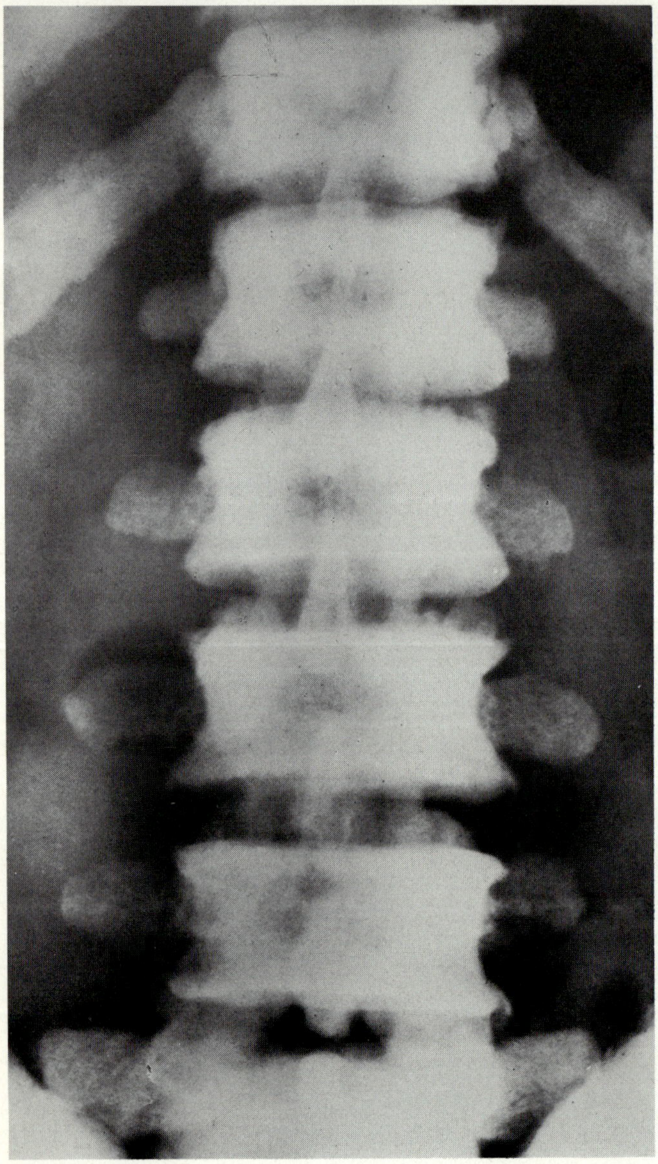

Fig. 2.5 Amorphous structure of vertebrae in a patient from Qatar with fluorosis.

Endemic fluorosis is prevalent in many areas of the world. In the tropics, the Persian Gulf states, Aden, Yemen, parts of North Africa and the Sahara, northern Tanzania, around Pretoria and in Turkey and the Punjab are well-recognised endemic zones.

The symptomatology is variable and is related to the extent of productive new bone. This can cause spinal rigidity or nerve root compression.

Radiologically there may be calcification of ligamentous structures or attachments, or bone density and contour alterations.

The ligamentous changes are seen in such areas as the linea aspera, the interossous membrane of the forearm (Grech & Latham, 1964; Soriano & Manchon, 1966), or the sacro-tuberous and sacro-spinous ligaments (Stevenson & Watson, 1957). The structures may eventually ossify. Gross exuberant calcification with subsequent ossification has been recorded in Spaniards who had been drinking wine contaminated with fluorides. Some of the illustrations show changes reminiscent of myositis ossificans (Soriano & Manchon, 1966).

Bone trabeculae may thicken, enlarge and show coarse trajectories (Fig. 2.4). The bones enlarge by accretion of peri-osteal new bone giving rough contours to areas of muscle and ligamentous attachments. Severe cases develop coalescence of trabeculae and a 'chalky' amorphous appearance of dense bone (Fig. 2.5).

Near joints hypertrophic new bone at the capsular attachments can simulate osteophytes. In fluorosis there is an increase in the incidence of Monckeberg arterial calcification.

REFERENCES

Eagers, R. Y. (1969) Toxic properties of inorganic fluorine compounds, Amsterdam: Elsevér.

Grech, P. & Latham, M. C. (1964) Fluorosis in the northern region of Tanganyika, *Transactions of the Royal Society of Tropical Medicine and Hygiene*, **58,** 566–574.

Kumar, S. P. & Kemp-Harper, R. A. (1963) Fluorosis in Aden, *British Journal of Radiology*, **36,** 497–502.

Soriano, M. & Manchon, F. (1966) Radiological aspects of a new type of bone fluorosis, periostitis deformans, *Radiology*, **87,** 1089–1091.

Stevenson, C. A. & Watson, A. R. (1957) Fluoride osteosclerosis, *American Journal of Roentgenology*, **78,** 13–18.

BONE INFECTIONS

Numerous causes of bone infection exist. The emphasis here is weighted towards some of the rarer and more exotic forms that are seen in tropical countries. However, we cannot entirely dismiss from consideration universal common lesions that quantitatively pose greater health problems than the diverse less common infections. Therefore we will briefly discuss pyogenic staphlococcal osteomyelitis and tuberculosis before describing the diseases resulting from other organisms.

Haematogenous osteomyelitis

Haematogenous osteomyelitis due to the staphylococcus is the most frequent acute bone infection. Trueta (1959) emphasised the importance of the patient's age and bone vascular development in determing the site of bone infection (Fig. 2.6).

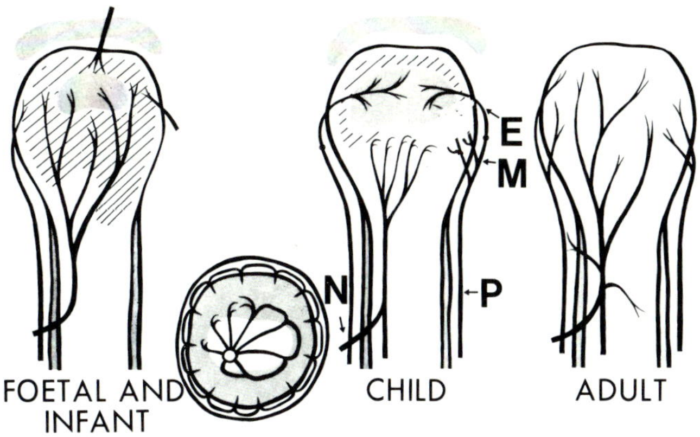

Fig. 2.6 Diagramatic representation of bone circulation at different ages. In the infant, vessels perfusing the epiphysis cross the growth plate. In the child the physis defines vascular territories. From the periosteal plexus P some perforating vessels M reach the metaphysis M and some through capsular attachments reach the epiphysis. In adults there is free ramification of vessels.

In infants under six months there are still large joints without formed growth plates at the extremities of long bones. At this stage branches of the nutrient artery cross to the epiphysis and there become end vessels. Organisms seem to preferentially lodge at this site where circulation is slow, and as the infective focus enlarges the joint cavity soon becomes implicated. Often the neonate has severe systemic septicaemic or chest disturbances so that the acute arthritis is easily missed. Thus by the time a radiograph is obtained there may be subluxation or dislocation of the joint with epiphyseal destruction—the opening act in a life-long disability. Often several joints are affected, with the hips and shoulders being the most frequent because of their anatomical arrangements.

In children and youths in the tropics classical haematogenous osteomyelitis differs in few respects from experience in the temperate world. However, it is more frequent and often presents at a later stage of development than is usual in industrialised parts of the world. Because of this there is rarely need to consider isotopic diagnosis by bone scan (even if available), as the clinical presentation and findings, and the radiological appearances, make the diagnosis obvious. Extensive diaphyseal destruction, sequestration and pathological fracture are not rare complications. In adults haematogenous bone infection is rare, whereas compound fracture will frequently lead to osteomyelitis. When present it may affect any part of the bone.

The specific infections of sickle cell disease are discussed later in this section. A useful radiological differential point between classical blood-borne osteomyelitis and the post-infarct bone infection of sickling is the location. Osteomyelitis is juxtametaphyseal whereas the sickling foci in long bones tend to be at a distance from the metaphysis in the intermediate fifth of the shaft (Bohrer, 1970).

REFERENCES

Bohrer, S. P. (1971) Fractures complicating bone infarcts and/or osteomyelitis in sickle cell disease, *Clinical Radiology*, **22,** 83–88.

Trueta, J. (1959) The three types of acute haematogenous osteomyelitis. A clinical and vascular study, *Journal of Bone and Joint Surgery*, **41B,** 671–680.

BONE AND JOINT TUBERCULOSIS

Tuberculosis is universal, but its incidence and manifestation differ greatly in the tropics from the textbook descriptions emanating nowadays from Europe and North America. It is not merely that the problem of bone tuberculosis is quantitatively greater, but that the sites affected and their evolution may confound those not familiar with the process in the tropics. As always in tuberculosis the patient's resistance is an important determinant of the behaviour of the disease. Lowered resistance and greater opportunities of exposure to tuberculosis doubtless account for many of the features of bone tuberculosis.

In reaching the correct diagnosis it is important to keep tuberculosis in the forefront of diagnostic possibilities. Proof can be difficult to obtain rapidly. An abnormal chest radiograph can be strong circumstantial evidence of tuberculosis. Adenopathy, synovial biopsy and aspirated material from an abscess can provide histologic or cultural material to establish the nature of the disease. At other times the therapeutic response provides telling evidence as to the presumed aetiology. The tuberculosis granuloma can be simulated by other granulomata, particularly certain dimorphic yeast infections and in histiocytosis X.

The spine is the most frequently affected part of the skeleton, though the proportion of cases with spinal disease varies from just above half to over 80 per cent in some series.

In classical Pott's disease the initial osteolytic focus is in a vertebral body that extends in a destructive manner to reach the intervertebral disc. This is no boundary to the extension of disease and the fibrocartilage disc rapidly becomes destroyed, unlike the process in dimorphic yeast infections where the disc is relatively preserved. In tuberculosis the granuloma extends to the next body and gradu-

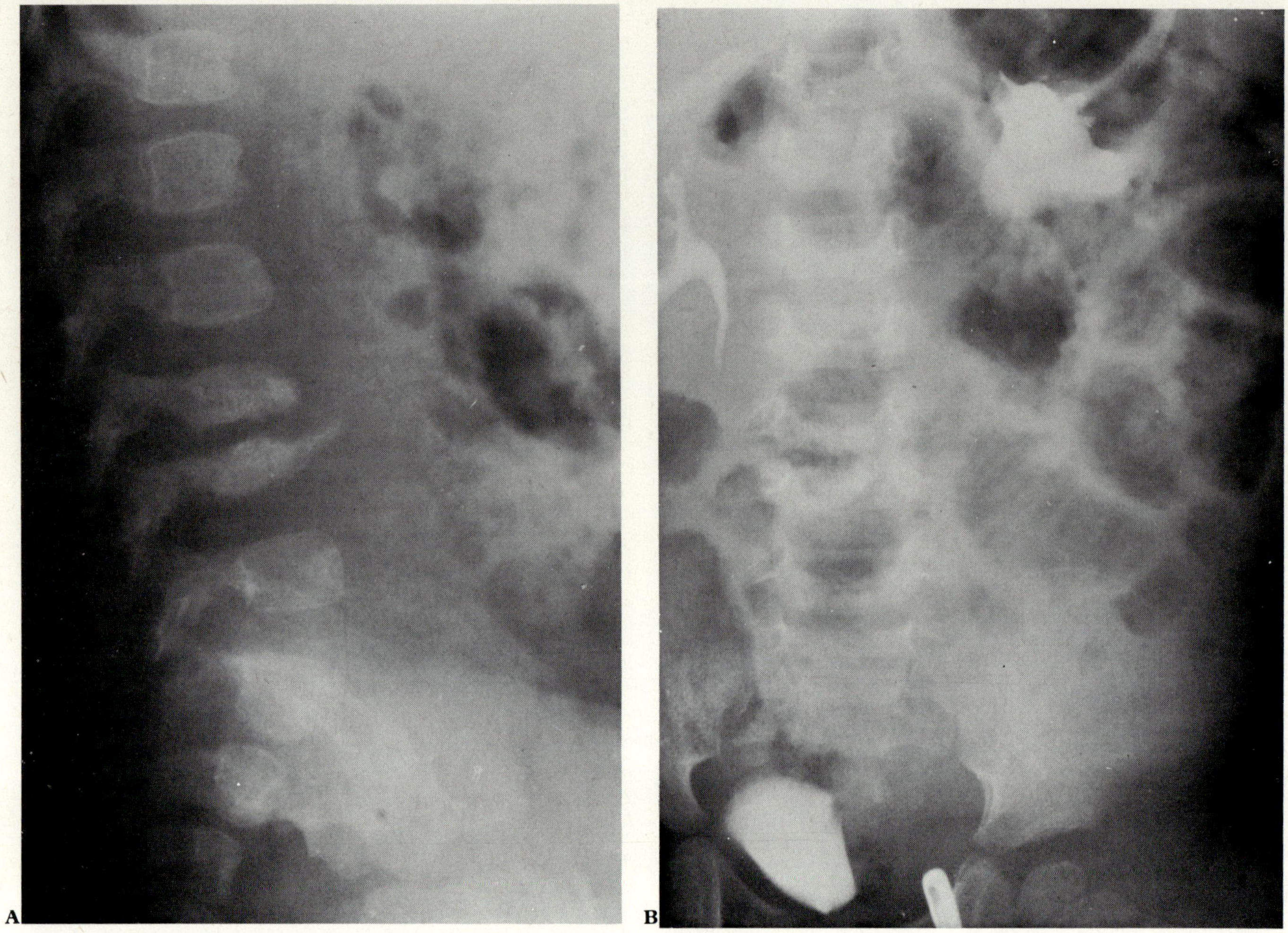

Fig. 2.7 A, B. Tuberculous uniform collapse of a vetebral body reminiscent of the Calvé type, though some disc narrowing is present. Bowel gas displaced forward by a paravertebral abscess which is seen to be causing obstructive uropathy and displacement of the bladder. (Courtesy of Dr. Peter Konstam.)

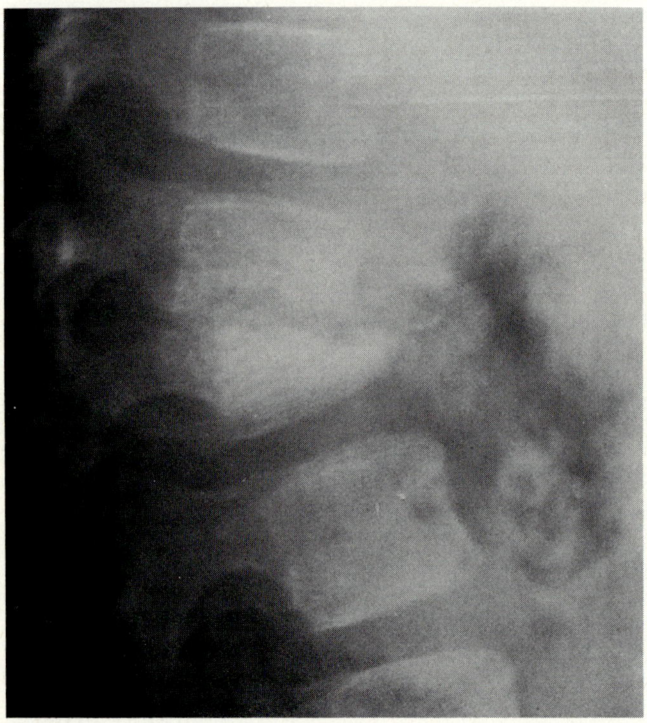

Fig. 2.8 Tuberculous destruction of contiguous surfaces of upper two lumbar vertebral bodies with disc destruction.

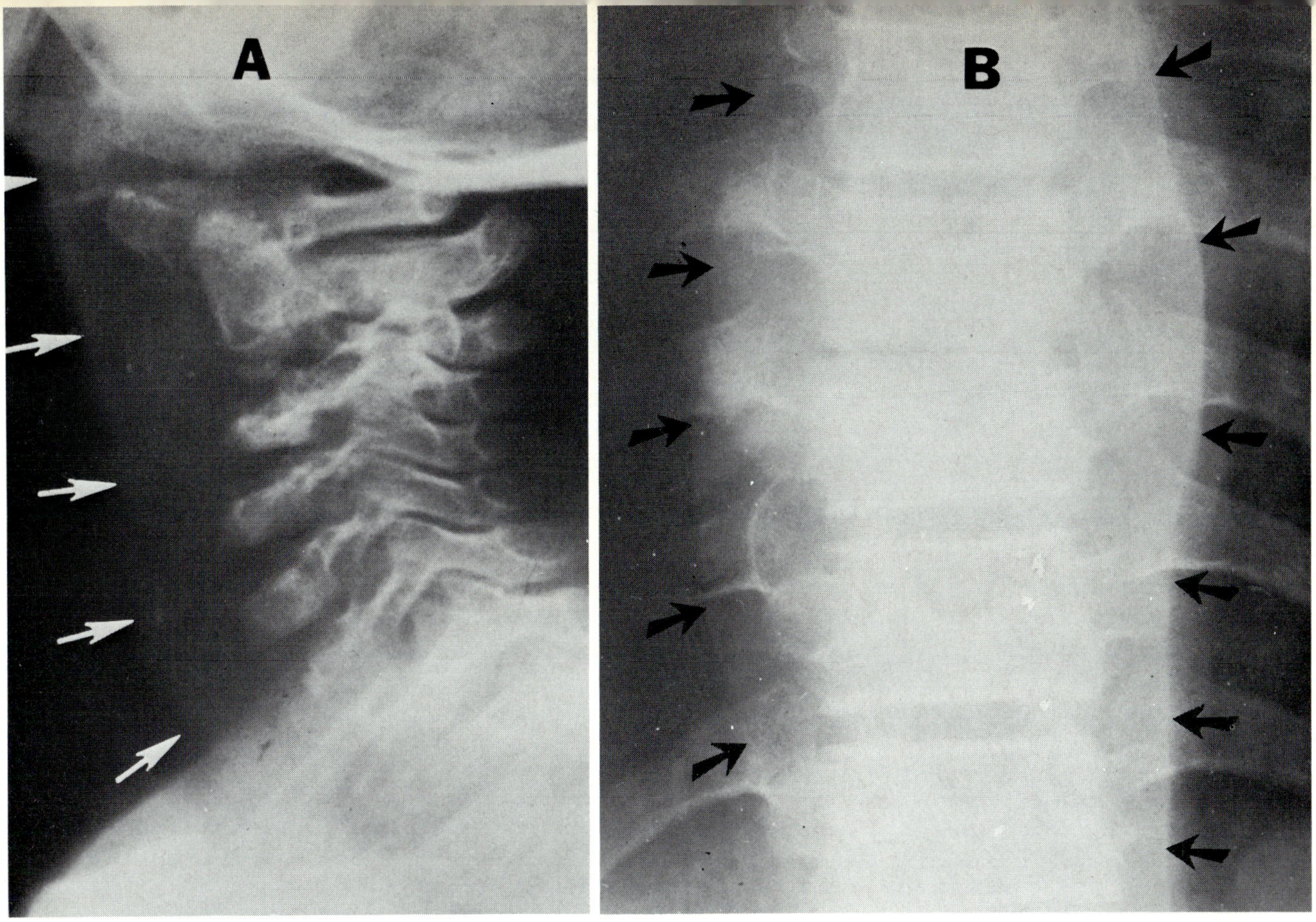

Fig. 2.9 **A.** Tuberculous collapse of bodies of CV3 with implication of bodies above and below. Atlanto-axial subluxation. Large anterior paravertebral abscess. White arrows indicate anterior limit of abscess. **B.** Antero-posterior view of dorsal spine focus. A disc space is narrowed and a large bilateral paravertebral abscess is defined by black arrows.

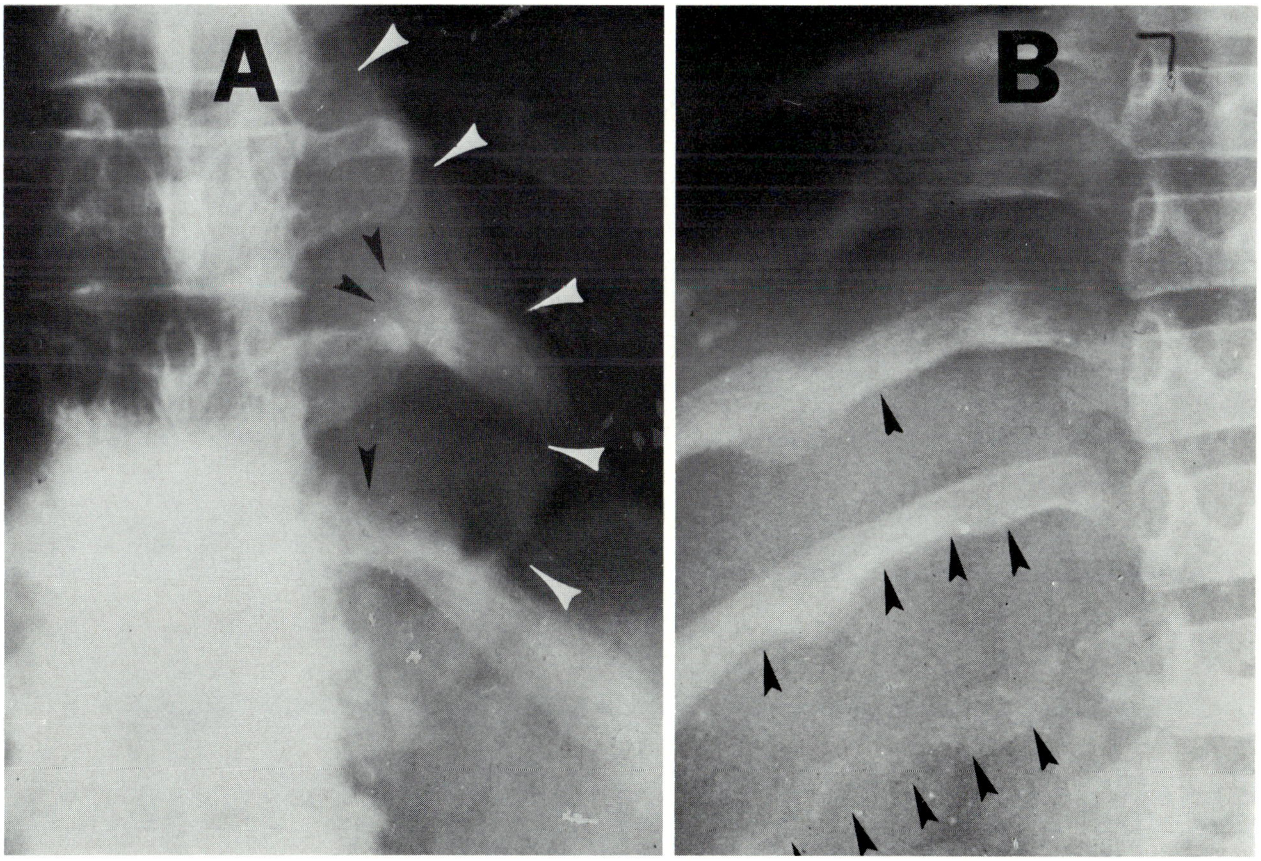

Fig. 2.10 **A.** Extensive tuberculous destruction of dorso-lumbar junction with kyhotic angulation. Large paravertebral abscess (white pointers). The left 11th and 12th ribs are eroded posteriorly and show upward subluxation. **B.** Extensive paravertebral abscess originating in right vertebral appendages of D12. Note how two ribs have been eroded on their inferior border and how the last rib is permeatively destroyed by granulation tissue.

ally the weakened bone collapses with angulation and extrusion of pus and debris into a paravertebral abscess (Figs. 2.7–2.10). In the spine typically the process does not occur initially at multiple discrete levels. The most affected segments of the spine lie between the bodies of D10 to L4 (Konstam & Konstam, 1958). The practical difficulties of dealing with very large numbers of patients led Konstam to experiment with treatment by chemotherapy and ambulant outpatient treatment of children in plaster of Paris casts (Konstam, 1963). Though the degree of angulation may be slightly greater than by other methods of therapy, the rapidity of compressive healing is impressive. Abscesses shrink and later may calcify. Surgical drainage and debridement is reserved for those with evidence of cord compression or of instability. A feature of repair in the Konstam regime is the formation of bridges of new bone along the antero-lateral spinal ligaments. It is believed that these consolidating bony bridges are excited by the presence of adjacent abscesses as well as by the ambulant regime. Vertebral foci of unusual type may be seen. A Calvé form of vertebra plana with collapse of a vertebral body and negligible disc involvement is not rare (Fig. 2.11). This may sometimes be associated with some sclerotic bone reaction which can be confusing. Involvement of neural arches and the pedicles are other perplexing presentations (Masel, 1966; Bell & Cockshott, 1971). The pedicular foci may be unilateral or bilateral, isolated or at multiple spinal segments (Fig. 2.12). Though disc changes may not be apparent, paravertebral abscesses are invariable. With chemotherapy reconstitution of the destroyed area occurs. Because of the close relationship to the cord compression, symptoms are not rare and may require surgical decompression.

Tuberculosis of flat bones such as the calvarium, sternum and pelvis typically simulate histiocytosis. The lesions may be more extensive but there are no clear-cut radiographic differentiating features, apart from abscesses, so that histological material is often necessary

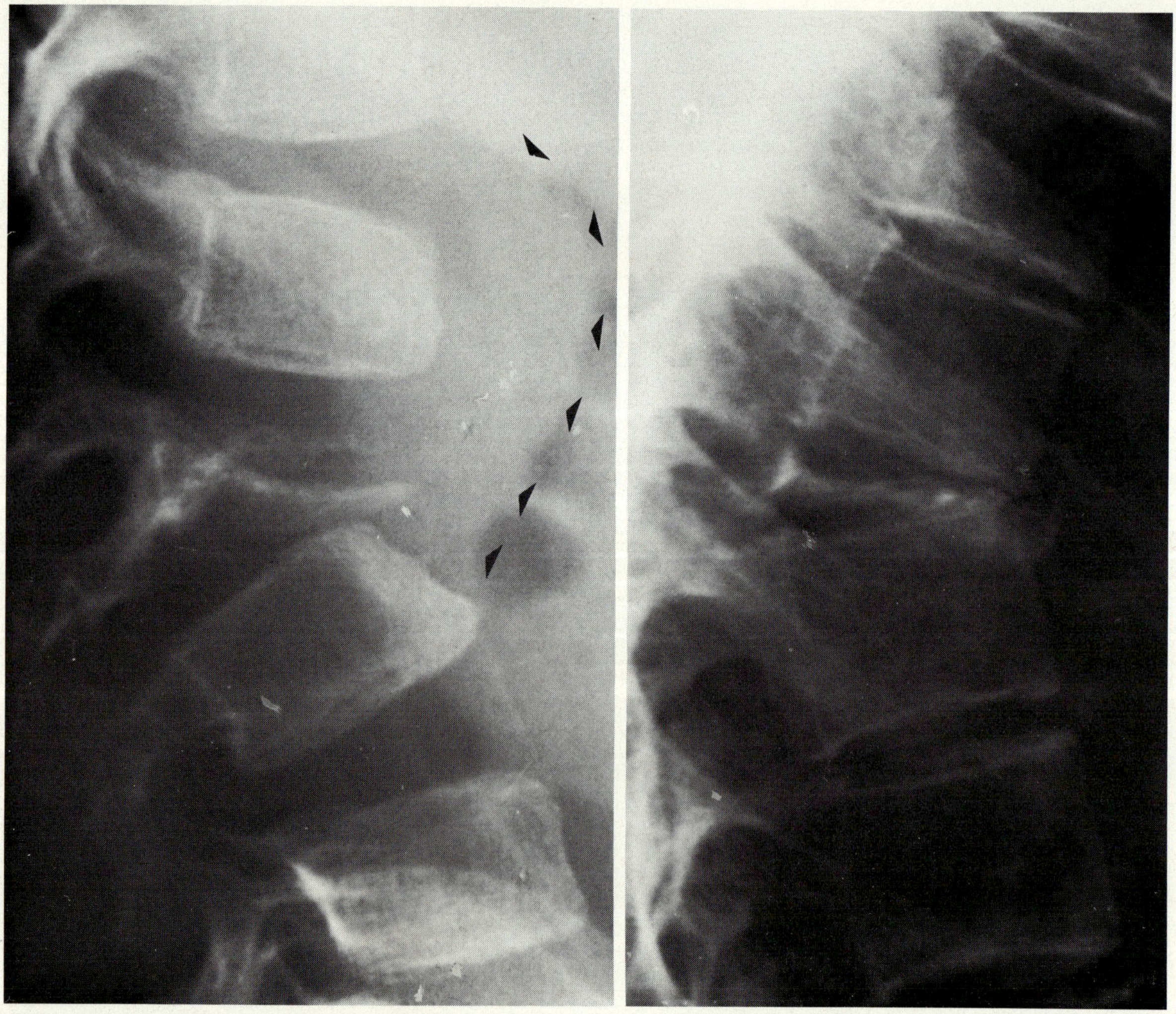

A B

Fig. 2.11 A, B. Two examples of Calvé type tuberculous vertebral body foci with compression. On right is a single body squashed with little disc involvement. The child on the left has two bodies compressed with some involvement of intervening disc. There is an anterior abscess.

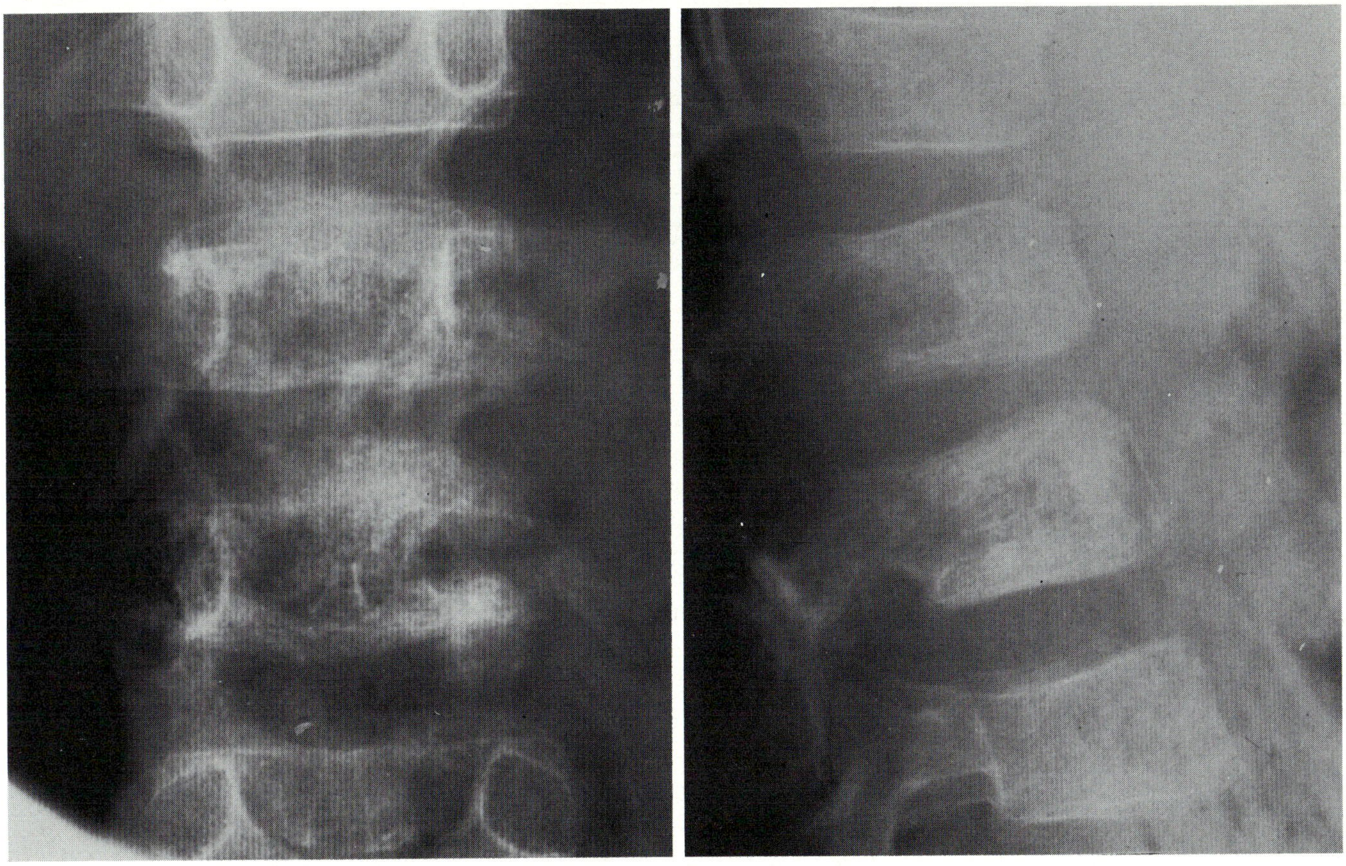

Fig. 2.12 **A, B.** Posterior vertebral body foci at adjacent levels implicating the pedicles. The disc spaces are preserved. Such permeative granulomata are often associated with abscesses and neuralgic symptoms. (Courtesy of *Radiology*.)

for proof of the aetiology. Such lesions initially have invasive ill-defined borders which later have sharper contours and may heal with sclerosis (Fig. 2.13) (Barton, 1961; Lea-Thomas & Reid, 1971).

Tuberculosis of the middle ear and mastoid soon leads to hearing loss and perhaps a discharging ear. In infants the well-defined rounded lesions have been said to be a form of primary tuberculosis reaching the mastoid through the eustachian tube. In adults the disease reaches the mastoid in a more usual fashion (Rousing, 1968).

Often it is difficult to determine the origin of joint tuberculosis. If no bony focus is evident, synovial disease is presumed. Extensive osteoporosis on both sides of the joint is obvious and loss of the subchondral plate 'white line' occurs later and is indicative of severe cartilage loss (Figs. 2.14 and 2.15). In other instances there may be a focal marginal bony lesion communicating with a joint. Less frequently a marked synovial inflammatory tuberculous hydrarthrosis causes well-defined bony erosion at the site of synovial reflections. These are mechanical and non-specific and do not necessarily reflect invasion of bone. In the shoulder joint caries sicca with well-defined erosive disease occurs—as the name indicates, with no outpouring of synovial fluid.

Multifocal diaphyseal tuberculosis of a pseudocystic type is sometimes seen (Clinton Thomas & Young, 1955; Cremin *et al.*, 1970). The distal diaphyseal lesions in the medulla erode the cortex which responds by periosteal reaction and expansion causing a local fusiform enlargement (Figs. 2.16–2.18). Though some writers have suggested confusion with sarcoid, the young age of patients

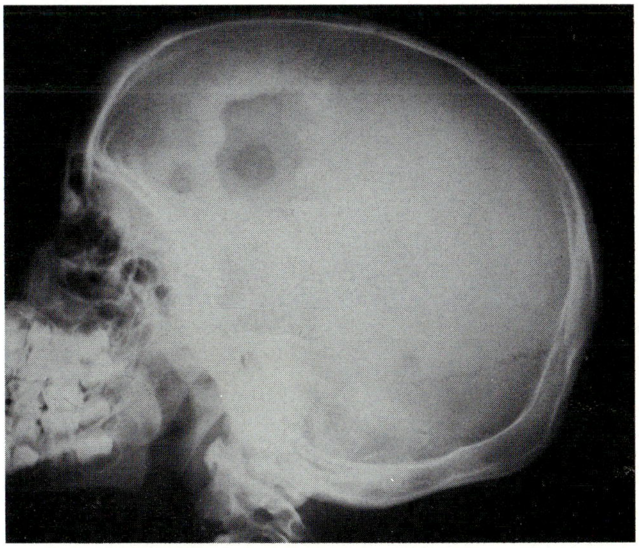

Fig. 2.13 Tuberculous destruction of calvarium.

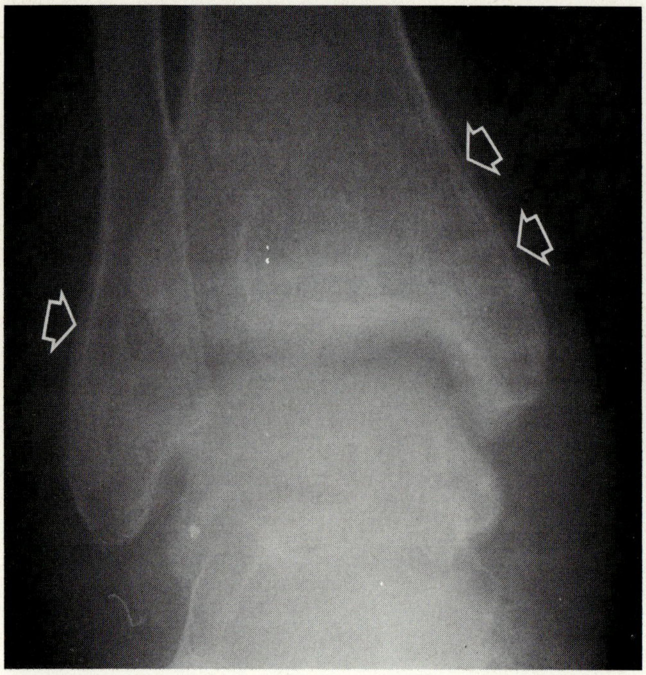

Fig. 2.14 Tuberculous arthritis of ankle. Loss of subchondral bone, osteoporosis and periosteal reaction (arrowed).

usually enables one to discount such a possibility. It has been suggested that this form of tubercle is due to early haematogenous dissemination to the marrow before primary immunity exist.

The extensive experience of Professor Cremin and his colleagues in Capetown has been recently published and provides an important reference in this field (Goldblatt & Cremin, 1978).

REFERENCES

Barton, C. J. (1961) Tuberculosis of the vault of the skull, *British Journal of Radiology*, **34,** 286–290.

Bell, D. & Cockshott, W. P. (1971) Tuberculosis of the vertebral pedicles, *Radiology*, **99,** 43–48.

Clinton-Thomas, C. L. & Young, W. B. (1955) Multiple pseudo-cystic tuberculosis of bone, *Journal of Bone and Joint Surgery*, **37B,** 624–631.

Cremin, B. J., Fisher, R. M. & Levinsohn, M. W. (1970) Multiple bone tuberculosis in the young, *British Journal of Radiology*, **43,** 638–645.

Goldblatt, M. & Cremin, B. J. (1978) Osteoarticular tuberculosis: Its presentation in coloured races, *Clinical Radiology*, **29,** 669–677.

Konstam, P. G. (1963) Spinal tuberculosis in Nigeria, *Annals of the Royal College of Surgeons of England*, **32,** 99–115.

Konstam, P. G. & Konstam, S. T. (1958) Spinal tuberculosis in Southern Nigeria, *Journal of Bone and Joint Surgery*, **40B,** 26–32.

Lea-Thomas, M. & Reid, B. R. (1971) Cranial tuberculosis presenting with proptosis, *Radiology*, **100,** 91–92.

Masel, J. P. (1966) Neural arch lesions in young people, *Australian Radiology*, **10,** 360–364.

Rousing, H. (1968) Tuberculose de l'oreille mise en évidence par la planigraphie et la tomographie, *Annales de Radiologie*, **11,** 587–598.

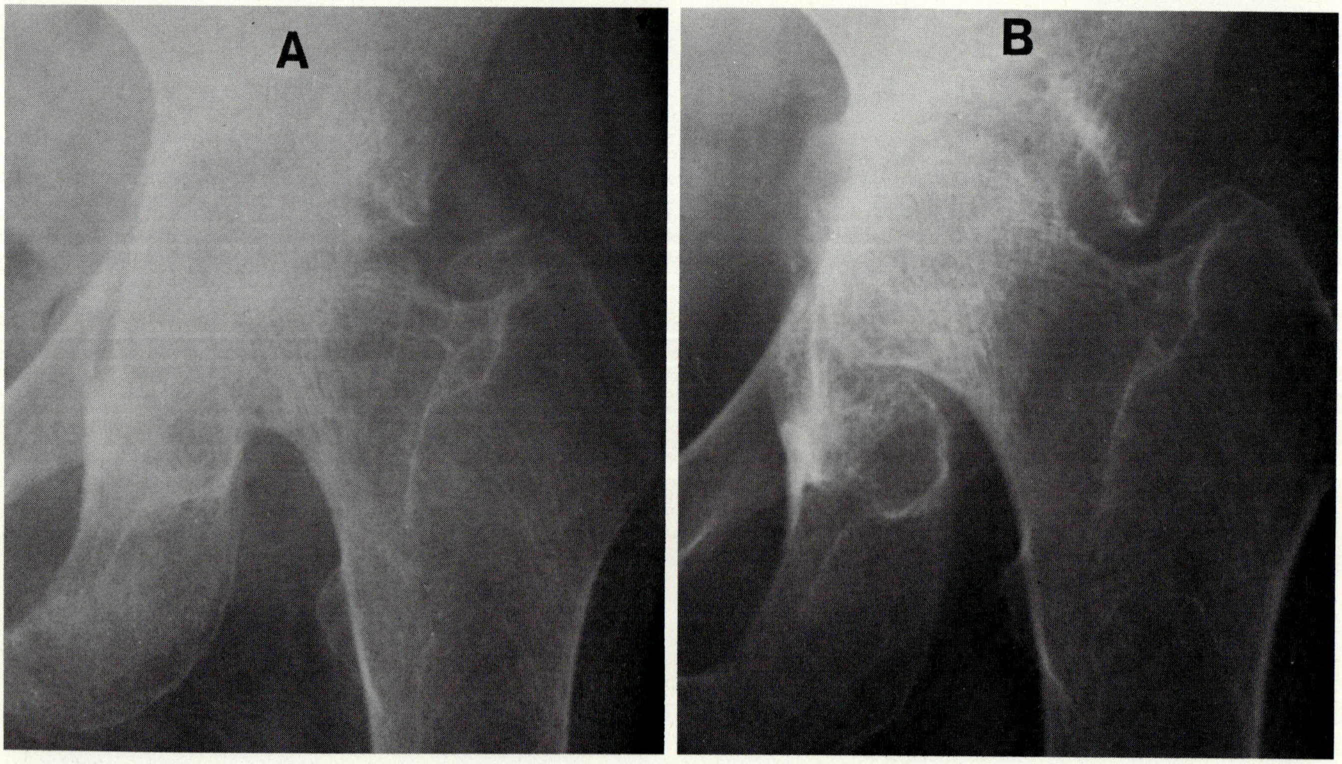

Fig. 2.15 Tuberculous arthritis of hip. **A.** In acute stage note loss of white line of articular subchondral bone indicative of cartilage loss. **B.** A year later there has been further bone loss and excavation.

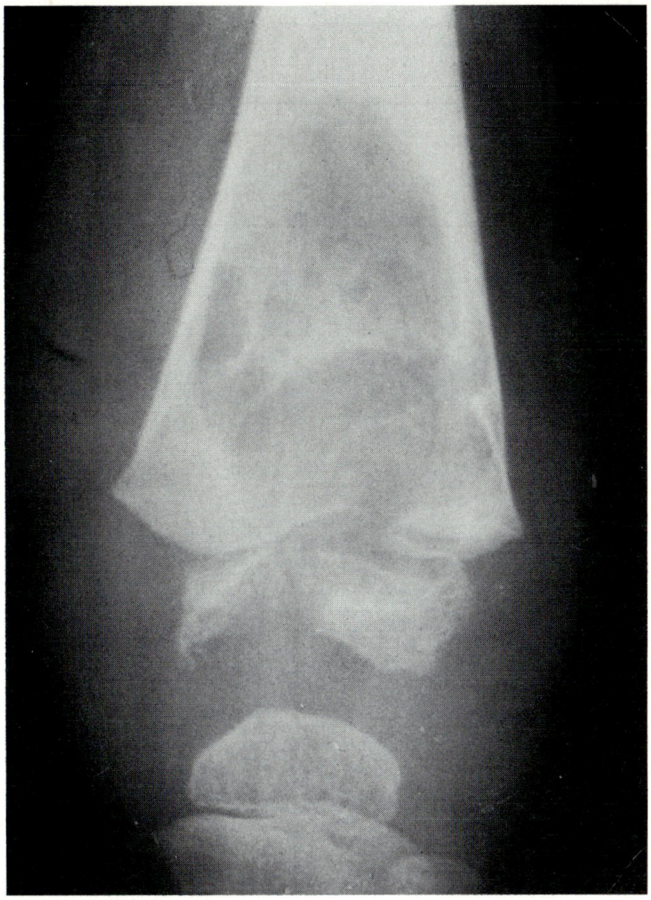

Fig. 2.16 Tuberculous destruction of lower femur of a Nigerian boy with extension of focus through growth plate into epiphysis. Fluid is present in the joint.

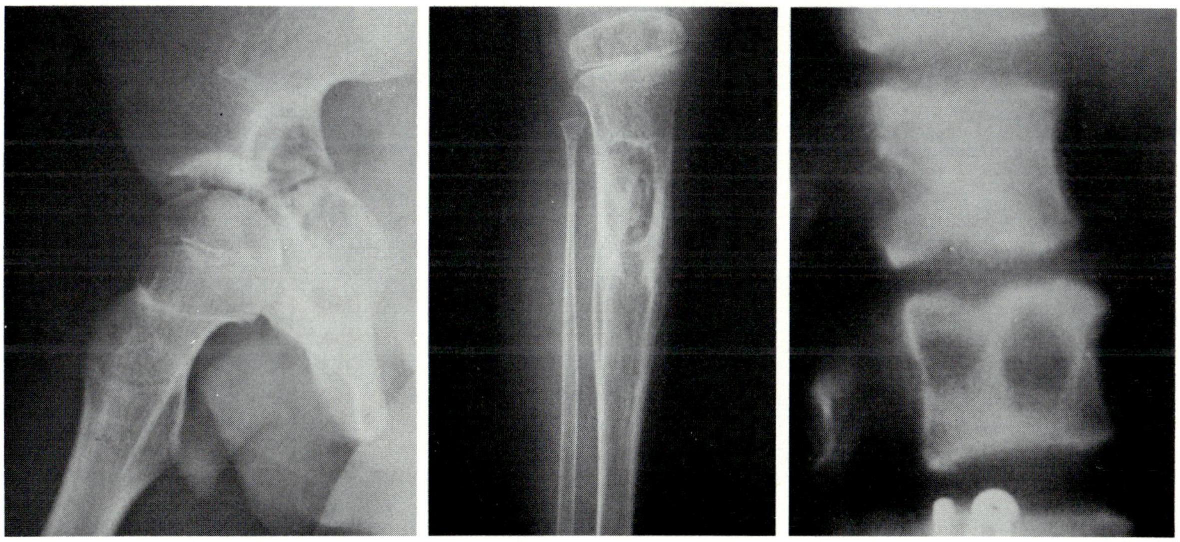

A B C

Fig. 2.17 A, B, C. Three examples of 'cystic' type of tuberculous granulomatous destruction in children. (Courtesy of Prof. B. Cremin, Capetown.)

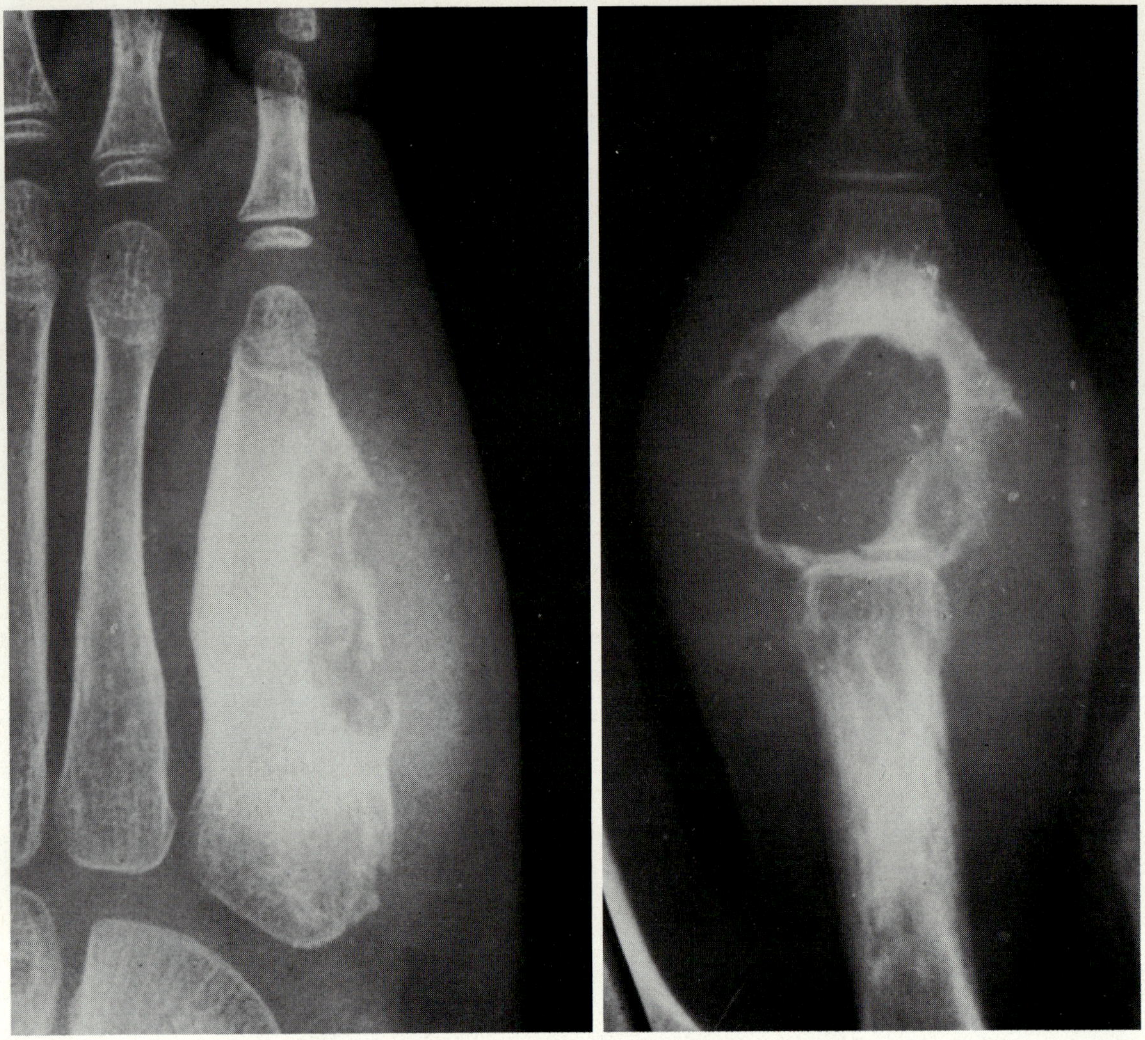

A B

Fig. 2.18 A, B. Tuberculous dactylitis can occur centrally or eccentrically in the diaphysis. It tends to occur in childhood or old age. Bone expansion can be severe. Diagnosis can be difficult.

TROPICAL ULCER

Tropical ulcers cause considerable disability in much of the humid tropics in labourers and others of poor economic status whose limbs are exposed to trauma. Lack of protective clothing, poor diet, anaemia and inadequate initial therapy are among the factors responsible for a high prevalence. In many rural clinics a significant proportion of the daily workload is concerned with the cleaning of ulcers and the application of dressings. Most of the lesions are below the knee involving the anterior aspect of the lower leg and foot. The initial pustular skin lesion breaks down to expose an extending necrotic slough that heals with granulations. But before this begins fascia, tendons and bone may become implicated in an indolent purulent lesion. The final skin cover on healing is often depressed, from cicatrisation, and paper-thin so that recurrence due to later trauma is not unusual. Epitheliomatous transformation of a long-standing lesion is a sad complication.

The bacterial flora is often mixed with haemolytic streptococci and Staphylococcus aureus, but Vincent's organisms often become obvious, perhaps by transference from a patient's mouth by saliva applied to the wound.

Radiological changes develop if the base of an ulcer approaches bone, so that lesions are most frequent where bone tissue is relatively superficial. Initially the response of bone to adjacent inflammation is the formation of a thin layer of periosteal new bone locally or extending some distance along the shaft. In young children, where there is a subacute process, productive periosteal bone may be lamellated (onion layering), or with exuberant spicules so that the accretion of investing new bone may reach 1·5 cm or more in thickness. With chronicity localised heaping

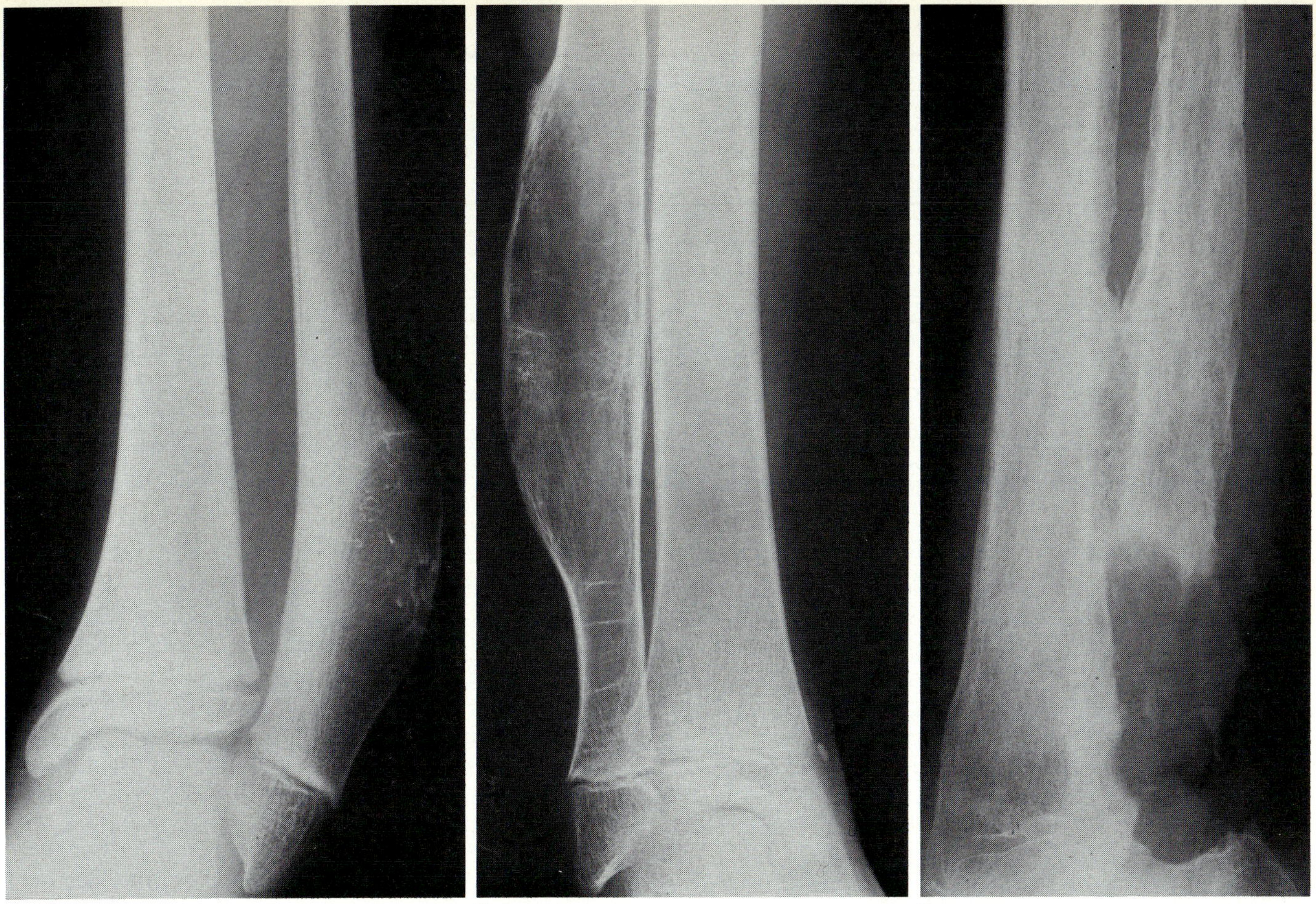

A B C

Fig. 2.19 **A & B** show large ulcer osteomas from leg ulcers of long duration. Note the deformity of the leg on the left. This tilting and bowing is due to disturbed weight stresses due to limping. **C.** The adult on the right has had chronic ulcer with infection for many years. Ephitheliomatous degeneration is destroying the fibula.

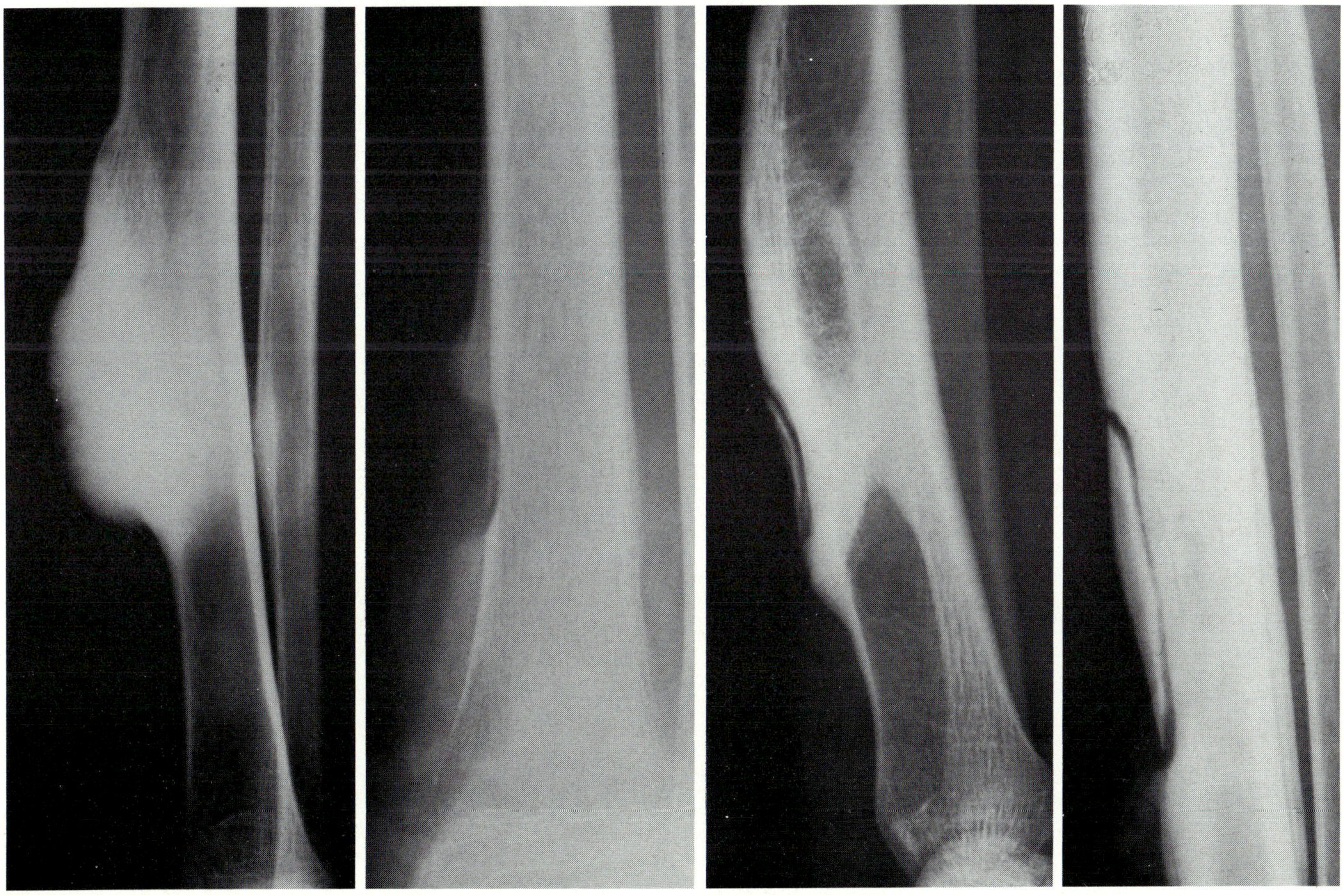

A B C D

Fig. 2.20 **A–D.** An ivory osteoma and three examples of flake cortical sequestra at base of ulcer.

up of new bone produces an osteoma-like protuberance—the so-called 'ulcer osteoma' (Fig. 2.19). This is usually cancellous in nature due to remoulding over a period of time, but denser types may develop.

Should the healing be interrupted with renewed exposure of bone in the floor of an ulcer, sequestration can occur with sloughing separation of a well-defined flake of cortex leaving a saucer-shaped depressed defect (Fig. 2.20) (Scott Brown & Middlemiss, 1956).

Ulcers in children can lead to distal bone deformities with the plane of the ankle joint tilting upwards laterally. It is thought that this results from the disturbed forces due to the limping gait rather than the consequences of any direct inflammatory effect on the growth plate. Altered lines of weight-bearing can also lead to bowing of the leg bones.

Malignant change can be suspected in long-standing ulcers by the appearance of the healing margins. Later as invasion of deeper structures occur, invasive bone destruction becomes evident radiographically (Fig. 2.19).

Other types of chronic ulcers may be present in the tropics, but these are usually distinct because of their appearance and site. Buruli ulcers due to Mycobacteria ulcerans have typical undermined borders; diphtheroid ulcers are multiple with greyish sloughs; and chromoblastomycotic lesions do not have a slough.

REFERENCE

Scott Brown, J. & Middlemiss, J. H. (1956) Bone changes in tropical ulcer, *British Journal of Radiology*, **29**, 213–217.

BRUCELLOSIS OF BONE

Brucellosis is a disease of animals which can be transmitted to humans. Because of its prevalence in Malta and its effect on the efficiency of the military personnel, a special Commission was set up which culminated in the discovery of the organism Brucella melitensis and the carrier, the goat, by David Bruce in 1887. It is now recognised that three forms of these gram negative organisms afflict man: B. melitensis with goat and sheep reservoirs; B. abortus with cattle predominantly infected; and B. suis which infects pigs. Transmission is from unpasteurised milk or cheese, or by direct contact. Hence herdsmen,

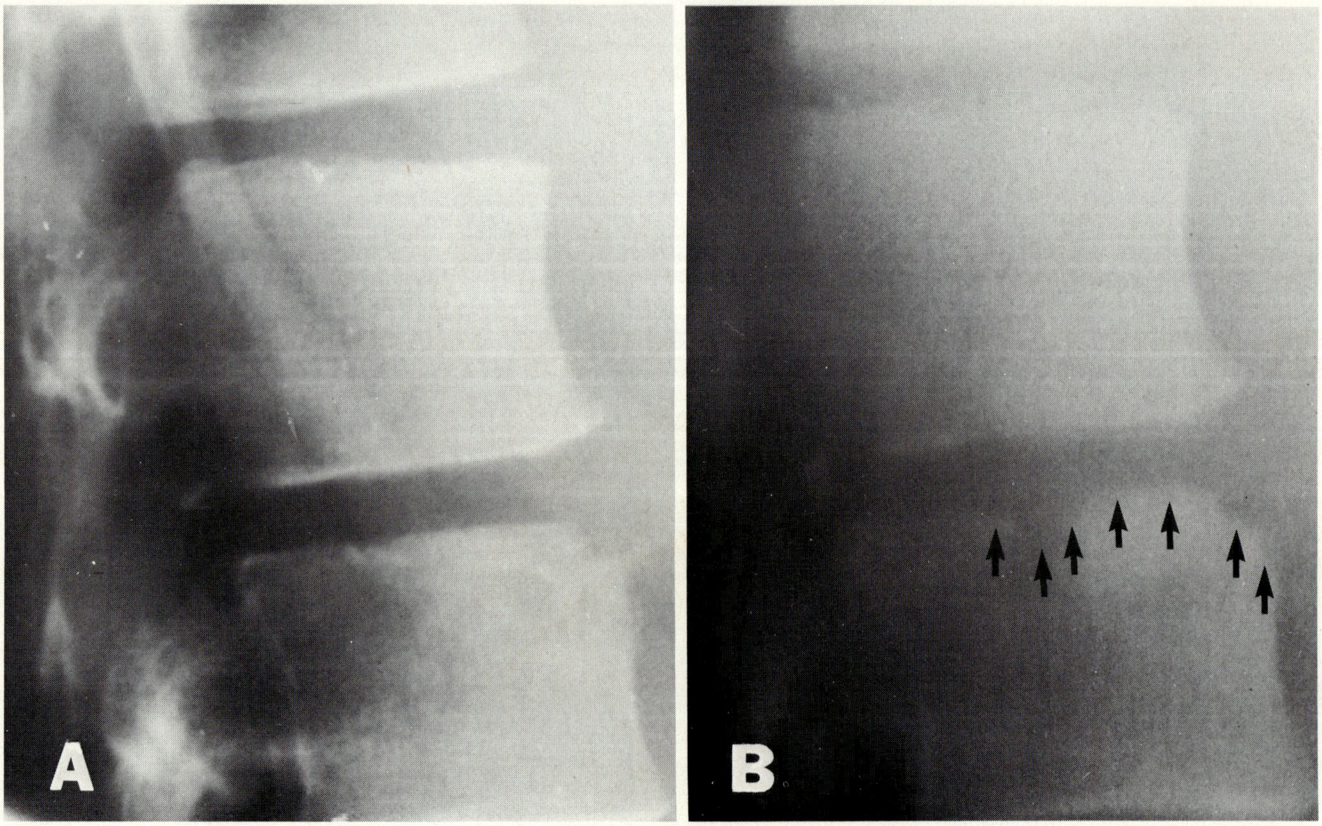

Fig. 2.21 Early brucellar spondylitis. There is bone destruction of the superior aspect of a vertebral body giving rise to an irregular erosive appearance from the anterior surface to the centrum. The disc space is not narrowed at this stage and the body above is spared. Eroded areas arrowed in tomogram B.

veterinary and abattoir workers are particularly at risk. The condition has a worldwide distribution, but the main centres are in Mediterranean areas, Central Europe and South America. Each species tends to have its own geographic pattern.

The incubation period is 10 to 14 days. Onset is ushered in by the development of an irregular fever, headache, joint aches and debilitation. Splenomegaly is frequent. Bone and joint complications with pain and muscle spasm develops in nearly 10 per cent of melitensis cases and nearly 2 per cent show neurologic disturbances (Ganado & Craig, 1958). The spine is the most often involved part of the skeleton, with increasing incidence at each level on descent from the cervical to lumbar area. Over half of the cases of spinal involvement are in the lumbar area. Two contiguous vertebrae are often implicated and several separate levels can be involved, though this is not frequent (Fig. 2.21).

The pathologic evolution suggests that there are many widespread bone marrow foci. Thus sternal marrow aspirates may grow the offending organism, despite repeated negative blood cultures. There are disseminate foci in the reticulo-endothelial system. The characteristic features are granulomata less than 5 mm in size with specific histologic features, widespread in bone marrow, but giving rise to few focal signs.

The evolution of vertebral lesions has been described in detail by Zammit (1961) and by Glascow (1976). As in other forms of bone infection there is a latent period between the clinical onset of a local lesion and radiographic evidence of any alteration. The usual initial change is bone destruction in the anterior portion of a vertebral body close to the disc cartilage plate (Figs. 2.21 and 2.22). Often this may be a self-limiting lesion that does not enlarge and becomes demarcated by a sclerotic zone, with perhaps proliferative anterior new bone formation (Fig. 2.22). At other times the erosive destructive process

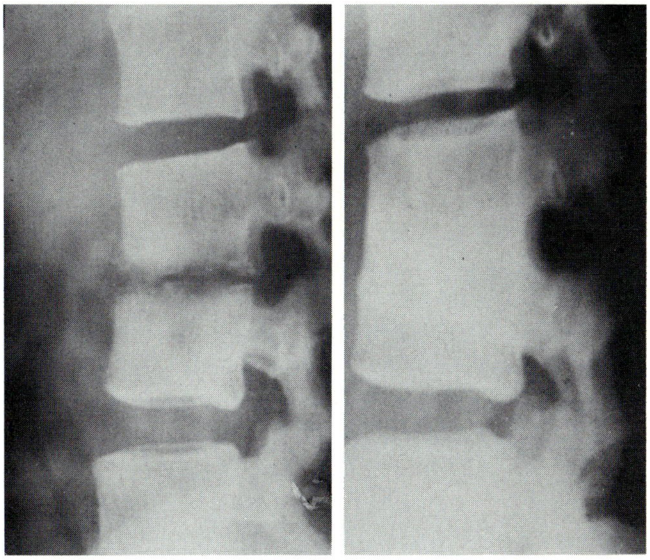

A B

Fig. 2.22 **A, B.** Three views to show progressive changes of third and fourth lumbar spine brucellar infection. The figures denote the intervals in weeks.

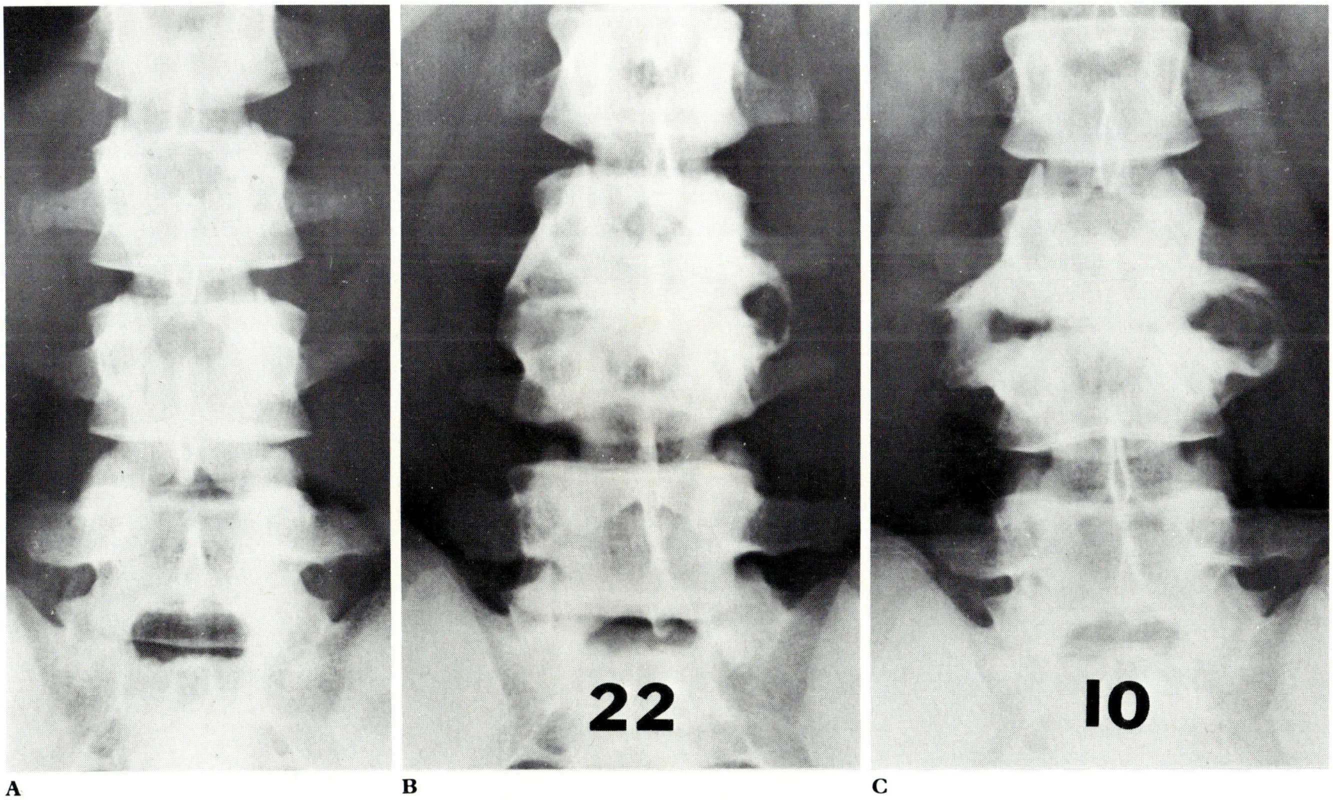

A B C

Fig. 2.23 **A, B, C.** Destruction and healing processes of brucellar spondylitis resulting in bony ankylosis. (Courtesy of Dr. F. Zammit, Malta.)

implicates the bone plate and invades the disc to spread to the adjacent vertebrae. The disc becomes narrowed or even destroyed anteriorly and as bone trabeculae are affected vertebral collapse and wedging may ensue. Healing is by production of sclerotic dense bone in the vertebral bodies; by antero-lateral new bone formation that may bridge the disc space; and in severe cases bony ankylosis anteriorly with disappearance of disc tissue (Fig. 2.23). Abscess formation is not a marked radiographic phenomenon though a slight bulge of the paravertebral shadow in the thoracic spine may occur, and small granulation masses and pustular collections can be seen at surgery.

Differentiation from tuberculous disease can be difficult from a single study but correlation with history and serial radiographs indicates that brucellosis has a more rapid course, both in development and in repair. Needle biopsy under fluoroscopic guidance is useful in securing material for culture when the serologic and blood culture tests are negative or equivocal.

Paraplegia can follow dural compression and any signs of this symptom warrant early myelography. Neurological symptoms and signs can develop from brucellar meningitis truly involving the spinal membranes in the absence of bone foci.

Bone lesions elsewhere may be due to synovial disease or small foci in marrow. The granulomata of brucellosis are widespread, but do not generally form significant bone lesions. Non-specific osteoporosis or effusions in joints, particularly hips and knees, are observed.

Under suitable drug therapy the lesions of brucellosis heal rapidly.

REFERENCES

Ganado, W. & Craig, A. J. (1958) Brucellosis myelopathy, *Journal of Bone and Joint Surgery*, **40A,** 1380–1387.

Glascow, M. M. S. (1976) Brucellosis of the spine, *British Journal of Surgery*, **63,** 283–288.

Zammit, F. (1961) Brucellosis. In *Tropical Radiology*, pp. 54–60. London: W. Heinemann.

MELIOIDOSIS PSEUDOMONAS PSEUDOMALLEI OSTEOMYELITIS

Melioidosis is an acute infective condition seen mainly in South East Asia. It can be fatal if not treated, and indeed the initial description of the disease from Rangoon was based on an autopsy series (Whitmore & Krishnaswami, 1912).

Melioidosis is a veterinary as well as a medical problem, since it can cause multiple abscesses in pigs and goats. Cases have been reported from Iran, Burma, Malaysia, India, Ceylon, Thailand, Guam, the Philippines, New Guinea, Queensland and Indonesia. Non-autochthonous examples have been seen in Africa (Tchad, Madagascar and South Africa) and various countries of Europe and the U.S.A. Most of the U.S. cases have been in Vietnam veterans. The condition is established in man and wild animals in Queensland and North Australia. Foci have been recorded in Panama and Aruba in the West Indies, but these are probably no longer active.

The source of the infection is probably varied. The organism has been recovered from rice paddies and river banks and it is well documented to have infected military and experimental wounds (Fournier, 1965). Rodents, dogs, rats, wallabies or monkeys in the wild have been found with the organism. Experimentally the rat flea and Aedes aegypti mosquitoes can transmit the disease (Nelson & Albright, 1967). Contamination of wounds, inhalation or ingestion may all be modes of infection.

The disease exists in two forms: a septicaemic acute process and an indolent chronic form. Subclinical infection may also exist, judging from antibody level surveys in endemic areas.

The clinical features are very variable. The rapid onset acute form can be difficult to differentiate from any other type of overwhelming septicaemia but non-specific pulmonary lesions may be seen. (See respiratory section.)

As we are here concerned with osseous manifestations the chronic form only will be described. Pathologically melioidosis causes multiple small abscesses that may coalesce and lead to chronic granulomata and draining sinuses. Infection may be acquired through a breach of the skin as in military wounds, but is more commonly blood-borne. This route can produce abscess localisation anywhere except the brain. The liver and lungs are frequently affected and then bone and soft tissues. The osteo-

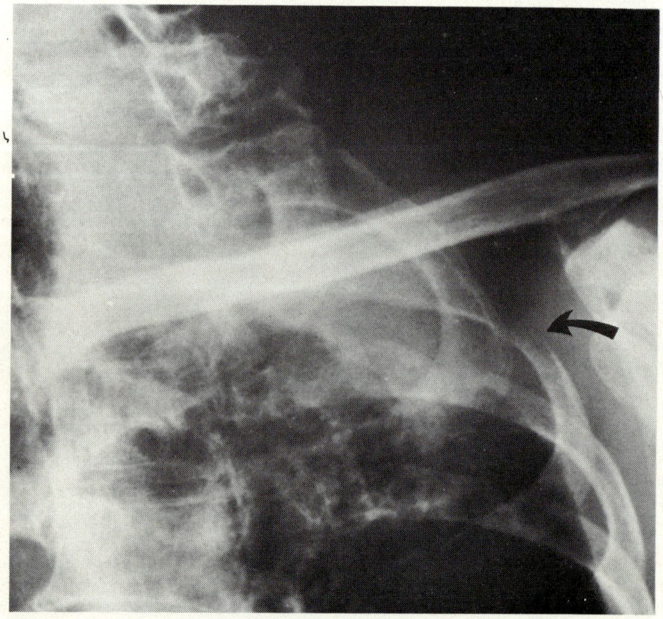

Fig. 2.24 Patient with left upper lobe infiltrate due to chronic melioidosis which has caused pleural granulomatous reaction and implicated the upper border of the third rib (arrow). (Courtesy Dr. W. B. Young, London.)

myelitis affects particularly red marrow areas—in adults the ends of long bones, the spine and ribs (Jones & Ross, 1963; Borchardt *et al.*, 1966; Sutherland & Dahlstrom, 1968). In certain situations, large abscesses may be present, and in the thorax a paravertebral abscess or an extrapleural soft tissue mass with rib involvement may be shown. The destruction is not well localised and reaction at its edges is slow in development so that the bone foci may resemble those of histiocytic or fungal granulomata (Fig. 2.24).

Bacteriological diagnosis is essential for confirmation. Under radiological control aspiration of an abscess or needle biopsy of bone foci can be of value in procuring suitable material for culture.

REFERENCES

Borchdardt, K. A., Stansifer, P. & Albano, P. M. (1966) Osteomyelitis due to Pseudomonas pseudomallei, *Journal of the American Medical Association*, **196**, 660–662.

Fournier, J. (1965) La Melioidose et le B. de Whitmore Controverses épidémiologiques et taxonomiques, *Bulletin de la Société de pathologie Exotique*, **58**, 753–765.

Jones, G. P. & Ross, J. A. (1963) Melioidosis, *British Journal of Radiology*, **36**, 415–417.

Nelson, R. N. & Albright, C. R. (1967) Melioidosis, *Oral Pathology*, **24**, 128–136.

Sutherland, J. D. & Dahlstrom, D. D. (1968) Melioidosis: Roentgen manifestations in a long bone, *Radiology*, **91**, 519.

Whitmore, A. & Krishnaswami, C. (1912) An account of the discovery of hitherto undescribed infective disease occurring among the population of Rangoon, *Indian Medical Gazette*, **47**, 262–267.

KLEBSIELLA OSTEOMYELITIS

A form of haematogenous osteomyelitis due to Friedlander's bacillus reported from South Africa provides sufficiently distinctive radiographic features that a correct aetiological diagnosis has been suggested from films on a number of occasions before the microbiological reports (Kopins *et al.*, 1950; Findlay & Skapinker, 1953). Osteomyelitis from a variety of unconventional organisms

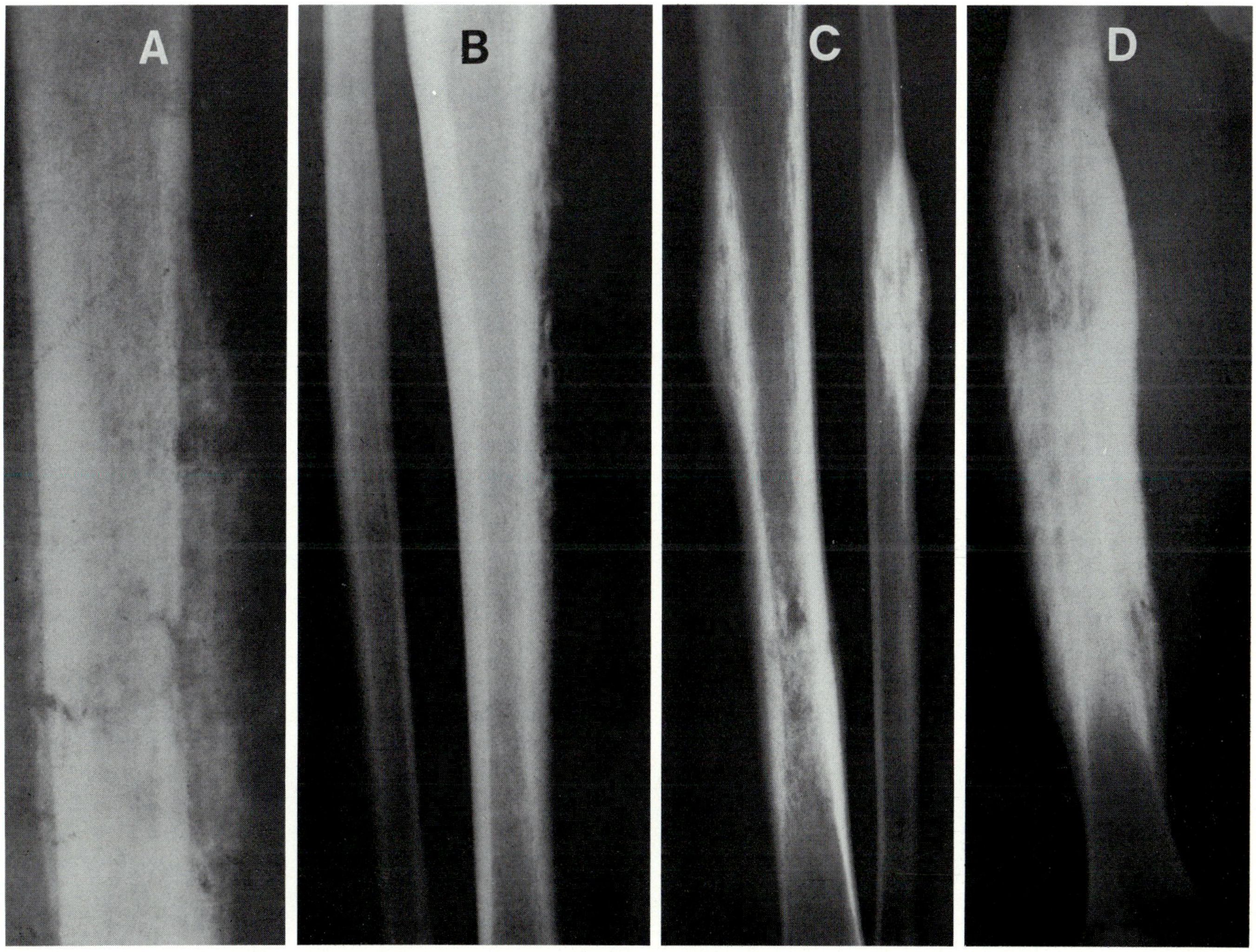

Fig. 2.25 Thighs (**A**, **D**) and leg (**B**, **C**) of patients with Klebsiella osteomyelitis. The diaphyseal location, the cortical erosion and proliferative investing periosteal new bone are characteristic. A pathological fracture is seen in **A.** (Courtesy of Prof. Solomon, Baragwarnath Hospital.)

including species of Klebsiella have been reported elsewhere in heroin addicts and other 'main liners' who use the intravenous route of administration. Then the spine seems to be the most common location (Kido *et al.*, 1973).

The condition is metatastic from a primary focus elsewhere such as pneumonia or prostatitis. Multiple bone involvement is characteristic with a definite predilection for symmetrical involvement of major long bones such as the femora and tibiae. An extensive segment of the diaphysis of the bone is involved with sparing of the proximal and distal segments so that joint involvement is not a feature. This distribution of the bone infection in the shaft and sparing of metaphyses may be related to the age of patients in the series recorded. Trueta (1959) has emphasised the importance of the vascular pattern in bone at different ages as the determinant of localisation.

The diaphyseal lesion begins subperiosteally, eroding the cortex over the middle third to two-thirds of the shaft. Exuberant periosteal new bone forms later as the cortical abscess strips the periosteum (Fig. 2.25). No sequestration ensues but the build-up of investing new bone causes considerable thickening of the shaft. 'Bone within bone' appearance may be noted due to remnants of the original cortical shaft lying within the expanded diaphysis. This cortical process resembles that seen in sickle cell anaemia apart from its more central position in the shaft. As in any other infective process causing bone destruction, pathological fracture may occur in the weakened area.

REFERENCES

*Findlay, M. & Skapinker, S. (1953) Further observations on Friedlander's osteomyelitis of long bones, *British Journal of Radiology*, **26,** 358–361.

Kido, D., Bryan, D. & Halpern, M. (1973) Haematogenous osteomyelitis in drug addicts, *American Journal of Roentgenology*, **118,** 356–363.

Komins, C., Skapinker, S. & Kay, S. (1950) Osteomyelitis of long bones caused by Friedlander's bacillus, *British Journal of Radiology*, **23,** 168–171.

Trueta, J. (1959) The three types of acute haematogenous osteomyelitis. A clinical and vascular study, *Journal of Bone and Joint Surgery*, **41B,** 671–680.

DONOVANOSIS
GRANULOMA INGUINALE OSTEOMYELITIS

Granuloma inguinale is a chronic granulomatous progressive infection usually affecting the skin and mucosa of the genital areas and perineum. Donovan originally demonstrated multiple intracellular capsulated organisms in mononuclear cells: the so-called Donovan bodies. The organism's taxonomic position has changed over the years and it is now termed Calymmatobacterium granulomatis.

Granuloma inguinale has been reported from many parts of the world and has a traditional association with seaports. It is endemic in parts of India, Indonesia, New Guinea, Northern Australia, West Africa, the Americas and the West Indies.

The lesion is usually transmitted in a venereal fashion but other modes of direct contact can lead to transmission. The initial lesion is generally a papule which breaks down to form an ulcer. This tend to spread with formation of peripheral satellite lesions and subcutaneous infiltration, so that dense scarring occurs with lymphatic involvement and localised lymphoedema, particularly of the vulva. Extragenital lesions may form by auto-inoculation or following systemic dissemination.

Bone can be invaded by direct spread from an ulcerating lesion, but blood-borne spread with multiple metastatic osseous lesions can present a difficult clinical and radiological problem.

The bone lesions are due to intra-osseous granulomata causing destruction arising in the medulla, usually near the end of a long bone (Kirkpatrick, 1970). Vertebral bodies and ribs may also be involved. The pattern of involvement suggests that the process occurs in cancellous bone areas where there is red marrow. The appearance is non-specific and can simulate histiocytosis or dimorphic yeast granulomata (Fig. 2.26). With appropriate antibiotic

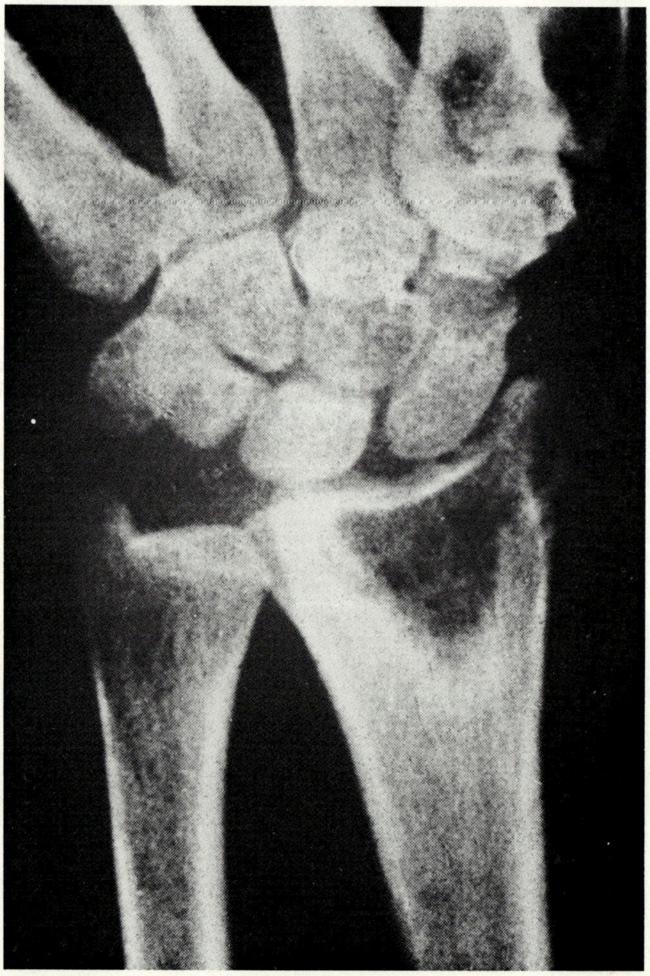

Fig. 2.26 Donovanotic destructive focus in distal radius of a teenage girl. (Courtesy of Prof. John Golding, University of the West Indies.)

therapy the bone defects heal. However, with spinal lesions surgery may be required. Bone lesions that expand and give rise to ulcerating granulomata have been described (Sieber, 1961).

REFERENCES

Kirkpatrick, D. J. (1970) Donovanosis (granuloma inguinale): a rare cause of osteolytic bone lesions, *Clinical Radiology*, **21,** 101–105.

Sieber, P. E. (1965) Granuloma inguinale with bone involvement, *American Journal of Roentgenologyy*, **95,** 515–517.

SALMONELLA VERTEBRAL OSTEOMYELITIS

Though not common haematogenous vertebral osteomyelitis from a variety of organisms may arise in adults. There are well-recognised relationships of spine infections to urinary tract infections, prostatic and pelvic surgery, iatrogenic infection by disc and lumbar punctures, and contaminated intravenous infections by heroin addicts. In tropical countries brucella, dimorphic yeasts, tuberculosis and salmonella also enter the differential diagnosis. The first three of these are considered in adjacent sections and this section is confined to salmonella spinal infections.

Salmonellosis can occur during intestinal infections and is also seen with increased incidence in the various haemoglobin-S syndromes, Bartonellosis (Oroya fever), and bilharzia.

Salmonella osteomyelitis has been a recognised complication of typhoid fever since Paget described it in 1876. In pre-chloramphenicol days this developed in between 0·18 to 2·7 per cent of cases (Stenstrom, 1958) and in more than half of these the spine was affected. The lumbar spine is involved in over 50 per cent of these and the relative incidence diminishes the higher the spinal level. The condition may not be manifest for a considerable interval after a known episode of typhoid, but in other instances the initial illness may not have been recognised. These factors render diagnosis difficult. The radiological changes are initially close to the vertebral end-plate. There, a destructive process begins which soon spreads to the disc and leads to reduction in disc space and involvement of the contiguous surface of the adjacent body. Paravertebral abscess formation is not a common feature. Healing takes place with permanent reduction of the disc space or even ankylosis of adjacent vertebral bodies and some sclerosis (Mills, 1964; Hunt, 1965). Confirmation of the diagnosis by serological methods may be difficult, but needle aspiration biopsy is a valuable way of obtaining material for culture. This is best performed under fluoroscopic control.

Salmonella infections are frequent when there is a HbS haemoglobinopathy, but a particular form of multilevel spondylitis, usually due to salmonella, has not received

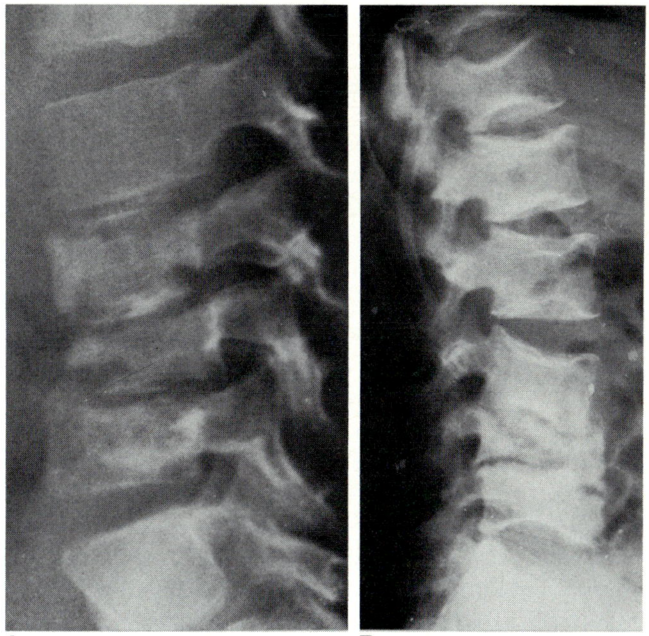

A B

Fig. 2.27 **A, B.** Salmonella multilevel vertebral osteitis of lumbar bodies in two Nigerian 'sicklers'.

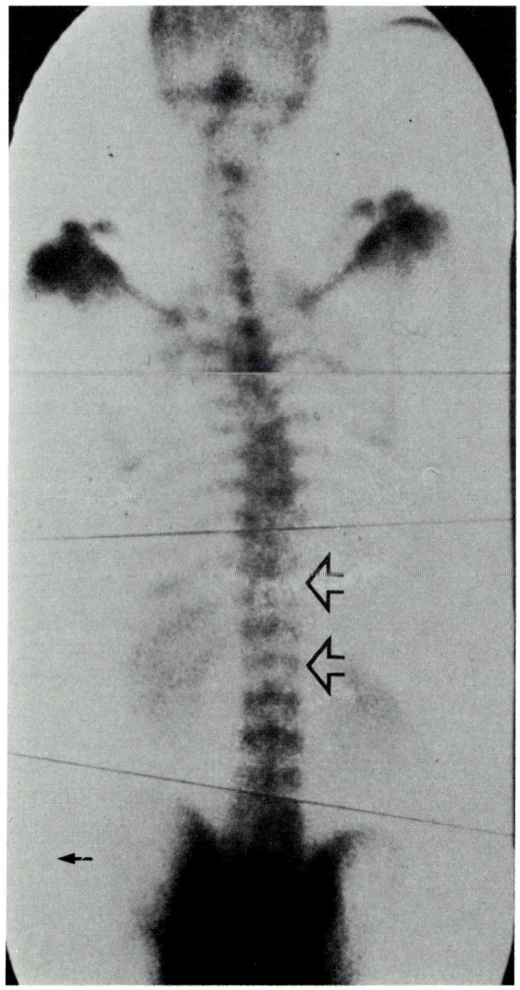

Fig. 2.28 D10 to L1 reduced isotope uptake in posterior isotope bone scan due to presumed vertebral infarction in a sickler. (Courtesy of Dr. Bob Cowan, Winston-Salem.)

great attention; yet its evolution is characteristic enough to suggest the diagnosis. The development of focal destructive processes near the vertebral end-plate is similar to that just described in typhoid except that several lumbar bodies are affected simultaneously (Fig. 2.27). Often a vertebral body is involved at both its superior and inferior disc borders. The destructive phase is followed by healing with permanent reduction in disc spaces. The etiology of this multilevel lesion is undoubtedly secondary infection of marrow infarcts. These have been seen at autopsy after labour (Shelley & Curtis, 1958). Lumbar pain from such infarcts is a recognised clinical feature of patients with sickle cell disease (Fig. 2.28). The probable pathogenesis is vena caval compression by the uterus leading to engorgement of the alternate paravertebral plexus pathway (Kerr *et al.*, 1964). This in turn results in stasis in lumbar vertebral marrow drainage leading to infarction of lumbar marrow. A similar process is probably responsible for the lumbar marrow infarct in soldiers with an S gene wearing tight belts in battle training courses (Jones *et al.*, 1970).

REFERENCES

Hunt, D. D. (1965) Cervical spondylitis caused by salmonella oranienburg, *Journal of Bone and Joint Surgery*, **47A,** 1243–1246.

Jones, S. R., Binder, R. A. & Donowho, E. M. (1970) Sudden death in sickle cell trait, *New England Journal of Medicine*, **282,** 323–325.

Kerr, M. C., Scott, D. B. & Samuel, E. (1964) Studies of inferior vena cava late in pregnancy, *British Medical Journal*, **1,** 532–533.

Mills, K. L. G. (1964) Osteomyelitis of spine due to salmonella muenchen, *Journal of Bone and Joint Surgery*, **46B,** 697–699.

Shelley, W. M. & Curtis, E. M. (1958) Bone marrow and fat embolism in sickle cell anaemia and sickle cell hemoglobin disease, *Bulletin of the Johns Hopkins Hospital*, **103,** 8–18.

Stenstrom, R. (1958) Spondylitis caused by salmonella typhimurium, *Acta Radiologica*, **49,** 355–359.

TREPONEMATOSIS
YAWS

A number of clinical syndromes throughout the world have been attributed to various treponema that are both morphologically and serologically indistinguishable: Treponema pallidum, T. pertenue and T. carateum. Though an aetiologically unitary concept of these disorders is held by many (Hudson, 1963), custom has resulted in acknowledging taxonomically the organisms responsible for the clinical presentations that show differences in modes of infection, clinical evolution and geographic distribution.

The non-venereal types of endemic treponematosis have numerous local names which indicate their regional endemicity as well as specific clinical features. Terms used include Bejel in the Euphrates valley, Pinta in Central America, Dichachwa in Bechuanaland, Siti in Ghana and endemic syphilis of Bosnia. In general the neurological and vascular complications of syphilis are not seen in this group of diseases. Bone infection may develop in all but is not a marked feature of pinta. In this section the radiological bone changes of yaws will be described to the neglect of other endemic disorders which are less frequent and have not been adequately characterised radiographically. The congenital and juvenile forms of syphilis that are so striking in radiological practice in Southern Africa are not considered. They have been well reviewed by Cremin & Fisher (1970).

Yaws infection is seen predominantly in children living in the humid tropics. Unlike syphilis, which is an urban disorder, yaws is largely a rural disease. Fortunately it is now rare as a result of eradication programmes conducted in many parts of the world under the aegis of W.H.O. Control has been achieved in many former endemic zones, but flare-ups in areas where surveillance may have lapsed indicate that eradication is not yet complete. Experience in Guinea suggests that certain monkeys may provide an animal reservoir.

Because of the progressive disappearance of the disease a clinical radiologist will not often encounter the acute phases of bone and skin infection but will see the adult deformities that can result from childhood infection by yaws.

Infection is probably through a skin cut or abrasion, but as treponema can pass through the intact skin of experimental animals this means of invasion also seems possible. Flies may provide a means of transmission by alighting on those with discharging sores. Congenital transmission is unknown.

The primary site superficial skin lesion is painless and may not be noticed by the individual affected. A few weeks or months later the secondary eruption develops over the trunk and limbs. These granulomata are sometimes raised and papillomatous and are termed frambesia. They tend to be self-limiting and come out in crops with eventual resolution. When the granulomata form subcutaneously on the sole of the foot they are painful and lead to alterations in gait called crab yaws. Fissuring of the feet with hyperkeratosis is frequent. Eventually tertiary lesions of the skin may appear. These are not infective but are progressive and may communicate with bone foci.

Though some authors have correlated the bone lesions by stages with the skin manifestations (Hackett, 1951), in practice the overlap and variability makes classification in this fashion of doubtful value.

The pathological process in bone is an osteoperiostitic granuloma of plasma cells, other mononuclear cells and fibroblasts combined with a cellular material. This granuloma infiltrates widely in bone and the radiographic appearance depends on the interplay between focal bone destruction and periosteal and endosteal reparative sclerotic processes. Generally speaking the later the phase of the disease the more pronounced the sclerosis.

The bone foci are first seen during the secondary skin lesions and affect several bones often in a partly symmetrical manner. The bones of legs, forearms and hands are

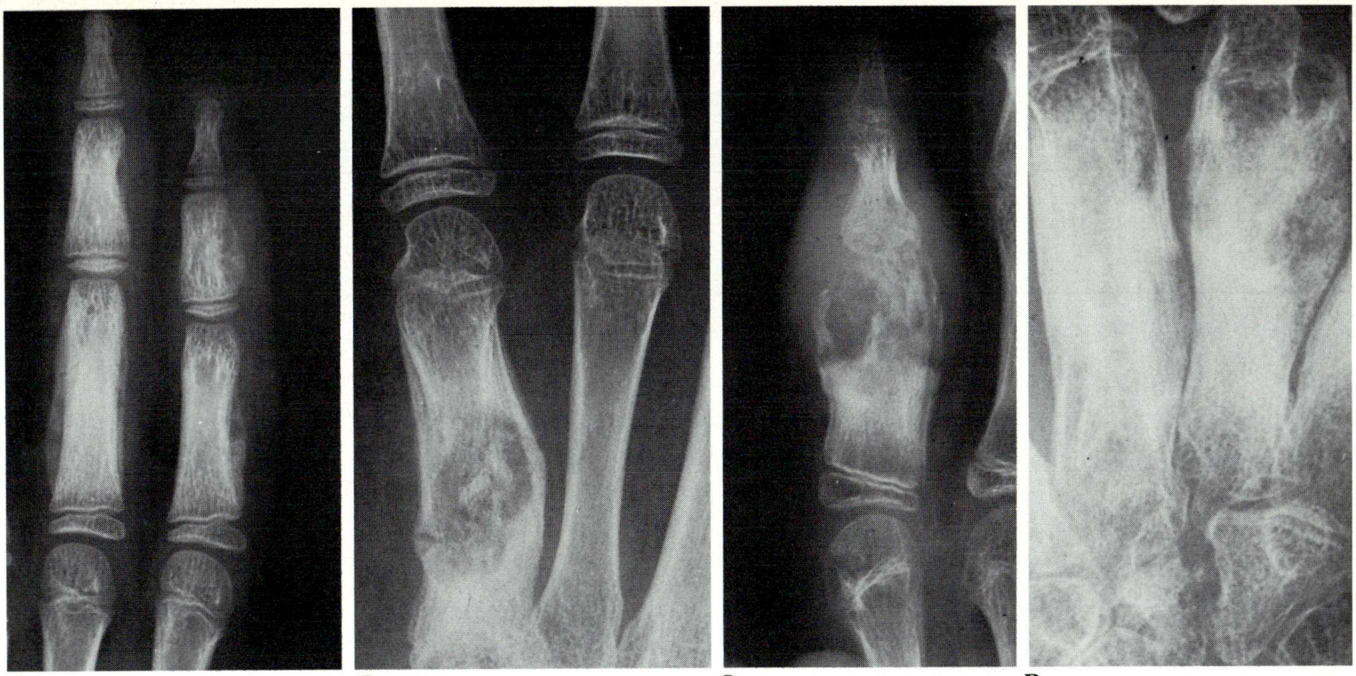

A B C D

Fig. 2.29 **A–D.** Yaws dactylitis showing cortical and medullary granulomata. All respond by periosteal new bone formation.

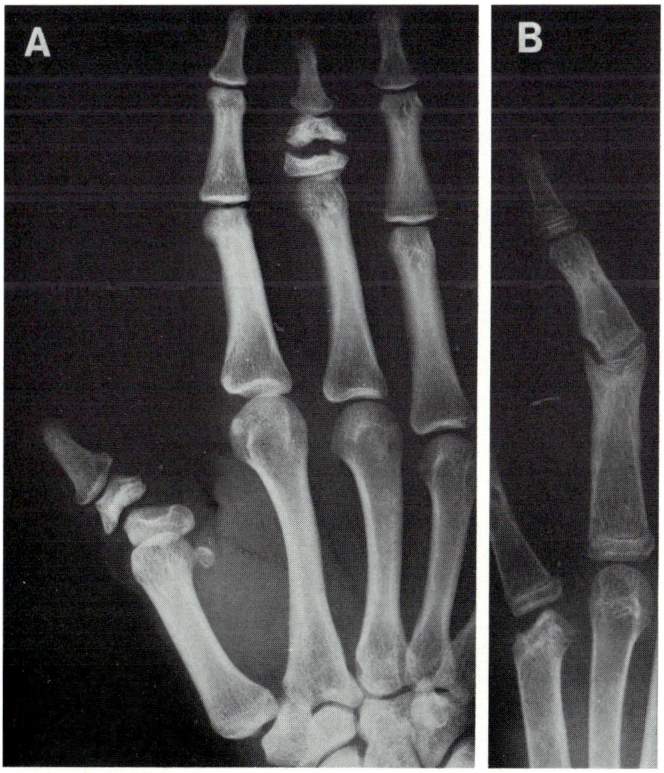

Fig. 2.30 Following childhood yaws persistent phalangeal fractures with pseudo-arthrosis have formed **A**. Unusual angulatory deformities have resulted from subarticular granulomata. (Courtesy of World Health Organisation.)

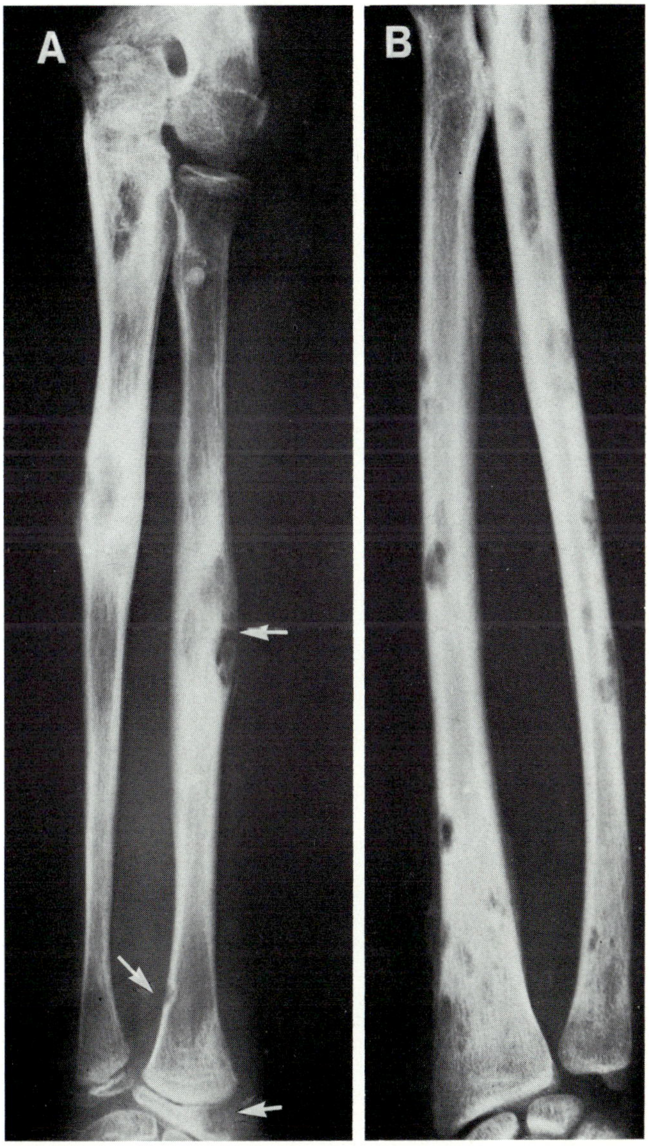

Fig. 2.31 Multiple cortical erosions of forearm bones in child and young adult. The periosteum is producing reactive new bone over foci. (Courtesy of World Health Organisation.)

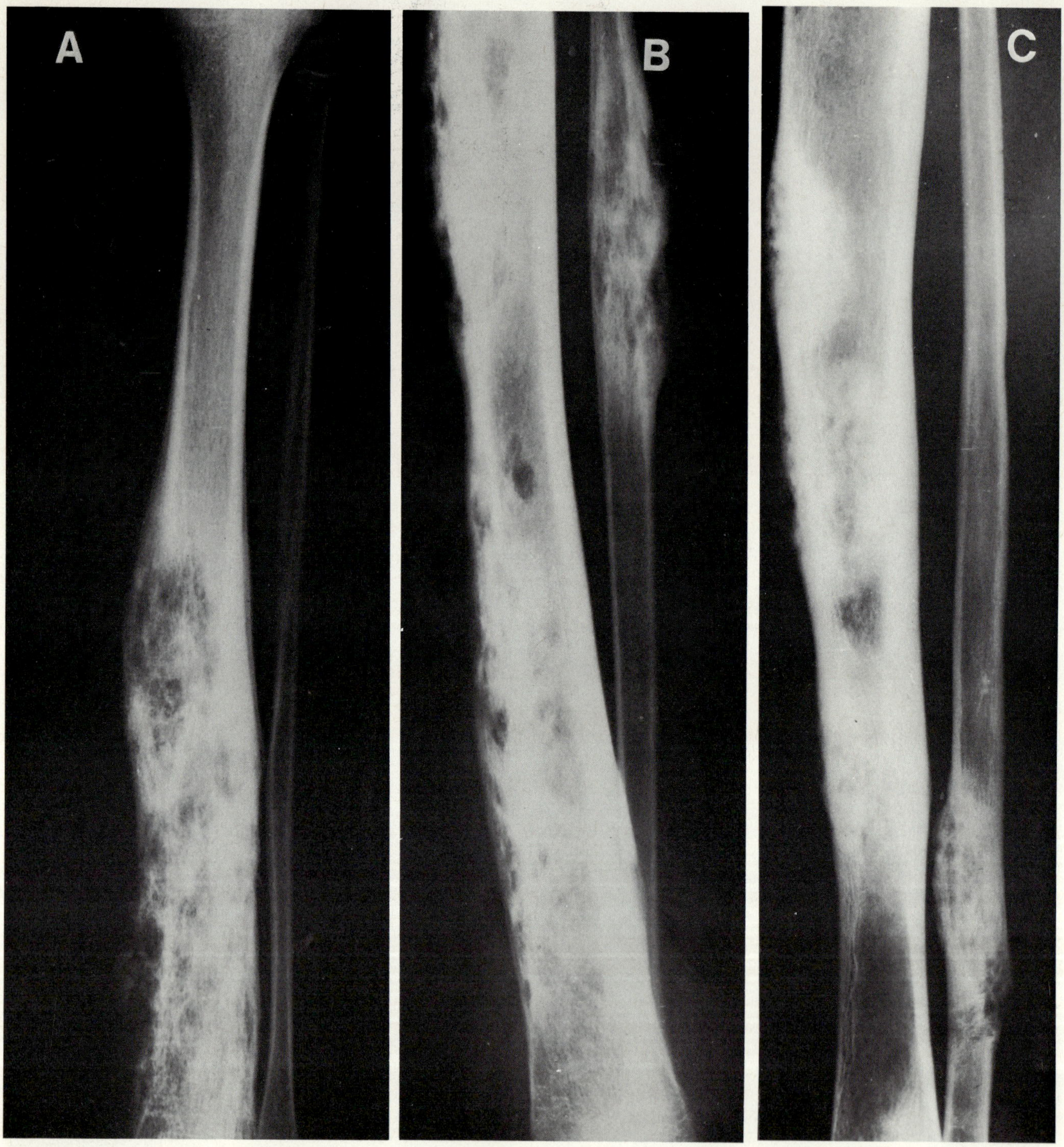

Fig. 2.32 Legs of child and two young adults with yaws osteitis. Sclerotic reaction due to healing is apparent in this later stage of yaws. The plasticity of bone is causing slight bowing.

the most frequently afflicted. If the periosteal new bone formation is exuberant obvious swelling of the part can be seen. There is often pain.

Radiologically the changes can be anticipated from the descriptive pathology. No rigid classification into secondary and tertiary lesions is usually feasible.

Dactylitis is common. Initially peri-osteal new bone diffusely surrounds the diaphysis of a phalanx or metacarpal. Usually several bones are affected and the radial side of the hand is the most involved (Fig. 2.29). In severe cases nearly all the short bones of the hands are affected, but generally the distribution of involvement is patchy and roughly symmetrical. Soft tissue swelling can be marked.

If the process affects the subarticular bone angular deformities can follow which later lead to bizarre finger deformities. Subluxations, arthropathies, shortening of bones from growth disturbances and pseudo-arthroses from fractures through gummatous areas also occur (Fig. 2.30) (Risebrough *et al.*, 1961). Focal areas of destruction which may be cortical and eccentric or medullary and central are caused by larger gummatous type foci (Fig. 2.31). Around such inflammatory infiltrates the bone often becomes sclerotic (Fig. 2.32).

Essentially similar but larger lesions can develop that produce massive exuberant partly ossified masses that clinically suggest the presence of a tumour (Fig. 2.33) (Cockshott & Davies, 1960).

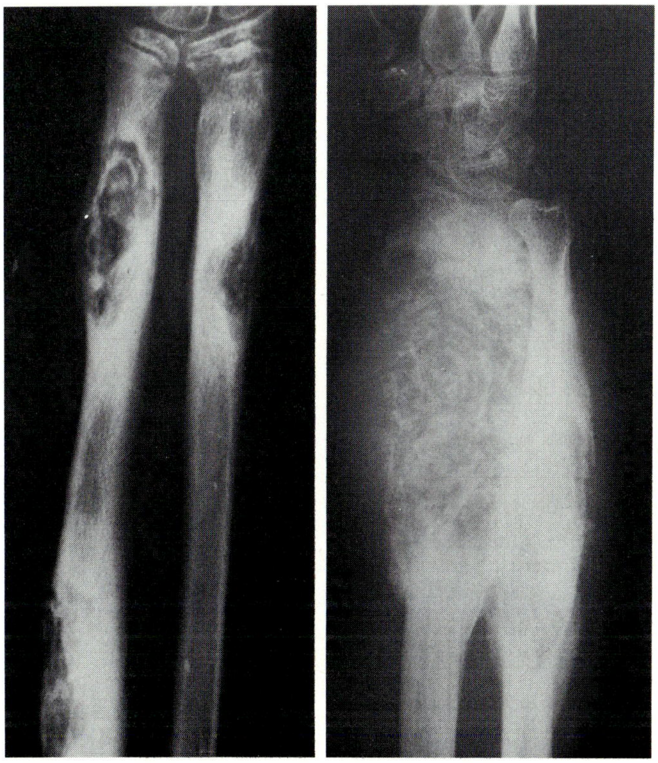

Fig. 2.33 Expansile yaws granulomata with coarse curvilinear whorls of new bone within the granulomata. The forearm of the adult has 'tumoural yaws'.

In the leg early lesions are characterised by thin periosteal new bone formation parallel to the diaphysis, which later thickens locally. Multiple foci of destruction can occur which may expand bone or lead to bowing due to bone 'softening'. Though the leg can be the clinical site of such a change (Hackett, 1936), the restriction of this syndrome to the aboriginal and its presence in those with negative serology suggests a more complex aetiology (Moodie, 1973).

Involvement of the skull is probably next in frequency. Three types of changes are described here: calvarial rounded gummatous destruction with adjacent sclerosis (Fig. 2.34); proliferative new bone around the root of the

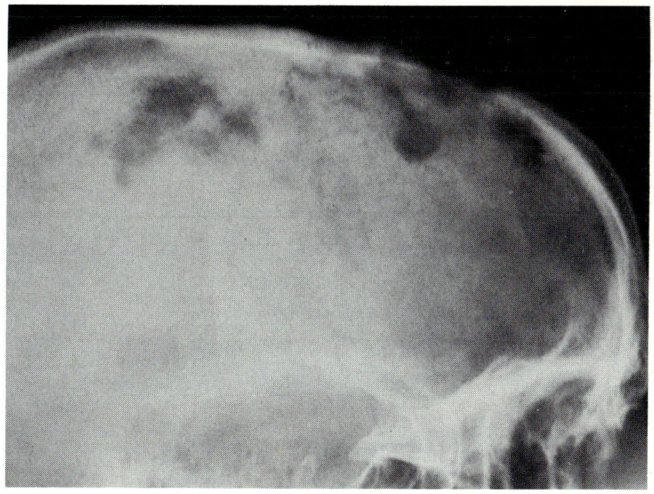

Fig. 2.34 Skull with lytic calvarial defects due to yaws granuloma.

nose termed 'goundou'; and erosive destruction of the premaxilla. The latter process causes considerable facial mutilation with loss of the nasal septum which is termed 'gangosa' in the tropical literature (Fig. 2.35).

Yaws differs from congenital syphilis in the perinatal period as it is not seen till a later age. Metaphysitis and dental changes of the Hutchinson or Moon type do not develop in yaws. However, the juvenile forms of syphilis show x-ray features that can by themselves be impossible to distinguish from yaws (Cremin & Fisher, 1970).

With antibiotic therapy in the acute stages there is rapid relief of clinical symptoms but radiographic resolution is slower in pace (Figs. 2.36 and 2.37).

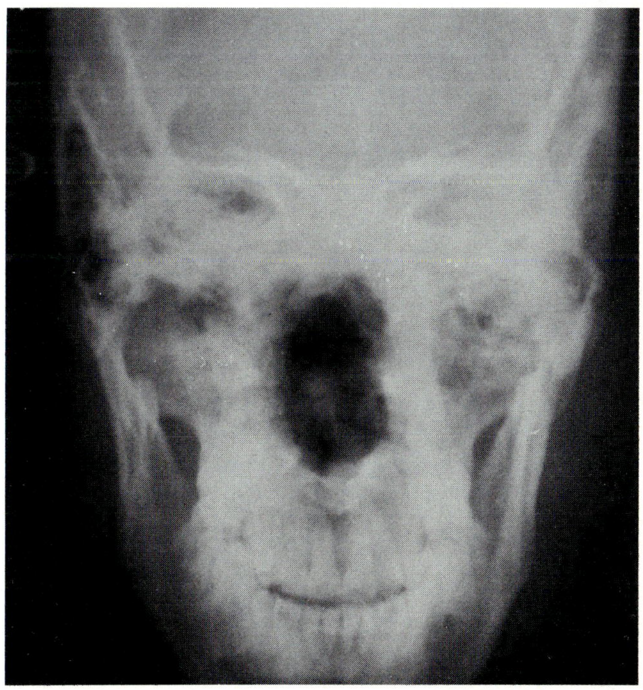

Fig. 2.35 Destruction of nasal septum and bridge of nose by yaws goundon.

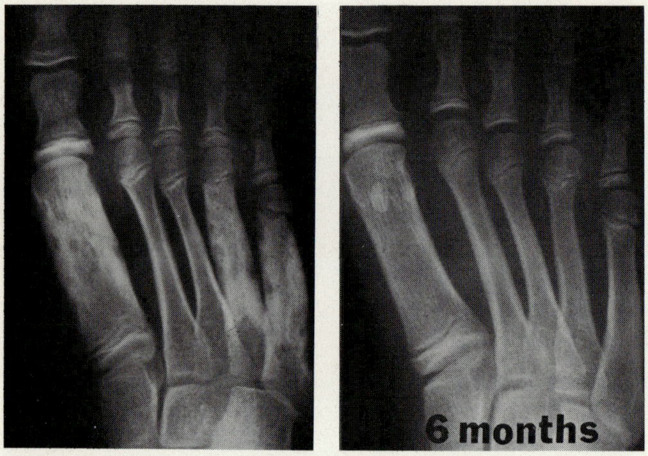

A B

Fig. 2.36 **A, B.** Dramatic response to specific yaws therapy over a period of six months.

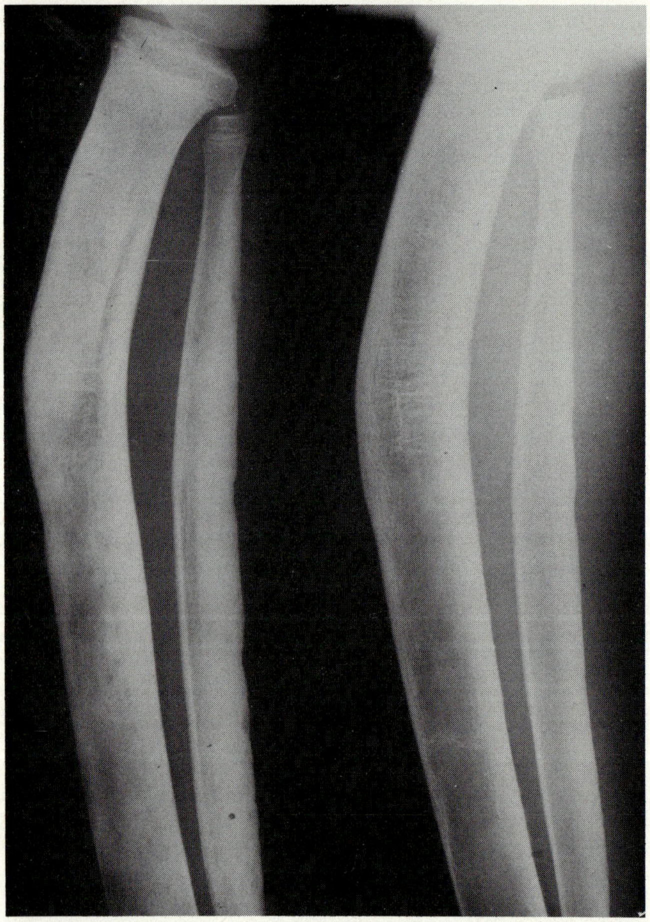

Fig. 2.37 Bilateral sabre tibiae in a youth due to spontaneously healed yaws.

REFERENCES

Cockshott, W. P. & Davies, A. G. M. (1960) Tumoural gummatous yaws, *Journal of Bone and Joint Surgery*, **42B,** 785–787.

Cremin, B. J. & Fisher, R. M. (1970) The lesions of congenital syphilis, *British Journal of Radiology*, **43,** 333–341.

Hackett, C. J. (1936) Boomerang leg and yaws in Australian aborigines, *Royal Society of Tropical Medicine and Hygiene Monograph*, **I.** London.

Hackett, C. J. (1951) *Bone Lesions of Yaws in Uganda.* Oxford: Blackwell Scientific Publications.

Hudson, E. M. (1963) Treponematosis and anthropology, *Annals of Internal Medicine*, **58,** 1037–1048.

Moodie, P. M. (1973) *Aboriginal Health*, pp. 133–134. Canberra: Australian National University Press.

Risebrough, A. W., Joske, R. A. & Vaughan, B. F. (1961) Hand deformities due to yaws in Western Australian aborigines, *Clinical Radiology*, **12,** 109–113.

LEPROSY

Leprosy is due to infection by Mycobacterium leprae. It is now rare in temperate climes and is found predominantly in the Far East, Polynesia, Micronesia, Africa, Central and South America. There are probably over 14 million lepers in the world. The organism has low infectivity and prolonged and intimate contact is usually necessary for the disease to be acquired. Precisely how the organism enters the body is unknown. Evidence from conversion rate of contacts suggests that transmission is much higher than is apparent from the clinical attack rate. Contacts of tuberculoid cases have a 70 per cent lower infection rate than those of lepromatous cases (W.H.O., 1977). The course of the disease is determined by the state of resistance of the host. If cell mediated immunity is well developed a less severe more focal form of leprosy, tuberculoid leprosy, evolves. The lepromin test is positive. Pathologically there may be caseation, and epithelioid tubercles. The skin lesions are well-defined hypopigmented anaesthetic areas. The nerves at palpable superficial exposed surfaces develop fusiform localised thickening.

In those with less resistance the more disseminate and progressive lepromatous leprosy becomes manifest. The skin shows extensive infiltrations with poorly defined macules. There is systemic dissemination with a multiplicity of lesions. Histologically organisms can be found subcutaneously and in the liver, lymph glands, testes, eyes and bone marrow. The nerve lesions are more symmetrical than in the tuberculoid form, evolve slowly, but inexorably with considerable sensory loss.

The classification into lepromatous and tuberculoid types is a convenience, but there is a continuum between the two forms. In between are types termed variously indeterminate, dimorphous and borderline leprosy. It has been noted that the organism replicates best at areas of low temperature, which probably accounts for the predominant involvement of skin and of nerves where they course superficially: the ulnar nerve at elbow; the lateral popliteal around the head of fibula; and the great auricular nerve. Similarly it accounts for bone granulomata in the hands and feet. The radiological changes in leprosy are confined to the face and the limbs.

The facial lesions have been redescribed by Moller-Christensen (1952) following a fascinating study that began from archaeological material derived from a medieval leprosaria burial ground in Denmark. Lepromatous granulomata erode the nasal spine of the maxilla and implicate the maxillary margin with possible loss of teeth (Fig. 2.38). If the condition progresses with septal destruction considerable nasal deformity may result.

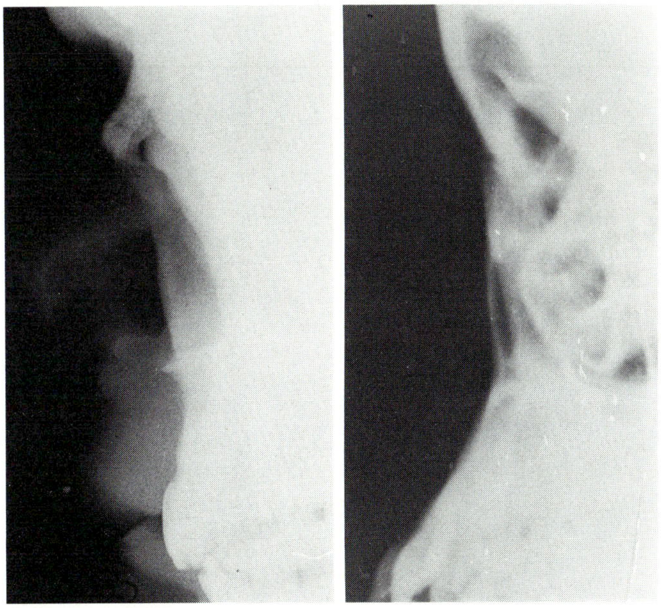

A B

Fig. 2.38 **A.** Early erosive disease of the maxilla. **B.** Advanced destruction with loss of the nasal spine of the maxilla.

The osseous lesions have been well documented in various papers from different parts of the world and the authors show considerable agreement (Paterson, 1955; Cave *et al.*, 1965; Enna *et al.*, 1971; Wastie, 1975). Obviously radiology is not the means of diagnosis, but useful to document progress and to provide a warning if there are changes suggestive of imminent catastrophic joint disintegration. Radiological findings, even in cases with severe mutilations, can then provide information which has management implications.

It is customary to consider bone alterations in two categories: those directly attributable to mycobacterial granulomata and those skeletal changes resulting from the interplay between the consequences of sensory loss, infection, loss of autonomic vascular regulation and the altered mechanics from changes in weight-bearing and muscular forces. A non-specific type of osteoporosis may occur in leprosy which is often attributed to disuse. Though this can occur consequent on therapeutic immobilisation or because of pain, it has no specific features. Focal destruction of trabeculae in phalanges and metacarpal or metatarsal heads result from bone marrow lepromatous granulomata. These are seen in cancellous bone and, when well defined, form geodes between 3 mm and 1 cm in size (Fig. 2.39). The granulomata can be less well defined with a

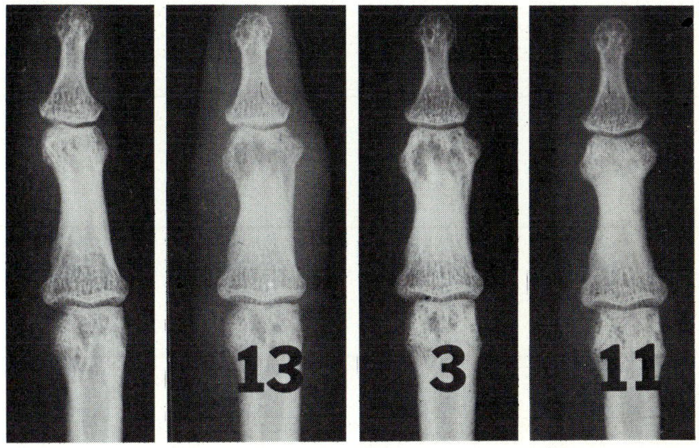

A B C D

Fig. 2.39 **A–D.** Osteitis leprosum. Films of phalanges of a patient taken at intervals—the black numerals indicate months between films. From the acute dactylitis obvious at 13 months, healing and resolution has gradually taken place with chemotherapy. (Courtesy of Dr. D. E. Paterson.)

permeative zone of destruction that can extend into the medullary portions. In these cases the medullary nutrient foraminae or apertures for emissary veins can be enlarged (Fig. 2.40). This can be difficult to assess, as the range of normal variation is large.

Should the zone of infiltrated lepromatous bone be subchondral this can lead to collapse of the articular surface with angulation or disorganisation (Fig. 2.40). The base of a phalanx implicated in this manner may expand and

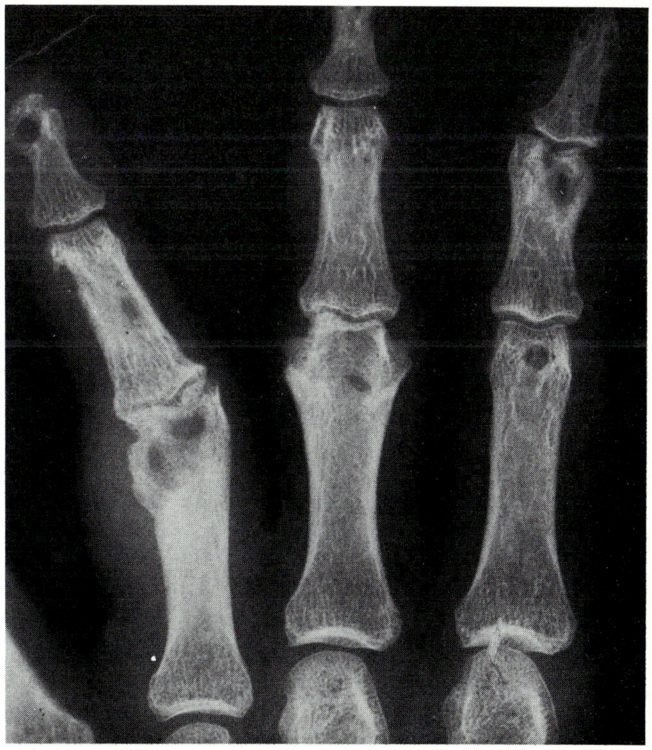

Fig. 2.40 Multiple lepra granulomata in bone with subarticular collapse and joint angulation. Enlarged nutrient foraminae are related to foci. (Courtesy of Dr. D. E. Paterson.)

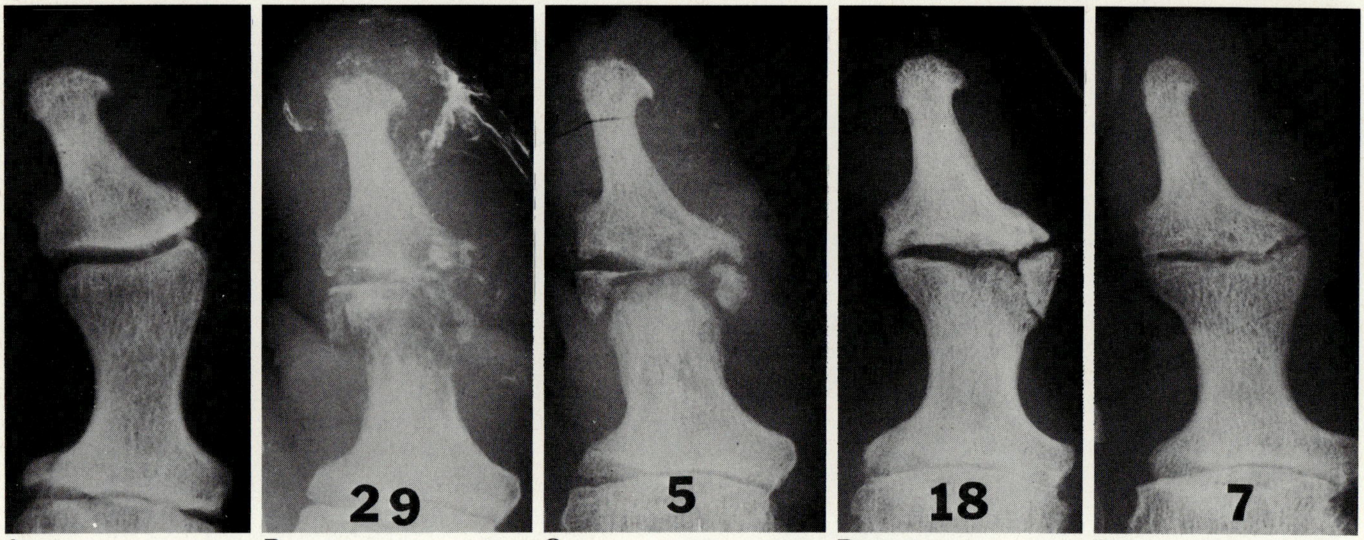

A B C D E

Fig. 2.41 **A–E.** Series of films of hallux of a patient treated and followed for five years. Despite the non-specific osteitis in this toe with sensory loss, careful management has resulted in healing with incorporation of fragments and an arthropathy. Numbers indicate months between films. (Courtesy of Dr. D. E. Paterson.)

broaden (Fig. 2.41). The deformities are exacerbated if there is capsular or ligamentous damage.

The development of linear investing periosteal new bone, usually over the lower tibia and fibula and less frequently the forearm bones, has been demonstrated histologically to be due to lepromatous infiltration. In patients with this reactive inflammatory change there is usually erythema nodosum of the overlying skin (Enna *et al.*, 1971). Infection arising from an ulcer may give rise to a similar appearance.

A rare pathognomic radiographic change directly attributable to lepromatous granulations is calcification of nerves. The calcium is thought to be deposited in caseous granulomata as a late dystrophic process. The calcium is deposited focally as an ovoid, but it can be arranged as linear flecks (Fig. 2.42) (Trapnell, 1965).

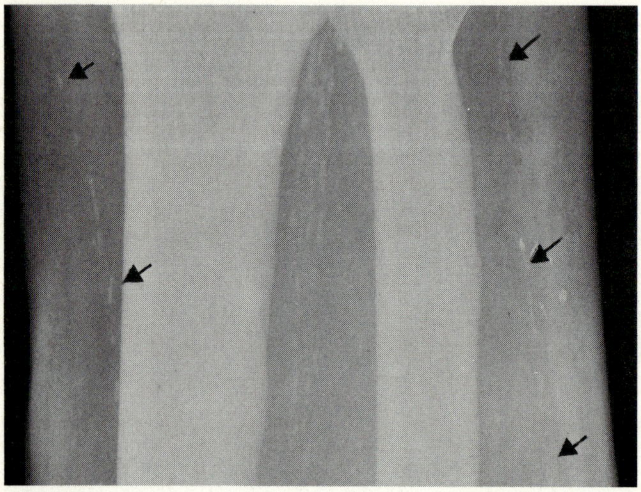

Fig. 2.42 Forearm showing thin flecks of calcium in line of nerves (arrowed). (Courtesy of Dr. David Trapnell and *British Journal of Radiology*.)

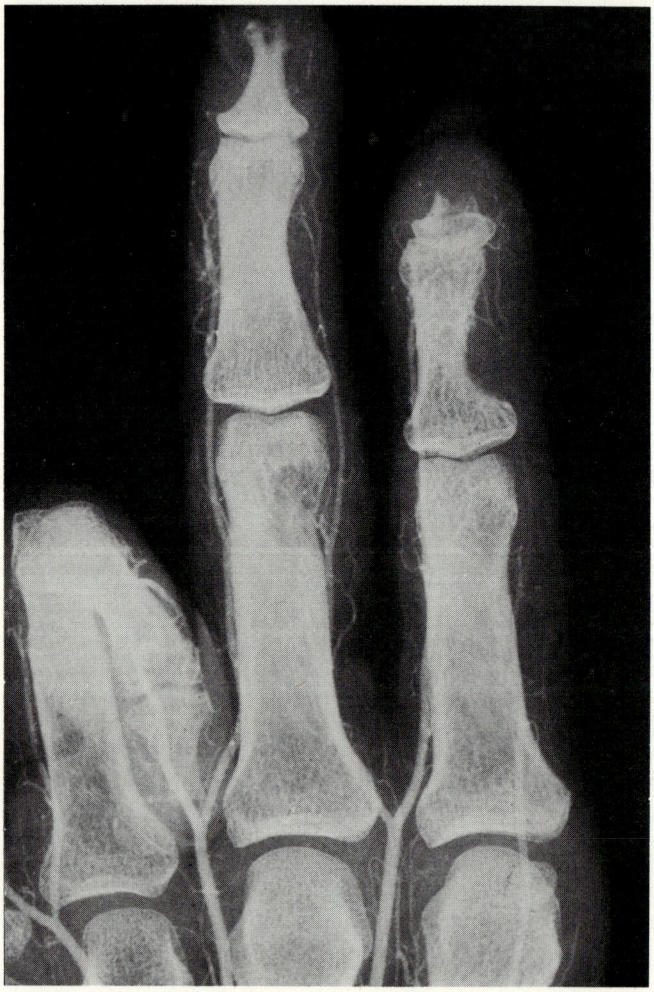

Fig. 2.43 Arteriogram in patient showing intra-osseous destruction and absorptive changes of terminal phalanges. Note interruption and attenuation of digital arteries. The osteolytic granuloma is closely related to an osseous branch of the digital vessel. (Courtesy of Dr. D. E. Paterson.)

The bony alterations of leprosy that remain to be described are more complex in pathogenesis. Loss of sensation *per se* results in Charcot-like joints. The development of perforating ulcers introduces infection as a complication. Yet there is a basic process of bone absorption that is not well understood. Vascular alterations have been proposed as an important determinant. Cave *et al.* (1965), Paterson (1965) and Johnson *et al.* (1978), have shown by angiography that circulatory changes occur in the hands and feet of lepers. Vessels can be of finer calibre than normal and considerable slowing of the circulation is evident in the lower limbs. Johnson and colleagues have shown in the lower limb that proximal diversionary shunting takes place in gastrocnemius and soleal muscles and that there is hyperaemia around foot ulcers which increase the functional ischaemia. They believe that diffuse deep-seated granulomata in the limb increases muscle compartment pressures to further reduce blood perfusion distally in the limb. Paterson emphasises the loss of the end vascular loops in the pulp of the fingers (Fig. 2.44). He and others reject the possibility of a specific leprosy arteritis. The consensus seems to be that the vascular disturbances are due to disuse, loss of reflex vasomotor arc and infection. Diminution in the blood supply by shunting and compartment pressure changes certainly delays the healing process and predisposes towards infection and trophic bone alterations, but does not of itself explain the mechanism of bone absorption or osteolysis.

Bone absorption in the absence of infection is characteristically clear-cut without an osteoporotic edge. Soft tissue absorption accompanies the bone loss. The tips of phalanges show the initial changes, but as the disease advances the bases of the phalanges and the metatarsal heads become implicated in a similar manner (Fig. 2.44). Bone loss is usually concentric and can lead to marked tapering of long bones. Cupping of the base of a phalanx distal to a pointed metacarpal or metatarsal is frequent (Fig. 2.44). In the hands the arthropathies are exacerbated by altered balance of tendon forces due to the palsies, whereas in the feet the additional effects of weight bearing add to the deforming process.

As the deformities develop, the trabecular trajectories in the tarsal bones, particularly the os calcis, do not seem to be able to realign to take the altered distribution of forces. Because of insensitivity the patient abuses the foot and receives many small injuries which are ignored. The calcaneus flattens with development of a reversed Bohler's angle. Once this change begins it proceeds rapidly and can lead to disintegration of the foot arches unless splint therapy is provided. Harris and Brand (1966) have pointed out the importance of the talo-navicular joint as the keystone of the arch. Small fractures on the dorsal surface

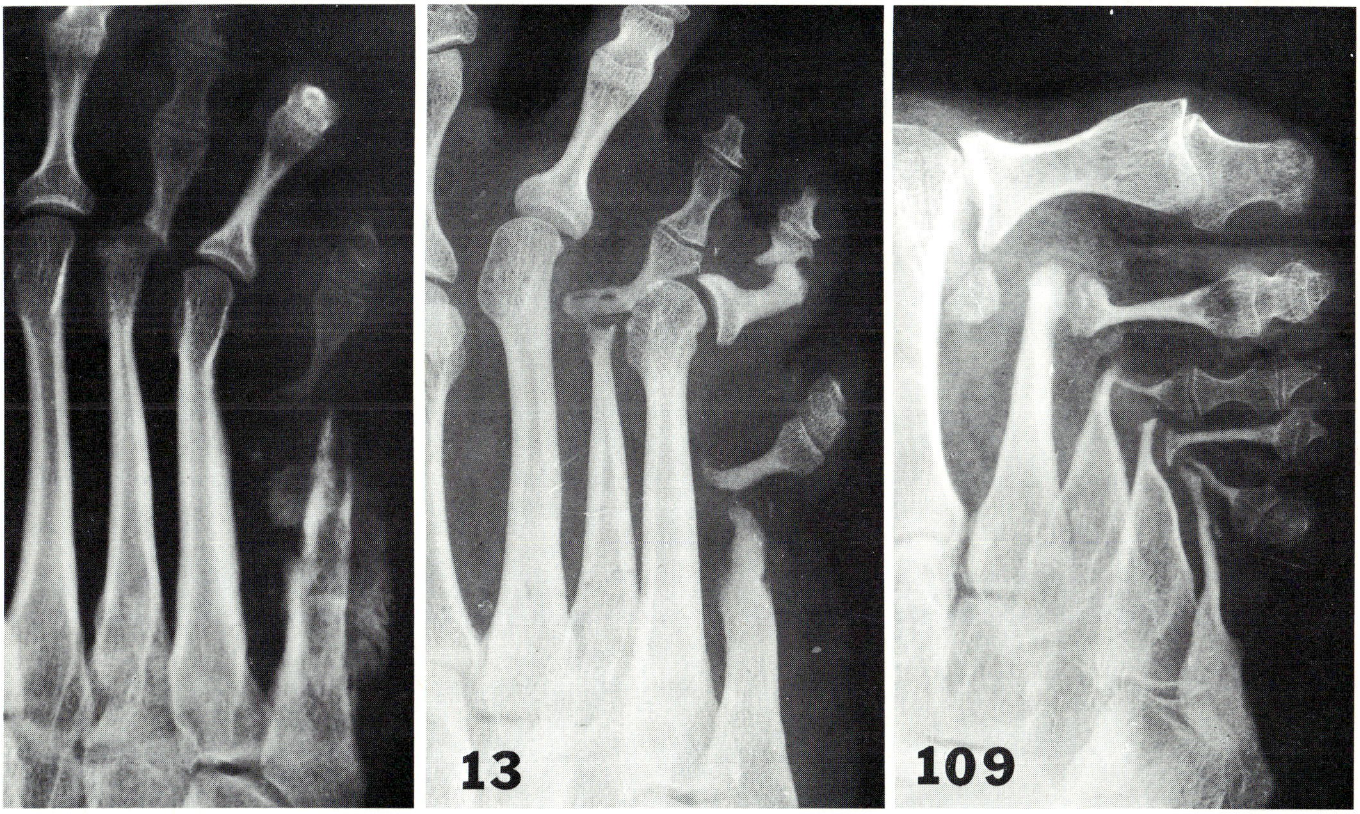

A B C

Fig. 2.44 A, B, C. Progression of foot changes over 122 months in a patient with plantar ulcer and sensory loss who received inadequate therapy. (Figures indicate interval in months between films.) (Courtesy of Dr. D. E. Paterson.)

indicate that unless there is prompt appropriate therapy a vicious progressive cycle of bone destruction will ensue (Fig. 2.45). These workers have noted that the skin overlying these areas is warm to palpation from the hyperaemia of repair. This would suggest that an isotope bone scan, though nearly always unavailable, would provide a very sensitive tool for monitoring the feet for the earliest infractions.

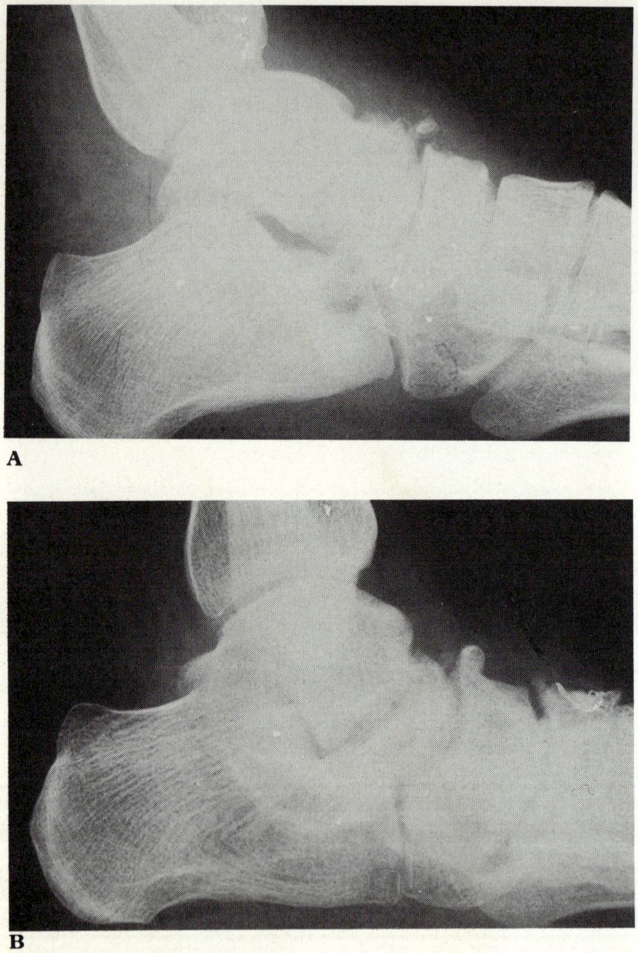

Fig. 2.45 A, B. Anaesthetic foot showing navicular marginal fracture and talar absorption with loss of keystone of the arch of the foot. Healing is taking place after bed rest and tendon transplant. (Courtesy of Dr. D. E. Paterson.)

Workers in Senegal (Basset *et al.*, 1969) and in Ibadan have performed neurography of the ulnar and lateral popliteal nerves in leprosy with ultra-fluid lipiodol. The contrast spreads in the perineural spaces and reveals the thickness of the nerve and the presence of intraneural granulomata (Fig. 2.46). These show up as areas of expansion with local filling defects. If they cause significant pressure they prevent the normal passage of contrast in the main trunk, and muscular branches become opacified. Since much of the course of the nerves can be palpated and the usefulness of decompression is uncertain, the clinical value of the procedure is not established.

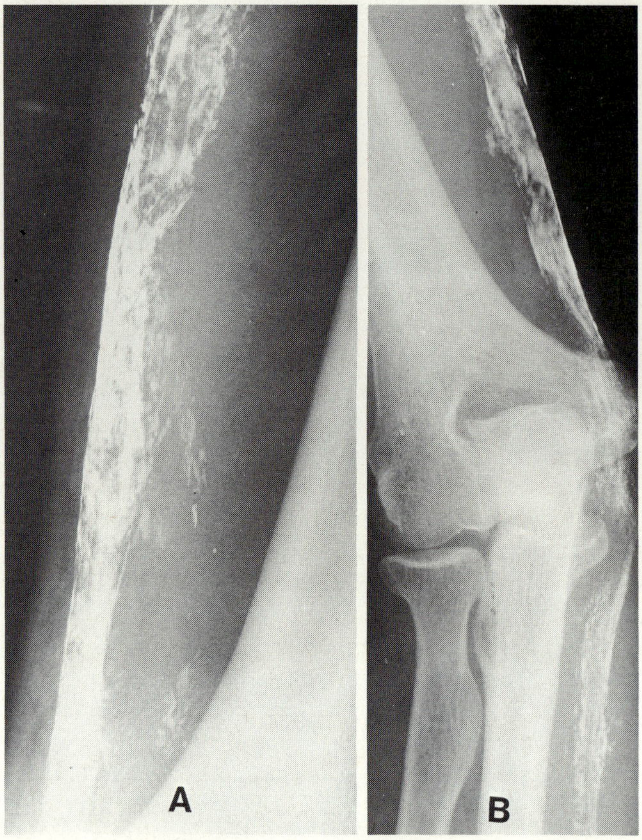

Fig. 2.46 Ulnar nerve neurography showing thickening of nerve and intraneural granulomatos reaction in upper arm. (**A**).

REFERENCES

Basset, A., Wackenheim, A. & Grosshans, E. (1969) La neurographie lipoidolée du nerf cubital, *Annales de Radiologie*, **12,** 565–570.

Cave, L., Fustec, R. & Basset, A. (1965) Radiologie de la lèpre, *Annales de Radiologie*, **8,** 61–76.

Enna, C. D., Jacobson, R. A. & Rausch, R. O. (1971) Bone changes in leprosy, *Radiology*, **100,** 295–306.

Harris, J. R. & Brand, P. W. (1966) Patterns of disintegration of the anaesthetic foot, *Journal of Bone and Joint Surgery*, **48B,** 4–16.

Johnson, A. C., Reddy, R., Johnson, S. & Everette James, A. (1978) Lower limb angiography in leprosy, *Radiology*, **126,** 327–332.

Lechat, M. & Chardome, J. (1957) Evolution radiologique des mutilations chez les lepreux traites par D.D.S., *Annales de la Société Belge de Médecine Tropicale*, **37,** 907–917.

Moller-Christensen, V., Bakke, S. N. & Melsom, R. S. (1952) Changes in anterior nasal spine and alveolar process of maxillary bone in leprosy, *International Journal of Leprosy*, **20,** 335–340.

Paterson, D. E. (1965) Radiological bone changes and angiographic findings in leprosy, *Journal of the Faculty of Radiologists*, **7,** 35–55.

Trapnell, D. M. (1965) Calcification of nerves in leprosy, *British Journal of Radiology*, **38,** 796–797.

Wastie, M. L. (1975) Radiological changes in serial x-rays of the foot and tarsus in leprosy, *Clinical Radiology*, **26,** 285–292.

W.H.O. (1977) *Expert Committee on Leprosy*. Fifth Report. Geneva: W.H.O.

FUNGAL OSTEITIS AND OSTEOMYELITIS

Many genera of fungi and actinomyceteceae can be pathogenic to man and involve bone in the course of an infection. Because of the diversity of aetiologic agents a description of disorders caused by each would be both chaotic and repetitive. In a clinical work such as this where recognition of the radiological patterns is important, we shall group entities together to stress the similarities of their pathological and radiological features, rather than use the complex controversial taxonomic relationships of the causative organisms.

In the simplest terms bone can be implicated by direct implantation of the organism from outside into bone or in the adjacent tissues, as with mycetoma or sporotrichosis; by dissemination from a pulmonary focus, as in various forms of blastomycosis; or by contact with an air passage, as is seen in rhino-entomophthora-mycosis and paranasal aspergilloma. In all these instances the infection generally involves a previously healthy individual and is not an opportunist invader of a debilitated host with an abnormal immunological status.

Haematogenous fungal osteomyelitis

There are several fungi with a yeast parasitic phase that may involve bone. Bone is implicated as a result of systemic haematogenous dissemination of a primary focus elsewhere, usually in the lungs. The causative organisms differ in their areas of endemicity and in the clinical entities they cause, but resemble each other in the pathological and radiological evolution of the bone lesions. For convenience the organisms are briefly described to indicate where they occur in the world, the mode of infection and the prevalence of bone involvement. Subsequently the pathology and radiology of the group will be considered together.

The organisms being grouped are largely dimorphic yeasts. These are fungi which have a mycelial phase and a parasitic yeast form in the tissues. Conversion from one phase to the other can be affected in the laboratory by modifications of the environment, notably temperature changes. Cryptococcus neoformans is included in this clinical grouping though it is a pure yeast with no mycelial stage.

Blastomyces dermatitidis

Blastomyces dermatitidis used to be termed North American blastomycosis, as cases were encountered in the United States in the Ohio and Mississippi valleys, the mid-Atlantic States and in eastern Canada. In recent years isolates from Mexico, Central and South America, Tunisia, the Congo and Uganda render the North American title obsolete.

The organism has been recovered from the soil. The portal of entry is normally inhalation of spores, but rare instances of direct cutaneous implantation have been documented. Since this last mode of infection can be discounted, as it is bizarre, one can assume that all patients will show evidence of either some pulmonary disease or of cutaneous or subcutaneous granulomata, or both. Between one-fifth to one-half of the patients with systemic dissemination have bone foci (Gehweiler *et al.*, 1970).

Coccidioides immitis

Coccidioides immitis is limited to the Americas, encompassing an area in the South-west (California, New Mexico, Nevada and Utah); Mexico, Paraguay, Venezuela and Argentina, where it was first found. The organism has been recovered from the soil and natural infection occurs amongst rodents. Infective arthrospores are inhaled and usually produce a mild illness that is not generally recognised. Skin sensitivity tests indicate that in endemic areas, such as the San Joaquim valley, a high proportion of agricultural workers respond in a positive fashion.

The pulmonary lesions may develop in a chronic manner and in some dissemination may occur. If in a miliary fashion, the meninges usually become implicated. Bone lesions occur in about 20 per cent of cases with dissemination (Iger & Larson, 1967; Dalinka, 1971). Isolated localised foci of involvement may occur in bone or synovia in the absence of widespread dissemination (Grebe, 1954; Pollock *et al.*, 1967).

Diagnosis is established by culture. This can be hazardous, as the arthrospores are highly infective. Histological sections suitably stained reveal typical sporangia and endospores in the tissues. Various types of immunological tests may also be of value.

Paracoccidioides brasiliensis

Paracoccidioides brasiliensis causes South American blastomycosis over a wide area of Brazil extending from Sao Paulo northwards through Venezuela, Central America to southern Mexico, but excluding the Amazon delta and equatorial valley. The organism has been found in the soil. As with the preceding organisms skin sensitivity tests reveal a high prevalence of infection in some areas (parts of Venezuela 53 per cent of the population), indicating that there are many subclinical cases (Rippon, 1974). The portal of entry is considered to be pulmonary inhalation and the frequent oral and cutaneous manifestations are probably metastatic rather than primary processes. Secondary foci develop in lymph glands, viscera: liver, spleen, adrenal and bowel more frequently than in bone, which is relatively spared.

Diagnosis is established by culture. The histological appearances with suitable staining can be characteristic.

Histoplasma capsulatum

Histoplasma capsulatum has a worldwide distribution, having been isolated from all continents. It exists in soil and is particularly associated with caves that have bat droppings and chicken runs, as it seems that the organism flourishes in such environments. It has endemic zones associated with river valleys such as the Ohio, Mississippi, St. Lawrence, Ganges, Amazon, etc. The organism was first described from Panama. It occurs in the Middle East, Egypt and sub-saharan Africa (Ajello *et al.*, 1977).

Man is infected by inhaling macro-conidia in the dust. Demolition of old buildings that have bird droppings and exploration of bat-infested caves have led to minor epidemics. In endemic areas skin sensitivity tests indicate a high prevalence of subclinical disease. Multiple calcified discrete granulomata in the lungs are also evidence of previous infection. Bone infection is rare with this organism, with only three cases recorded and one of H. capsulatum synovitis (Allen, 1959). All known bone cases had lung and visceral involvement.

Histoplasma duboisii

Histoplasma duboisii has the most restricted habitat of any of the organisms being discussed. Autochthonous cases are confined to an 'equatorial band' between the Sahara desert in the North and the Kalahari in the South. All patients seen in Europe and America have lived in Africa. It is presumed that the organism exists in the soil and that there is a pulmonary portal of entry. However, in practice evidence of lung infection is not obtainable in most clinical cases who present with skin and subcutaneous lesions or bone granulomata. Generalised visceral involvement also occurs. In such cases evidence of interstitial lung disease can be detected radiologically and shown histologically.

The African form of histoplasmosis is noteworthy not only for its paucity of evidence of lung disease but also for the great frequency of bone involvement—probably in 80 per cent of cases. This is in complete contrast to H. capsulatum, where the lung disease is universal and involvement of bone is unusual (Cockshott & Lucas, 1964).

Diagnosis is established by culture. Histologically the appearance of the large intracellular yeasts in giant cells is sufficiently characteristic to make the diagnosis. Skin sensitivity test to histoplasmin shows such variable responses that it has limited and epidemiological value.

Cryptococcus neoformans

Cryptococcus neoformans is a cosmopolitan encapsulated yeast that has been recovered from the soil. It is also associated with areas containing pigeon droppings and is a hazard to those who clean out pigeon lofts. This affinity to bird excrement has been shown to be related to guano's high content of creatinine which selectively C. neoformans uses as a nitrogen source (Ajello, 1968).

C. neoformans is an opportunistic invader of compromised hosts and widespread systemic spread, particularly to the meninges and brain, is frequent. Thus infection is seen in patients with reticuloses, leukaemia, and those receiving steroids and immuno-suppressive drugs. Though bone may be involved in these patients, the main attention is focused on the life-threatening visceral manifestations so that its presence there may well be overlooked.

Individual infective organisms are sufficiently small to reach the lung alveoli. There in most cases a non-progressive subclinical reaction occurs, or the disease may become established with the production of a localised focus or a more infiltrative process. If dissemination develops bone foci occur in about 8 per cent to 10 per cent of patients (Gosling, 1956; Cowen, 1969; Chleboun & Nade, 1977). A further clinical form is seen in which no lung lesions can be demonstrated and a single bone marrow focus evolves in an otherwise healthy individual.

Pathology

Inhalation is considered to be the normal mode of infection, usually producing a subclinical self-limiting disorder that may not be noticed. In some cases the pulmonary lesions evolve and at any time spread may occur to other tissues. When this happens a granulomatous and/or suppurative focus develops with initially a polymorphonuclear response and later, as the granuloma forms, a histiocytic and giant cell response. In some instances the yeast may be seen in giant cells. Special stains (Silver, P.A.S., etc.) may be needed for clear detection of the yeasts. In exudates india ink may be helpful to reveal the capsule of the organism.

The granulomata may be in skin or subcutaneously where bone may be implicated by continuity from without. This obviously can occur where bone is closely related to the subcutaneous tissues, but similar extension by continuity is seen from 'cold' abscesses. Thus paraspinal abscess and granulomata can erode the vertebral portions of adjacent ribs.

More frequently bone granulomata occur within the cancellous part of the bone in adults and in the medulla in children. It appears that the organisms lodge and parasitise the red marrow. Thus, in young children in a long bone the infection will develop—often in multiple areas and with a striking symmetry—in the central diaphysis. As adolescence is reached the site of predilection moves to the juxtametaphyseal area. In adults when long bones are affected the cancellous former epiphyses and apophyses are most likely to be involved. The vertebrae are frequent sites, as are flat bones as ribs, calvarium, sternum and pelvis. The cuboidal bones of the carpus and tarsus, which harbour red marrow, can also be implicated. A convenient *aide mèmoire* as to the likely sites of involvement in an adult is to consider a pyrophosphate Tc bone scan: those areas of normally high pick-up are the most likely to be affected. Whether the degree of vascular perfusion of bone or the location of the red marrow is the important determinant is an academic question, since the two go hand in hand.

This behaviour of location in bone is not unique to these fungal disorders. Another granulomatous condition, histiocytosis X, exhibits the same characteristics, as also do the skeletal sites of election for Burkitt's tumour.

Because of the location in the proximal and distal ends of long bones, penetration into joints would be expected to occur. Articular cartilage, unlike that of the physis, resists this form of extension so that fungal arthritis is uncommon. Joint involvement by haematogenous synovial seeding has been recorded without organisms in joint aspirates (Pollock *et al.*, 1967).

RADIOLOGY

The essential pathological process in bone in all these conditions is a granuloma in the marrow. Consequently the lesions are characterised initially by trabecular destruction in cancellous bone in a vascular area of bone that has red marrow (Figs. 2.47 and 2.48). In a child diaphyseal lesions of striking symmetry may be noted (Fig. 2.49). Also in children, much more readily than in adults, the granuloma can expand, and erode in a scalloped fashion, the cortex from within. The periosteum may be reached and elevated, giving rise to varying degrees of periosteal new bone that can be lamellated or have an 'inflammatory' Codman's triangle (Fig. 2.49). Pathological fractures may develop in the weakened areas (Fig. 2.50). In children and adolescents granulomas may readily cross the cartilaginous growth plate (Fig. 2.50). Then because of interference to the physis growth disturbances develop (Cockshott & Lucas, 1964). In deep-seated lesions the periosteum may be breached and cold abscesses form. If the bone is superficial, sinuses or ulcerating granulomata that are in continuity with bone may be seen. Fortunately most long bone lesions remain localised and confined. Despite the frequent foci close to joints, particularly in adults, a fungal arthritis is rare and articular cartilage often remains intact even when there is extensive subchondral destruction. Extension from one bone to another is most unusual. A patient's resistance probably has a bearing on whether the process remains focal with perhaps a reactive sclerotic margin or whether it extends. Under the influence of appropriate therapy, such as Amphotericin B, foci gradually fill in and heal.

In the tarsus and carpus essentially the same process occurs. Flat bones, apart from the pelvis, are relatively superficial. Sometimes they may be eroded by a subcutaneous granuloma penetrating the outer cortical bone, but generally they develop foci within their diploe or medulla. However, if they extend a subcutaneous granuloma forms. Then it can be difficult to determine

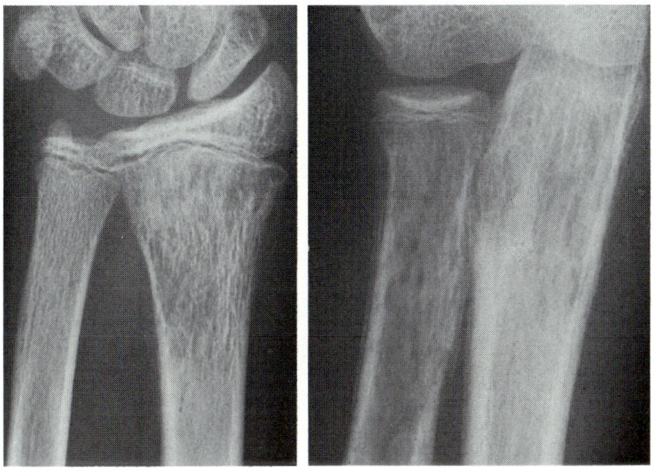

A B

Fig. 2.47 A, B. Permeative calcaneal cancellous destruction from Histoplasma duboisii granuloma of diaphyses and metaphyses.

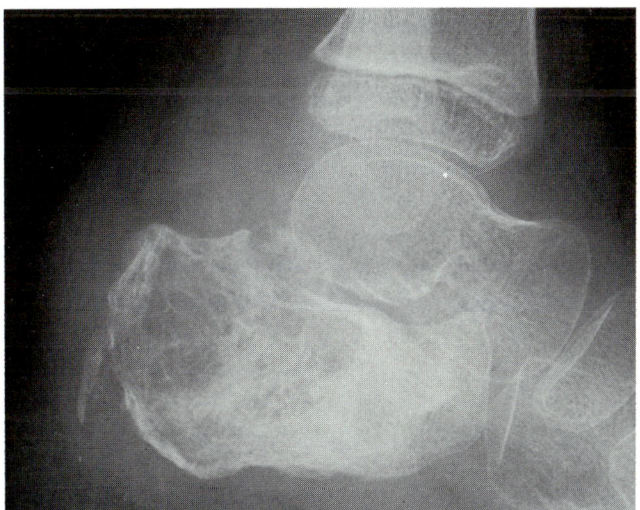

Fig. 2.48 Permeative granuloma of os calcis due to H. duboisii.

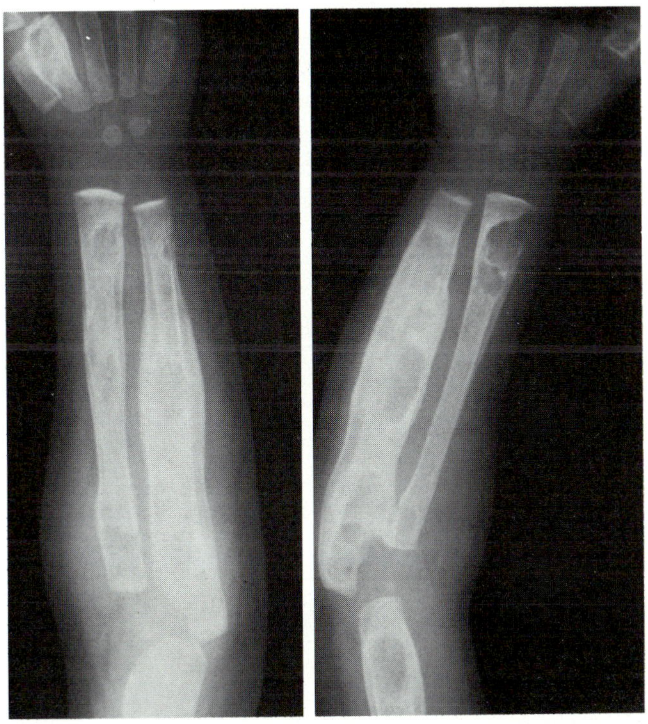

A B

Fig. 2.49 A, B. Multiple granulomata of H. duboisii expanding diaphyses and inciting considerable periosteal reaction in forearms of Nigerian child.

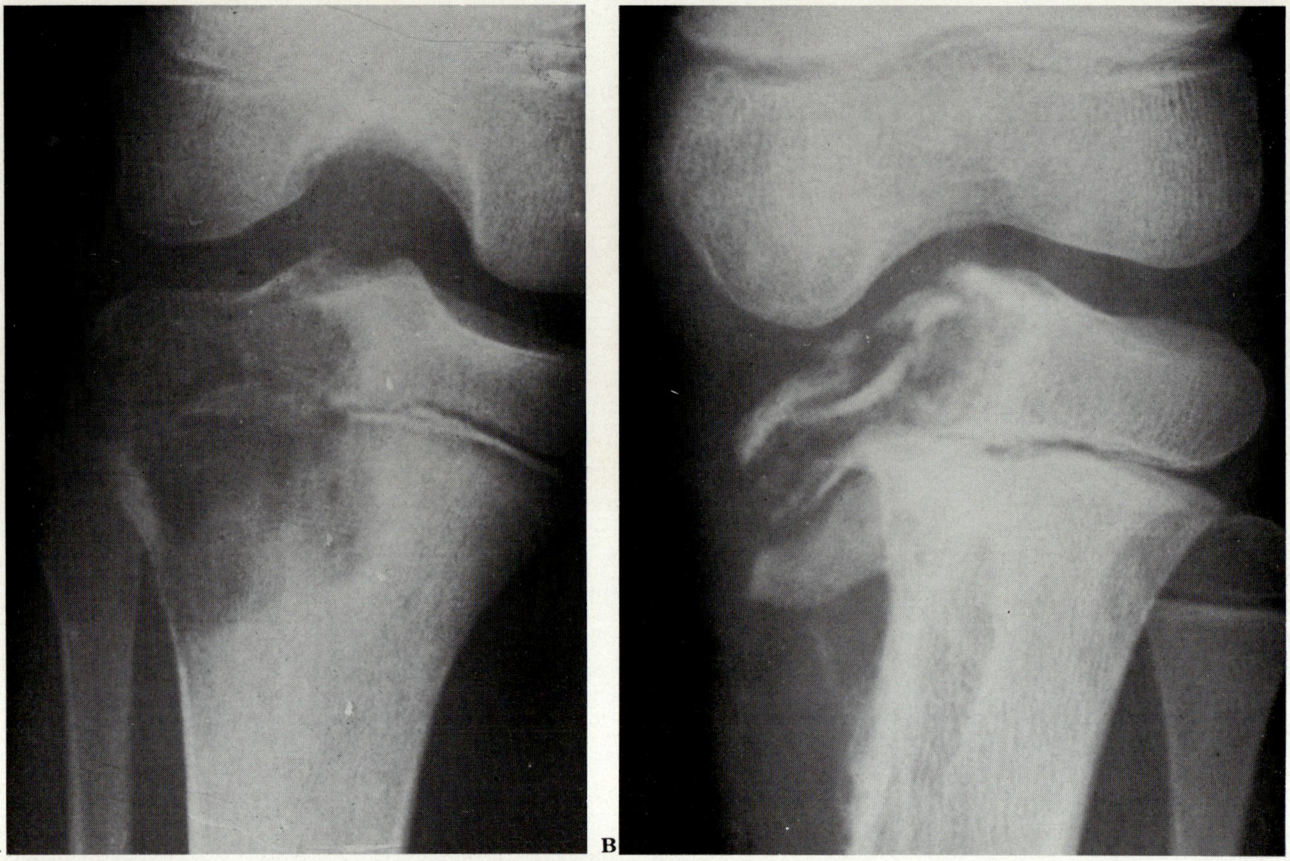

A B

Fig. 2.50 Fungal granulomata crossing growth cartilage. **A.** Lesion due to C. neoformans. **B.** Lesion due to H. duboisii.

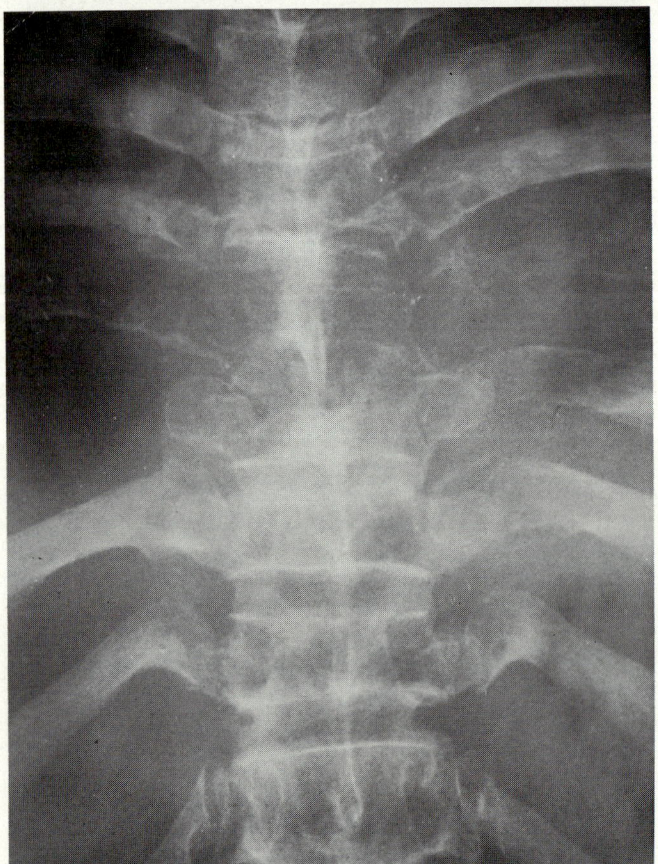

Fig. 2.51 Extensive H. duboisii multilevel vertebral bone destruction with paravertebral abscesses. Unlike tuberculosis most disc spaces are preserved despite diffuse vertebral body granulomata.

where the original process started. Subcutaneous granulomata are readily demonstrated because of their contrasting density with fat (Fig. 1.18). Ribs can be involved by extension from a spinal or paravertebral granuloma. This gives rise to erosive lesions and perhaps upward displacement of the neck of a rib due to disturbance of the ligaments and the pull of the intercostal muscles. This sequence of change also occurs in tuberculosis.

Vertebrae are frequently involved and unfortunately, if not recognised, a focus can rapidly progress to cause extradural compression and paraplegia. The destructive lesions in a vertebral body show early collapse and angulation. Paravertebral abscess or masses may be seen. Pedicle destruction, even as an isolated process, is not rare. Generally the sparing of the intervertebral disc space is in contrast to the collapsing destroyed vertebral bodies (Fig. 2.51). Sometimes in B. dermatitidis infections the disc spaces may be destroyed. Sclerotic vertebral bodies have been reported in coccidioidomycosis (Eller & Siebert, 1969).

It can be seen that any bone, including sesamoids, may be involved. The differential diagnosis is considerable and it is impossible to cover all eventualities. Suffice to say that histiocytosis X and tuberculosis are the most important differential conditions to consider. The former for long bones and flat bones and the latter for the spine and small bones such as the tarsus (Figs. 2.52–2.54).

Since the radiological manifestations are so similar in all these entities, one can only make an intelligent guess as to which specific etiological agent is responsible if there are epidemiological and geographical aids. Histology and microbiology provide specific identification, but unless an

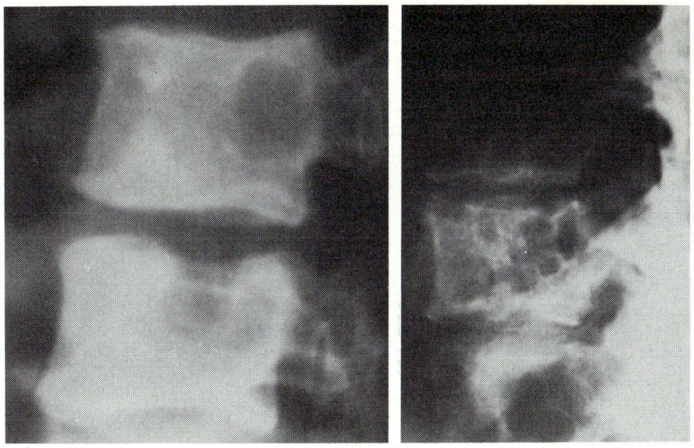

A B

Fig. 2.52 A, B. Coccidioidal vertebral granulomata. Note the maintenance of disc spacing. (Courtesy of Dr. Jack Campbell, Los Angeles.)

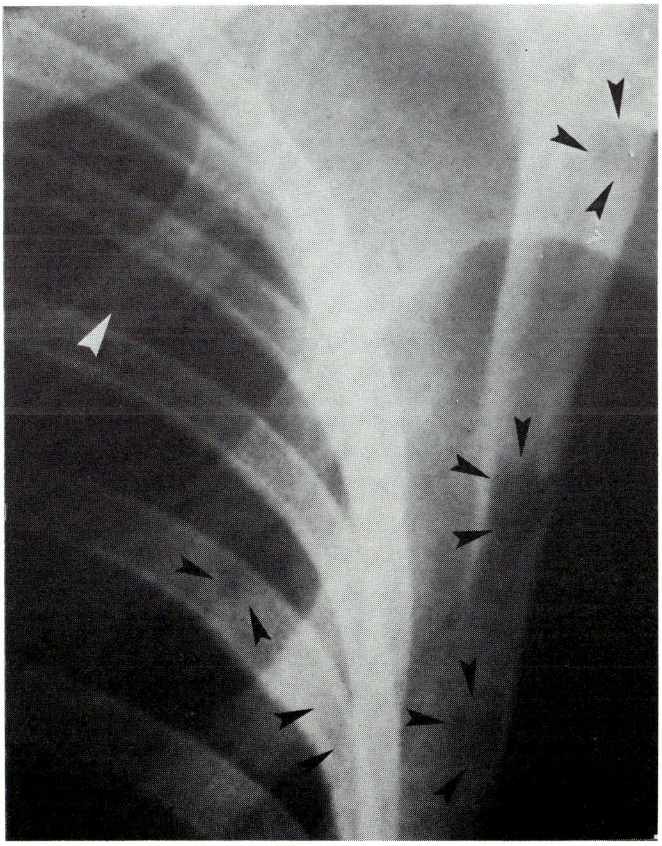

Fig. 2.53 Scapula of Brazilian showing lytic granulomatous defects due to South American blastomycosis in ribs and scapula.

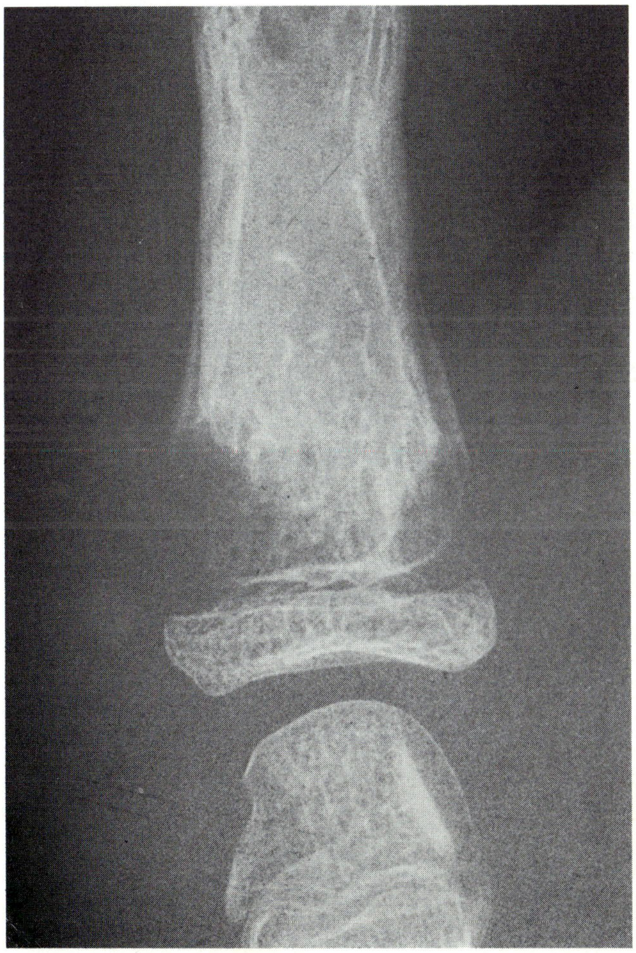

Fig. 2.54 Juxtametaphyseal granulomata in 14-year-old with H. duboisii infection.

informed eye suggests from the radiograph a possible fungal etiology the appropriate culture methods and stains may not be sought.

Radiological features can be modified by unusual modes of infection such as synovial disease in coccidioidomycosis and direct implantation by thorns or cacti. Obviously the latter type of patient is not likely to show an abnormal lung radiograph, though this is frequent in most of the other yeast infections except H. duboisii and C. neoformans.

REFERENCES

Ajello, L. (1968) In *Systemic Mycoses*, pp. 133. London: J. & A. Churchill.

Ajello, L., Kuttin, E. S., Beemer, A. M., Kaplan, W. & Padhye, A. (1977) Occurence of Histoplasma capsulatum Darling, 1906 in Israel, with a review of the current status of histoplasmosis in the Middle East, *American Journal of Tropical Medicine and Hygiene*, **26**, 140–147.

Allen, J. H. (1959) Bone involvement with disseminated histoplasmosis, *American Journal of Roentgenology*, **82**, 250–254.

Chleboun, J. & Nade, S. (1977) Skeletal cryptococcosis, *Journal of Bone and Joint Surgery*, **59A**, 509–514.

Cockshott, W. P. & Lucas, A. V. (1964a) Histoplasmosis duboisii, *Quarterly Journal of Medicine*, **33**, 223–238.

Cockshott, W. P. & Lucas, A. V. (1964b) Radiological findings in histoplasma duboisii infections, *British Journal of Radiology*, **37**, 653–660.

Cowen, N. (1969) Cryptococcosis of bone, *Clinical Orthopaedics*, **66**, 174–182.

Dalinka, M. K., Dinnenberg, S., Greendyke, W. H. & Hopkins, R. (1971) Roentgenographic features of osseous coccidioidomycosis and differential diagnosis, *Journal of Bone and Joint Surgery*, **53A**, 1157–1164.

Eller, J. L. & Siebert, P. E. (1969) Sclerotic vertebral bodies: an unusual manifestation of disseminated coccidioidomycosis, *Radiology*, **93**, 1099–1100.

*Gehweiler, J. A., Capp, M. P. & Chick, E. W. (1970) Observations on the roentgen patterns in blastomycosis of bone, *American Journal of Roentgenology*, **108**, 497–510.

Gosling, H. R. & Gilmen, W. (1956) Skeletal cryptococcosis, *Journal of Bone and Joint Surgery*, **38A**, 660–668.

Grebe, A. A. (1954) Monostotic coccidioidal infection, *Journal of Bone and Joint Surgery*, **36A**, 859–862.

Iger, M. & Larson, J. (1967) Coccidioidal osteomyelitis. In *Coccidioidomycosis*. Ed. Ajello, L. pp. 89–90. U.S.A.: University of Arizona Press.

Pollock, S. F., Morris, J. M. & Murray, W. R. (1967) Coccidioidal synovitis of the knee, *Journal of Bone and Joint Surgery*, **49A**, 1397–1407.

Rippon, J. W. (1974) In *Medical Mycology*, pp. 396. Philadelphia: W. B. Saunders & Co.

MYCETOMA

Mycetoma is a chronic granulomatous process due to the implantation of various fungi and actinomycetes into tissues with the development of grains in tissues and the formation of sinuses. The condition has been frequently referred to as Madura foot, which is an inappropriate term emphasising an exclusive geographic and anatomical location.

The condition can occur virtually anywhere on the body surface and occurs in most tropical countries but is rare in the temperate world.

Mycetoma is a clinical entity due to a very wide variety of organisms which are generally divided into the actinomycetes and the maduromycetes. The former are gram positive filamentous bacteria and the latter septate hyphal organisms with well-defined cell walls. There are numerous genera that have been implicated, often the same species receiving different names over the years, but all the organisms form grains in tissues. Grains are aggregates of organisms gathered together as discrete colonies that are large enough to be readily visible to the naked eye. The grains may be pigmented brown, black, yellow, or red, and each species possesses characteristic morphology on histologic study. Determination of the responsible

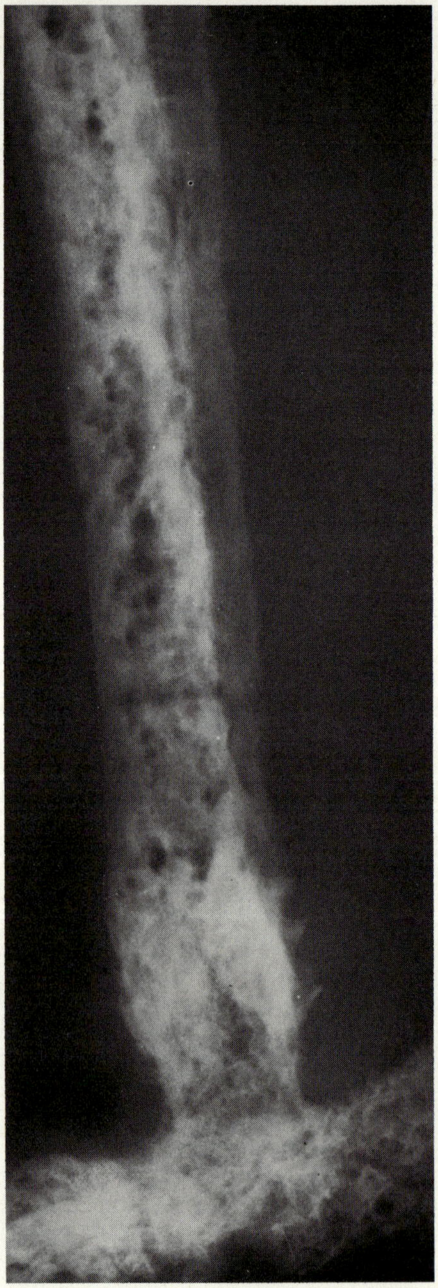

Fig. 2.55 Nocardial mycetoma in a Bedouin. The multiple microabscesses are typical.

organism is of value in assessing both prognosis and in the selection of the appropriate, if any, chemotherapeutic agents. Serological diagnosis has some differentiating capabilities but is not highly specific due to cross reactivity (Mahgoub & Murray, 1973).

It is unlikely that all possible etiological agents have yet been identified; doubt exists on the pathogenicity of some isolates; and other isolates appear under a variety of synonyms so that a comprehensive listing of all micro-organisms responsible for mycetoma is a formidable taxonomic task. The table designates the important organisms and indicates whether they are bacterial or fungal. The term fungi imperfecta was applied to all the fungal agents in mycetoma, but is no longer appropriate since some are now identified in their perfect sexual forms.

The geographic distribution of the organisms is complicated to describe because of their variety. However, broadly speaking M. mycetomi, L. senegalensis and N. brasiliensis are frequent isolates in the hot, dry areas of Africa, the Middle East, India and Mexico. In addition S. somaliensis and S. pelletieri are common isolates in desert areas of the Sudan, Arabia and the Sahara. In the Sudan the prevalence of mycetoma is so high that it poses a substantial medical and socio-economic problem.

The initial implantation of the organism is thought often to be by a thorn or puncture wound, and thorns abound in many endemic areas. Mycetoma organisms have been isolated from thorns and, more particularly, the soil. Hence the common occurrence of the disorder in the foot in populations where many walk unshod.

The pathological behaviour following implantation is determined to varying extents by the initial location, the virulence of the infective agent, the duration of the process, and whether secondary infection is present.

The site of the initial lodgment in relation to tissue planes is of considerable importance, particularly with an organism such as M. mycetomi that tends to form local accumulations of grains. Thus a subcutaneous implant can cause a superficial nodule whereas a lesion with a well-defined tissue boundary (plantar fascia or thick skin or the heel) tends to remain for a long while in that tissue compartment. By contrast, at the other extreme, granulomata due to S. pelletieri rapidly transgress tissue planes to spread in an invasive fashion to adjacent structures, bone and lymph glands. If secondary infection from sinuses occurs this introduces additional factors that can alter the behaviour. The late stage of the disease results in similar features of a densely scarred swollen area with sinuses.

In radiographs the initial soft tissue lesions can be recognised in low kilovoltage films obtained with suitable orientation to show displacement or blurring of fat and fascial boundaries such as the plantar aponeurosis. In late cases the indurated scarred areas show a homogeneous appearance without evidence of normal anatomic structures.

Bone is usually invaded from without. In the Actinomy-

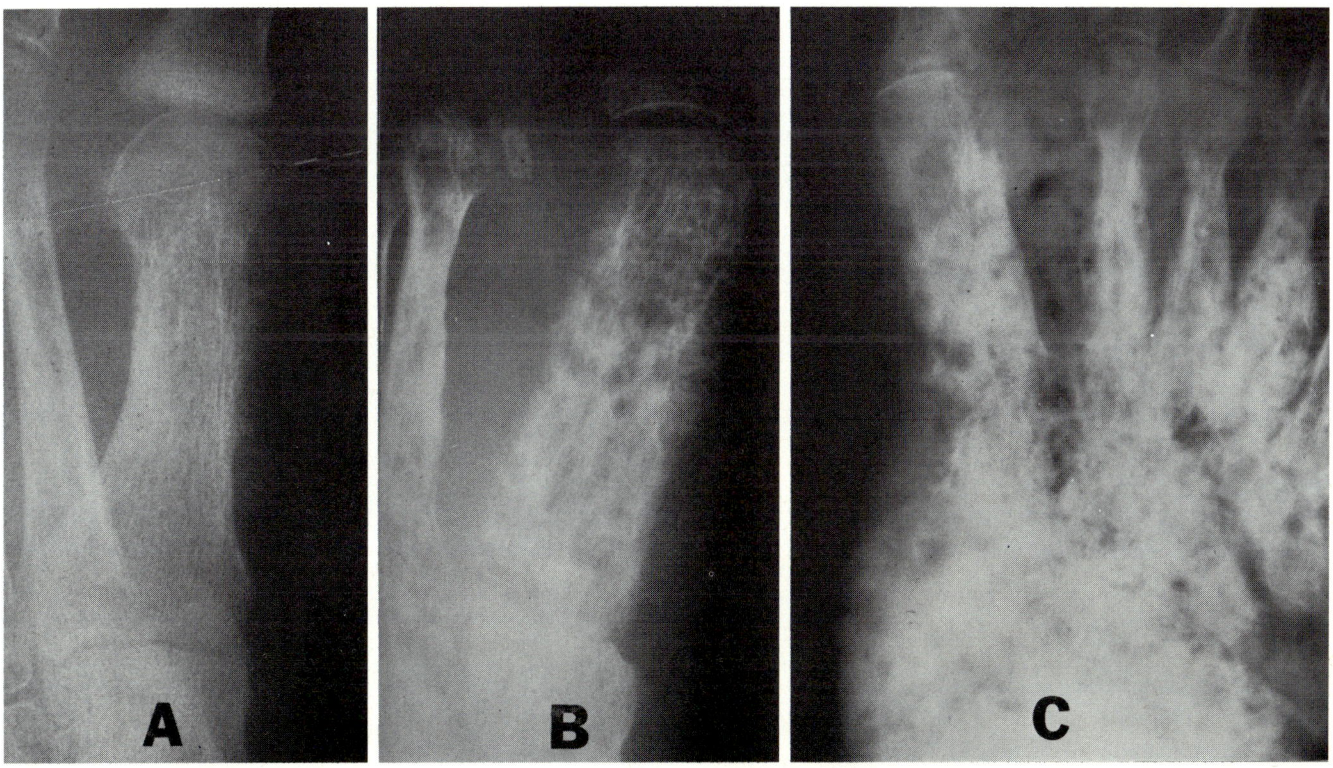

Fig. 2.56 Invasive Nocardia brasiliensis and Streptomyces mycetoma. The inflammatory process from these organisms do not respect tissue planes, articular cartilage or ligaments but extend by continuity in all directions.

cetes, some fungal infections and all secondarily infected mycetomata, the bones develop significant sclerosis. The bone density is partly periosteal accretion but in addition there is a pan osteitis leading to dense bone formation perhaps interspersed with small areas of bone destruction—micro-abscesses (Figs. 2.55 and 2.56). With S. pelletieri and S. madurae this feature is marked. In some instances there is an initial diffuse loss of bone with invasion across joint surfaces, which gives rise to what Davies (1958) has likened to a 'melting snow' appearance. This invasion across joints rapidly destroys cartilage and can result in bony ankylosis (Figs. 2.57 and 2.58). Eventually bone loss with attenuation of phalanges can be seen, which is suggestive of trophic disorders (Fig. 2.58).

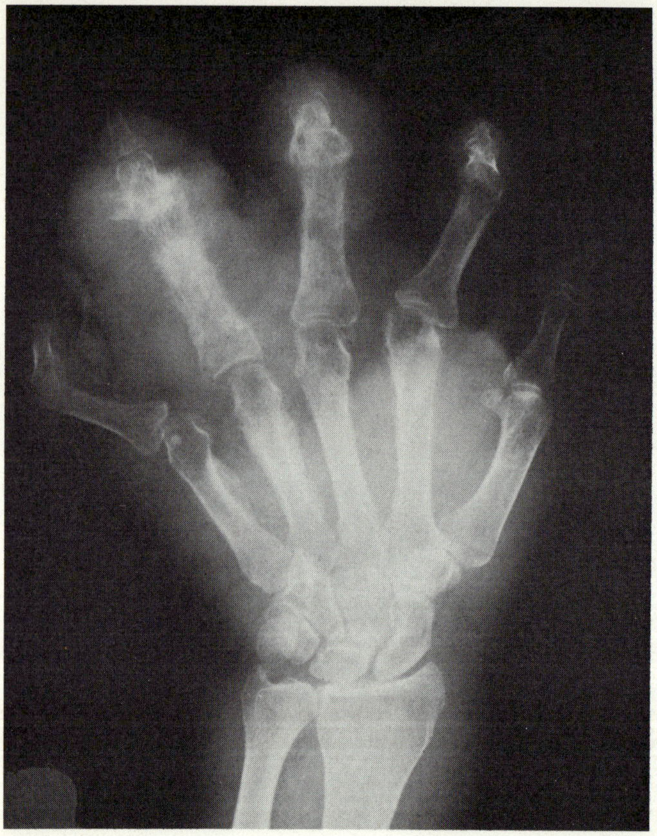

Fig. 2.57 Nocardial hand mycetoma with soft tissue involvement and early phases of bone disease before reactive sclerosis. Chemotherapy resulted in healing.

Bone can be invaded along the medullary canal once the endosteum has been breached. In M. mycetomi infections this leads to focal destructive areas of about 1 cm in diameter where there are the black grain accumulations that are characteristic of this organism (Fig. 2.59). Its tendency to remain localised is observed when the tibia or the calcaneus has a direct intra-osseous implant and a large expanding destructive zone develops which can be 10 cm or more in diameter. On incision it is found to be stuffed with grains (Grantham Hill, 1931; Abbott, 1956; Cockshott, 1956) (Fig. 2.60).

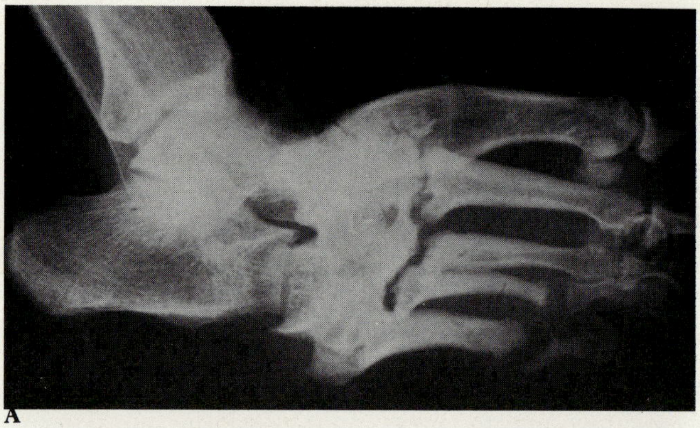

A

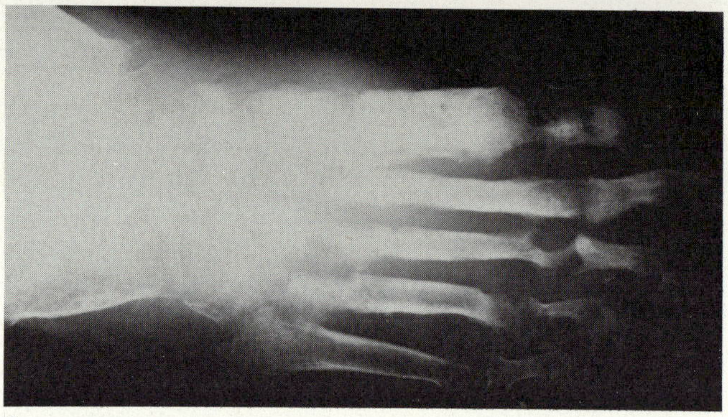

B

Fig. 2.58 **A, B.** Late stages of mycetoma with sclerosis, bony ankyloses, and distal metatarsal and phalangeal alterations simulating trophic changes.

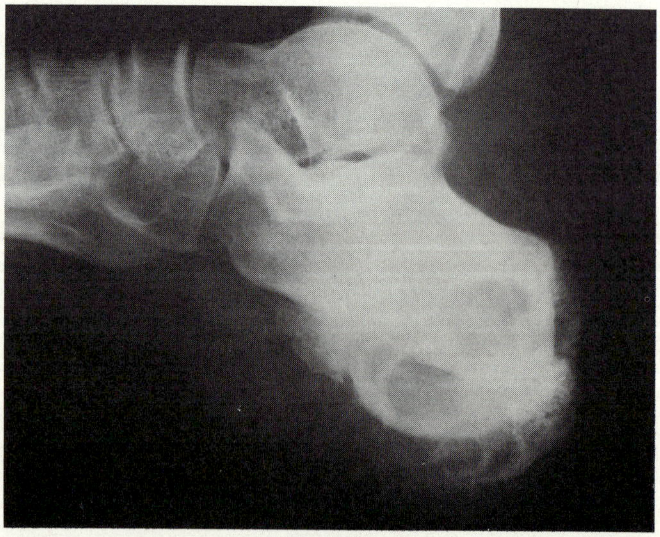

Fig. 2.59 Mycetoma. Typical geodes due to accumulation of large black grains of Madurella mycetomi. The os calcis is expanded and peri-osteal new bone extends from posterior and plantar surfaces.

Now that some organisms are susceptible to chemotherapy (Cockshott & Rankin, 1960; Mahgoub & Murray, 1973), radiology has a role in monitoring the healing process. Periosteal new bone and sclerotic reaction resolves with time in N. brasiliensis infections.

Table 2.1 Organisms of mycetoma

	Grain colour	*Invasiveness*	*Relative frequency*
Fungi			
Madurella mycetomi	Black	+	+++
Madurella grisea	Brown		
Leptosphaeria senegalensis	Black	+	++
Pyrenochaeta romeroi	Brown		
Phialaphora jeanselmei	Black		
Allescheria boydii	White	+	+
Cephalosporium species	White/yellow		
Actinomycetes			
Nocardia brasiliensis	White/yellow	++	+++
Streptomyces madurae	Yellow	+	++
Streptomyces somaliensis	Yellow	++	+
Streptomyces pelletieri	Red	+++	

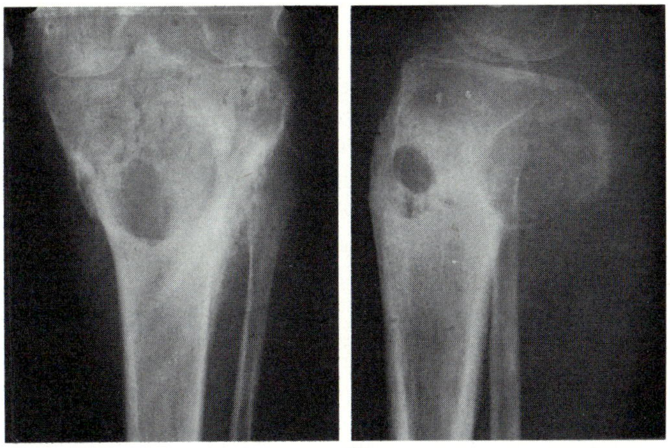

A B

Fig. 2.60 A, B. Madurella mycetomi expansile lesions in upper tibia of a Yemeni.

REFERENCES

Abbott, P. H. (1956) Mycetoma in the Sudan, *Transactions of the Royal Society of Tropical Medicine and Hygiene*, **50,** 11–24.

Cockshott, W. P. & Rankin, A. M. (1960) Medical treatment of Mycetoma, *Lancet*, **2,** 1112–1114.

Cockshott, W. P. (1956) *Mycetoma.* M.D. Thesis Edinburgh University.

Davies, A. G. M. (1958) Bone changes of Madura foot. Observations on Ugandan Africans, *Radiology,* **70,** 841–847.

Grantham-Hill, C. (1931) Some clinical observations on mycetoma, *Transactions of the Royal Society of Tropical Medicine and Hygiene*, **25,** 39–48.

Mahgoub, El S. & Murray, I. G. (1973) *Mycetoma.* London: William Heinemann.

Mahgoub, El S. (1977) Mycoses of the Sudan, *Transactions of the Royal Society of Tropical Medicine and Hygiene*, **71,** 184–188.

SPOROTRICHOSIS

Sporotrichosis is a worldwide, but uncommon, cutaneous and subcutaneous infection due to Sporotrichum schenckii. The fungus is a ubiquitous saprophyte that has been isolated from vegetation and timber. The usual portal of entry is through an abrasion or puncture wound, usually of the dominant upper limb. Agricultural workers, florists and miners are frequent occupations of affected persons. In the Rand goldfields infection once reached epidemic proportions from infected pit props. In Guadalajara, Mexico, sporotrichosis is the most frequent mycosis (Mariat, 1968).

The initial lesion is a small abscess or granulomatous nodule which may later ulcerate. Extension along the course of thickened lymphatics with the formation of satellite nodules is characteristic. The disease does not usually progress beyond this stage and since iodide therapy is effective further clinical forms are rare. However, the process can extend and affect bone directly from a cutaneous ulcer where bone is superficial, or theoretically, bone may be involved by metastatic extension. A case of Dr. Lurie in South Africa caused extensive calvarial destruction but the lesion may have been a direct inoculation rather than metastatic (Fig. 2.61).

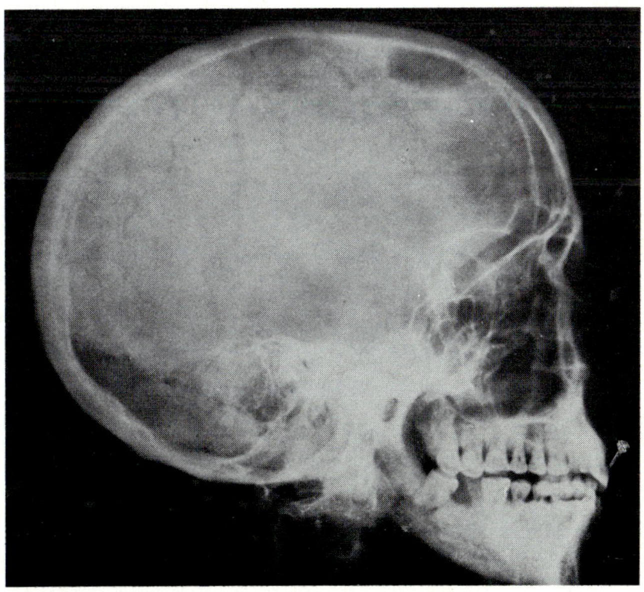

Fig. 2.61 Skull with a lucent defect due to a sporotrichosis granuloma. (Courtesy of Dr. Lurie, S. Africa.)

Involvement of the knee joint in the absence of a primary lesion elsewhere may indicate direct inoculation of S. schenckii into the joint (Webster & Willander, 1957; Rhangos & Chick, 1964).

Radiologically osteoporosis and non-specific cartilage destruction producing joint space narrowing is seen.

REFERENCES

Mariat, F. (1968) Sporotrichosis and its epidemiology. In *Systemic Mycoses*, pp. 150. London: J. & A. Churchill.

Rhangos, W. C. & Chick, E. W. (1964) Mycotic infections of bone, *Southern Medical Journal*, 57, 664–674.

Webster, F. S. & Willander, D. (1957) Chronic sporotrichal synovitis of the knee, *Journal of Bone and Joint Surgery*, **39A**, 207–215.

ASPERGILLUS BONE INFECTIONS

Aspergillus species involve bone in two clinical forms: an aspergillus paranasal sinuses granuloma seen predominantly in the Sudan; and a rare but ubiquitous type, often involving vertebrae, which has a probable respiratory portal of entry. These two clinical forms occur in healthy individuals and are not opportunist infections. Such infections occasionally are also seen in compromised hosts.

Aspergilloma infections of paranasal sinuses

In otherwise healthy individuals aspergilloma infection of the paranasal sinuses has been reported from many parts of the world as single case presentations, but reports from Khartoum indicate that there it is of frequent occurrence (Miloshev *et al.*, 1966; Green *et al.*, 1969; Veress *et al.*, 1973; Rudwan & Sheikh, 1976; Mahgoub, 1977). The patients, usually adult males, came from hot, dry, dusty desert conditions. The organism responsible, A. flavus, is a common saprophyte that has locally been cultured from the soil and thatch (Mahgoub, 1971; Veress *et al.*, 1973). It has also been recovered from nasal secretions of those without disease. Perhaps the dry sandy soil provides environmental conditions that encourages nasal encrustations and predispose to the development of invasion by a normal commensal.

The granuloma behaves aggressively and by spread from the maxillary antra or the ethmoid cells causes proptosis after breaking through into the orbital cavity. In the Sudan the granuloma is the most common cause of unilateral proptosis. Because of the initial clinical behaviour and radiographic evidence of bone destruction these patients can readily be mistaken as cases with malignant disease. Fortunately surgical excision of the firm rubbery granuloma results in cure (Martinson *et al.*, 1970). Diagnosis is established by histological and cultural study of surgical material.

Madurella mycetomi has been recorded as invading the paranasal sinuses with a fatal outcome (Muyunga-Kasengulu *et al.*, 1971).

Aspergillus osteomyelitis

Aspergillus osteomyelitis is generally secondary to dissemination in individuals with compromised immune mechanisms, but has been known to develop in fit indivi-

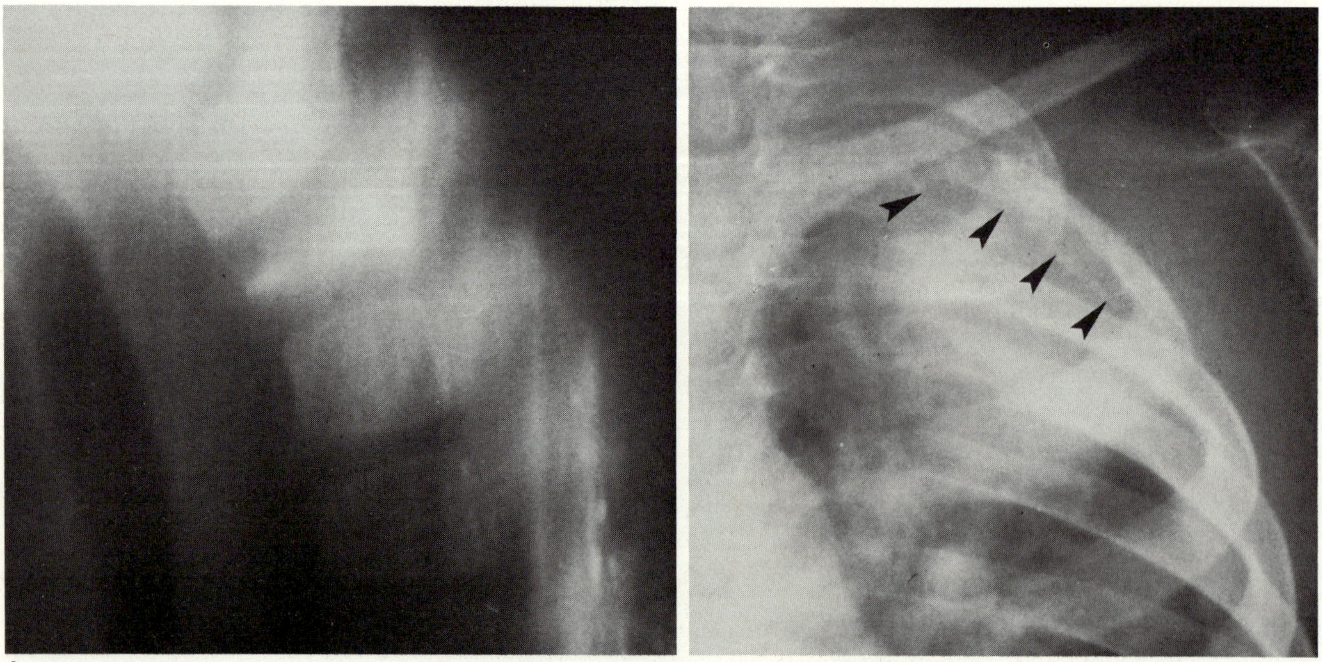

A B

Fig. 2.62 A, B. Examples of aspergillar osteitis. Collapse of vertebral body with little disc implication and lytic destruction of second rub with expanded periosteal shell shown by black arrows.

duals. There may be evidence of a previous lung infection and the vertebrae are the most common bones to be involved (Seres *et al.*, 1972; Grossman, 1975). This was certainly so in our two cases, both of whom had previous lung infiltrates of undetermined origin. However, dissemination to vertebrae from aspergillus osteomyelitis of a finger due to a foreign body has, among several reports of metastatic bone lesions, also been reported (Shaw & Warthen, 1936).

Aspergillus in bone causes a granuloma that spreads by destructive continuity. When it reaches ribs from the spine it may extend and expand the rib. In the vertebrae the lesions lead to collapse and wedging, but usually the disc space is preserved (Fig. 2.62). Because of extension of the granuloma around ribs large extrapleural opacities may form. Nerve complications such as Horner's syndrome and cord compression have been reported.

REFERENCES

Green, W. R., Font, R. L. & Zimmerman, L. E. (1969) Aspergillosis of the orbit, *Archives of Opthalmology*, **82**, 302–313.

*Grossman, M. (1975) Aspergilloma of bone, *British Journal of Radiology*, **48**, 57–59.

Mahgoub, El S. (1971) Mycological and serological studies on aspergillus flavus isolated from paranasal aspergilloma in Sudan, *Journal of Tropical Medicine and Hygiene*, **74**, 162–165.

Mahgoub, El S. (1977) Mycoses of the Sudan, *Transactions of the Royal Society of Tropical Medicine and Hygiene*, **71**, 184–188.

Martinson, F. D., Alli, A. F. & Clark, B. M. (1970) Aspergilloma of the ethmoid, *Journal of Laryngology and Otology*, **84**, 857–861.

Miloshev, B., Davidson, C. M., Gentles, J. C. & Sandison, A. T. (1966) Aspergilloma of paranasal sinuses and orbit in Northern Sudanese, *Lancet*, **1**, 746–747.

Muyunga-Kasengulu, C., Bastin, J. P., Gatti, F. & Vanbreuseghem, R. (1971) Invasion of paranasal sinuses by Madurella mycetomi in a Congolese child, *Annales de la Société Belge de Medécine Tropicale*, **51**, 247–254.

Rudwan, M. A. & Sheikh, H. A. (1976) Aspergilloma of paranasal sinuses: a common cause of unilateral proptosis in the Sudan, *Clinical Radiology*, **27**, 497–502.

Seres, J. L., Ono, H. & Benner, E. J. (1972) Aspergillosis presenting as spinal cord compression, *Journal of Neurosurgery*, **36, 221–224.**

*Veress, B., Malik, O. A., El Tayeb, A. A., El Daoud, S., Mahgoub, El S. & El Hassan, A. M. (1973) Further observations on the primary paranasal aspergillus granuloma in the Sudan: a morphological study of 46 cases, *American Journal of Tropical Medicine and Hygiene*, **22**, 765–772.

RHINOPHYCOMYCOSIS RHINO-ENTOMOPHTHOROMYCOSIS

Acute phycomycotic infections of the paranasal sinuses in sick individuals, particularly diabetics, have been known for many years. In the last two decades a chronic phycomycosis due to *Entomophthora coronata* developing in otherwise healthy individuals has been widely recognised throughout the tropics. In Africa cases are recorded from Nigeria, Cameroun, Zaire, Ghana, Senegal, Tchad, Ivory Coast, Kenya and Uganda; in Asia, Iran, India and Burma; Indonesia and New Guinea; and in the New World in Brazil, Colombia, Cayman Islands, Puerto Rico and the United States. The organism has been isolated in Texas, where it causes nasal granulomata in horses; and in Kenya in a wild chimpanzee (Roy & Cameron, 1972). In nature the organism can be found parasitising insects and associated with decaying vegetation (Clark, 1968).

The term rhinophycomycosis was used by Martinson (1963) in Nigeria to differentiate the entity from subcutaneous phycomycosis. Clinically it behaved differently and later, when Clark showed that E. coronata and not Basidiobolus meristoporus was responsible, the separation of the two phycomycoses was vindicated.

The early lesion is in the nasal mucosa close to the anterior aspect of the inferior turbinate. Presumably it begins at the site of a traumatic implant. The granuloma from there extends by the line of least resistance to occlude unilaterally the nose and spreads submucosally to involve the paranasal sinuses. Then by extending through bony foraminae it can burrow deep to the facial muscles leading to facial deformities. Firm masses are fixed to the deeper tissues but the overlying skin remains mobile, in contrast to the findings in subcutaneous phycomycosis where the indurated mass is fixed to the skin. Most of those afflicted are adults with a male preponderance, once again differing from subcutaneous phycomycosis.

Clinically the superficial masses are obvious but radiological examination is helpful in showing the extent of sinus involvement. The sinuses are invariably implicated on the same side as the nasal obstruction. The ethmoid cells and maxillary antra are usually affected but the exact location is best shown by tomography (Fig. 2.63) (Cockshott, *et al.*, 1968). Bone destruction does not develop, which is a helpful differential sign from malignancy and from paranasal aspergillus granuloma. Extension to the retropharyngeal space can occur and the condition then presents radiologically as a soft tissue density intruding on the nasopharyngeal airway (Fig. 2.63).

Biopsy and culture confirms the diagnosis. The therapeutic response to iodide therapy and sulphamethoxazole with trimethoprin is effective (Martinson, 1971; Fromentin & Ravisse, 1977).

Rare infections by Drechslera hawaiiensis can produce a very similar clinical picture (Young *et al.*, 1978).

REFERENCES

Clark, B. M. (1968) Epidemiology of phycomycosis. In *Systemic Mycoses*, pp. 179–192. London: J. & A. Churchill Ltd.

Cockshott, W. P., Clark, B. M. & Martinson, F. D. (1968) Upper respiratory infection due to Entomophthora coronata, *Radiology*, **90**, 1016–1019.

Fromentin, H. & Ravisse, P. (1977) Les entomophthoromycoses tropicale, *Acta Tropica*, **34**, 375–394.

Martinson, F. D. (1963) Rhinophycomycosis, *Journal of Laryngology and Otology*, 77, 691–705.

Martinson, F. D. (1971) Chronic phycomycosis of the upper respiratory tract—Rhinophycomycosis entomophthorae, *American Journal of Tropical Medicine and Hygiene*, **20**, 449–455.

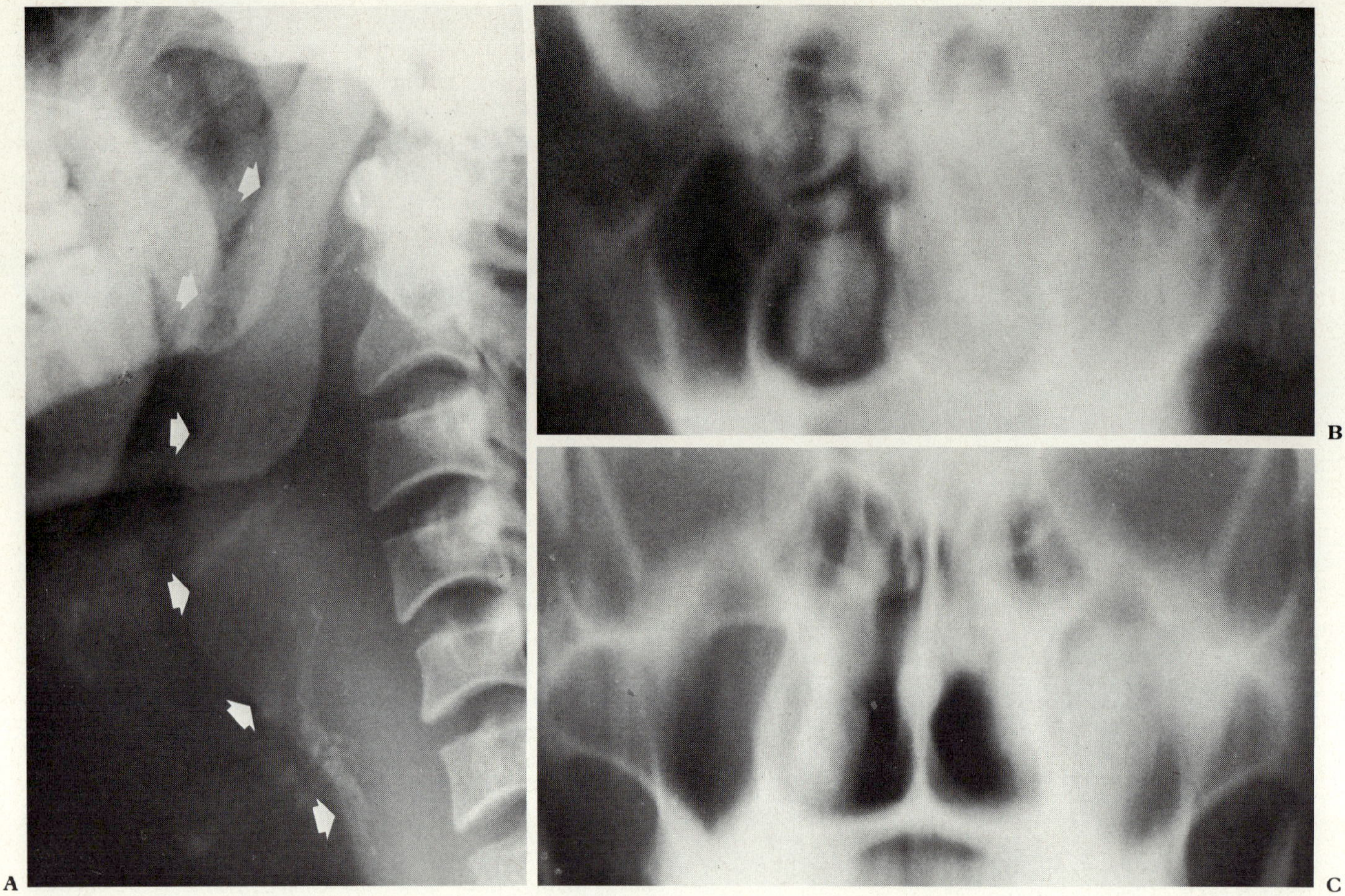

Fig. 2.63 **A.** Prevertebral soft tissue mass (arrowed) in a patient where the granuloma has extended. **B, C.** Tomogram of another patient shows soft tissue masses in sinuses and occluding the nasal airway unilaterally.

Roy, A. D. & Cameron, H. M. (1972) Rhinophycomycosis entomophthorae occurring in a chimpanzee in the wild in East Africa, *American Journal of Tropical Medicine and Hygiene*, **21**, 234–237.

Young, C. N., Swart, J. G., Ackerman, D. & Davidge-Pitts, K. (1978) Nasal obstruction and bone erosion caused by Drechslera hawaiiensis, *Journal of Laryngology and Otology*, **92**, 137–143.

RHINOSCLEROMA

Rhinoscleroma is a chronic ulcerating condition of the nasopharynx. It occurs in Eastern Europe, India, Indonesia, New Guinea, the West Indies, Central and South America, and has been recorded throughout Africa (Barten, 1956; Kouwenaar, 1956; Bhagwandeen, 1977).

The condition is due to a bacillus (Klebsiella rhinoscleromatis of von Frisch), which causes a spontaneous, painless, chronic growth of the nostrils and in the nasal cavity. This may ulcerate, causing destruction of the adjacent skin and mucous membrane. Whether ulcerating or not it extends to destroy the cartilage of the nasal septum, the uvula, and may involve the bone of the maxilla, the hard palate and the nasal septum. It sometimes progresses to affect the larynx and trachea. It may start in childhood or adult life, and many members of the same family are sometimes seen with the condition. It may pass into a quiescent phase only to become reactivated subsequently. There is usually involvement of the regional glands but the general health of the affected person is often unaffected while the disease is confined to the nasal cavity.

Radiologically there may be complete destruction of the nasal septum or local invasive destruction of the alveolar border of the maxilla by the granuloma (Fig. 2.64). In either case the destruction is total and there is no evident bone reaction. If the destruction is extensive and involves the hard palate as well as the nasal septum a 'gangosa-like' appearance may exist. Indeed, some cases of gangosa may be due to rhinoscleroma. Cases have also been confused with maxillary carcinoma.

REFERENCES

Barten, J. J. C. (1956) Scleroma respiratorium in Indonesia, particularly scleroma endemic in North Celebes, *Documenta de Medicina Geographica et Tropica*, **8**, 101–116.

Bhagwandeen, S. B. (1977) Klebsiella rhinoscleromatis, *Tropical and Geographical Medicine*, **29**, 288–290.

Khouwenaar, W. (1956) Rhinoscleroma, a review of present situation, *Documenta de Medicina Geographica et Tropica*, **8**, 13–22.

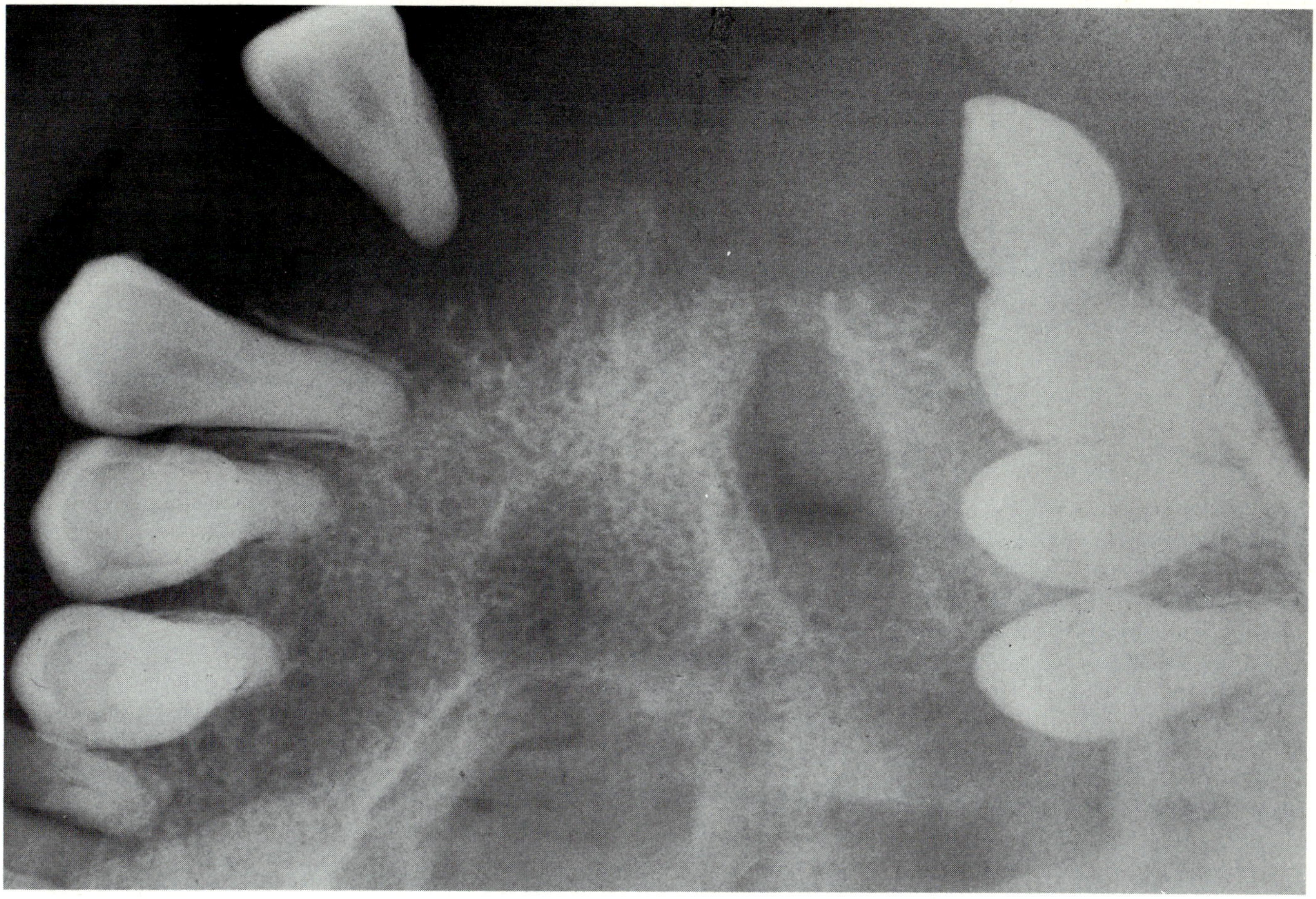

Fig. 2.64 Rhinoscleroma. Destruction of anterior maxillary alveolar ridge with loss and displacement of teeth by granuloma. (Courtesy of Dr. G. Davies, Kampala.)

VIRAL BONE INFECTIONS

Osteotropic viruses may infect bone *in utero* after transplacental passage as with rubella and cytomegalic viruses, or may be acquired after birth as with vaccinia, variola, encephalitis and other unidentified viruses.

The congenital forms are not discussed here, as the features in tropical environments do not differ from those recorded elsewhere (Merten & Gooding, 1970; Whalen *et al.*, 1974).

Without question our present knowledge of virus infections of bone is deficient. This is partly due to the lack of suspicion regarding the possibility of a virus etiology in bone, especially children and young persons, with arthralgia and unusual transient low-grade periosteal reactions occurring in clusters of cases. Viral study of such cases may be rewarding (Markowa, 1961, 1962).

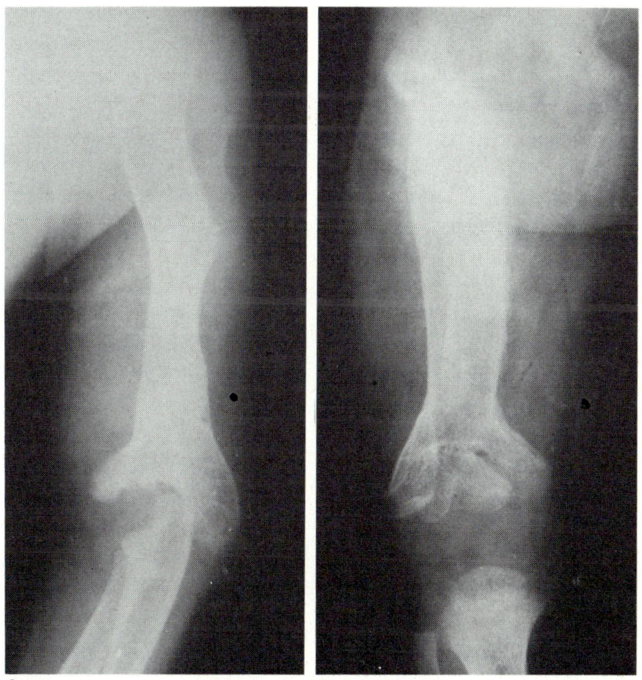

A B

Fig. 2.65 **A, B.** Left humerus and right femur of young child after vaccinial osteitis. The metaphysitis has resulted in considerable deformity of distal growth plates.

Vaccinial osteomyelitis

There have been over ten cases recognised of this entity (Elliott, 1959; Cockshott, 1965). The condition develops in young children within one to two weeks after vaccination. The onset is insidious with no systemic upset. Swelling and failure to use a joint is usually the earliest evidence that anything is amiss. Radiologically the lesions are initially destructive. The metaphysis is first affected, and this can lead to growth disturbances. Later the shaft of the affected bone thickens by apposition of new periosteal bone (Fig. 2.65). The bones of the upper limb are more often affected than those of the lower limb. The lesions can be symmetrical. If there is epiphyseal involvement this serves to differentiate the process from Caffey's disease (i.e. infantile cortical hyperostosis).

Osteomyelitis variolosa

Now that smallpox has been virtually eradicated this entity will fast become a historical curiosity. The condition develops in 2 to 5 per cent of children who have smallpox. The onset is insidious at the time the crusts of the exanthem are separating. The child develops, usually at the elbows or the feet, marked swelling and loss of function. The condition is often symmetrical (Cockshott & MacGregor, 1958, 1959). The virus usually involves bone close to the growth plate to cause a transverse metaphysitis associated with joint effusions (Fig. 2.66). The destructive process can result in displacement of epiphyseal centres or gross alteration in their growth potential so that bizarre deformities ensue (Figs. 2.67 and 2.68). Involvement is often patchy, especially in the dactylitis of the hands and feet. Marked periosteal reaction can follow along the shafts of bone. This can be exuberant even in the absence of any secondary pyogenic infection (Fig. 2.66). If the latter occurs fibrosis or bony ankylosis of the adjacent joint is not unusual, particularly at the elbows (Figs. 2.69 and 2.70).

Radiologically the importance of the condition is recognition of the aetiology of bone changes that may be seen in radiographs many years after the attack of smallpox. Joint deformities, often associated with bones, show-

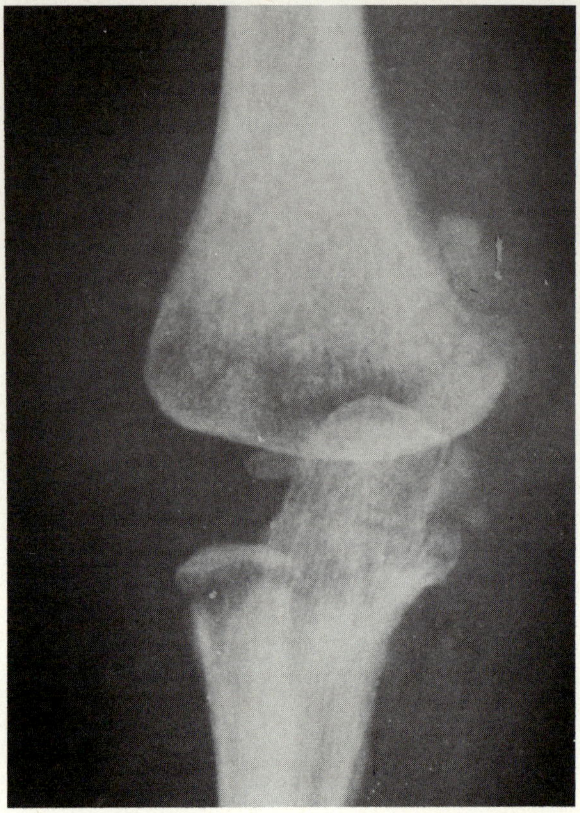

Fig. 2.66 Disorganised joint two and a half weeks after onset. Large effusion with disrupted articular relationships. Transverse metaphysitis can still be seen. Periosteal reaction present lower end of humerus. Case complicated by secondary infection.

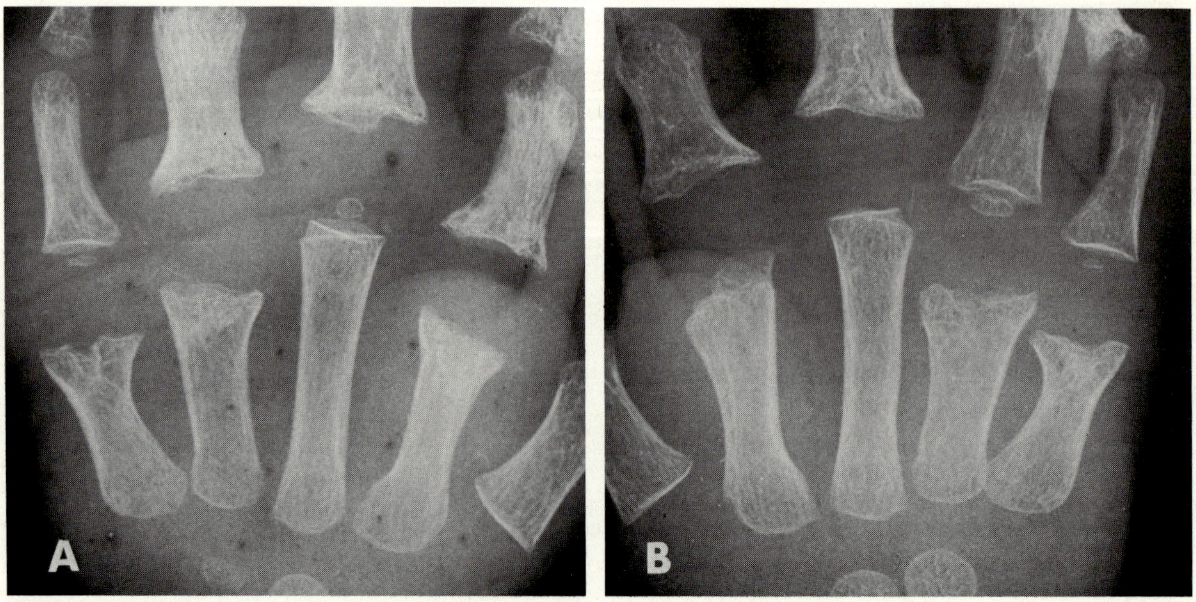

Fig. 2.67 Hands of child showing the result of smallpox metaphysitis. Involvement is almost symmetric. Considerable growth disturbance is already evident and some epiphyses have vanished. (Courtesy of *British Journal of Radiology*.)

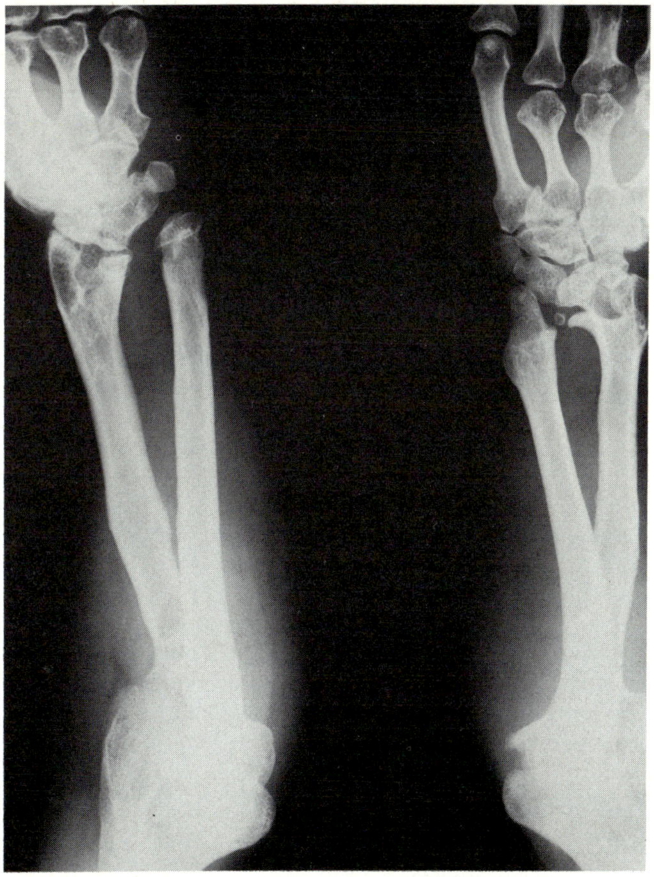

Fig. 2.68 Telescoped forearms and abbreviated metacarpals consequent on osteomyelitis variolosa.

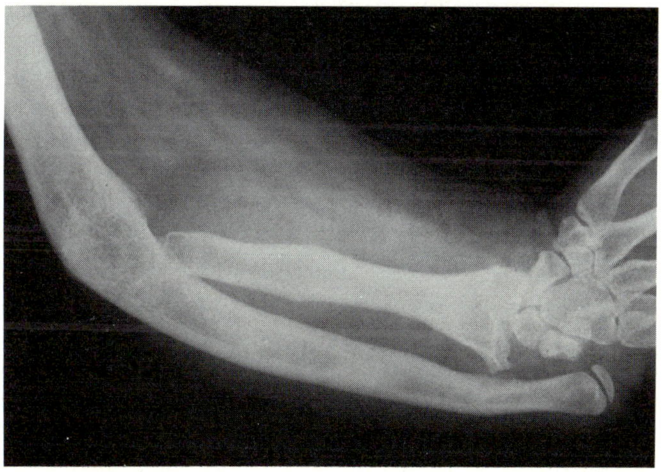

Fig. 2.69 Ankylosed elbow and shortened radius with dislocation of distal radio ulnar joint after childhood smallpox.

ing growth disturbances and absent epiphyses, around the elbows, hands or feet, should suggest the diagnosis.

REFERENCES

Cockshott, W. P. (1965) Osteomyelitis variolosa, *Tropenmedizin und Parasitologie*, **16,** 199–206.

Cockshott, W. P. & MacGregor, M. (1958) Osteomyelitis variolosa, *Quarterly Journal of Medicine*, **27,** 369–387.

Cockshott, W. P. & MacGregor, M. (1959). The natural history of osteomyelitis variolosa, *Journal of the Faculty of Radiologists*, **10,** 57–63.

Elliott, W. D. (1959) Vaccinial osteomyelitis, *Lancet*, **2,** 1053–1055.

Markowa, J. (1961) Acute osteitis of undetermined origin with neuro infection, *Journal of Bone and Joint Surgery*, **43B,** 95–99.

Markowa, J. (1962) Osteitis produced experimentally in mice by the virus of tick borne encephalitis, *Journal of Bone and Joint Surgery*, **44B,** 722–734.

Merten, D. F. & Gooding, C. A. (1970) Skeletal manifestations of congenital cytomegalic inclusion disease, *Radiology*, **95,** 333–334.

Whalen, J. P., Winchester, P., Krook, D. U. M., O'Donohue, N., Dische, R. & Nunez, E. (1974) Neonatal transplacental rubella syndrome, *American Journal of Roentgenology*, **121,** 166–172.

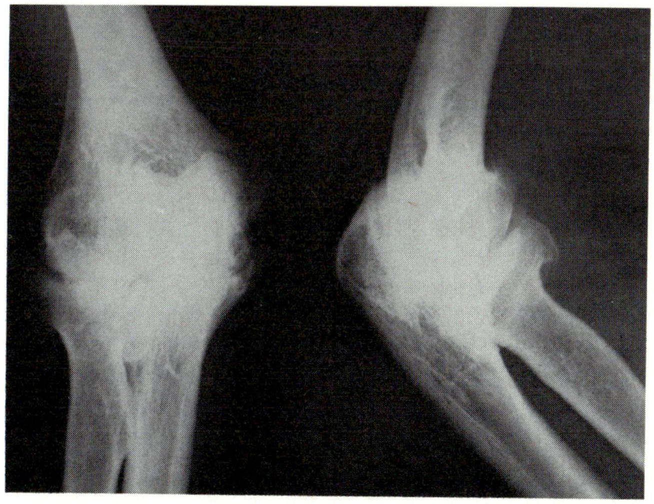

Fig. 2.70 Extensive arthritis following smallpox joint involvement in childhood.

PARASITIC BONE INFECTION

Apart from hydatid disease, bone infection by parasites are rare and are due to ectopic localisation. We have seen a sinus in relation to an eroded rib from which eggs of S. haematobium were recovered and at surgery worms were found in the marrow cavity of the rib (Fig. 2.71). However, apart from this bizarre example, a trematode abscess of the retro-auricular tissues with erosion of the mastoid has been noted with sufficient frequency to be worthy of mention.

Originally reported from eastern Nigeria by Yarwood and Elmes (1943) and later from the Congo (Vandepitte *et al.*, 1957) and in western Nigeria (Oyediran *et al.*, 1975), the condition has also been seen in Sarawak (Wong & Lie, 1965) and in China. There is doubt as to the nature of the worm, as only the eggs are usually recovered. The trematode eggs are operculated and could represent a paragonimus (possibly P. uterobilateralis or Poikilorchis congolensis). Detailed discussion of these possibilities is made in the excellent review by Oyediran *et al* (1975) and even more recently by Beaver *et al.* (1977), who suggest that Achillurbania species may be responsibile. In these infections there is a retro-auricular cyst that contains a clay-like material. The cyst implicates the mastoid directly and destroys bone. Sclerotic reaction may be slight or marked

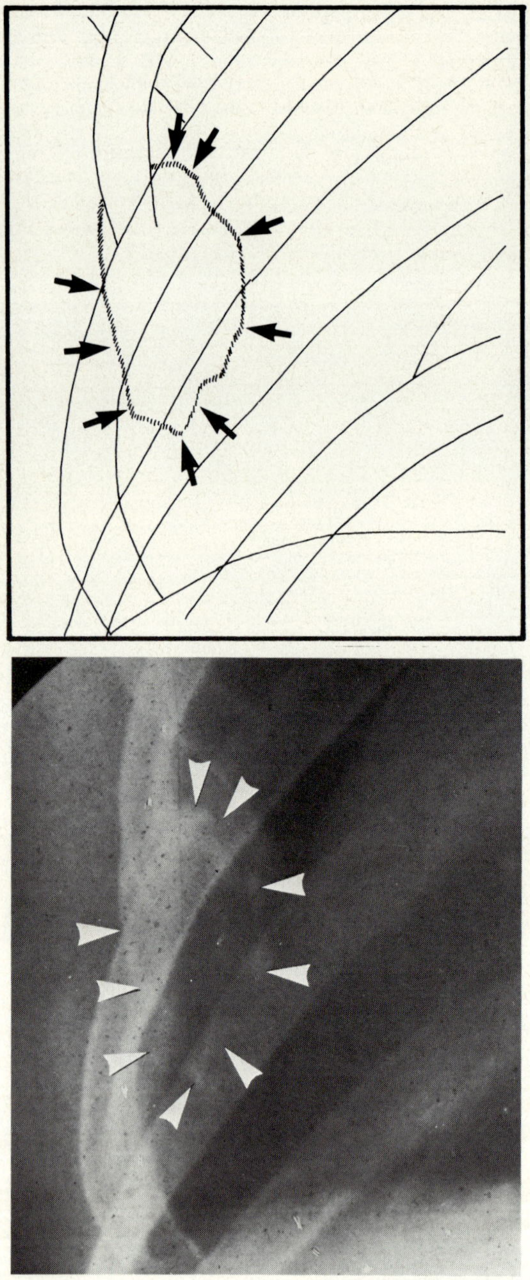

Fig. 2.71 Arrows indicate lytic lesion of anterior rib which has become expanded. This was the site of lodgment of aberrant schistosomes.

and can involve air cells and the petro-mastoid (Oyediran *et al.*, 1975). Examination of the excised tissues reveals granulation tissue and operculated eggs. Surgical therapy is successful.

In the Caribbean and Central America twelve cases of neck abscesses, which may involve the mastoids, have been reported due to Lagochilascaris minor. Eggs and worms can be identified in the pus of the lesions (Oostburg, 1971).

REFERENCES

Beaver, P. C., Duron, R. A. & Little, M. D. (1977) Trematode eggs in the peritoneal cavity of man in Honduras, *American Journal of Tropical Medicine and Hygiene*, **26**, 684–687.

Oostburg, B. J. F. (1971) Thiabenzole therapy of Lagochilascaris minor infection in Surinam, *American Journal of Tropical Medicine and Hygiene*, **20**, 580–583.

Oyediran, A. B. O. O., Fajemisin, A. A., Abioye, A. A., Lagundoye, S. B. & Olugbile, A. O. B. (1975) Infection of the mastoid bone with a paragonimus-like trematode, *American Journal of Tropical Medicine and Hygiene*, **24**, 268–273.

Vandepitte, J., Job, A., Delaisse, J. & Tabary, M. J. (1957) Quatre cas d'abscès rétro-auriculaires chez des Congolais, produit par un nouveau distome, *Annales de la Société Belge de Médecine Tropicale*, **37**, 309–316.

Wong, S. K. & Lie, K. J. (1965) Another peri-auricular abscess in a Dyak boy in Sarawak probably caused by a trematode of the genus Poikilorchis, *Medical Journal of Malaya*, **19**, 229–230.

Yarwood, G. R. & Elmes, B. G. T. (1943) Paragonimus cyst in a West African native, *Transactions of the Royal Society of Tropical Medicine and Hygiene*, **36**, 347–351.

HYDATID DISEASE OF BONE ECHINOCOCCOSIS

Hydatid disease of bone is uncommon, occurring in about 2 per cent of those with echinococcosis. The cysts reach bone by arterial dissemination, usually from larvae that have bypassed both the liver sinusoids and the pulmonary vascular bed and entered the systemic arterial circulation (for details of life history and epidemiology see liver section). There are two main species involved: E. granulosus and E. multilocularis. They differ in their life history, areas of endemicity and pathological response. E. multilocularis, or alveolar disease, often behaves as an invasive tumour with poorly defined limits. The ectocyst laminar layer is undeveloped, allowing permeative spread due to the unrestricted exogenous budding of small alveoli from the germinal layer.

E. granulosus cysts in bone do not have a well-developed outer host adventitial layer which is characteristic of cysts developing in viscera. The enlarging hydatids cause pressure atrophy of trabeculae and spread along the line of least resistance—usually extending along the medullary spaces of long bones. This feature of insinuating daughter cysts proliferating through the diaphysis because of the lack of a host restraining membrane leads to the production of an intra-osseous multilocular system, the components of which are much larger than those of E. multilocularis.

The cortex can be thinned from within but, when the periosteum is reached, a limiting reaction is excited that walls off the process. Consequently there may be endosteal bone absorption, internal scalloping, multilocular cyst formation and areas of expansion with periosteal new bone borders (Fig. 2.72) (Latham, 1953).

Fracture of the weakened bone often leads to the patient first presenting (Figs. 2.73 and 2.74). Usually a single bone is involved, though contiguous invasion of adjacent vertebral bodies or of a rib and a vertebral appendage may be seen.

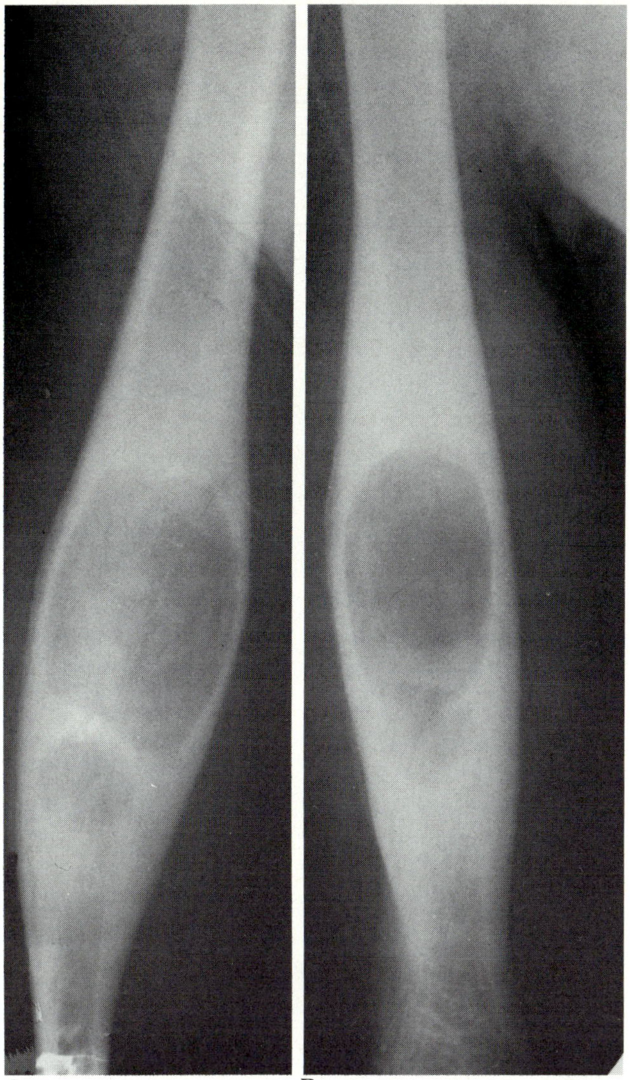

A B

Fig. 2.72 **A, B.** Hydatid cyst expanding humerus.

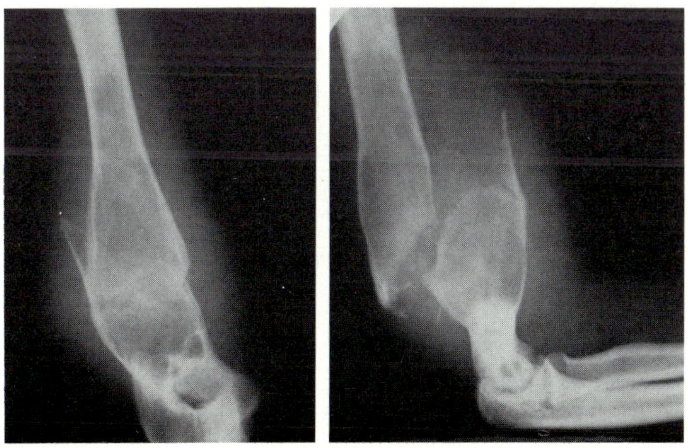

A B

Fig. 2.73 **A, B.** Pathological fracture of humerus through a hydatid cyst.

Over 40 per cent of cases involve vertebrae and nearly a quarter the pelvis. The remaining cases involve the femora, tibiae, humeri and skull in descending order of frequency (Jaffe, 1972).

The radiological appearances can be most suggestive and the possibility of this condition needs to be considered in endemic zones. The differential diagnosis is considerable, but since the condition is pleomorphic depending on the site involved there is no point in listing the various possibilities here. The Casoni and complement fixation tests may be helpful. A search should be made for possible cysts in other sites such as the liver or the lungs.

Though the disease progresses slowly its management poses a great challenge to surgical therapy since ablation is the only effective treatment.

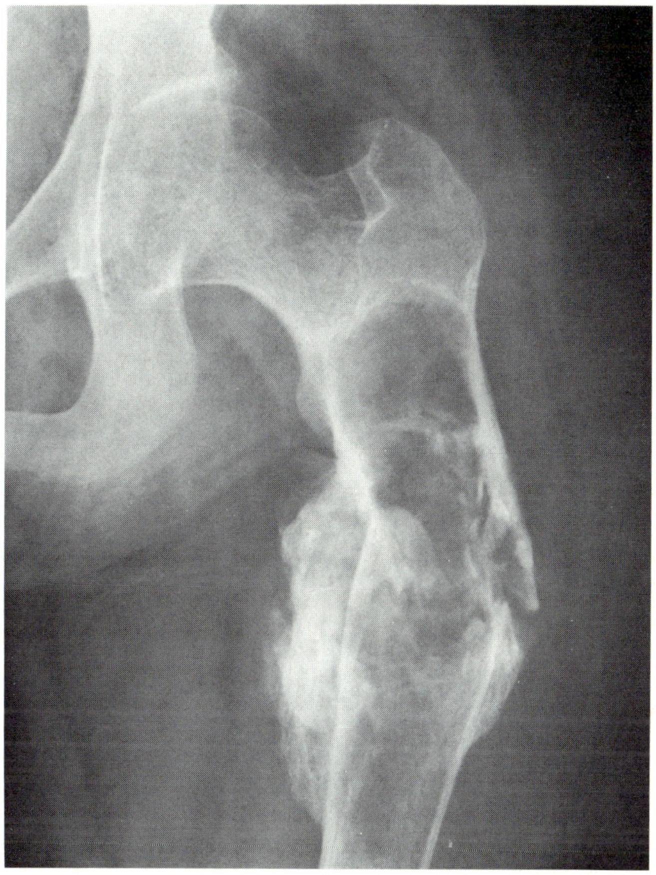

Fig. 2.74 Healing pathological fracture due to hydatid disease.

REFERENCES

Jaffe, H. L. (1972) *Metabolic Degenerative and Inflammatory Diseases of Bones and Joints*, p. 1073. Philadelphia: Lea & Feibiger.

Latham, W. J. (1953) Hydatid disease, *Journal of the Faculty of Radiologists*, **5**, 65.

TETANUS—FRACTURES

In many areas in the tropics tetanus still takes its toll. In some studies in Africa incidence has been as high as 100 cases per 100 000 births. Mortality diminished from 52 per

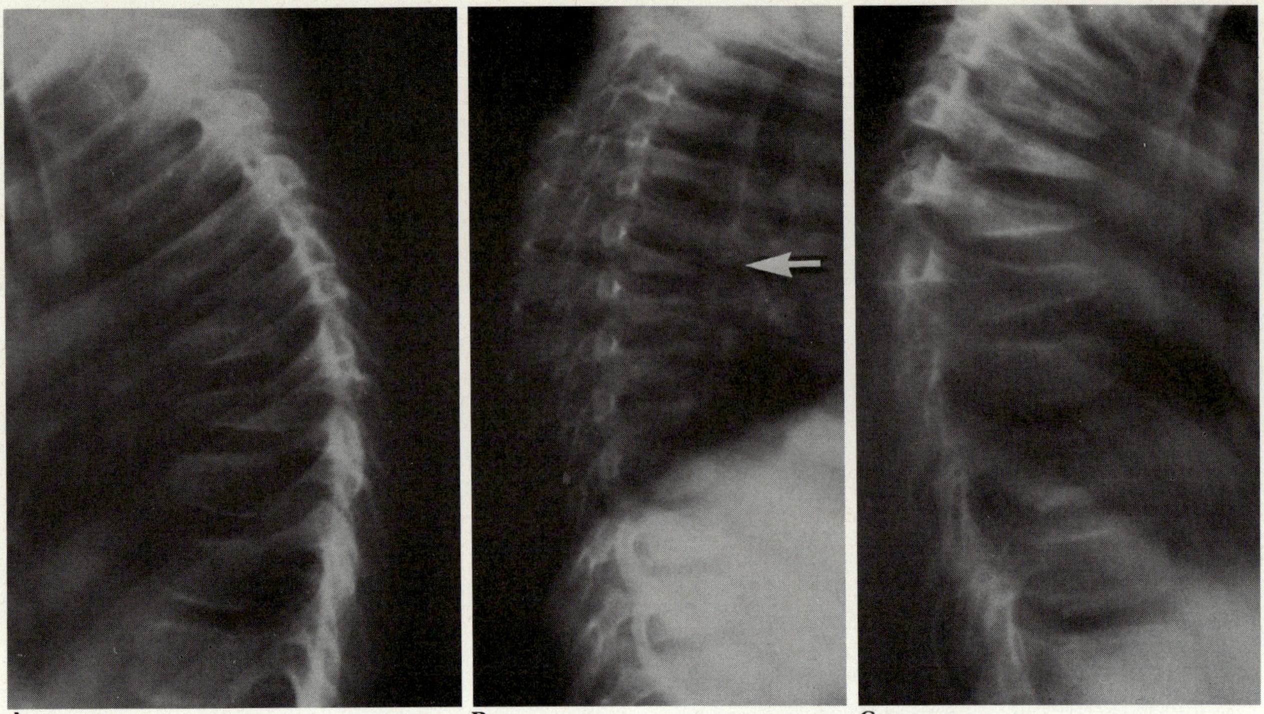

Fig. 2.75 **A, B, C.** Tetanus fractures. Three examples of the typical compression fractures of the upper dorsal spine.

100 000 in the 0 to 4 years of age group, to below 40 per 100 000 for the entire population (Bourgeade *et al.*, 1974; Kadio, 1974). In infancy the main portal of entry is probably the umbilical cord from contamination during the cutting or from later applications to the stump. Other aetiologies include intramuscular injections, foot and other wounds, delivery and abortion, and even circumcision and ear piercing. Adult infections are mainly from wounds sustained by agricultural workers.

Bone changes follow the combined results of increased muscle tone, trismus, and the spasmodic contractions that cause opisthotonus. These uncoordinated forces exert tremendous pressure on bone so that compression fractures of the vertebral bodies, and less often fractures of long bones, may occur. In addition para-articular subluxations and avulsions can lead to crippling myositis ossificans in about 1 per cent of survivors (Diop Mar & Sow, 1973).

The spinal fractures are most often seen in males, particularly in children and young muscular youths. Characteristically they involve the thoracic spine between D4 to D8 with the most severe deformities developing at D5–6 (Bohrer, 1965; Davis & Rowland, 1965). The vertebral bodies are primarily compressed and flattened, though slight anterior wedging and kyphosis may be manifest (Fig. 2.75).

The vertebral appendages stay intact. The disc spaces remain normal though some nuclear protrusion into the bodies may develop in 7- to 14-year-olds. The lesion does not generally affect the growth potential of the vertebral body, so that with time, correction of spinal deformity and shape may take place.

Bohrer has explained the paradox of how anterior compression fractures develop in the spine in a disease where the strongest forces are developed during the arching of the back in opisthotonus. In the segment of the thoracic spine involved, the posterior spinal extensor muscles are

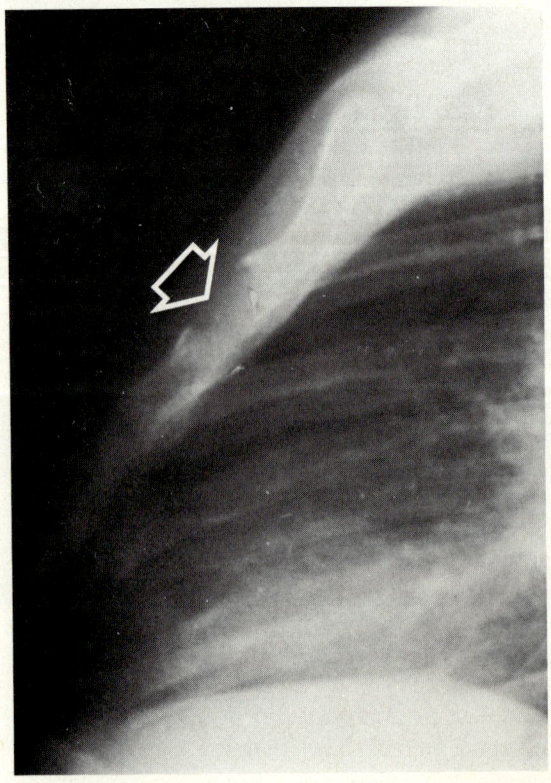

Fig. 2.76 Avulsion fracture of sternum in child due to tetanic spasm.

relatively weaker than their anterior antagonists, so that during simultaneous contractions and increased tone a compressive force is exerted on the thoracic vertebral bodies.

Transverse bowing or avulsion fractures of long bones and the sternum develop due to imbalance between antagonists (Fig. 2.76). We have also seen an avulsion fracture of the olecranon in a patient with tetanus.

REFERENCES

Bohrer, S. P. (1965) Spinal fractures in tetanus, *Radiology*, **85,** 1111–1116.

Bourgeade, A., Kadio, A. & Vincent, N. (1974) Tragedie: le tetanos aprés injection intra musculaire, *Annales de l'Université d'Abidjan*, **8,** 177–178.

Davis, P. R. & Rowland, H. A. K. (1965) Vertebral fractures in West Africans suffering from tetanus: a clinical and osteological study, *Journal of Bone and Joint Surgery*, **47B,** 61–71.

Diop Mar, I. & Sow, A. (1973) Les osteopathies para-articulaires du tetanos, *Abstracts Ninth International Congress of Tropical Medicine and Malariology, Athens*, 195.

Kadio, A. (1974) Contribution á l'étude epidémiologique du tetanos á Abidjan en Cote-d'Ivoire, *Annales de l'Univertié d'Abidjan*, **8,** 179.

AINHUM

Ainhum is an acquired self-limiting disorder usually affecting the fifth toe by a constricting fibrosing groove that leads to auto-amputation of the toe below the neck of the proximal phalanx.

The lesion is seen predominantly in those of the negro race, particularly West Africans, where the incidence may reach 2 per cent (Cole, 1965). It is less common in the Congo—0·25 per cent (Browne, 1965), and Bantu areas. In Brazil, particularly the Bahia area, Central America, the West Indies, and the United States, it is seen occasionally (Fetterman *et al.*, 1967). Isolated instances in those of non-African ancestry are recorded, as in India and Polynesia, but such an event is exceptional. The sex incidence is approximately equal and the condition is seen in all ages from five onwards, with the greatest frequency in the third decade. There is no obvious familial factor.

Ainhum is often bilateral and can progress to the fourth toes. Finger involvement is rare though recorded (Earle, 1944; Browne & McLoughlin, 1962).

The patient may complain of the appearance of a constricting band, but pain rather than the cosmetic blemish is the usual reason for seeking a medical opinion. Often the pain is attributable to infection or ulceration of the groove and band. Hyperkeratosis may be noted. Though many descriptions of the entity have been from leprologists there is no association between the two entities.

The radiological findings consist of evidence of the soft tissue groove at the level of the neck of the proximal phalanx of the fifth toe. Deep to this the bone gradually becomes thinner and becomes sclerotic, losing the normal trabecular pattern (Fig. 2.77). At this stage a fracture may develop or the process goes on to eventual further attenuation of the bone and auto-amputation. Evidence of bone infection is not a feature.

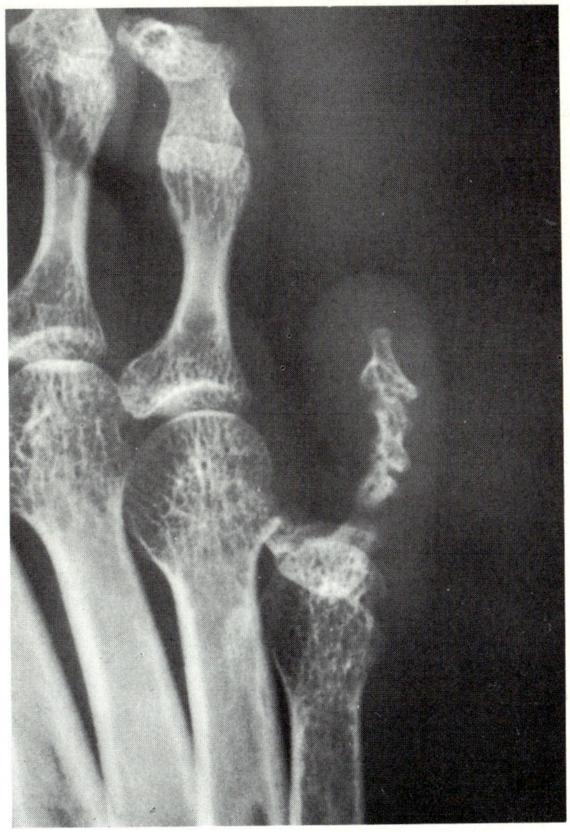

Fig. 2.77 Ainhum with transection of proximal phalanx of small toe at site of constriction.

REFERENCES

Browne, S. G. & McLoughlin, D. (1962) A case of ainhum of the finger, *West African Medical Journal*, **11,** 168–171.

Browne, S. G. (1965) True Ainhum: its distinctive and differentiating features, *Journal of Bone and Joint Surgery*, **47B,** 52–55.

Cole, C. J. (1965) Ainhum: an account of fifty-four patients with special reference to etiology and treatment, *Journal of Bone and Joint Surgery*, **47B,** 43–51.

Earle, K. V. (1958) Ainhum of the fingers: a case from Sierra Leone, *Transactions of the Royal Society of Tropical Medicine and Hygiene*, **52,** 570–573.

Fetterman, L. F., Hardy, R. & Lehrer, H. (1967) The clinico-roentgenologic features of Ainhum, *American Journal of Roentgenology*, **100,** 512–522.

MISCELLANEOUS SKELETAL TOPICS

In this section several subjects are discussed that do not readily fit in previous categories.

Anatomic anomalies

These are to a large extent under genetic control so that

their incidence varies widely in different communities. At times a mutation conferring no significant disadvantage can become prevalent in an isolated closed community. Much of the literature on minor variations is to be found in anthropological writings. Since some anomalies may prove to be useful genetic markers, interest is increasing in anatomical variations that can be readily detected. Radiology provides a useful tool for the study of skeletal variations. Not many such anomalies have medical significance and so few are mentioned here in what is intended to be a clinical work.

Carpal fusions

Carpal fusions, or more properly congenital failure of separation of mesenchyme to form a joint, are of great frequency in parts of Africa. A conjoined lunate and triquetrum exists in 0·05 per cent to 0·14 per cent in Japanese and Caucasian populations but levels up to 9·5 per cent in West African Hausas and 8·3 per cent in Yorubas in Nigeria have been recorded (Cockshott, 1963). The anomaly is frequent throughout West Africa but even in Uganda in East Africa 3·8 per cent of people are affected. The joined bones have a tendency to fracture transversely at the point where there is usually a joint so that a fracture there can readily be missed, particularly if there is separation of fragments. Recognition is important since non-union is inevitable without treatment (Fig. 2.78). In much of West Africa a joined capitate and hamate occurs in a little under 1 per cent of the population but we have not seen fractures at this site (Fig. 2.79).

Congenital dislocation of the hip

Congenital dislocation of the hip is rare in those of African ancestry (Roper, 1976). Some have attributed this to the practice of carrying babies with legs spread out around the mother's back. It seems unlikely that this procedure is the cause of the negligible clinical incidence of hip dysplasia, since in certain African communities and most

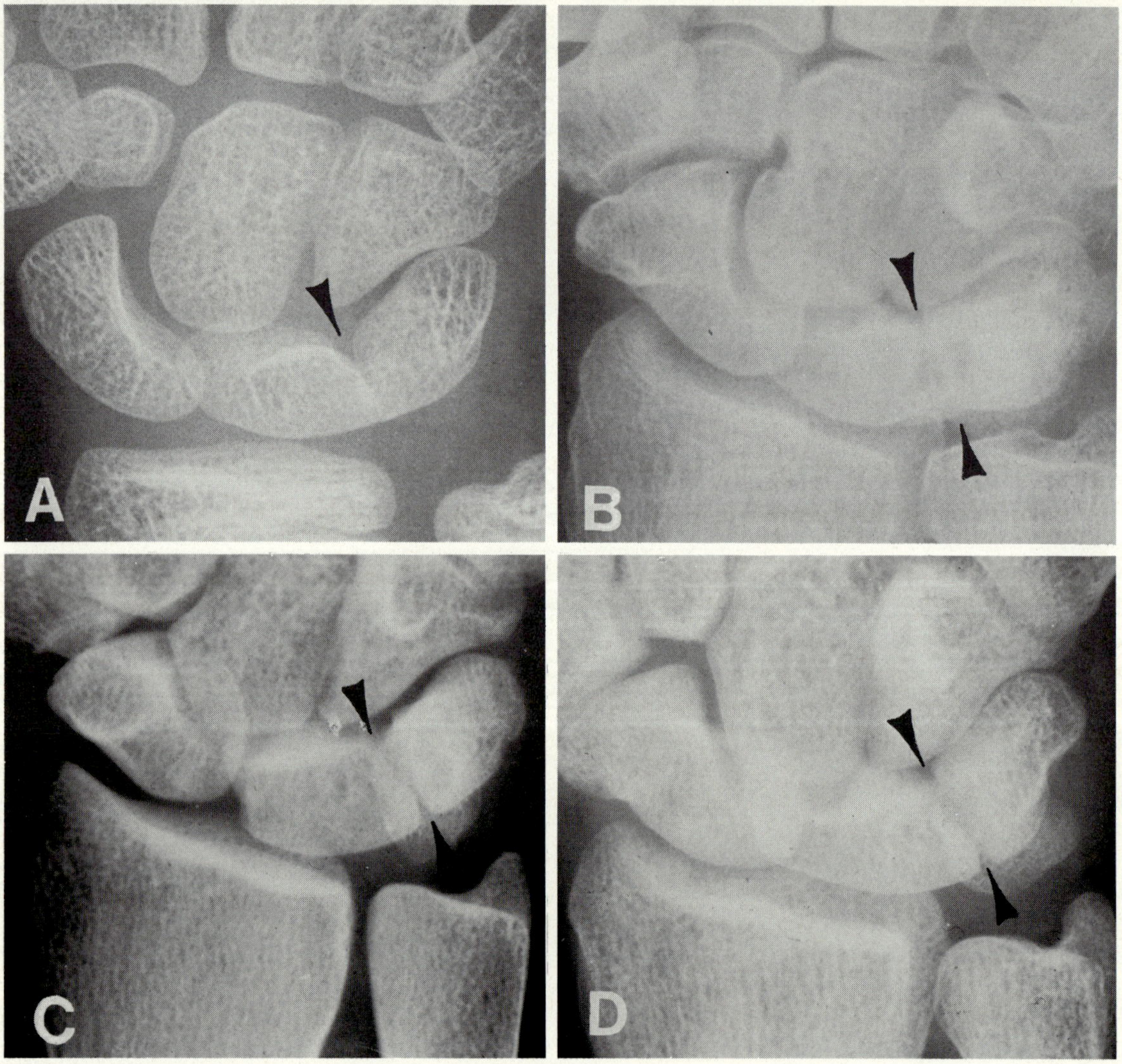

Fig. 2.78 Os lunato triquetrum. In **A** arrow points to cleft formed during fusion of ossific centres. In **B**, **C** and **D** arrows indicate fractures with chronic non-union of os lunato triquetrum. (Courtesy of *American Journal of Roentgenology*.)

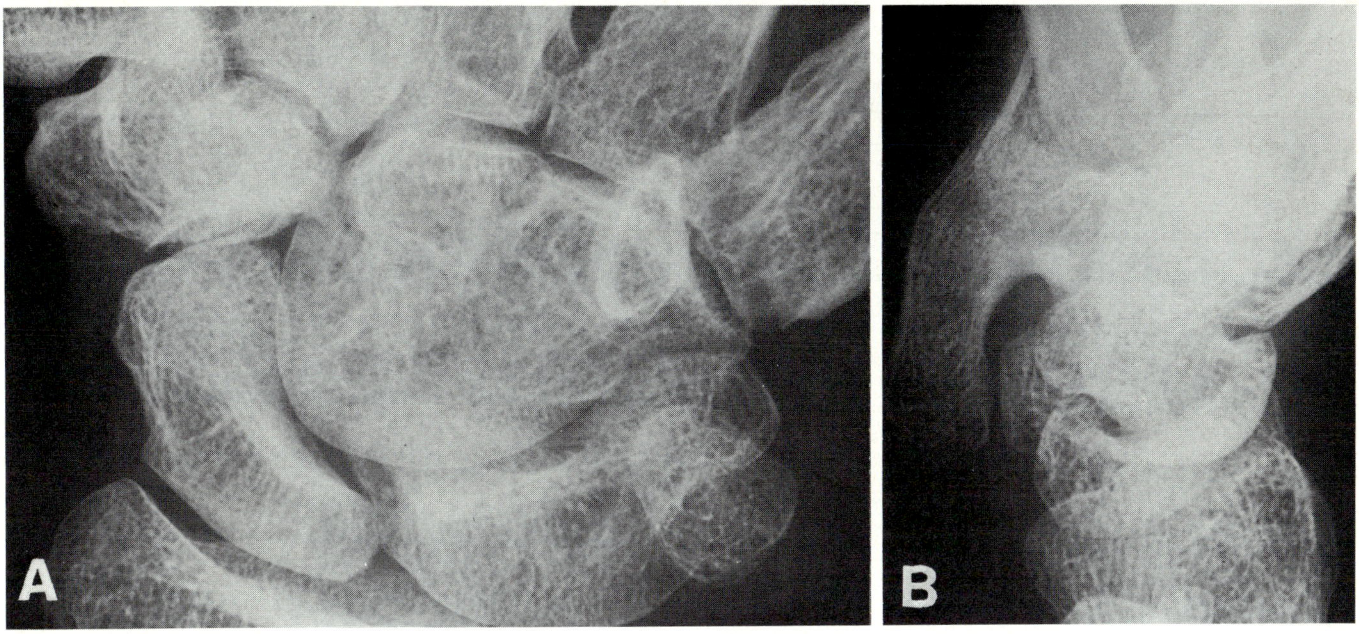

Fig. 2.79 **A.** Os lunato—triquetrum and capitate—hamate in West African. **B.** Junction of pisiform and hamate in a Nigerian.

Caribbean groups babies are not carried on the back and in these communities there is also a great rarity of congenital hip dislocation.

Hallux valgus

Hallux valgus becomes symptomatic and progressive with the wearing of tight shoes. Those who walk unshod or in sandals rarely develop significant deformity. Anatomically some hallux valgus may be seen in those who have not worn shoes (Barnicot & Hardy, 1955). Some workers have indicated that the deforming action of shoes and even socks is important for the development of symptoms and that broad shoes or sandals with straps fixed appropriately will stop the deformity from becoming symptomatic (Wheeler, Haines & McDougall, 1954).

Blount's disease or tibia vara

Blount's disease causes bow legs. Knock knees and bow legs secondary to the plasticity of bone induced by rickets is not rare in parts of the developing world, due to environmental factors or religious and social practices. A non-rachitic type of tibia vara is seen in West Africa, the Caribbean, and South and Central America (Bateson, 1966). The condition may be unilateral or bilateral. At birth slight bow leg angulation is normal but this is transient and normally changes to a degree of knock knees. Early walking, particularly with a heavy child, can allow the bow leg stage to persist. Weight-bearing increases the loading forces on the medial aspect of the tibia. This results in thickening of the cortex medially to buttress the load. The growth cartilage responds by angulation and may even fragment medially because of the deformity stresses. Once established the process of maldistribution of weight-bearing forces tend to exacerbate the deformity,

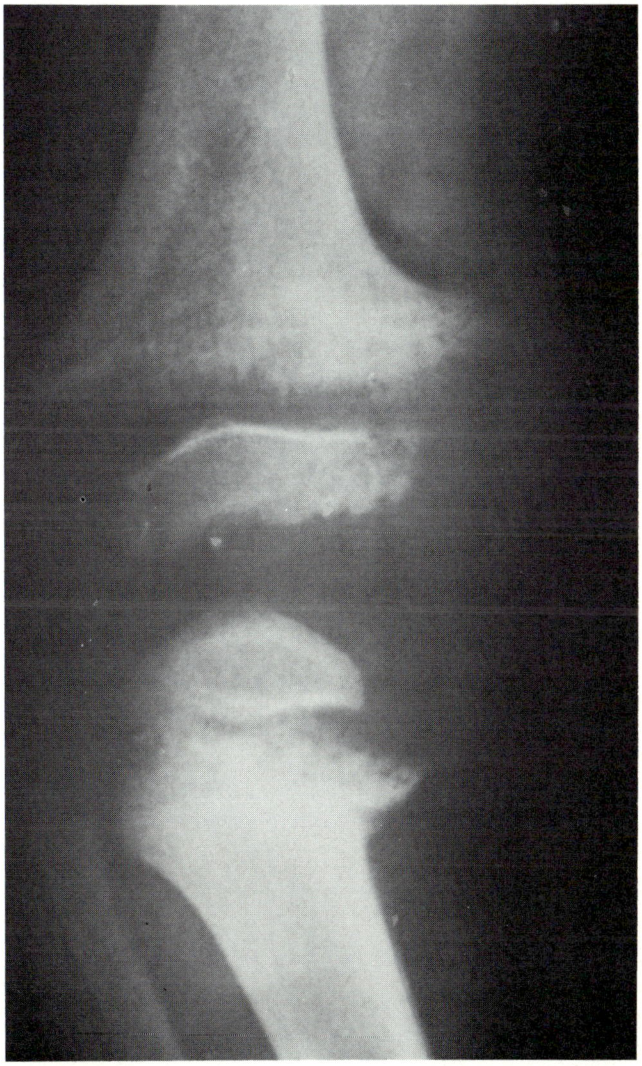

Fig. 2.80 Blount's disease combined with rickets showing typical deformity. Normally there is no radiological evidence of rickets.

since the bony response is adaptive and not corrective (Bateson, 1968). We have seen similar progression following healed rachitic deformities of the knee (Fig. 2.80). It would appear that the appearance of Blount's disease is not specific and can follow any knee deformity whatever was the initiating factor. Less frequently an analogous process occurs on the lateral side of the tibia with knock knee deformity. The majority correct themselves by growth adaptation and show little residual deformity by the time adolescence has been reached. The staying hand of the radiologist on the chisel of the enthusiastic orthopaedic surgeon can be of importance.

Ectopic nasal dentition

Ectopic nasal dentition is a rare developmental anomaly which, apart from dental deformity, is of some relevance since it may be associated with purulent nasal obstruction and long-standing unilateral maxillary sinusitis. There have been reports from many parts of the world, including India, Malaysia, Ghana and Nigeria (Hong, 1971). In one hospital in the latter country 12 cases were annotated (Cockshott & Martinson, 1972). Radiologic diagnosis is easy, as the ectopic tooth, readily recognised by the dense enamel of the crown, lies in the nasal cavity close to the inferior turbinate. The antrum on the same side as the ectopic tooth is opaque. Removal of the tooth is curative.

Pregnancy pubic changes

Pubic changes due to considerable activity in the later stages of pregnancy are common in communities where women carry loads or do heavy work throughout pregnancy. Minor changes are invariably seen in all pelvic radiographs obtained following pregnancy, but the severity of changes is much greater in those who have been physically active, working in the last trimester of pregnancy. The earlier age of first pregnancy and degree of multiparity seen in agricultural and nomadic people exacerbate the symphyseal reactive changes. The pubic ligaments become lax in late pregnancy and this is associated with increased vascularity and subchondral pubic bone resorption. The combination of the increased mobility of the symphysis and the haemorrhage that may occur in the symphyseal clefts at delivery result eventually in narrowing of the symphysis, sclerotic irregular edges and marginal new bone reactive changes, particularly posteriorly. Sometimes persistent widening causes marked pelvic instability. The excessive range of pubic movements can be documented by taking radiographs of the pubis with the patient standing on one leg then the other. In obstructed labour the foetal parts may cause pressure necrosis on soft tissues if delivery becomes impacted. Vesico-vaginal fistulae develop and infection may reach the symphysis leading to inflammatory destructive changes followed by pubic ankylosis (Cockshott, 1973).

Frontal mucocele

These may reach large proportions and enlarge to cause severe proptosis. The radiological appearances are characteristic (Figs. 2.81 and 2.82). The enlarging obstructed frontal sinus at first destroys by pressure the superior orbital margin, then distorts the anterior ethmoids on the medial aspect. The superior margin migration and the anterior protrusion of the frontal bone develop later—probably as the bone is thicker there. The margin between the frontal bone remains initially well defined and may be sclerotic. The mucocele casts a less dense shadow than

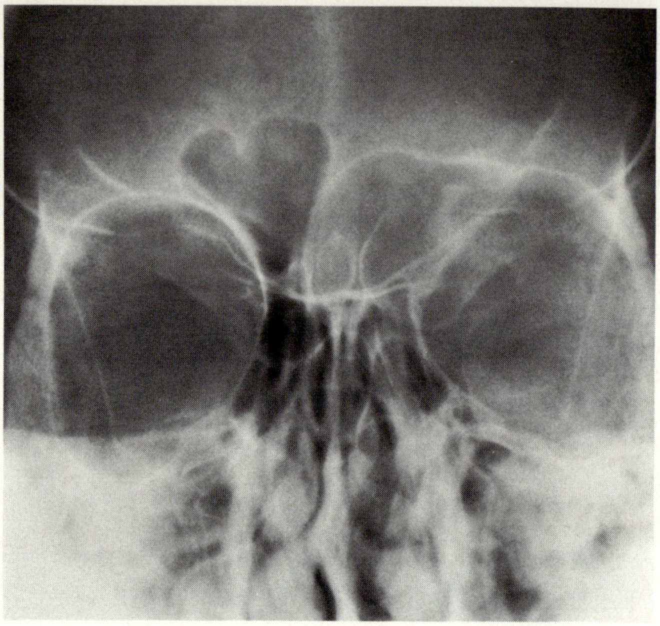

Fig. 2.81 Large left mucocele deforming left orbit and causing proptosis.

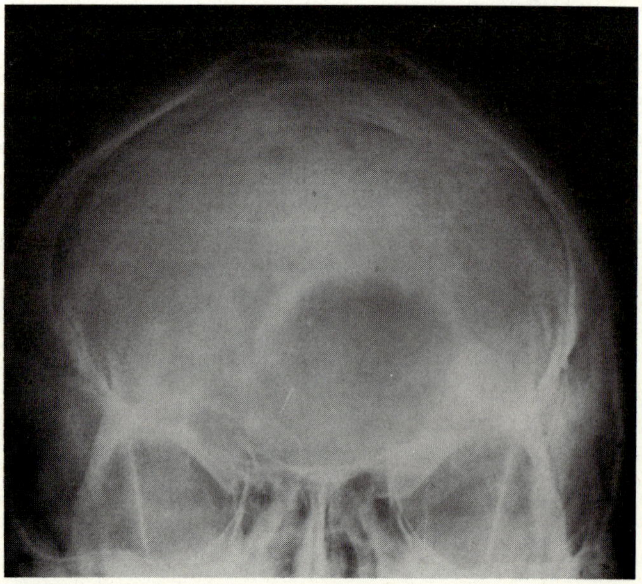

Fig. 2.82 Mucocele with secondary infection leading to ill-defined borders and sclerosis of frontal bones.

might be expected and may even be more translucent than the adjacent part of frontal sinus, as cholesterol is usually present. Often there is evidence of pansinusitis.

REFERENCES

Barnicot, N. A. & Hardy, R. H. (1955) The position of the hallux in West Africans, *Journal of Anatomy (London)*, **89,** 355–361.

Bateson, E. M. (1966) Non-rachitic bow leg and knock knee deformities in Jamaican children, *British Journal of Radiology*, **39,** 92–101.

Bateson, E. M. (1968) The relationship between Blount's disease and bow legs, *British Journal of Radiology*, **41,** 107–114.

Cockshott, W. P. (1963) Carpal fusions, *American Journal of Roentgenology*, **86,** 1260–1271.

Cockshott, W. P. (1973) Pubic changes associated with obstetric vesico vaginal fistulae, *Clinical Radiology*, **24,** 241–247.

Cockshott, W. P. & Martinson, E. (1972) Ectopic nasal dentition, *Clinical Radiology*, **23,** 451–454.

Hong, C. Y. (1976) Ectopic nasal tooth, *Medical Journal of Malaysia*, **30,** 239–240.

Roper, A. (1976) Hip dysplasia in the African Bantu, *Journal of Bone and Joint Surgery*, **58B,** 155–158.

Wheeler Haines, R. & McDougall, A. (1954) Shoe design and toe formation, *Lancet*, **2,** 1308–1311.

HAEMOGLOBIN DISEASES

Over 100 variants of normal adult haemoglobin—haemoglobin A (HbA)—are known. These are designated by alphabetical titles—haemoglobins S, C, D, E, etc.—or by place names—Hb Massachusetts, Hb Hyderabad, etc. Most are of little clinical significance, but HbS, HbC and HbE are associated with disease processes.

At birth normal infants have foetal haemoglobin (HbF) and continue to manufacture it for approximately the first three months of life. All haemoglobins are under genetical control and HbF is under a different genetical control from HbA. If for any reason during the period when the production of HbF would normally diminish, the parallel increased production of HbA does not take place, then the erythropoietic system continues to manufacture HbF.

Like other protein molecules, the globin of haemoglobin consists of intertwined polypeptide chains—a pair of alpha-chains and a pair of beta-chains. Each chain is a coiled string of 140 to 150 amino acids. The immense variety of all the proteins in nature is achieved with only about twenty amino acids as building blocks by varying the number and order of those that are built into the chains. While haemoglobin is being made in the young red cells, the amino acids are added on in the right order, an order prearranged by the individual's genetic constitution. But if there is a mutation in the genetic template at one point, it will mean that at just one particular point in the chain the wrong amino acid will be put in; and this is what an abnormal haemoglobin is. For example in HbS, a single amino acid, valine, replaces the glutamic acid normally present in HbA in position six of the beta polypeptide chain, whereas in HbC the glutamic acid is replaced by lysine in that same position.

But haemoglobin production can go wrong for other reasons than the incorporation of wrong amino acids. The synthesising mechanism may be perfect but the genetic message may not come through to the site of synthesis so that there is a failure to produce, say, the alpha-chains or the beta-chains. This is the defect that underlies thalassaemia and, if the defect is inherited in a homozygous manner, the result is more disastrous than if there is merely an aberrant haemoglobin, because the red cells lacking haemoglobin are non-viable and are liable to be destroyed as soon as formed (Weatherall, 1965). The marrow hypertrophies but its efforts at erythropoiesis are ineffective.

Some of the haemoglobinopathies do not produce an anaemia, but those that do, and they are the common ones, all do so because the life span of the red cells containing the abnormal haemoglobin is reduced, often very drastically, from an early stage of infancy. To say that the red cell life-span is reduced is the modern definition of a haemolytic anaemia and to indicate that the bone marrow will be called on to replace red cells at an increased rate, which may reach six to ten times the normal rate. To do this, the marrow hypertrophies.

In addition HbS causes red cells to become elongated and adopt a sickle shape at low oxygen tensions. In sickle cell anaemia (homozygous SS disease) nearly all the individual's haemoglobin is HbS and sickling occurs quite readily in the capillaries and marrow sinusoids; but so long as the circulation is not blocked the cells can 'unsickle' when they pass on to better oxygenated regions (Serjeant *et al.*, 1972). In the heterozygous SC and S/thalassaemia states when the proportion of HbS in the red cells may be over 50 per cent, sickling may also occur readily; further in Hb SC disease there is increased blood viscosity (Serjeant *et al.*, 1973a). In bone, in the marrow sinusoids where circulation may be slow and oxygen utilisation high, all these factors may lead to packing of the sinusoids with sickled cells, further reduction of oxygen tension and more sickling, thus proceeding to thrombosis, infarction and necrosis. A further complication is that wherever typhoid/paratyphoid diseases are common, infarcts tend to become infected by these organisms and this leads in turn to salmonella osteitis (Bohrer, 1971).

The S gene is the only variant of adult haemoglobin to cause the sickling phenomenon and so is the only one to cause infarction.

Carriers of the S gene appear to have an increased resistance to the malaria parasite. This applies to infants and children in the sub-Sahara belt of Africa where it is thought this genetic mutation first occurred. It is not clear at present whether other haemoglobin variants confer similar advantages (Huehns & Shooter, 1965).

The S gene occurs across the tropical belt of Africa and wherever people have migrated to from that area, e.g. the

Mediterranean coast, the Arabian peninsula, the Caribbean, North, Central and South America.

The E gene has its highest incidence in Bengal, both in India and Bangladesh, and also occurs in Burma, Thailand, Indonesia and elsewhere in South East Asia.

The thalassaemia genes occur around the Mediterranian coast, in Kuwait, Bengal, throughout South East Asia and South China and sporadically with migrants in West Africa, Mozambique and the New World.

The skeletal changes that may occur radiologically depend on whether or not an S gene is present.

If an S gene is present then the features of infarction followed by necrosis and repair will be apparent, the extent of repair depending on the age of the individual at the time of the episode. In the carrier state (HbAS) the individual possesses the one functioning A gene to enable him to manufacture normal haemoglobin and no stigmata occur, whereas if the same individual had inherited a thalassaemia gene it would have inhibited the production of HbA and he would have suffered from S/thalassaemia disease.

The second radiological feature is marrow hyperplasia and the extent of this is dependent on how profound the haemolytic anaemia is. In homozygous thalassaemia, for example, the condition is not compatible with prolonged life and outside the Western world, where diagnostic facilities and repeated transfusions may not be readily available, it is rare for such an individual to reach adolescence, whereas in Hb SC disease the haemolytic anaemia may be minimal and the resulting marrow hyperplasia not overtly manifest. These conditions occur predominantly in parts of the world where other causes of anaemia are not uncommon and undernutrition folic acid deficiency, repeated pregnancies and a high hookworm load may all contribute to the occurrence of haemolytic crises more frequently than occurs to individuals endowed with a similar gene pattern in industrialised countries.

The third group of skeletal radiological features are due to complications added to or arising from the infarcts or marrow hyperplasia, e.g. growth defects, disorganisation of joints, salmonella osteitis, extramedullary haemopoietic tissue producing spinal block leading to paraplegia, etc.

Sickle cell anaemia (Hb SS disease)

Infarction in the small bones of the hands and feet is especially common in infancy and childhood—the 'hand/foot syndrome'. The metacarpals and phalanges are commonly involved. The response is an attempt at repair resulting in hyperaemia, especially of the arteriolar penetrating branches from the periosteum (Middlemiss, 1958). This produces slight elevation of the periosteum causing a periosteal reaction. The aseptic necrosis is followed by osteoclastic resorption showing as zones of translucency in the affected bone. Infarction of the diaphysis of a long bone usually occurs in the intermediate fifth at either the proximal or distal end (Bohrer, 1970). This is sufficiently characteristic that infection in bone at this site is very suggestive of a sickling state (Fig. 2.83A). If the metaphysis of a growing bone is affected, growth in epiphyseal cartilage ceases during the repair process with resultant deformity (Cockshott, 1963).

The hyperaemia due to the repair process may bring about premature fusion of the epiphysis further reducing growth (Fig. 2.85B).

Infarction may occur in an epiphysis; for example, the femoral head or humeral head, where the line of cleavage separating the infarcted area, which is usually segmental, from the viable bone, may be clearly seen radiologically (Fig. 2.84A). In such cases the repair process usually buttresses adjacent subcortical bone and bone adjacent to the line of cleavage, producing sclerosis. In the long bones, as always, radiological signs lag behind the clinical presentation and, as always, it is the repair process that produces changes (Fig. 2.83C). Osteoclastic resorption of necrotic bone produces translucent zones, occasionally with some calcification of debris within the translucent area, and osteoblastic activity produces a sclerotic rim sealing off the affected area (Ennis *et al.*, 1973). The so-called 'bone-within-a-bone' sign in which an apparent 'cortex' lies within the true cortex, producing a 'tram-line' effect within the medulla parallel to the cortex, is possibly due to infarction of a long segment of the shaft during the years of growth. It appears that in such a case the repair process is unable to absorb the necrotic cortex in its entirety, but that this subsequently almost certainly becomes re-vascularised and is not left as a sequestrum. Meanwhile a new cortex is laid down by the periosteum as an involucrum

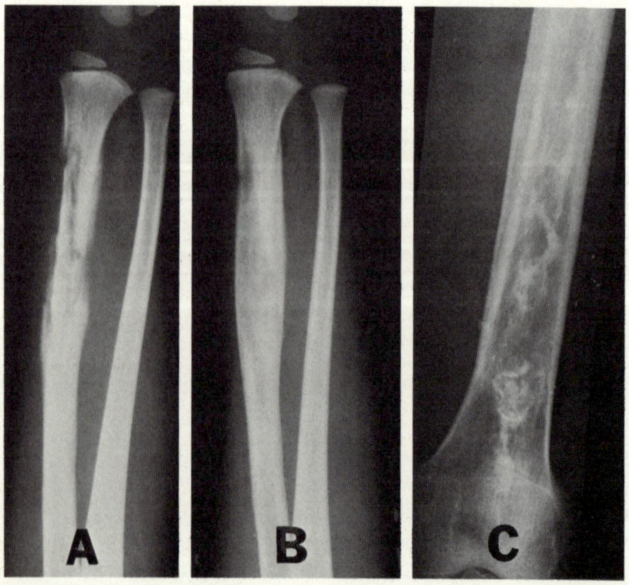

Fig. 2.83 **A.** Infarction in the distal half of left radius with periosteal new bone (repair) and absorption of necrotic bone (SS disease). **B.** Same case four weeks later. **C.** Infarction in the distal half of the femur with absorption of necrotic bone, calcification of debris and peri-osteal new bone. The 'bone within a bone' appearance is shown (S/thalassaemia).

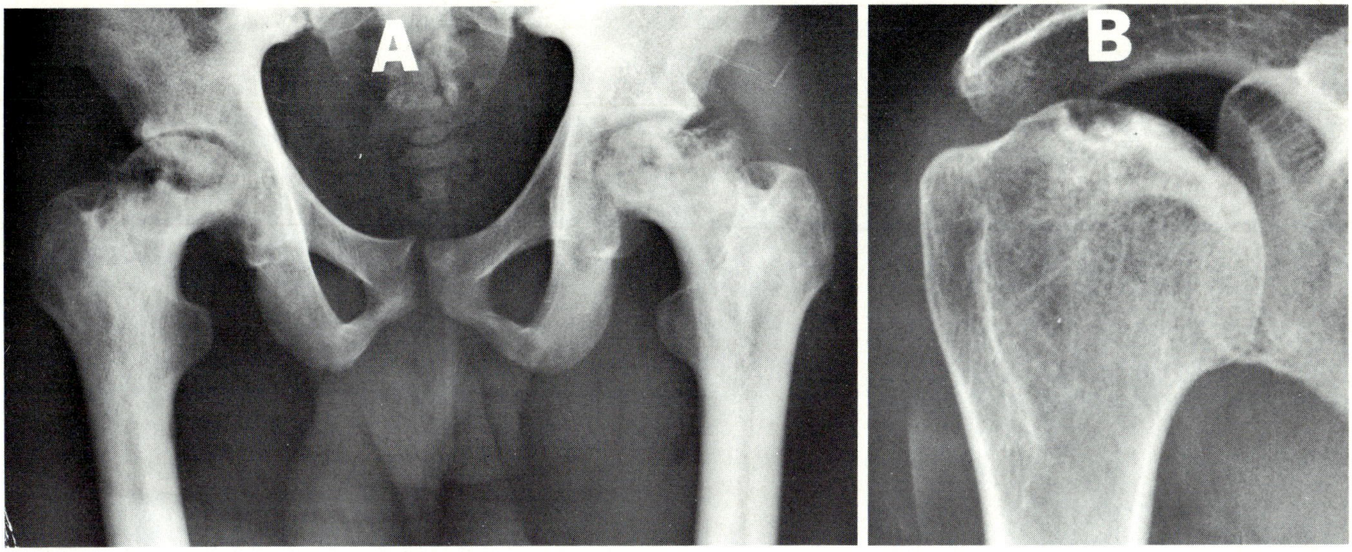

Fig. 2.84 **A.** Infarcts in both femoral heads of a 'non-complaining' Jamaican with SC disease. **B.** Absorption of necrotic bone in an infarct in the head of the humerus (SC disease).

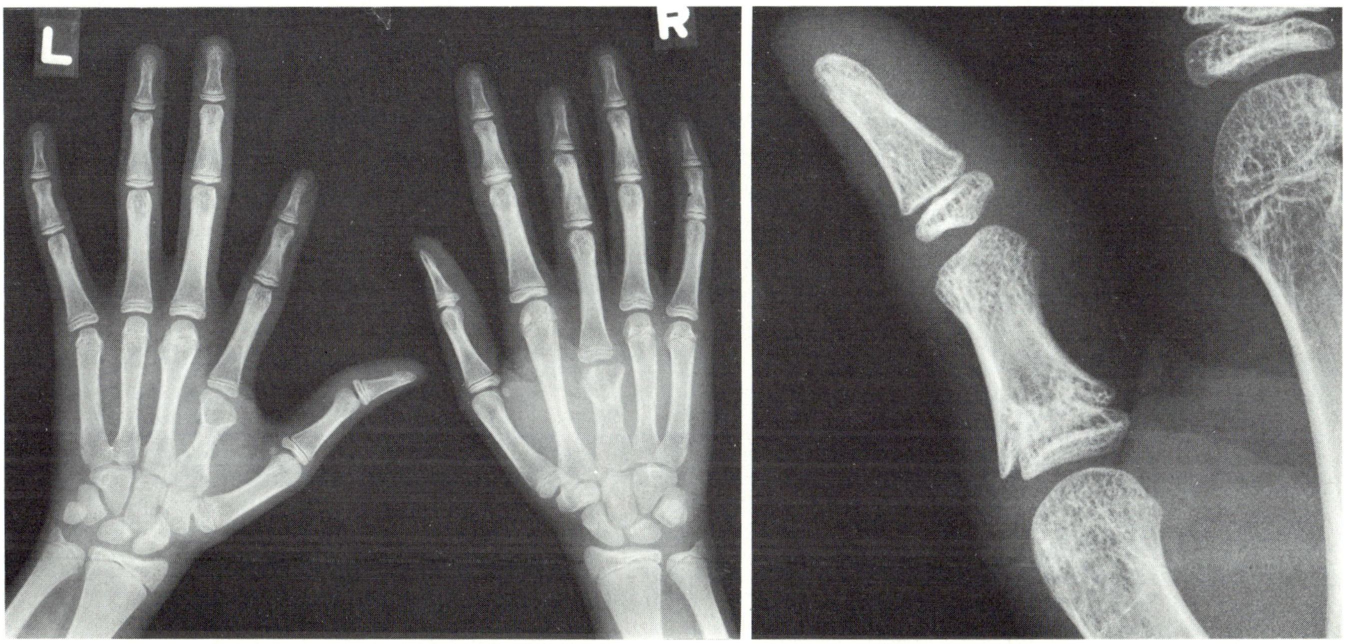

Fig. 2.85 **A.** The end result in adulthood of metaphyseal infarction in the distal ends of the left second and right third metacarpals (SC disease). **B.** Infarction in the proximal end of the proximal phalanx of the thumb. The repair hyperaemia is causing premature epiphyseal fusion and thus cessation of growth (S/thalassaemia).

which with the following years of growth is remodelled, retaining entombed the old cortex (Bohrer, 1970). We have observed at least one case following this pattern in its entirety.

Marrow hyperplasia produces generalised increased translucency of bones, especially of the small bones of the hands and feet, and of the vertebrae. Analysis of the increased translucency shows it to be due to widening of the medulla, widened intertrabecular spaces and narrowing of the cortex (Fig. 2.86A). The vertebral bodies may show a bi-concave deformity with a widened bulging nucleus pulposus between them. This may affect the whole spine (Fig. 2.89). In some vertebrae a 'step' sign may occasionally be seen in which a small segment of the upper cortex appears to be depressed into the medulla with loss of continuity at its anterior and posterior margins. This has been interpreted as due to growth disturbances or minimal fractures during weight-bearing or muscular activity through areas of subclinical infarction in hyperplastic marrow.

Characteristic appearances may occur in the skull producing, clinically, frontal bossing. The appearances are

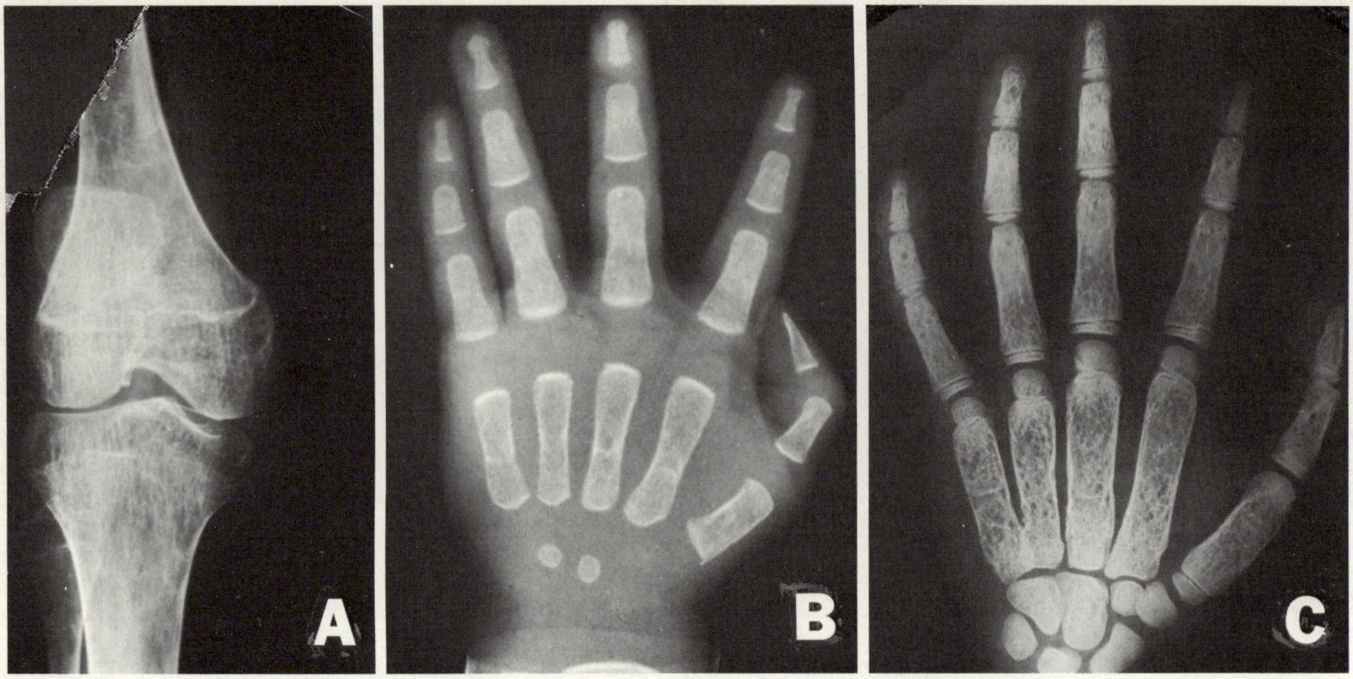

Fig. 2.86 **A.** Marrow hyperplasia in SS disease. **B.** Marrow hyperplasia in a 2-year-old with homozygous beta-thalassaemia. **C.** Marrow hyperplasia in a juvenile with homozygous beta-thalassaemia.

due to widening of the diploae; in long-standing cases there may be thickening of the frontal and parietal bones with thinning of the outer tables and a radial arrangement of new trabeculae (Fig. 2.87) (Barton & Cockshott, 1962; Olufemi-Williams *et al.*, 1975).

Salmonella osteitis

As mentioned in the opening part of this section, the aseptic necrosis tends to become infected by typhoid/paratyphoid organisms resulting in salmonella osteitis. Radiologically the lesions differ little from pyogenic osteomyelitis, but extension of the infective process is usually somewhat slower and response to specific drugs is slow (Bohrer, 1971). The process may destroy epiphyseal cartilage, unlike pyogenic osteomyelitis, and often the periosteal reaction and involucrum formation is minimal (Fig. 2.88). The clinical severity of the condition is sometimes mild when radiological features are quite marked.

It has been suggested that the hand/foot syndrome may be due to salmonella osteitis and certainly there may be occasions when these organims are implicated; equally certainly the condition can occur without there being any likelihood of an infective element.

Spontaneous fractures

We have drawn attention previously to the tendency to spontaneous fracture in this condition, suggesting that the diminished resilience of bone demineralised possibly by marrow hyperplasia and/or the undernutrition that may occur in the communities affected, probably contributes to this factor (Fig. 2.88) (Middlemiss, 1958). More recently attention has been drawn to the fact that such cases of spontaneous fracture almost certainly occur through areas of infected bone where there is salmonella osteitis (Bohrer, 1971).

Hb SC disease

In Hb SC disease the acute infarcts seen in childhood in homozygous Hb SS disease are less common. However, the chronic infarcts that occur in the femoral and humeral heads, the growth defects and the large medullary infarcts in long bones occur with equal frequency in Hb SC disease and differ in no way from those seen in the homozygous state (Fig. 2.84). They are often found incidentally in uncomplaining individuals who on persistent questioning will sometimes admit to 'aches and pains'. They are often bilateral and extensive (Serjeant *et al.*, 1973).

Marrow hyperplasia is never so great in this condition, presumably because haemolysis is not so profound (Barton *et al.*, 1962). It may however occur and a feature sometimes noted owing to the late clinical presentation of individuals is widened vascular channels in the phalanges and possibly metacarpals, presumably due to the altered haemodynamics associated with the production of red cells in bones not normally associated with haemopoiesis.

In the *homozygous CC state*, lacking an S gene, no infarction takes place; and the increased haemolysis is so slight that the majority of individuals of this genotype suffer from little or no disability and rarely present clinically as having a disease entity. There are no specific radiological features associated with the condition.

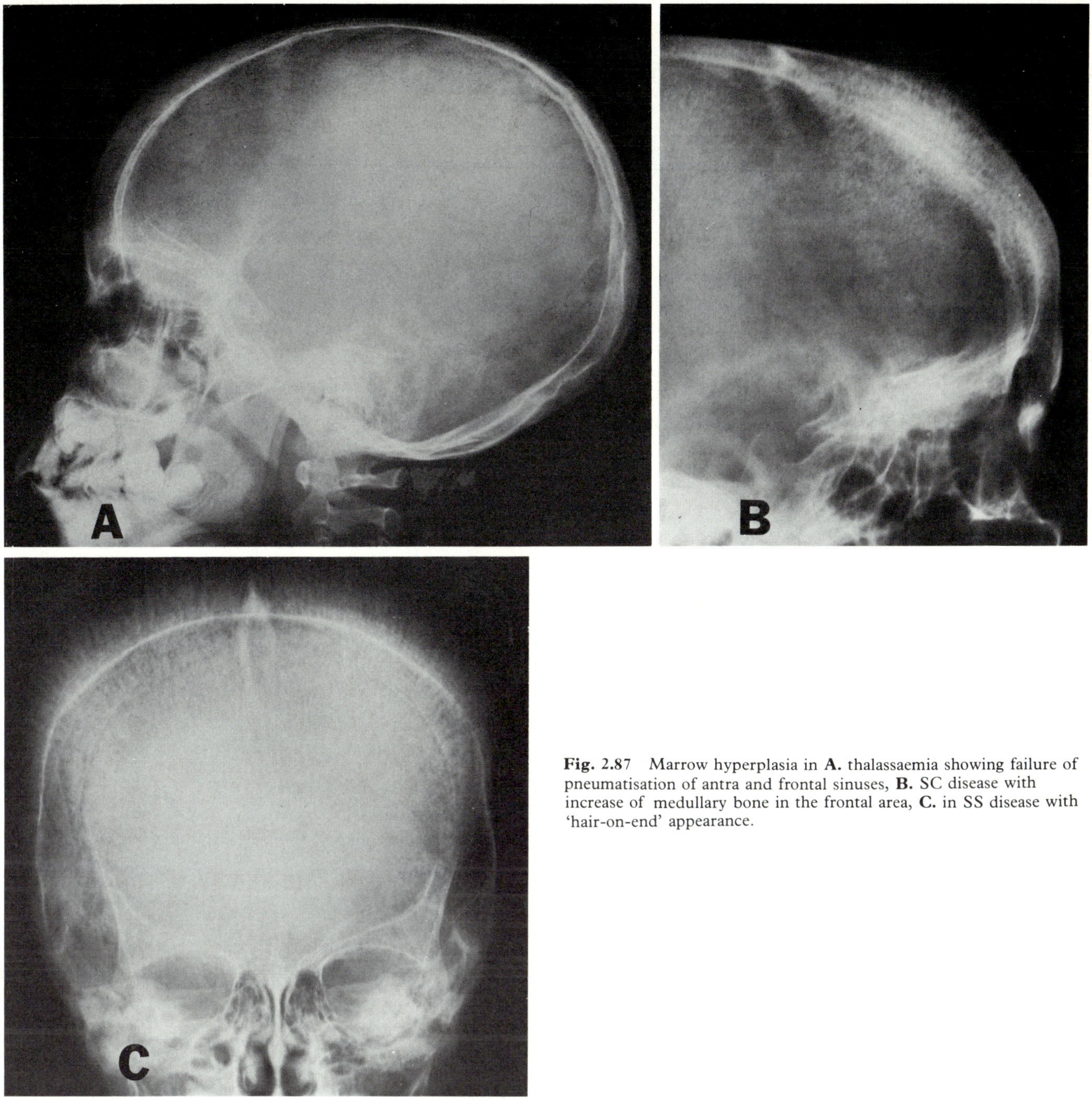

Fig. 2.87 Marrow hyperplasia in **A.** thalassaemia showing failure of pneumatisation of antra and frontal sinuses, **B.** SC disease with increase of medullary bone in the frontal area, **C.** in SS disease with 'hair-on-end' appearance.

Thalassaemia

Whether the inherited failure to manufacture the polypeptide chains effects the alpha-chains or the beta-chains, the outcome is the same. The homozygous state is not compatible with prolonged life. In either case haemolysis is profound, probably more profound than in any other condition known to mankind, and marrow hyperplasia is consequently extensive. Erythropoiesis takes place wherever it is possible; every part of medullary bone is mobilised, and the mobilisation takes place at an early stage in life, affecting certain aspects of growth and development. The metacarpals and phalanges, not normally the site of haemopoiesis, now become actively the site of this process—the medulla widens, the cortex narrows, the intertrabecular spaces are occupied by red-cell-producing tissue and so are widened, haemodynamics are altered and so vascular channels are enlarged, modelling of bone in the years of growth is interfered with and so the bones appear 'swollen' (Fig. 2.86). Similar changes take place in the ribs with widening of the ribs. The long bones, pelvis and vertebrae are affected. In the skull, similar changes to those described in homozygous SS disease occur but usually greater in extent. Also in the skull the air sinuses often fail to pneumatise and become occupied

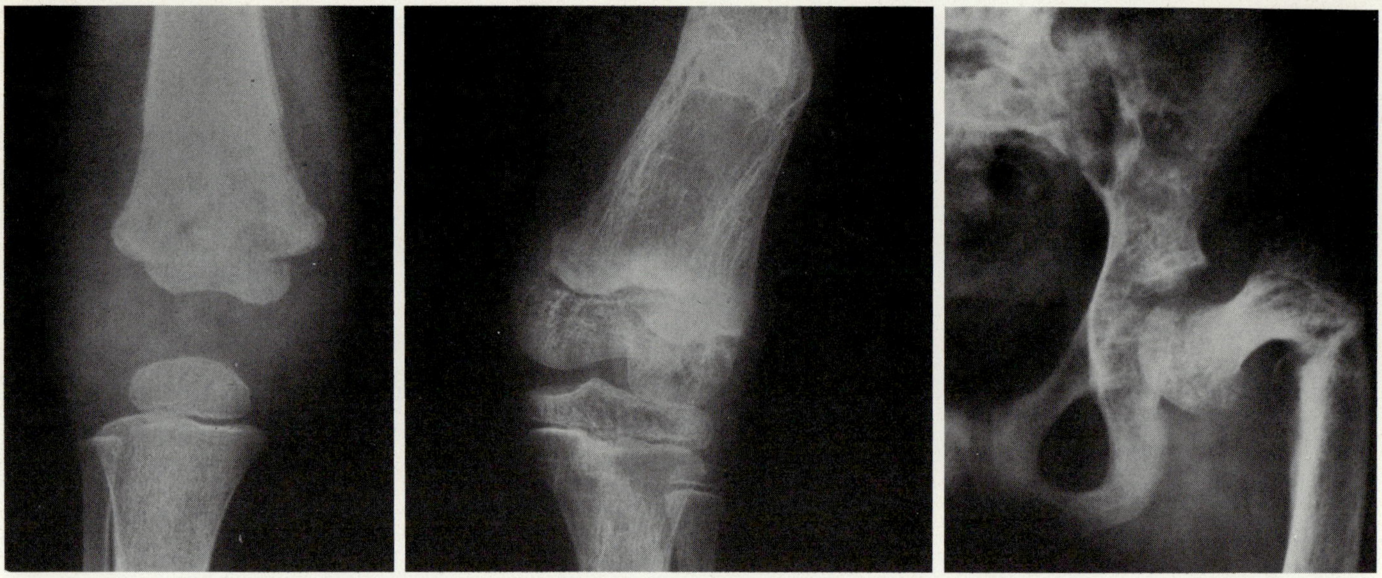

A B C

Fig. 2.88 **A.** Salmonella osteitis in a case of SS disease with destruction of the growth plate. **B.** Healed pathological fracture of the femur in SS disease. Note marrow hyperplasia. **C.** Healed pathological fracture in the upper femur with coxa vara deformity in SS disease. Note the marrow hyperplasia.

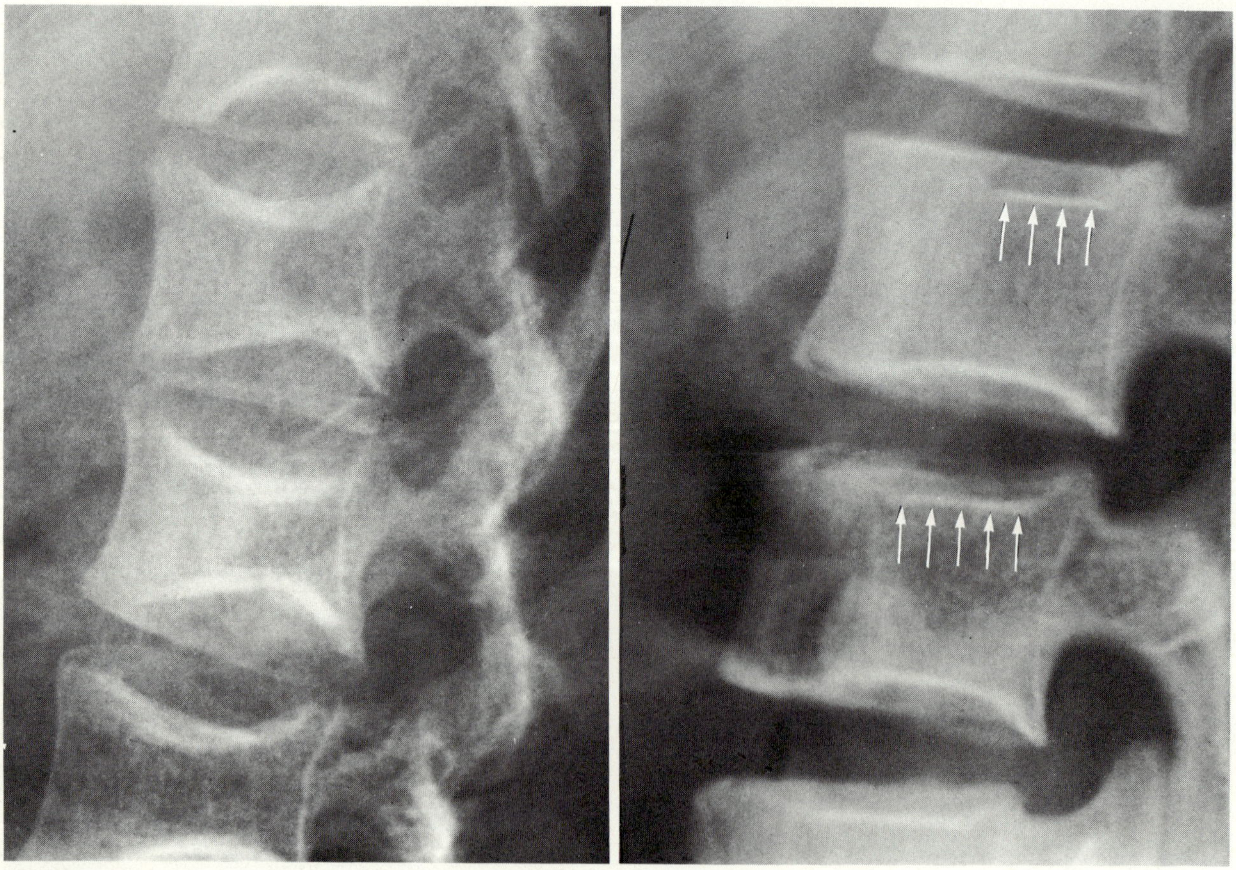

A B

Fig. 2.89 Spinal deformities: **A.** bi-concave deformity due to marrow hyperplasia, **B.** 'the step sign' possibly due to vascular compromise during growth.

by haemopoietic tissue—appearing radiologically as of bony density with wide intertrabecular spaces (Fig. 2.87) (Middlemiss *et al.*, 1966). Extramedullary haemopoietic tissue develops in certain sites—in the spleen, for example, producing splenomegaly, and beneath the periosteum of long bones and metacarpals and metatarsals, producing 'scalloping' of the cortex from the periosteal side; it also occurs in the paravertebral gutter, producing enormous soft tissue masses which may be seen in the chest film as large often symmetrical paravertebral tumours throughout the thorax, occasionally as retrocardiac masses (Fig. 2.90) (Korsten *et al.*, 1970). These paravertebral masses of haemopoietic tissue have been known to extend through the intervertebral foramina into the spinal canal, causing paraplegia. This is described elsewhere in this book.

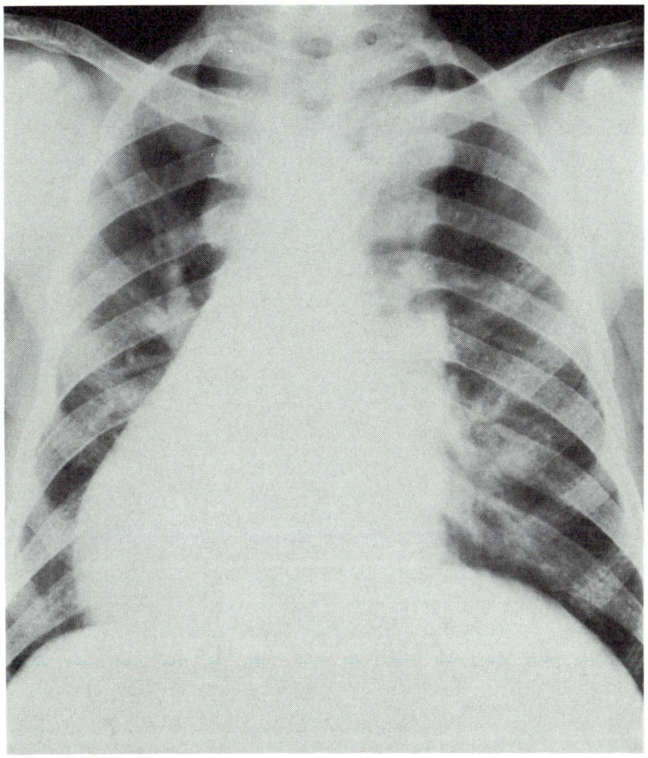

Fig. 2.90 Extramedullary haemopoietic tissue producing paravertebral gutter soft tissue masses in E/thalassaemia.

Hb E/thalassaemia disease

The homozygous Hb E state produces no clinical haemoglobinopathy. Hb E occurs in about 4 per cent of the population of Bengal and to a lesser extent throughout Burma, Thailand, Indonesia and South China. The thalassaemia gene occurs in almost identical proportions throughout those same geographical areas. It is to be expected therefore that intermarriage will produce the Hb E/thalassaemia state and this does occur; in this the prognosis is not so grave and affected individuals do progress into adult life, albeit with repeated haemolytic crises (Chatterjea, 1965). Radiologically the features seen in this condition are those that have been described under homozygous thalassaemia, the difference being that they are seen in adult life. These individuals are known, in the geographical areas of South East Asia affected, to live to the ages of 40 and 50 years, and in some Western countries to which some have migrated they are known, under medical supervision and care, to have had a normal life-span.

Hb S/thalassaemia disease

The heterozygous HbS/thalassaemia state does occur in some communities. It has been described in West Africa and North and South America. Serjeant *et al.* (1973b) described the skeletal changes in a (mostly adult) group of 70 uncomplaining cases in Jamaica traced through family studies. Skeletal changes were common, most individuals having some stigmata; they were similar to a group in the same study with Hb SC disease, there being many examples of infarction, and few with great evidence of marrow hyperplasia. None had the excessive marrow hyperplasia associated with Hb E/thalassaemia disease, though we have seen some evidence of extramedullary haemopoiesis in this condition (Middlemiss, 1966).

In all the haemoglobinopathies described in this section we have seen anaemic dilatation of the heart (described elsewhere) and in all we have seen splenomegaly (Fig. 3.60) (see chapter 3). In addition in all those conditions described here with an S gene there may be a raised incidence of pigment gall-stones (see chapter 3) and there may be episodes of necrotising papillitis with or without haematuria (Fig. 6.13) (described in chapter 6).

REFERENCES

Barton, C. J. & Cockshott, W. P. (1962) Bone changes in Hb SC disease, *American Journal of Roentgenology*, **88**, 523–532.

Bohrer, S. P. (1970) Acute long bone diaphyseal infarcts in sickle cell disease, *British Journal of Radiology*, **43**, 685–697.

Bohrer, S. P. (1971) Fractures complicating bone infarcts and/or osteomyelitis in sickle cell disease, *Clinical Radiology*, **22**, 83–88.

Chatterjea, J. B. (1965) Some aspects of haemoglobin E and its genetic interaction with thalassemia, *Indian Journal of Medical Research*, **53**, 1–23.

Cockshott, W. P. (1963) Dactylitis and growth disorders, *British Journal of Radiology*, **36**, 19–26.

Ennis, J. T., Serjeant, G. R. & Middlemiss, J. H. (1973) Homozygous sickle cell disease in Jamaica, *British Journal of Radiology*, **46**, 943–950.

Huehns, E. R. & Shooter, E. M. (1965) Human haemoglobins, *Journal of Medical Genetics*, **2**, 48–90.

Korsten, J., Grossman, H., Winchester, P. H. & Canale, V. C. (1970) Extramedullary haematopoiesis in patients with thalassemia anemia, *Radiology*, **95**, 257–263.

Middlemiss, J. H. (1958) Sickle cell anaemia, *Journal of the Faculty of Radiologists*, **9**, 16–24.

Middlemiss, J. H. & Raper, A. B. (1966) Skeletal changes in the haemoglobinopathies, *Journal of Bone and Joint Surgery*, **48B**, 693–702.

Olufemi-Williams, A., Lagundoye, S. B. & Johnson, C. Lent (1975) Lamellations of the diploe in the skulls of patients with sickle cell anaemia, *Archive Diseases of Childhood*, **50**, 948–952.

Serjeant, G. R. & Serjeant, B. E. (1972) A comparison of erythrocyte characteristics in sickle cell syndromes in Jamaica, *British Journal of Haematology*, **23**, 205–213.

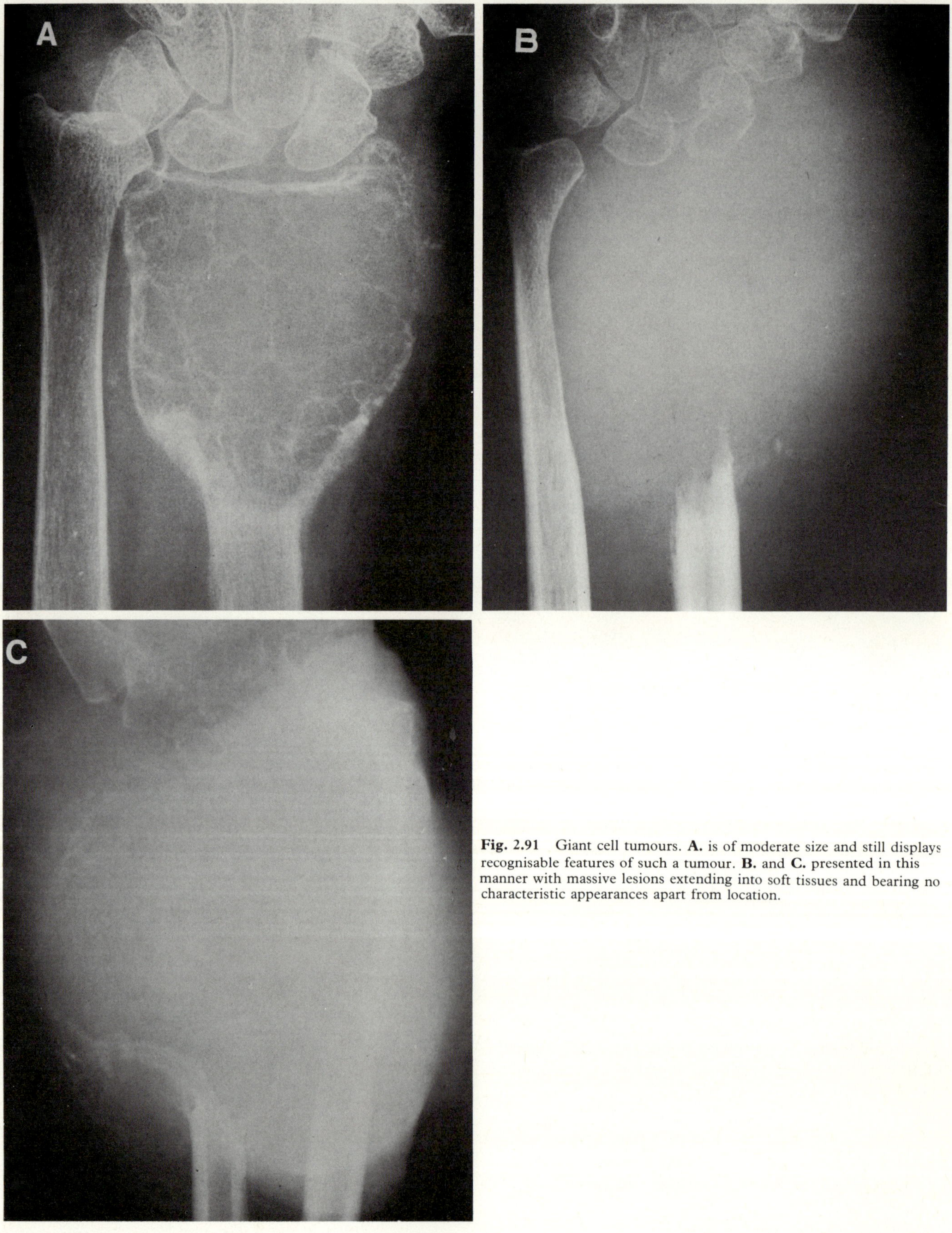

Fig. 2.91 Giant cell tumours. **A.** is of moderate size and still displays recognisable features of such a tumour. **B.** and **C.** presented in this manner with massive lesions extending into soft tissues and bearing no characteristic appearances apart from location.

Serjeant, G. R., Ennis, J. T. & Middlemiss, J. H. (1973a) Haemoglobin SC disease in Jamaica, *British Journal of Radiology*, **46,** 935–942.
Serjeant, G. R., Ennis, J. T. & Middlemiss, J. H. (1973b) Sickle cell B thalassaemia in Jamaica, *British Journal of Radiology*, **46,** 951–959.
Weatherall, D. J. (1965) In *The Thalassaemia Syndromes*. Oxford: Blackwell Scientific Publications.

BONE TUMOURS

The advanced stage of many bone tumours when they first present for medical attention makes precise diagnosis difficult, since many of the classic radiographic features may be lacking. The sheer local bulk of the lesions effaces characteristic signs upon which the radiologist relies so that biopsy is, as always, an important part of the work-up. This aspect is exemplified by the illustration of three large giant cell tumours (Fig. 2.91). The first retains fine bony septa within the expanded radius, but in the larger tumours all vestige of bone has vanished and the soft tissue mass has actually produced pressure erosion of the ulnae.

At present there are few bone tumour registries in the tropics so that the data base is too restricted for comparative comments. Suffice it to say that forms of osteogenic sarcoma are the most frequent, followed closely by giant cell tumour. Certain categories are rare, including osteoid osteoma.

Burkitt's lymphoma

Since this lymphoma is a multi-organ multifocal malignancy, it is probably semantically correct not to consider this form of malignancy a primary bone tumour. Burkitt's tumour is found in parts of the tropics where malaria occurs, possibly because it shares a vector with similar needs to the malarial mosquito to transmit the Epstein-Barr virus, or because the effect of malaria on a child's reticulo-endothelial system sets the stage for the virus to initiate the lymphoma. Many consider that both factors operate.

The tumour is seen in all races and affects children—those between 3 and 13 years being the most vulnerable. Cases have been reported from East and West Africa, New Guinea (ten Saldam, 1966), Malaysia (Ramanathan, 1972) and Brazil. Cases from the U.S.A., Europe and other temperate climates have many similarities histologically and immunologically, but the clinical presentations and location of deposits differ somewhat from those seen in the tropics.

The initial bone foci are permeative in the marrow, destroying smaller trabeculae before eroding and penetrating cortical bone and elevating the periosteum. Deposits develop in areas of red marrow so that in younger children bone destruction may occur almost anywhere in a long bone, by the age of six or older bone destruction

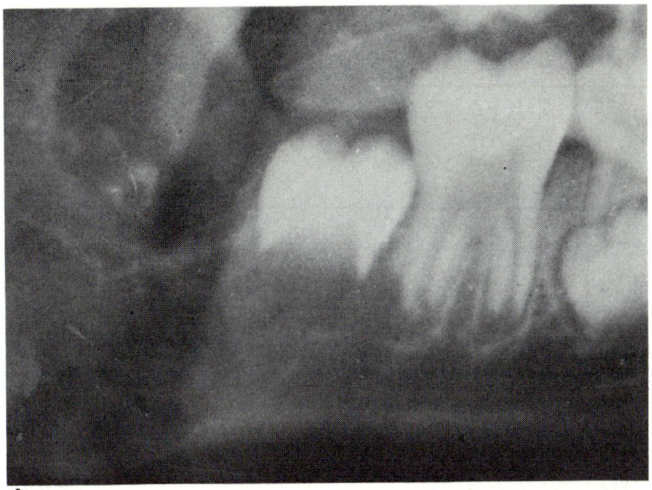

A

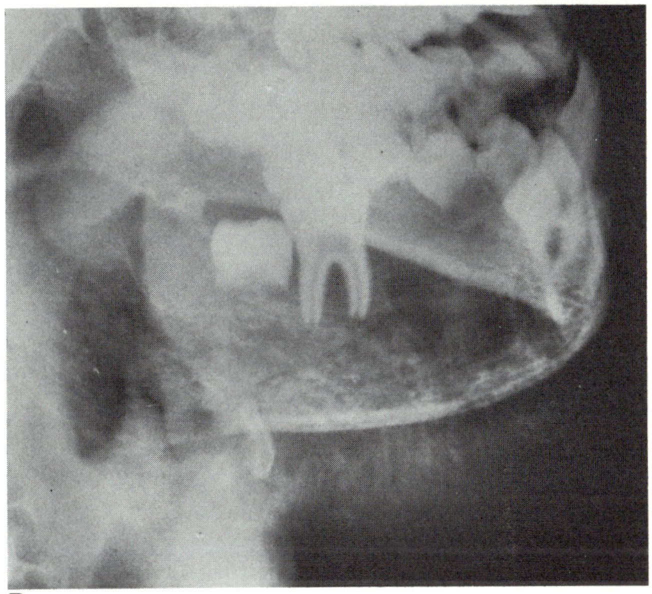

B

Fig. 2.92 Burkitt's tumour. The upper film **A** shows focal loss of lamina dura around the germinal follicle of lower 8, roots of 7, and posterior part of 6. There is also loss of trabecular structure. The lower view **B** reveals greater permeative cortical destruction, loss of teeth and periosteal new bone development.

is juxtametaphyseal in the proximal and distal ends of long bones. Pathological fracture at the site of a deposit is infrequent. In flat bones bone destruction may be difficult to appreciate radiographically. In the mandible of a child non-screen film or high detail intensifying screens provide films of optimum quality. Spreading deposits in the jaws erode the lamina dura around some tooth sockets, cause frank osteolytic defects, and may displace teeth and germinal follicles with tooth buds (Fig. 2.92) (Cockshott, 1965). Views tangential to the surface of flat bones will reveal either 'spiculated' or 'onion layer' types of peri-osteal new bone production (Figs. 2.93–2.96).

In the calvarium diploic deposits cause multiple osteolytic defects which as they enlarge and coalesce can penetrate the outer table and excite periosteal new bone formation and a mass. Suture diastasis raised intracranial

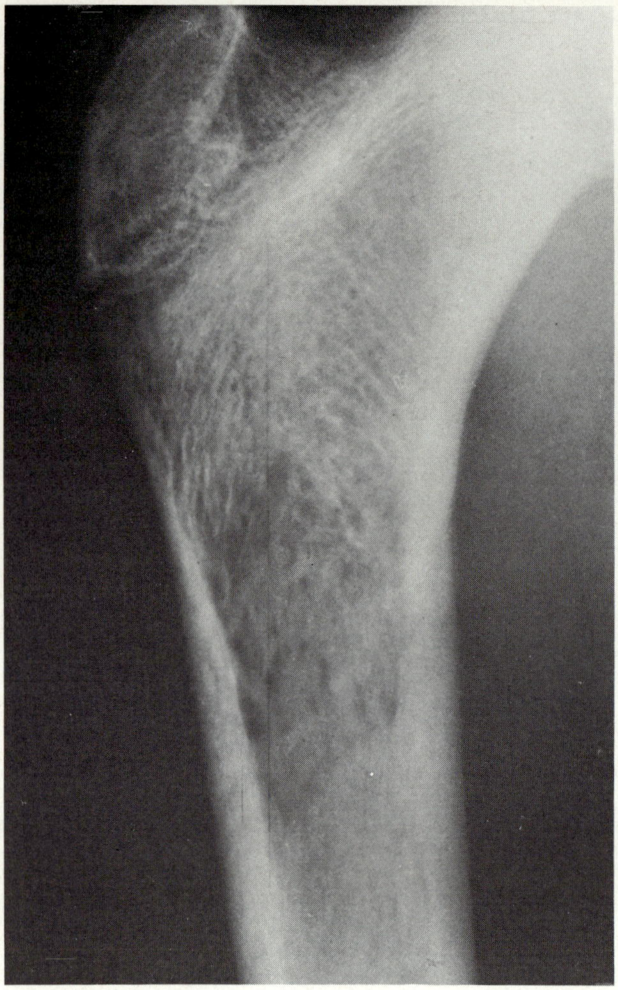

Fig. 2.93 Burkitt's tumour. Permeative bone destruction destroying trabecular structure of femur and eroding cortex.

pressure is normally the result of meningeal and intracerebral perivascular tumour infiltrates. Vertebral and paravertebral foci are discussed in the section on the nervous system.

Because of the nature of the destructive process extending from foci in the marrow, other diseases that behave in a similar fashion may cause diagnostic confusion in an area where Burkitt's lymphoma is frequent. Neuroblastoma marrow metastases can be puzzling, as abdominal masses may also be present as they are in the lymphoma. The multiplicity of foci helps to exclude Ewing's tumour. Histiocytosis X, particularly in younger children with multiple lesions, can be confusing in the early stages of a bone lesion, but in this histiocytic granuloma foci tend to be more locally destructive as the disorder progresses.

Jaw tumours

Jaw tumours are frequent in Africa even if Burkitt's lymphoma is excluded. It has been suggested that as many of the jaw tumours are benign slow-growing lesions, they have accumulated in countries that lack medical facilities; but rate figures suggest that though such a statement accounts for large lesions it does not account for the frequency. In a four-year period in Ibadan, Nigeria, 135 malignant jaw tumours were seen (102 of these were Burkitt lesions) and there were 121 benign jaw tumours (40 per cent ameloblastoma and 50 per cent fibro-osseous lesions) (Anand *et al.*, 1967).

Ameloblastoma comprised 2·5 per cent of all tumours seen in Ibadan, 1·5 per cent in Dakar, 1·3 per cent in the Sudan in comparison with 0·07 per cent for U.S. whites and 0.15 per cent for U.S. blacks.

Ameloblastomas were twice as common in males as in females, and though sometimes seen in adolescence or even earlier were most frequent in the third and fourth decades. Out of 49 tumours only one developed in the upper jaw. The predilection for the lower jaw is seen in all series but not to such an extent in Uganda and South Africa (Anand *et al.*, 1967).

Radiologically these lesions are multilocular expanding destructive process that greatly distort the normal anatomy and displace teeth. An early lesion may appear as a small cyst but more become multilocular with fine septa (Braband, 1965). Some of the trabeculae coursing through a lesion may be thickened in a response to stresses rather than bone infection. In a large lesion the soft tissue component may dominate, with teeth lying in the cellular

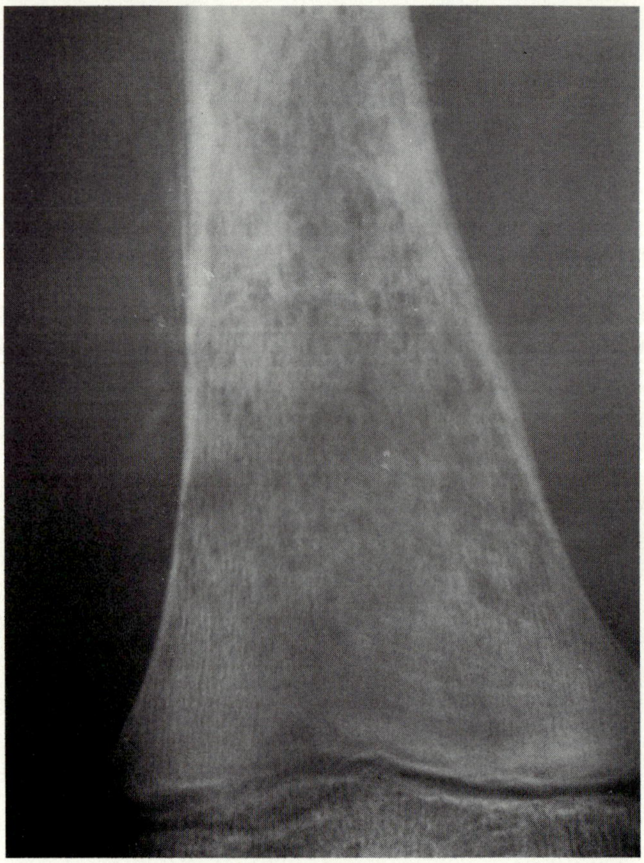

Fig. 2.94 Erosive permeative Burkitt destruction from marrow cavity exciting multilayer lamellated periosteal new bone.

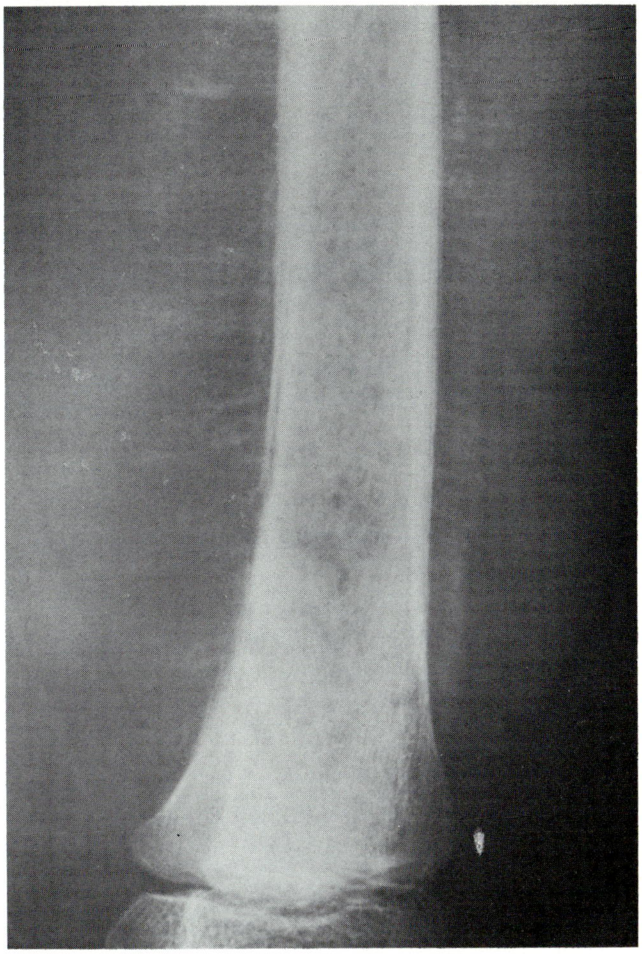

Fig. 2.95 Burkitt's lymphoma leading to periosteal new bone spicules at right angles to diaphysis.

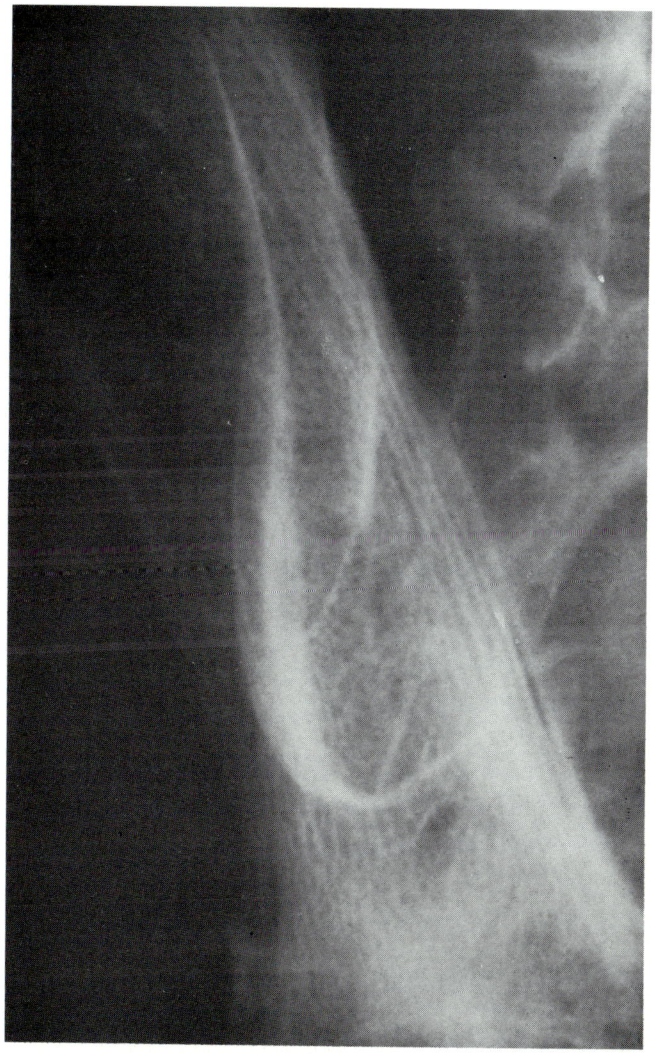

Fig. 2.96 Parallel layers of new bone in tangential view of iliac bone in a case of Burkitt lymphoma. (Kind permission of *British Journal of Radiology*.)

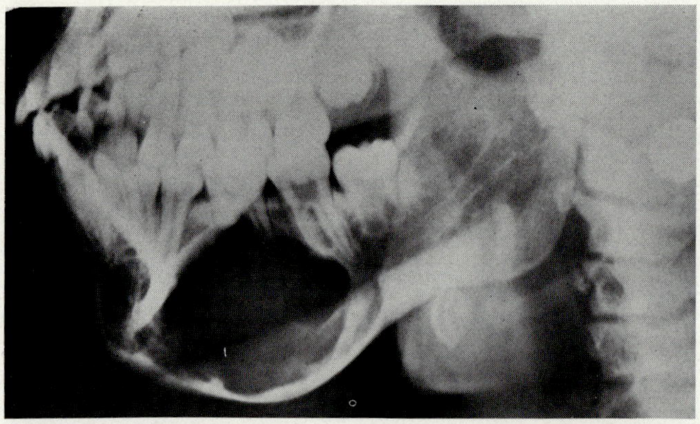

A

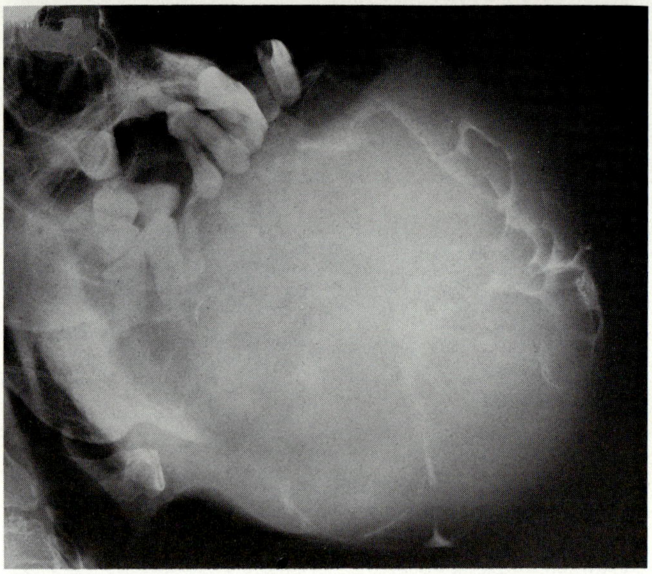

B

Fig. 2.97 **A, B.** Two examples of adamantinoma to show a large expanding cyst which has eroded apices of molar root lower 6 and an enormous multiseptate tumour that has completely distorted dentition.

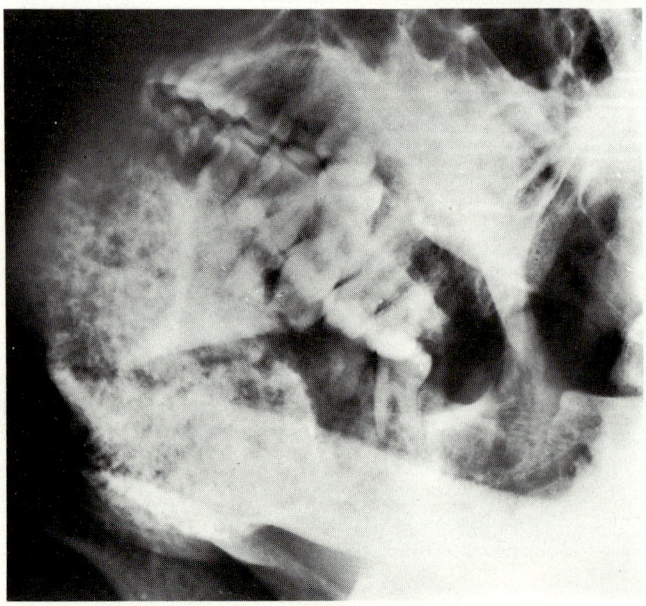

Fig. 2.98 Massive lower jaw fibro-osseous tumour.

matrix without any evidence of a bony tooth socket (Fig. 2.97).

Fibro-osseous lesions of the jaw are a vexing problem in classification and subdivision, not only because of the difficulties of interpretation of histological and radiological features, but because of confusion between tumours and dysplasias, and application of embryological hypotheses to designations. However, there is one type that is usually readily recognised—the ossifying fibroma. Unlike the adamantinoma it is more frequent in females, occurs about a decade earlier and is equally distributed between the upper and lower jaws.

Radiologically the tumours are often well defined externally, as they may have a thin bony capsule or because of calcification in the soft tissues. The calcium is often finely granular but larger amorphous deposits may be seen (Fig. 2.98). Large osteolytic lesions with little calcium can resemble ameloblastomas.

Secondary tumours

In many parts of the tropics where primary liver carcinoma is common bronchial carcinoma is rare. Consequently the relative frequency of the primary tumour responsible for osteolytic metastases may be in this order: hepatoma, renal carcinoma, thyroid neoplasia and then bronchial carcinoma and other cancers (Fig. 2.99).

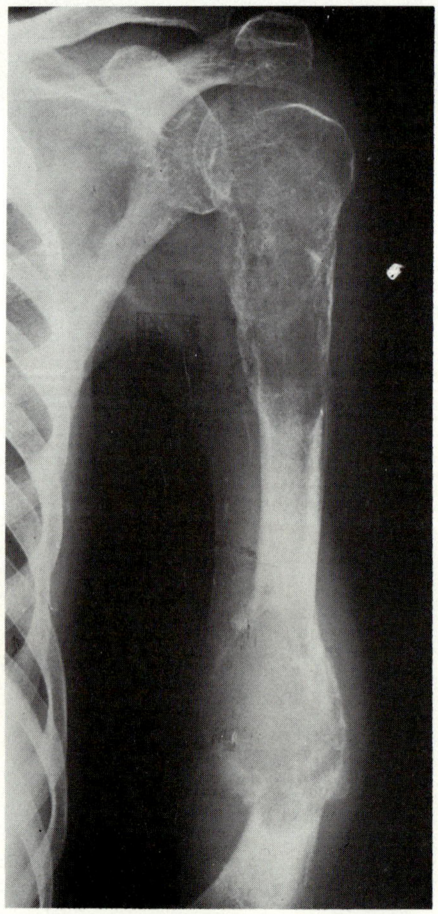

Fig. 2.99 Osteolytic secondary hepatoma.

REFERENCES

Anand, S. U., Davey, W. W. & Cohen, B. (1967) Tumours of the jaw in West Africa, *British Journal of Surgery*, **54,** 901–917.

Braband, H. (1965) Problems der Rontgendiagnostik des Ameloblastoms in West Africa, *Fortschritte Röntgenstrahlen*, **102,** 310–319.

Cockshott, W. P. (1965) Radiological aspects of Burkitt's tumour, *British Journal of Radiology*, **38,** 172–180.

Ramanathan, K. (1972) Burkitt's lymphoma in West Malaysia, *South East Asian Journal Tropical Medicine and Public Health*, **3,** 249–254.

ten Saldam, R. E. J., Cooke, R. & Atkinson, L. (1966) Childhood lymphoma in the territories of Papua and New Guinea, *Cancer*, **19,** 437–446.

SEPTIC ARTHRITIS

S. P. Bohrer

This is primarily a disease of the young in tropical countries, occurring commonly before one year of age. The disordered growth which pyogenic arthritis causes is, perhaps, the most common cause of severe limping in developing countries. The hip and the shoulder are the most frequently involved joints and most cases are secondary to osteomyelitis at these sites, rupturing into the joint. Haematogenous spread from a distant focus of infection also occurs. In the neonate, a septic umbilicus may be the source of infection and in patients with kwashiorkor, skin sepsis may be the site of origin. Multiple joint involvement is also common.

Staphylococcus aureus and pyogenes are frequently the infecting organisms.

Initial clinical findings such as malaise, fever and irritability are non-specific. The earliest radiographic features are widening of the joint space due to fluid and soft tissue swelling with displacement of the peri-articular fat lines, although surrounding oedema often obscures this finding. Osteomyelitis of the adjacent metaphysis may also be evident (Fig. 2.100).

Cartilage and bone destruction develop rapidly. This may be due to ischaemia secondary to the raised pressure within the joint and bacterial enzymes which destroy cartilage. The epiphysis may become completely separated from the metaphysis and can float freely within the joint space or, if the pyo-arthrosis ruptures, the separated epiphysis may migrate out of the joint space (Fig. 2.100). Alternatively, the epiphysis may remain in normal position and the metaphysis may become severely displaced. If treatment begins too late or is inadequate, the ossified epiphysis may disappear radiographically or may appear fragmented. A disappearing epiphysis may later reappear.

Late radiographic manifestations include delay in appearance or non-appearance of the epiphysis, incomplete epiphyseal development, avascular necrosis of the epiphysis, distortion of the femoral neck, coxa vara or valga, pseudo-acetabulum, ankylosis, and growth disturbances such as uneven growth and shortening.

REFERENCE

Kolawole, T. M. & Bohrer, S. P. (1972) Acute septic arthritis in Nigeria, *Tropical and Geographic Medicine*, **24,** 327–338.

Guinea worm arthritis

This process may be initially aseptic, but if secondary pyogenic infection develops the lesion is more serious. Rarely the female worm reaches a joint cavity and deposits larvae within the synovial cavity. A gross synovial effusion forms. Larvae can be found in the aspirated fluid (Reddy & Sivaramappa, 1968; Reddy, 1970) (Figs. 2.101 and 2.102).

Septic arthritis can presumably be a consequence of the events just described, but more frequently follows the death and dissolution of a female close to a joint. In the acute phase the radiological features are merely those of acute arthritis, swelling and oedema, effusion and progressive cartilage and subchondrial bone destruction. It is only later that calcified remnants of Dracunculus become visible close to the joint.

Worms may enter bursae and there fragment and eventually calcify. At other times, a cyst appears to form, containing mobile calcified parasitic fragments. We are not sure whether this is always due to guinea worm or whether a yet undefined parasite can produce a similar appearance.

REFERENCES

Reddy, C. R. R. M. (1970) Pathology of guinea worm synovitis, *Journal of Tropical Medicine and Hygiene*, 73, 28–32.

Reddy, C. R. R. M. & Sivaramappa, M. (1968) Guinea worm arthritis of the knee joint, *British Medical Journal*, **1,** 155–156.

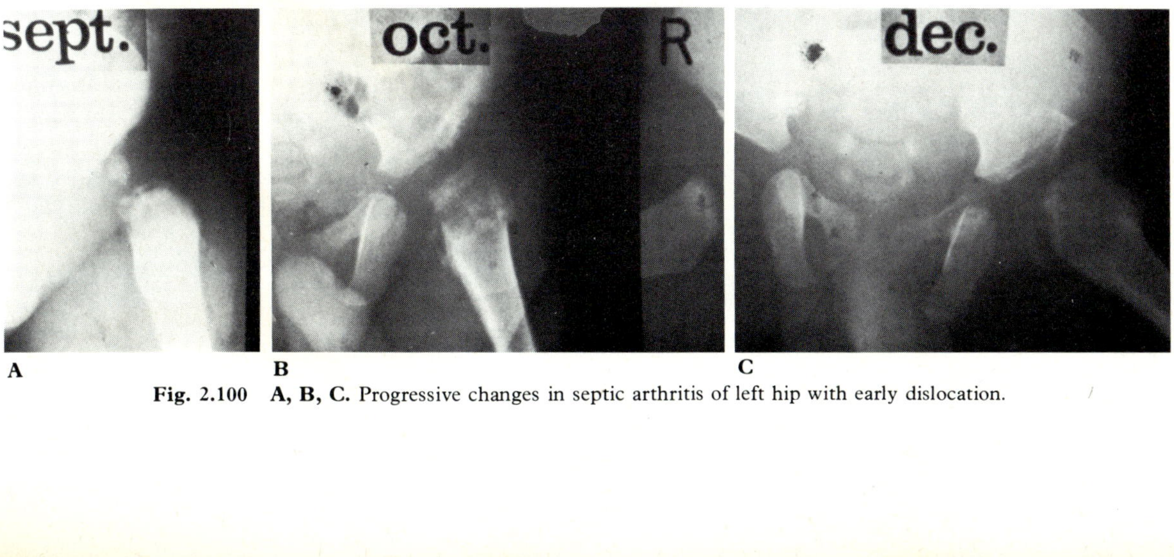

Fig. 2.100 A, B, C. Progressive changes in septic arthritis of left hip with early dislocation.

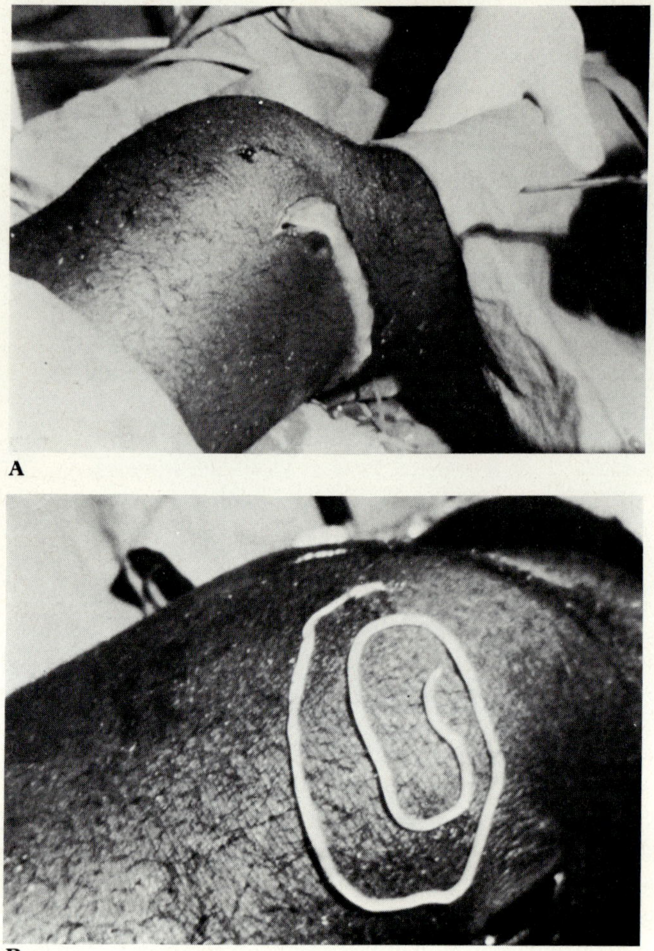

A

B

Fig. 2.101 A, B. Pyogenic arthritis due to guinea worm, showing drainage of pus and worm that was extracted.

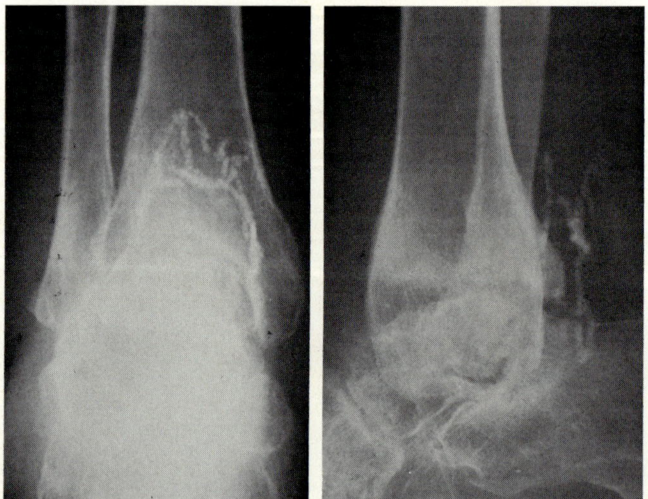

A B

Fig. 2.102 A, B. Old destructive arthritis of ankle due to a long-standing guinea worm joint infection. Note remnants of calcified worms in the soft tissues.

RHEUMATOID ARTHRITIS

S. P. Bohrer

Rheumatoid arthritis is a worldwide disorder, that shows considerable variations in incidence and expression in different parts of the world. Thus the ratio of new rheumatoid arthritis patients to new hospital admissions differs widely, as in England it is 1/125, in Japan 1/167, in Singapore 1/245, in Malaysia 1/638, and in Nigeria 1/2344 (Tay, 1976). Even in the same area in multiracial communities differences in racial frequency are observed. In Singapore the disorder is more frequent in the Chinese than in Malays or Indians.

Clinical accounts from all over sub-saharan Africa emphasise the low incidence of rheumatoid arthritis and the diminished severity of its presentation and evolution in comparison to the disease known in Europe. In Africa it rarely progresses to chronic deformity and crippling polyarthritis, being milder, usually controlled by salicylates, and often proving to be a self-limiting process. In Malaysia and Singapore the disease manifests itself less severely than in temperate climates.

In Africa, the larger joints are involved more commonly than the smaller ones; the wrists being the most common site affected. There it can be severe without manifestations in other joints of the hand. The ankle and knee joints are next in frequency of involvement, followed by the proximal interphalangeal joints and the metacarpophalangeal joints. Often these are normal in radiographs but at worst show only minor marginal erosions in cases with radiological findings.

The many manifestations of small vessel disease such as rheumatoid skin nodules, pulmonary nodules, neuritis and arteritis are not seen in African and Malaysian rheumatoid arthritis (Greenwood, 1969; Toh *et al.*, 1973).

There is much evidence to suggest that the modified form of the disease in Africa is due to altered immunological responses of this population because of chronic malaria and other parasitic infections (McGregor, 1974). In Nigeria it has been found that normal controls have high levels of IgG and IgM immunoglobulins relative to levels in developed countries. They also have high levels of heterophile antibody and rheumatoid factor. These levels decrease when the African lives in a developed country or regularly takes anti-malarial medication. Blacks in America have levels similar to Whites in America and rheumatoid arthritis like Whites in America. The rheumatoid factor is not helpful for diagnostic assessment in Nigeria, as it is no higher in Nigerians with rheumatoid arthritis fulfilling the criteria of the American Rheumatism Association, than in healthy controls (Greenwood, 1968; Greenwood & Herrick, 1970). In Malaysia tests for RF factor are higher in cases than in the general population but still lower than for R.A. cases in temperate climates (Toh *et al.*, 1973).

REFERENCES

Greenwood, B. M. (1968) Autoimmune disease and parasitic infections in Nigerians, *Lancet*, **2**, 380–382.

Greenwood, B. M. (1969) Polyarthritis in Western Nigeria. I. Rheumatoid arthritis, *Annals of Rheumatic Diseases*, **28**, 488–495.

Greenwood, B. M. & Herrick, E. M. (1970) Low incidence of rheumatoid factor and autoantibodies in Nigerian patients with rheumatoid arthritis, *British Medical Journal*, **1**, 71–73.

McGregor, I. A. (1974) Immunity and malaria in man, *Tropical Doctor*, **4**, 104–109.

Tay, C. H. (1976) Rheumatoid arthritis in Singapore, a clinical study, *Singapore Medical Journal*, **17**, 160–166.

Toh, B. H., Sengupta, S., Ang, A. H., White, J. C. & Lau, K. S. (1973) Pattern of rheumatoid arthritis in West Malaysia, *Annals of Rheumatic Diseases*, **32**, 151–156.

ACUTE TROPICAL POLYARTHRITIS

S. P. Bohrer

An acute form of non-specific, non-migratory polyarthritis is seen in Africa. Primarily large joints are involved; the knees, ankles, wrists, elbows and shoulders. Patients have an elevated sedimentation rate and may be febrile. There is no eosinophilia. X-rays are normal or merely reveal evidence of some soft tissue swelling. No bone changes are seen. Laboratory tests for specific arthridities such as uric acid estimations, A.S.O. titres, etc. are not helpful.

The disease usually resolves in several weeks with salicylate therapy only.

The etiology is, at present, unknown. It may turn out to be a viral arthritis as did O'Nyong-Nyong fever in East Africa or possibly an allergic manifestation to another infection.

REFERENCE

Greenwood, B. M. (1969) Acute tropical polyarthritis, *Quarterly Journal of Medicine*, **38**, 295–306.

3. Alimentary System

CANCRUM ORIS

Cancrum oris is a gangrenous ulcerative, mutilating condition of the mouth which extends to the soft tissue of the lips, nose and cheek and causes dreadful disfigurement and severe disability in eating, drinking and retaining saliva. It is seen in debilitated or malnourished children of two to five years of age. These children have often just suffered from a severe infection such as measles.

Cancrum begins suddenly in the molar or premolar area and rapidly spreads to a line of demarcation and then subsides. In the acute stage Vincent's organisms can be recovered but it is doubtful if they are the initiators of the ulcerating destructive process. Bone of the alveolar ridge, palate, antra, orbit may be exposed but the soft tissue destruction is extensive and greater, often reaching the tonsillar area and the tissues around the tempero-mandibular joint. Healing of ulcers, once the sloughs have separated, is rapid but leaves appalling visible tissue defects and, of as great consequence, invisible areas of extensive fibrosis.

Radiology is of little value in the early stages. Later, once healing has taken place, it will indicate if any bone has sequestrated. It is particularly useful to display fully the mandible, palate and the alveolar ridge tooth-bearing areas. Though these can be seen clinically, the full extent of loss of developing, erupting teeth, secondary dentition and germinal follicles can be better assessed radiographically. Dental disturbances, if allowed to take their course, result in such severe alterations that the Dakar workers have used the apt phrase of 'anarchie dentaire' to signify their inability to describe the situation which they have now classified (Reynaud *et al.*, 1974). Another factor that is of concern to the plastic surgeon is the inability to move the jaw. Cicatricial fibrosis is the main element in the trismus but radiological study of the tempero-mandibular joint will show whether it is deformed or ankylosed. Bone may form within the fibrous tissue in the pterygoids, masseter or temporalis muscles to produce a form of myositis ossificans. Because of the abnormal cicatricial tethering stress on the growing jaw, various malformations may develop. The mandible on the affected side may become hypoplastic with mandibular recession and there may be compensatory hypertrophy of the coronoid process (Lagundoye & Oluwasanmi, 1975). Septic arthritis may have destroyed the temporo-mandibular joint. Tomographic study is often of value in elucidating the radiographic changes in these children who have limited jaw mobility. Cancrum auris is occasionally seen and then the T.M. joints are usually implicated.

Cancrum is preventable. When it develops it poses severe nutritional, surgical, and social problems. These can be overcome within a plastic surgery service, as has been shown by Michael Tempest (1971).

REFERENCES

Lagundoye, S. B. & Oluwasanmi, J. O. (1975) Radiologic examination of trismus as a complication of cancrum oris, *Oral Surgery, Oral Medicine, Oral Pathology*, **39**, 812–820.

Reynaud, J., Diop, L. S. & Medji, L. A. (1974) Les types anatomocliniques des gangrènes par noma et de leur séquelles, *Bulletin et Mémoires de la Faculté de Médecine de Dakar*, **22**, 44–49.

Tempest, M. N. (1971) Cancrum oris, *Tropical Doctor*, **1**, 164–169.

CHAGASIC MEGA-OESOPHAGUS

It has been known for many years that in endemic areas of Chagas' disease there were a large number of patients with mega-oesophagus. From two towns in Minas Gerais state of Brazil with populations under 50 000, 1514 and 2000 cases of mega-oesophagus have been published. In another part of Brazil 85 per cent of patients with mega-oesophagus had a positive complement fixation test (Andrade & Andrade, 1971). Conversely a very high proportion of patients with antibodies to T. cruzi by the Machado–Guerreiro reaction have disturbed oesophageal motility (Brasil, 1955; Ferreira-Santos, 1961).

Mega-oesophagus at autopsy show a few or no ganglion cells in Auerbach's parasympathetic myenteric plexus, and patients dying of chronic Chagas' disease without mega-oesophagus invariably have a reduction in nerve cells (Koberle, 1963). Whether this process is due to a cytotoxin released by the disruption of leishmanoid trypanasomes or by an auto-antibody process is not agreed. The parasite favours muscle, so that in addition the oesophageal wall may have a focal myositis that contributes to the motility disturbances. The wall of the oesophagus gradually hypertrophies, suggesting that the unbalanced autonomic activity leads to obstructive increase in tone of the lower oesophagus as well as to the aperistalsis. Nevertheless as the condition progresses and the dilated redundant oesophagus attains grotesque proportions, with a capacity of several litres, the distended wall is ultimately thinned.

The incidence of this condition in Chagas' disease is variable, but figures as high as 30 per cent have been reported for patients in the chronic phase.

Koberle believes that the stasis may lead to oesophageal cancer, as such an association was present in 10 per cent of autopsy cases (Hutt *et al.*, 1973; Camara-Lopes, 1961).

Radiologically the earliest changes are disturbances of motility with poor peristaltic stripping waves and hold-up at the cardio-oesophageal junction. In asymptomatic cases this is all that may be evident. Gradually the hold-up becomes more marked and there are often food residues. The oesophagus slowly becomes dilated and because of retained food and fluid it is visible as a retrocardiac density. In gross cases the oesophagus begins to overlap the right heart border and is visible up into the upper mediastinum.

However, a concomitant cardiomegaly may conceal a large oesophagus in a poorly penetrated anterior film.

Chest apparatus has been used in a crude screening way to assess the amount of oesophageal problem in a community. A more penetrated film than usual is taken and films are obtained after a liquid barium swallow at the end of swallowing and at three, five and thirty minutes. A typical positive response is illustrated (Fig. 3.1).

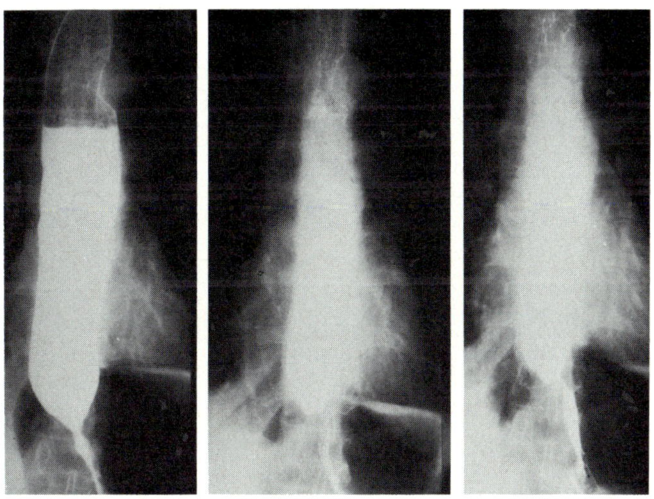

A B C

Fig. 3.1 A, B, C. Chagasic mega-oesophagus. Films were obtained erect immediately after swallowing, at five minutes and half an hour. The dilatation and considerable emptying delay are demonstrated. (Courtesy of Prof. L. Prata, Bahia, Brazil.)

REFERENCES

Brasil, A. (1956) Etiopatogenia da aperistalsis do esôfago, *Revista Brasilia Medica*, **13**, 577–590.

Camara-Lopes, L. H. (1961) Carcinoma of the oesophagus as a complication of megaesophagus, *American Journal of Digestive Diseases*, **6**, 742–756.

Ferreira-Santos, R. (1961) Aperistalsis of the oesophagus and colon (megaoesophagus–megacolon) etiologically related to Chagas' disease, *American Journal of Digestive Diseases*, **6**, 700–726.

Hutt, M. S. R., Koberle, F. & Salfelder, K. (1973) In *Tropical Pathology*. p. 394. ed. Spencer, H. Heidelberg: Springer.

Koberle, F. (1963). Enteromegaly and cardiomegaly in Chagas' disease, *Gut*, **4**, 399–405.

CORROSIVE OESOPHAGEAL STRICTURES

Accidental ingestion is a much more frequent cause of caustic oesophagitis than suicidal attempts. For various local industrial and domestic needs, clear acid or lye may be kept in unlabelled bottles, or with the same result a labelled bottle is picked up by an illiterate. As a rule children are the unfortunate victims. Lye may be kept for making soap or dyeing indigo, whilst acid is used for car batteries, by goldsmiths, and in rubber plantations (Durenne & Navigue, 1972).

Initially there are obvious peroral burns and involvement of the larynx, oesophagus and stomach. The burnt surface is denuded so that repair is by granulation tissue. This inevitably results in stricture formation.

In the acute stage radiologic investigation beyond a chest film is generally unnecessary. There may be aspiration changes in the lungs which being chemical in type can lead to severe alveolar type consolidation. Free perforation of the oesophagus or stomach rarely occurs but oesophago-tracheal fistulae, usually at the level of the carina, is a complication which is demonstrable by barium studies. Because of pain on swallowing at this semi-acute stage it may be difficult to obtain patient co-operation. The oesophagus is of generally reduced calibre at this stage due to spasm, and because of the small amount of barium swallowed there is no bolus distension. This should not be confused with strictures which occur later. The usual site is just below the carina. If the stricture is tight, dilatation of the upper segment is marked. This dilatation may be asymmetric with the narrow distal portion continuing eccentrically (Fig. 3.2).

Lesions of the stomach may develop, particularly with acid corrosives (Fig. 3.3). These are usually combined with oesophageal lesions. Antral strictures with pyloric obstruction can develop as rapidly as four weeks (Lambeth & Somasundram, 1970).

Following bouginage or other instrumentation, oesophageal perforation may occur with development of midiastinitis, pleural effusions or pyopneumothorax. Well-penetrated chest films can then be of great assistance.

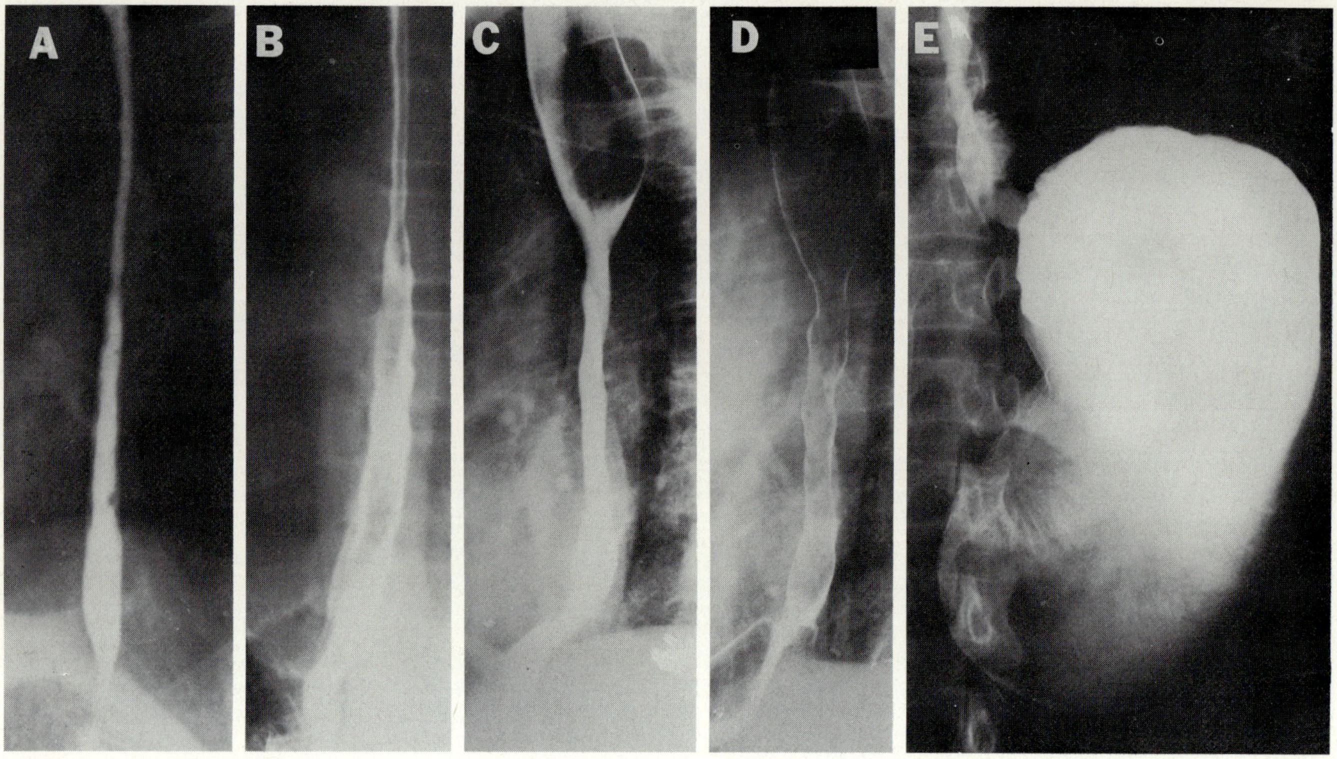

Fig. 3.2 Corrosive strictures. **A** and **B** show very long narrow stricture in single and double contrast. **C**, **D** and **E** are from another patient who had both a considerable oesophageal corrosive stricture and also gastric outlet obstruction from extensive caustic scarring. (Courtesy of Prof. H. E. Engelbrecht, Durban.)

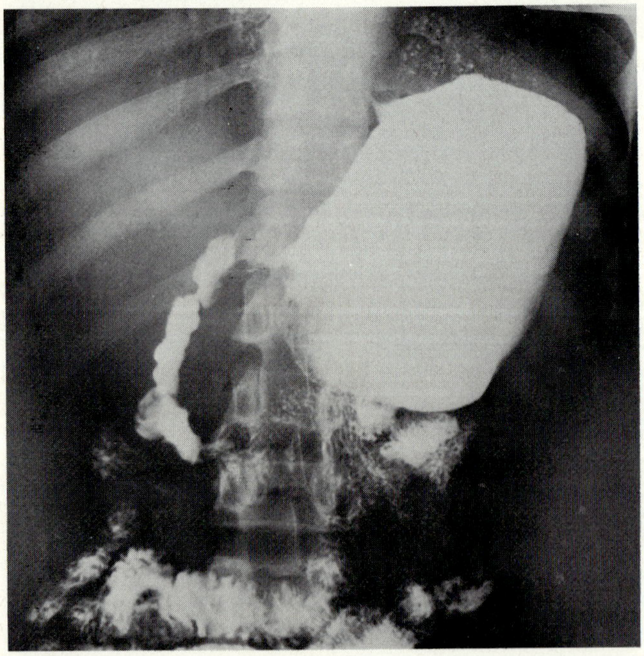

Fig. 3.3 Gastric outlet obstruction from swallowed corrosive. (Courtesy of Prof. S. P. Bohrer.)

REFERENCES

Durenne, J. M. & Navigué, C. (1974) Propos sur les brulures caustique de l'œsophage chez l'enfant Africain, *Annales de la Société Belge de Médecine Tropicale*, **52,** 499–500.

Lambeth, J. T. & Somasundram, K. (1970) Pyloric obstruction due to formic acid ingestion, *Medical Journal of Malaya*, **24,** 187–189.

PEPTIC ULCERATION

The radiological features of peptic ulcer in some areas of the tropics differ from the disorder described in standard textbooks in the location and complications of ulcers.

It is not known whether the high proportion of ulcers found in barium studies in some communities indicates wise selection of patients where radiological facilities are scarce or overburdened, or whether the figures merely reflect a high prevalence of ulceration in the population. Thus in Nigeria in one series 49 per cent of barium meals on referrals had ulcers, and in Southern India 32 per cent of those examined showed an ulcer (Paterson & Hancock, 1960). In a prospective autopsy investigation 15 per cent of Ugandan males and 4·7 per cent of females showed evidence of present ulceration or scars of previous active disease (Raper, 1958).

Duodenal ulcers are much more frequent than gastric ulcers in most tropical communities (Table 3.1). The duodenal ulcers are typically posterior wall and close to the apex of the bulb. They show a marked tendency to scar excessively and so obstructive symptoms are common. By contrast perforation is most infrequent, perhaps due to the location of the ulcer. Haemorrhage is also seen much less often than in Europe.

The technique of study obviously can influence diagnostic yield. With double contrast barium meals far more higher lesser curve and fundal gastric ulcers are detected. However, the magnitude of the difference in incidence between D.U.s and G.U.s, as well as surgical experience, indicate that variations in incidence in different areas are not spurious. Perhaps contrary to expectations, in much of the tropics the disease is primarily a disorder of the rural population.

The extensive scarring shortens and deforms tissues, so that at times the precise location of an ulcer can be difficult to define (Paterson & Hancock, 1958). A relatively high proportion of post-bulbar ulcers have been recorded from Southern India and various parts of Africa.

Table 3.1 Duodenal to gastric ulcer ratio

Predominant D.U.	
Cameroons	155–1 S
Nigeria, Lagos	123–1 S
Zanzibar	108–1 S
Morocco	90–1 S
Dahomey	60–1 S
India, Mysore	64–1 R
Uganda, Kampala	49–1 R
India, Madras	20–1 S
Ghana, Accra	17–1 R
Ivory Coast, Abidjan	17–1 R
Senegal, Dakar	14–1 R
Kenya, Nairobi	12–1 R
Scotland, Glasgow	12–1 R
Tanzania, Dar-es-Salaam	7–1 R
Rhodesia, Bulawayo	6–1 S
England, Plymouth	1·4–1 R (D.C.)
New Zealand	1–1 R (D.C.)
Predominant G.U.	
Peru (light altitude)	1–21
Turkey & Chile	1–12
Rwanda	1–11 S
Rwanda	1– 4 R
New Guinea, Goroka	1– 4 R
Autopsy series	
Uganda	6·6–1
Scotland	2–1
Java (Chinese)	1–2
Javanese	2–1

Letters R indicate radiological series; S, surgical and (D.C.) double contrast studies.

(Data from Dempster, 1957; Payet *et al.*, 1959; Konstam, 1959; Bretland, 1961; Cleave, 1962; Tovey, 1972, 1974; Hamber & Von Bergen, 1973; Ghoti, 1974; Djedje & Lesquerre, 1974; Sims, 1974; Wagner, 1975; Stevenson, 1977.)

Gas in the biliary tree is sometimes noted (Fig. 3.4). This is usually the result of an ulcer perforating into the common bile duct (Fig. 3.5) (Barton & Cockshott, 1961; Pineau *et al.*, 1962; Lewis & Bohrer, 1969). Barium usually spontaneously displays the biliary tree as the fistula is widely patent. Less often barium may reflux through a sphincter of Oddi rendered incompetent by the extensive cicatrisation seen in this disease (Pineau *et al.*, 1962).

In most of the world gastric ulcers occur less often than duodenal ulcers, but in a few areas the reverse is true. In an area in Rwanda and around lake Kivu in Zaire, gastric ulcer is seen eleven times more often than duodenal (Hamber & Von Bergen, 1973). Gastric ulcer is three times more frequent than duodenal in Goroka in the New

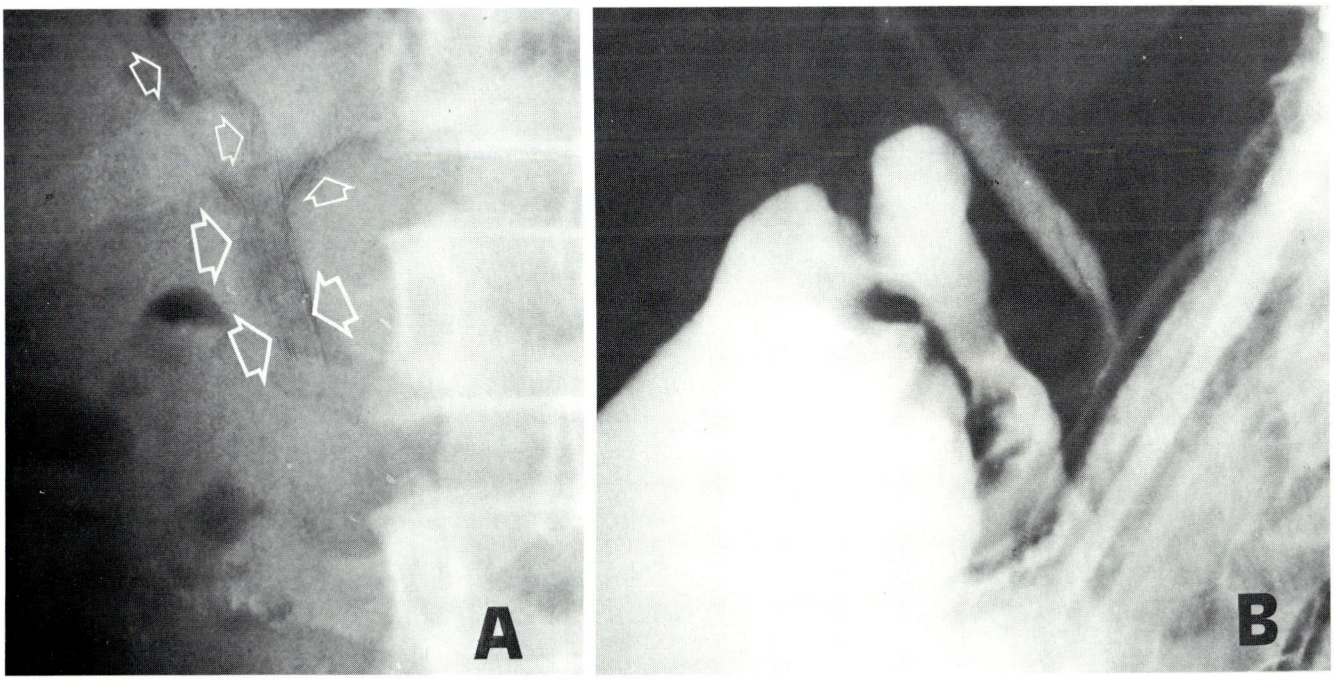

Fig. 3.4 **A.** Plain film shows gas in biliary tree. **B.** Barium is seen to outline the common bile duct in this patient with a post-bulbar ulcer. In this instance the papilla and sphincter have been rendered incompetent by scarring.

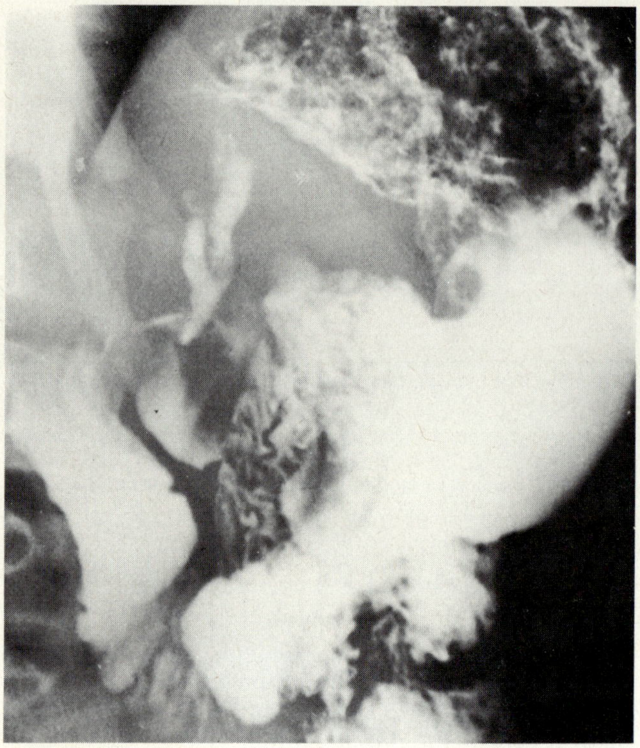

Fig. 3.5 Duodenal ulcer perforating into common bile duct.

Guinea highlands, whereas in adjacent low-lying Papua gastric ulcers are only slightly more frequent than duodenal, and then only in males (Wagner, 1975; Muirden, 1976).

The relation of ulcers to stress is no clearer in the tropics than elsewhere. In a careful study in Johannesburg it was found that duodenal ulcers were more frequent in urbanised better educated individuals than in matched controls (Segal *et al.*, 1978). Such studies are difficult to design and undertake, but it would be of interest if the findings were confirmed in other settings of working-class mobility.

REFERENCES

Barton, C. J. & Cockshott, W. P. (1961) Post bulbar duodenal ulceration in Nigeria, *British Journal of Radiology*, **34,** 216–220.

Bretland, P. (1961) Personal communication, Accra, Ghana.

Dempster, W. H. (1957) Radiological survey of gastro-intestinal lesions during a twelve month period at the Southern General Hospital, Glasgow, *British Journal of Radiology*, **30,** 31–34.

Djedje, A. T. & Lesquerre, C. L. (1974) Bilan statistique de 6 ans de radiologie digestive au CHU de Treichville, *Annales de l'Université d'Abidjan*, **8,** 116–121.

Fraser-Ross, W. & Harington, L. P. 1963) Geographical pathology—Central Africa, *Clinical Radiology*, **14,** 187–192.

Ghoti, M. (1974) Notre attitude dans le traitement de l'ulcère gastroduodenal, *Journal de Médicine du Maroc*, **10,** 161–163.

Hamber, G. & Von Bergen, M. (1973) Gastric ulcer in tropical Africa, *Tropical and Geographic Medicine*, **25,** 1–7.

Konstam, P. G. (1959) Peptic ulcer in India, *Indian Journal of Medical Sciences*, **13,** 486–492.

Lewis, E. A. & Bohrer, S. P. (1969) Choledochoduodenal fistula complicating chronic duodenal ulcer, *Gut*, **10,** 146–149.

Muirden, J. C. (1976) A radiological survey of upper gastrointestinal lesions in Port Moresby, *Papua and New Guinea Medical Journal*, **19,** 149–152.

Paterson, D. E. & Hancock, D. M. (1958) Duodenal stenosis due to postbulbar ulcer. A comparison of radiological and surgical findings, *British Journal of Radiology*, **31,** 660–665.

Payet, M., Pellegrino, A. & D'Assomption, U. (1959) Un an de radiologie gastro-duodénale en milieu Africain à Dakar, *Bulletin de la Société Médecine d'Afrique Noire*, **4,** 369–390.

Pineau, P., Serafino, X. & Pouye, I. (1962) Signification de l'opacification spontanéee des voies bilaires en radiologie gastroduodenale, *Bulletin de la Société Médecine d'Afrique Noire*, **7,** 127–136.

Raper, A. B. (1958) The incidence of peptic ulceration in some African tribal groups, *Transactions of the Royal Society of Tropical Medicine and Hygiene*, **52,** 535–546.

Segal, I., Dubb, A. A., Ou Tim, L., Solomon, A., Sottomayor, M. C. C. G. & Zwame, E. M. (1978) Duodenal ulcer and working class mobility in an African population in South Africa, *British Medical Journal*, **1,** 469–472.

Stevenson, G. (1978) Personal communication, Hamilton, Canada.

Tovey, F. I. (1972) Duodenal ulceration in Mysore, characteristics and aetiological factors, *Tropical and Geographic Medicine*, **24,** 107–117.

Tovey, F. I. (1974) The geographical distribution and possible factors in the aetiology of peptic ulcer, *Tropical Doctor*, **4,** 17–21.

Wagner, F. (1975) Incidence of peptic ulcer in Goroka 1973–74, *Papua New Guinea Medical Journal*, **18,** 45.

INFECTIVE AND INFLAMMATORY LESIONS

Anisakiasis

Anisakiasis is an infection of the gastro-intestinal tract by Anisakis marina, a parasite that passes its adult stage in whales, dolphins, porpoises and possibly seals, and a larval stage in many species of fish, including the herring, mackerel, cod, salmon, haddock and pollack. The larvae lie in the fish's peritoneum but, if not promptly gutted, they migrate into the muscles.

The initial cases described from Holland (Kuipers *et al.*, 1960) had eaten lightly salted infected herring, whilst most Japanese cases resulted from having Sashimi—a raw fish dish. A case has been reported from Honolulu (Ashby *et al.*, 1964). In Thailand, where raw fish is a popular dish, parasitism by gnathostomiasis is a more common disorder. According to Petter (1969) a sardine nematode of Thynnascaris species is responsible for an eosinophilic granuloma in man seen in Brittany. These facts indicate that the full nature and extent of this type of disorder is still inadequately known.

Common to all these parasitisms are the histological features. Some parts of the alimentary tract show an oedematous connective tissue stroma diffusely infiltrated with eosinophils in the submucosa and possibly extending through the muscle layer to the muscularis mucosae and even to the serosa. The mucosa itself is intact except for a minute aperture where a worm may be gaining entry to the deeper tissues.

The worms are about 1 mm in diameter and 15 to 28 mm long. It is believed that the eosinophilic phlegmon is a hyperergic reaction to the presence of the larva in an individual who has become sensitised by a previous exposure (Kuipers, 1964).

The location of lesions differs somewhat in the Dutch cases with predominant ileal disease, whereas in 92 Japanese patients the site of greatest involvement was the stomach and the ileum was implicated in only 30 per cent (Yokogawa & Yoshimura, 1967).

Clinically the gastric cases present subacutely with features of recent onset suggestive of peptic ulcer or gastric malignancy. Those with small bowel disease have a

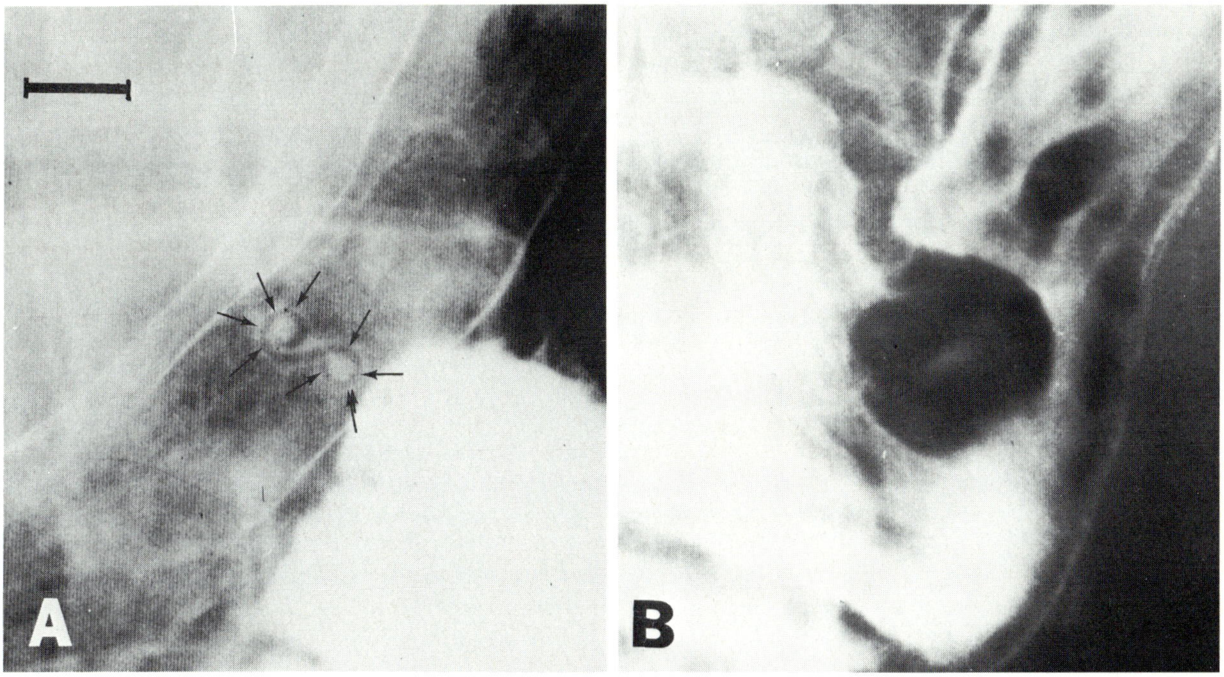

Fig. 3.6 Thirty-four-year-old female with recent abdominal pain and vomiting. In **A** an anisakiasis worm is shown by double contrast. In **B** a well-defined eosinophilic antral phlegmon has caused an intramural inflammatory mass. (Courtesy of Dr. Masayoshi Namiki.)

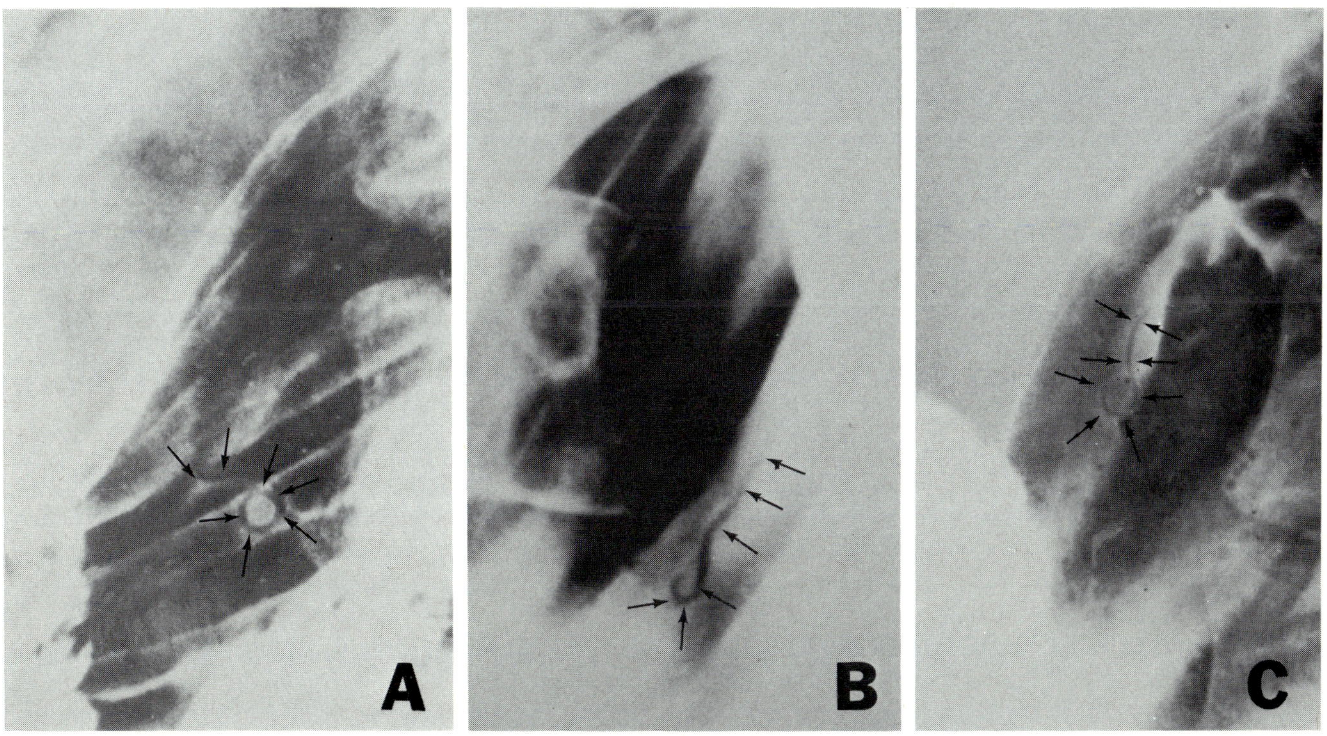

Fig. 3.7 Anasikiasis worms in double contrast barium meals. **A** and **B** is stomach of 54-year-old female who had eaten cod fish sashimi six hours before. **C** was a 33-year-old female who had two days of epigastric distress and vomiting after eating raw mackerel. The worms were removed by fibre optic endoscopy. (Courtesy of Dr. Kazuo Nagano and Dr. Tatsuya Yamada.)

more acute onset with obstructive elements or with appendiceal symptomatology.

Stool testing is of little value. A mild eosinophilia is present.

The radiological findings can be difficult to interpret but on occasions barium studies can provide an almost definitive diagnosis.

In the stomach a submucosal mass lesion with an intact but stretched mucosa can be shown. This is most often in the body of the stomach but the antrum and pylorus are involved in about a quarter of the gastric cases. In a double contrast study, in addition to the intramural mass, a worm may be outlined (Figs. 3.6 and 3.7).

The ileal lesions, particularly if in the terminal portion, show segmental narrowing that can be difficult to differentiate from Crohn's disease or Yersinia infections (Richman & Lewicki, 1973). The intact mucosa may help to eliminate the former possibility.

Biopy of lesions and removal of worms by endoscopy has been carried out in Japan (Nagano, 1977).

REFERENCES

Ashby, B. S., Appleton, P. J. & Davison, I. (1964) Eosinophilic granuloma of gastrointestinal tract caused by herring parasite Eustoma rotundatum, *British Medical Journal*, **1**, 1114–1145.

Kuipers, F. C., Van Thiel, P. H., Rodenburg, W., Wielinga, W. J. & Roskam, R. Th. (1960) Eosinophilic phlegmon of the alimentary canal caused by a worm, *Lancet* **2**, 1171–1173.

Kuipers, F. C. (1964) Eosinophilic phlegmonous inflammation of the alimentary canal caused by a parasite from the herring, *Pathologia et Microbiologia*, **27**, 925–930.

Petter, A. M. (1969) Enquête sur les nématodes des Poissons de la région Nantaise, *Annales de Parasitologie*, **44**, 559–580.

Richman, R. H. & Lewicki, A. M. (1973) Right ileo colitis secondary to anisakiasis, *American Journal of Roentgenology*, **119**, 329–331.

Yokogawa, M. & Yoshimura, H. (1967) Clinico pathologic studies on larval anisakiasis in Japan, *American Journal of Tropical Medicine and Hygiene*, **16**, 723–728.

Nagano, K. (1977) Personal communication, Hokkaido, Japan.

HOOKWORM
ANKYLOSTOMA DUODENALE
NECATOR AMERICANUS

Though A. duodenale was once predominantly found in Europe and the Middle East and N. americanus in America and Africa, they are now both so widespread that the former geographic boundaries have become blurred. The infection can be a serious cause of iron deficiency anaemia through chronic blood loss. Each worm when attached to the duodenal or jejunal mucosa pumps through its digestive tract between 0·03 ml (N. americanus) to 0·34 ml (A. duodenals) of blood a day. Since there may be hundreds of worms it is obvious that serious consequences can sometimes develop. It has been clearly shown that the degree of anaemia is dependent on the iron content of the diet, the state of the iron reserves, and the duration and intensity of the infection (Gilles *et al.*, 1964). Where the iron content of the diet is low, as in Mauritius, a small worm load will be serious, whereas in Nigeria a state of haemostasis can be maintained with as many as 800 worms, since food contains a lot of iron.

The adult worms measure under 1 cm and are attached to the villi of the upper small bowel. The site of attachment does not ulcerate or bleed except through the alimentary tract of the worm.

Infection is acquired from soil contaminated by stools containing ova. These ova hatch a larva which undergoes moults in the soil to become a filariform larva that can pierce the skin of man to enter small vessels and be carried by the venous system to the lungs. There they then reach the alveoli and passively reach the bronchi, pass up the trachea, down the epiglottis to reach the small bowel one day to a week after penetrating the skin. After some further maturation they copulate and the female discharges large quantities of ova.

Many radiological changes have been attributed to hookworm infection. The most severe is anaemia. Radiologically this can manifest itself by a high output failure and dilated heart (discussed in cardiac section) and by the development of a hyperplastic marrow that expands the medullary cavity of bones. The combination of anaemia, and the sometimes associated folic acid deficiency, contribute to delay in the skeletal maturation of children.

The gastro-intestinal changes have often been commented upon, but like Rowland we doubt their specificity (Rowland, 1966).

Patients with heavy worm burdens are not only anaemic but also can have hypo-albuminaemia due to the protein as well as iron loss from the parasites. This can cause nonspecific swelling of the upper bowel mucosa. Peptic ulceration and duodenitis do not appear to be related to hookworm. Probably the malabsorption pattern described in barium studies of patients with hookworm are attributable to the hypo-albuminaemia. Histologically and by gross pathology no changes have been demonstrated in the bowel apart from the minute portion of mucosa sucked into the parasites' buccal apparatus. Further, careful metabolic studies have not revealed malabsorption in hookworm patients (Da Costa, 1971).

Exceptionally a worm can migrate through the bowel wall to cause a localised abscess (Elmes & McAdam, 1954).

In conclusion we believe that barium studies are of no value in the investigation of hookworm infection unless some concurrent condition is a diagnostic possibility, since the infection *per se* does not give rise to any specific changes. The majority of individuals with hookworm have no symptoms and are not anaemic.

REFERENCES

Da Costa, L. R. (1971) Small intestinal cell turnover in patients with parasitic infections, *British Medical Journal*, **3**, 281–283.

Elmes, B. G. T. & McAdam, I. W. J. (1954) Helminthic abscess, a surgical complication of oesophagostomes and hookworms, *Annals of Tropical Medicine and Parasitology*, **48**, 1–7.

Gilles, H. M., Watson-Williams, E. J. & Ball, P. A. J. (1964) Hookworm infection and anaemia, *Quarterly Journal of Medicine*, **33**, 1–24.
Rowland, H. A. K. (1966) Dyspepsia, duodenitis and hookworm infection, *Transactions of the Royal Society of Tropical Medicine and Hygiene*, **60**, 481–485.

STRONGYLOIDIASIS OF THE ALIMENTARY (TRACT)

Strongyloides stercoralis is a widespread nematode in the warmer climates in the Far East, Africa, India, South and Central America, Northern Australia and New Guinea, and the Caribbean. It occurs in temperate zones and high incidences have been reported from institutions for the mentally deprived. The incidence in some population groups may be high but clinical presentations directly attributable to an infestation are scanty. Nevertheless there is no doubt that the parasitism can be responsible for chronic ill health and severe disease. Usually the organism causes gastro-intestinal symptomatology but it can produce protean manifestations in patients who are debilitated, have an altered immune state, or are receiving corticosteroid therapy. The pulmonary manifestations are described elsewhere.

In a clinical study Jones (1950) found that the most common symptom was upper abdominal discomfort and pain in nearly 80 per cent of his patients. Nausea, weight loss, vomiting and diarrhoea were, in descending order, the next most frequent features. A sprue-like syndrome with malabsorption and atrophic jejunal villi is a recognised manifestation, though some workers consider that the malabsorption syndrome is usually due to concomitant malnutrition rather than to the parasite itself (Bartholomew *et al.*, 1977; Garcia *et al.*, 1977). Paralytic ileus and obstructive symptoms have been well documented by several authors (Louisy & Barton, 1971; Cookson *et al.*, 1972).

S. stercoralis is an unusual parasite in that it can pass a sexual stage outside of a host in warm moist ground. However, the usual cycle is for rhabditiform larvae passed in the stool to the soil to moult into the filariform infective

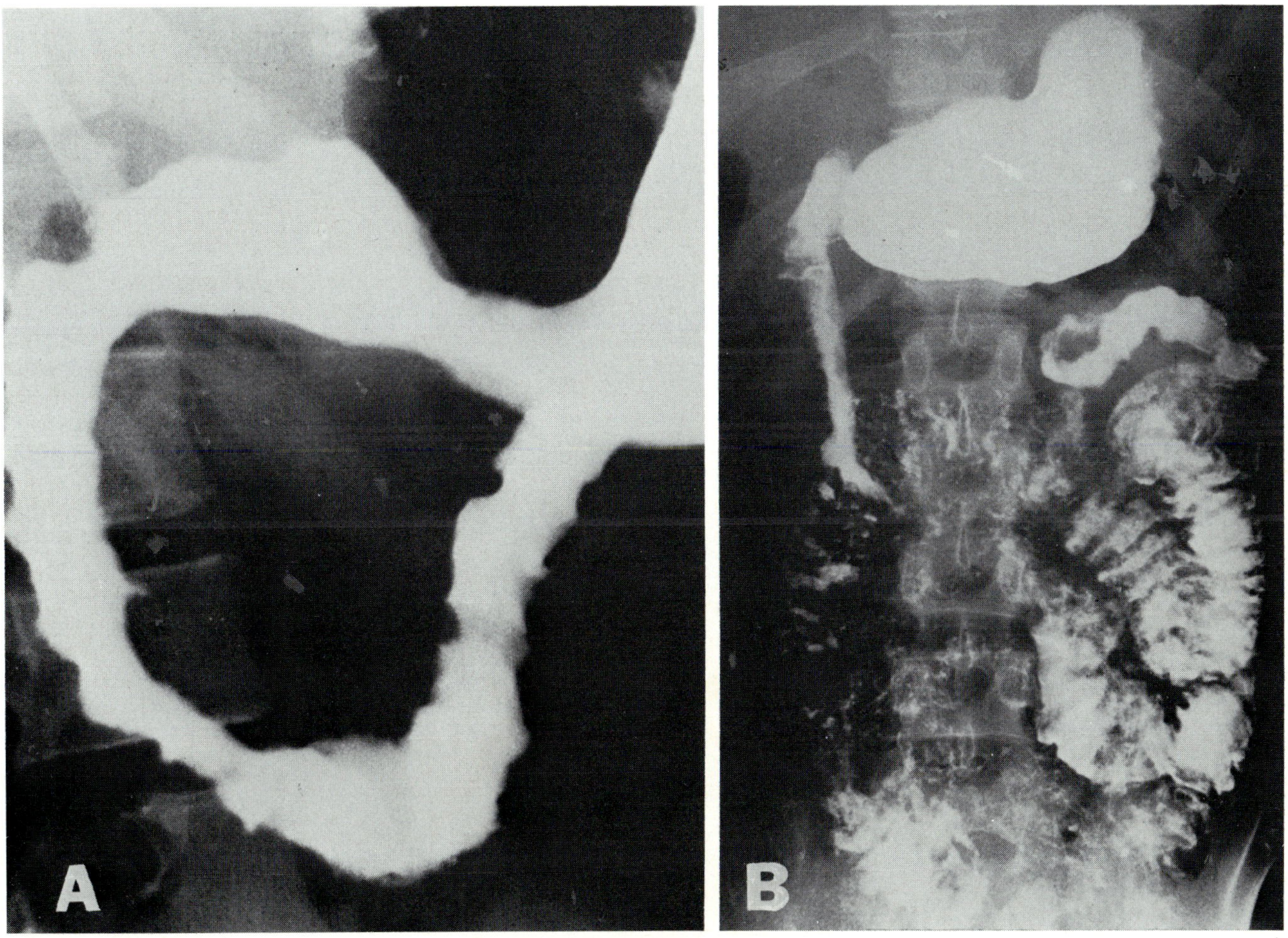

Fig. 3.8 Strongyloidiasis. **A** demonstrates extensive generalised duodenal inflammation which at the later stage of the study, **B,** is shown to be accompanied by jejunal dilation, large mucosal folds and segmentation. (Courtesy of Dr. C. J. Barton, Jamaica.)

stage. These pierce the skin, giving rise to a temporary local itch and perhaps urticarial reaction, and then enter vessels or lymphatics. From there they may travel to the lung, where they mature and fertilise before undergoing the obligatory ritual of passing retrogradely up the respiratory passage and thence down the oesophagus. The females burrow into the duodenal and jejunal mucosa. An inflammatory reaction takes place leading to partial villous atrophy, bowel wall thickening, oedema of the mesentery and enlargement of mesenteric lymph glands. Within these filariform larvae may be found. This form of auto-infection from maturing rhabdoid larvae in the intestine can lead to severe infestation.

The radiological features are readily understood in terms of the pathological process just described. The main alterations are noted in the duodenum and the jejunum, though ileal and colonic ulceration may be present in severe cases (Drasin *et al.*, 1978). Louisy and Barton (1971) describe two forms: one in which dilatation of the duodenum is present and the other where it is narrowed. In both forms there is disturbance in transit of the barium (Fig. 3.8). In the first form hold-up proximal to the ligament of Treitz results in duodenal ileus with some reverse peristalsis. At surgery the thickened mesenteric root around the superior mesenteric artery is seen to mechanically impede the transmission of bowel contents. The mucosal folds of the duodenum are somewhat effaced and the jejunal folds are coarse, thick and fleshy (Patterson, 1958) (Fig. 3.9). The inflammatory reaction in the bowel wall and the oedema consequent on the frequently accompanying hypo-albuminaemia are largely responsible for the mucosal abnormalities.

In the second form of duodenal involvement the calibre is reduced, there is lack of peristalsis, and a fine irregular border to the lumen with no trace of normal mucosal pattern is noted.

We have not seen the erosive type of apthous ulcers that are characteristic of a number of conditions, including Crohn's in strongyloidiasis. Reflux of barium into the common bile duct is sometimes seen and is presumably due to involvement around the sphincter of Oddi.

When the infection results in obstructive clinical features in the small bowel the presence of distended jejunal loops and fluid levels presents radiographic features indistinguishable from a high small bowel mechanical obstruction with ileus. Stool examination and study of aspirated duodenal contents confirms the diagnosis of strongyloidiasis.

REFERENCES

Bartholomew, C., Butler, A. K., Bhaskar, A. G. & Jankey, N. (1977) Pseudo obstruction and a sprue like syndrome from strongyloidiasis, *Postgraduate Medical Journal*, **53,** 139–142.

Bras, G., Richards, R. C., Irvine, R. A., Milner, P. R. A. & Ragbeer,

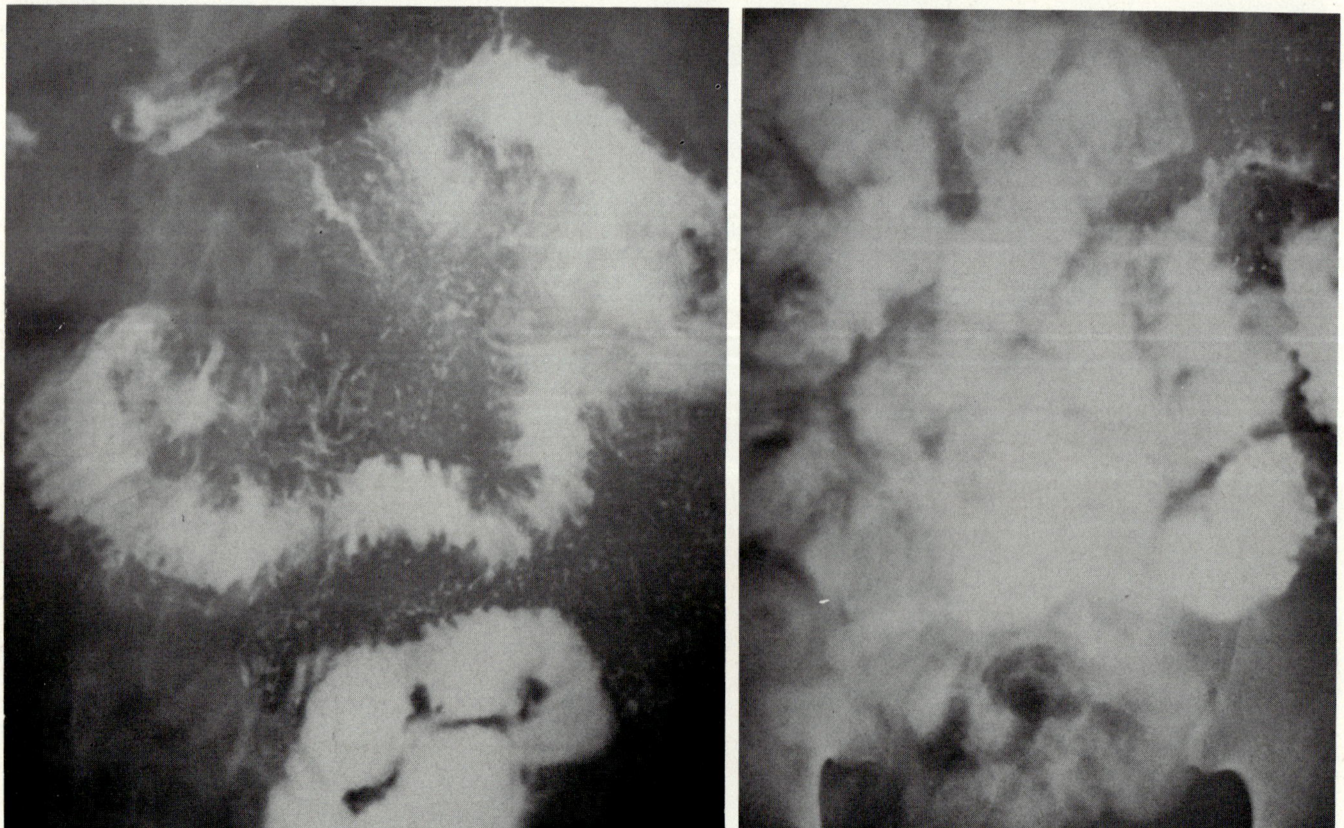

A B

Fig. 3.9 A, B. Small bowel follow-through studies demonstrating gross malabsorption patterns in strongyloidiasis. (Courtesy of Dr. C. Louisy, Jamaica.)

M. M. S. (1964) Infection with Strongyloides stercoralis in Jamaica, *Lancet*, **2**, 1257–1260.

Cookson, J. B., Montgomery, R. D., Morgan, H. V. & Rudor, R. W. (1972) Fatal paralytic ileus due to strongyloidiasis, *British Medical Journal*, **4**, 771–772.

Drasin, G. F., Moss, J. P. & Cheng, S. H. (1978) Strongyloides stercoralis colitis: findings in four cases, *Radiology*, **126**, 619–621.

Garcia, F. T., Sessions, J. T., Strum, W. B., Schweistris, E., Tripathy, K., Bolanos, O., Lotero, H., Dugue, E., Ranelli, D. & Mayoral, L. G. (1977) Intestinal function and morphology in strongyloidiasis, *American Journal of Tropical Medicine and Hygiene*, **26**, 859–865.

Jones, C. A. (1950) Clinical studies in human strongyloidiasis. I. Semeiology. *Gastroenterology*, **16**, 743–756.

Louisy, C. L. & Barton, C. J. (1971) The radiological diagnosis of Strongyloides stercoralis enteritis, *Radiology*, **98**, 535–541.

Paterson, D. E. (1958) Strongyloides infestation of the jejunum, *British Journal of Radiology*, **31**, 102–103.

ASCARIASIS

This is the commonest alimentary parasitism, with hundreds of million people infected. In many parts of the tropics the presence of Ascaris lumbricoides in a barium study is so prevalent that it scarcely invites comment.

Ascariasis is associated with inadequate sanitary facilities and is prevalent in deprived socio-economic areas in the humid tropics and subtropics. Though associated with overcrowding it is seen more in rural areas than in cities with sewage services. Man is infected when contaminated objects or soil reach the mouth, so that the incidence of infection is higher in children than adults. The ova have a characteristic morphology with differences between the fertile and unfertilised eggs. When a fertile egg is passed in the stool and remains on suitable moist soil where it is not exposed to extremes of temperature and sunlight, it segments and a rhabtidiform larva develops within the chitinous covering of the egg. On ingestion by man this outer covering is dissolved by the gastric juice and the larva emerges in the small bowel from the inner vitelline capsule. There, the larva pierces the mucosa to enter the portal system or lymphatics. By the former route the larvae pass through the hepatic sinusoids, hepatic veins and vena cava to reach the pulmonary capillary bed. With the lymphatic route the lung capillaries are attained via the thoracic duct and subclavian vein. With either pathway the journey may not be completed, giving rise to eosinophilia and localised self-limiting granulomatous reactions.

From the capillaries the larvae enter the alveolar air spaces where they excite an outpouring of eosinophils and fluid as they moult. The reaction depends on the intensity of the infection, the immune state of the host and whether there has been a previous sensitising infection. The lung radiological aspects are considered in the pulmonary section.

The surviving maturing larvae ascend the air passages and from the hypopharynx pass down the oesophagus to reach the lumen of the small bowel. There they take several months to attain sexual maturity and have a lifespan of about one year. The adult males are smaller than the females (males 15–30 cm long by 3 mm wide and females 20–35 cm by 4 to 6 mm wide). The anterior end is blunt and the posterior tip is pointed. It has been observed at fluoroscopy in barium studies that worms actively maintain their position with their heads directed against the current in a manner analogous to a fish staying on station in a flowing stream (Makidono, 1956). Because of their active propulsion against displacement they are particularly active when meeting an obstruction or narrow passage such as the appendix, Meckel's diverticulum or the biliary and pancreatic passages (Milroy Paul, 1972). This can result in various surgical problems.

Worms can cause pressure atrophy and perforation of a Meckel's diverticulum. Protrusion through the tip of an appendix is probably due to propulsive movements of the worm and pressure necrosis. Ascarids have been reported free in the peritoneal cavity without any evident perforation.

The large majority of ascarids reside in the jejunum. The worm load may be a few (10 or less), particularly in adults, but in children immense numbers have been recorded. Indeed, it has been claimed by a surgeon that 5000 worms can be accommodated without symptoms (Louw, 1956). However, the presence of that many would entail such a considerable dietary protein loss that even should no mechanical symptoms ensue, the nutritional sequelae would be serious.

In plain films an isolated worm can sometimes be seen

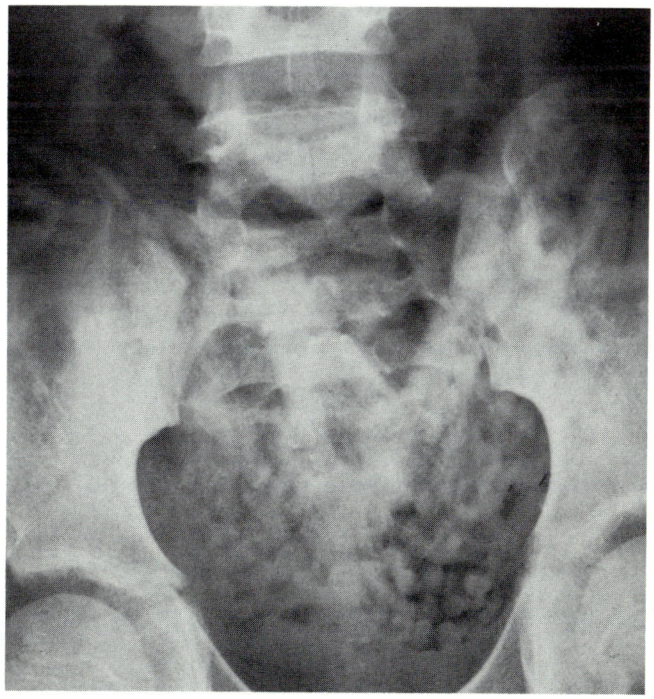

Fig. 3.10 Plain abdominal film showing vast numbers of tangled ascaris worms outlined by gas.

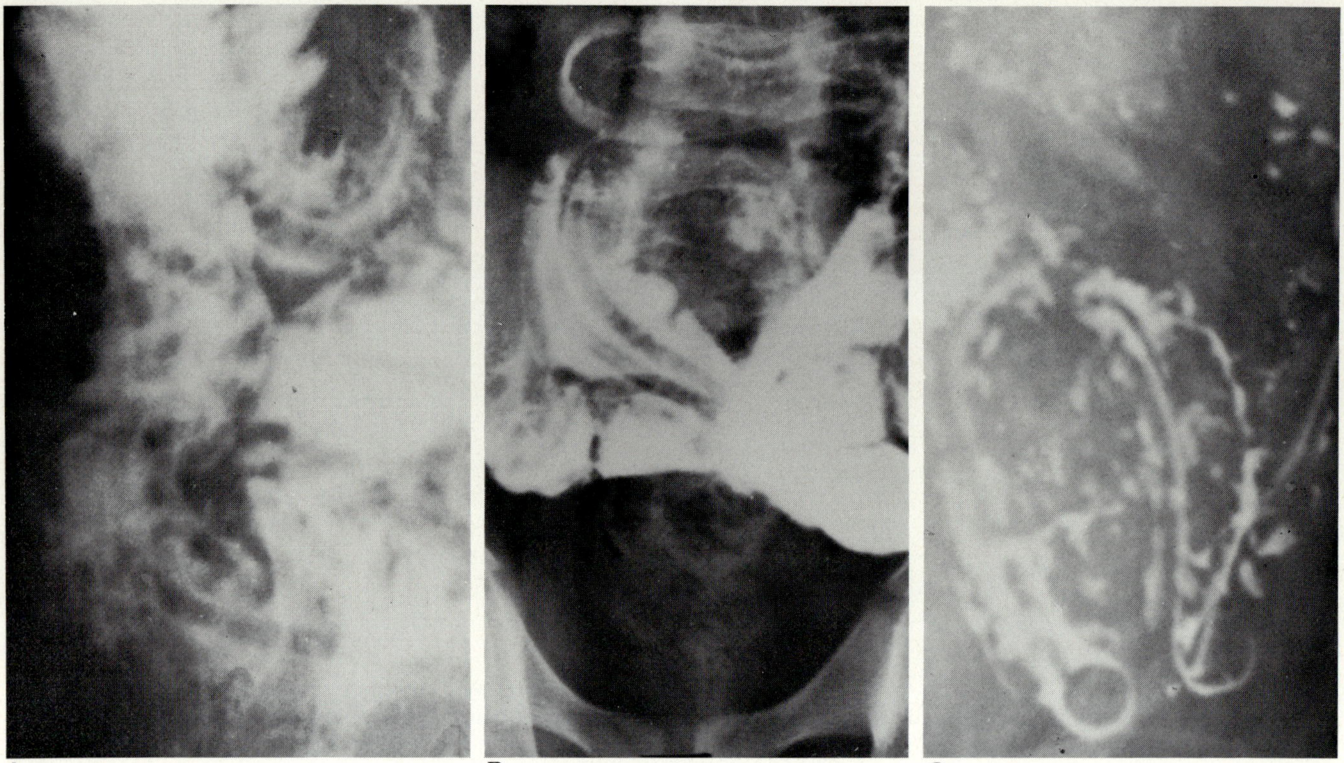

A B C

Fig. 3.11 Ascaris worms in barium small bowel studies: filling defects and on right opacification of the worm's alimentary tract.

silhouetted by surrounding luminal gas. When there are a large number of matted worms plugging the lumen and causing subacute obstruction, with local gas accumulation, many interlocked coiled worms may be partially outlined resembling a skein of wool or a bundle of macaroni (Balikian & Garabedian, 1964) (Fig. 3.10). When confronted with a child with colicky pain this can be a useful finding, particularly if there is a history of a recent administration of a purge of vermifuge. The site of impaction can extend from the duodenum throughout the small intestine (Cole, 1965). With this form of obstruction there is often a local inflammatory reaction with peritoneal fluid which is sometimes detectable radiologically. The severity of this complication can be gauged in that in Capetown at a large children's hospital surgical unit 13 per cent of all abdominal emergencies were related to ascariasis and that ascariasis accounted for 38 per cent of the deaths in a series of 731 acute abdominal cases (Louw, 1966). In barium studies several appearances are noted, depending on the stage of the study. Initially worms are seen as tubular filling defects but later, when the parasites' alimentary tract has ingested opaque material, it is outlined as a 1/2 mm linear track centrally disposed within the outlined worm (Fig. 3.11). Later still, after the barium bolus has passed, persisting residual linear density of barium in the intestinal apparatus of the worm is noted.

Sometimes worms are seen in the colon, where they are often coiled or U-shaped. This is because they are either dead or find difficulty combating peristalsis in the colonic pultaceous environment which differs from their normal liquid surroundings in the small bowel. Worms can be detected in the stomach, duodenum and in gastro-enterotomy stomas. Less frequently they are visualised in the biliary passages if there is reflux of barium. This is discussed in the liver section of this work.

Lagundoye has noted that a high proportion of cases show a malabsorption pattern and considers that the mechanism deserves further study (1972).

REFERENCES

Balikian, J. P. & Garabediam, M. M. (1964) A roentgenographic study of intestinal ascariasis, *Lebanese Medical Journal*, **17**, 377–399.

Cole, G. J. (1965) Surgical manifestations of Ascaris lumbricoides in the intestine, *British Journal of Surgery*, **52**, 44–447.

Lagundoye, S. B. (1972) Disordered small bowel pattern in ascariasis, *Tropical and Geographical Medicine*, **24**, 226–231.

Louw, J. H. (1966) Abdominal complications of Ascaris lumbricoides infestation in children, *British Journal of Surgery*, **53**, 510–521.

Makidono, J. (1956) Observations on Ascaris during fluoroscopy. *American Journal of Tropical Medicine and Hygiene*, **5**, 699–702.

Milroy Paul (1972) The movements of the adult Ascaris lumbricoides. *British Journal of Surgery*, **59**, 437–442.

GIARDIASIS

This protozoan flagellate parasite is found throughout the world. Though there is no doubt about its pathogenicity, nevertheless it often seems to behave as a commensal—particularly in areas of high endemicity. Children are more prone to harbour the parasite than adults. Poor socio-economic conditions usually parallel areas of high prevalence. Thus Faust and Gonzales-Mugaburu (1965) recorded a 47 per cent incidence in a poor urban community in Colombia.

Though commoner in the tropics, cases and outbreaks develop in temperate climes. For travellers Leningrad is particularly notorious in this respect. Epidemics due to water contamination have developed in resorts in Colorado, Utah, New Hampshire and in cruise liners.

As an opportunist invader giardiasis is associated with depressed immune states such as dysgammaglobulinaemia.

Parasites appear in the stools about nine days after infection and acute symptoms begin three or four days later in a proportion of infected individuals. Onset is often manifested by explosive foul diarrhoea, excessive flatus, abdominal distension, cramps and nausea.

A subacute form with less dramatic symptomatology may follow, which passes on to a chronic phase with fewer symptoms but there are occasional relapses. Spontaneous cure may occur if there is no reinfection. Specific therapy is highly effective in eradicating the parasite.

The characteristic motile trophozoites can be recovered from duodenal aspirate and upper jejunal biopsies, but in the stools the cyst form is more common. The trophozoites are microscopic and generally do not invade the mucosa to which they are attached by a sucking disc. Biopsy has shown that in heavy infections with G. lamblia present in mucosal crypts, the villi may show considerable flattening as in malabsorption states. Histologically invasion is exceptional though superficial epithelial ulcers can develop. The mechanisms by which malabsorption occurs in this disorder are not understood (Wright *et al.*, 1977).

The infective form of G. lambia, the cyst, forms in the distal small bowel and large bowel.

The radiological features are usually negligible but in circumstances of high parasite load, possibly low host resistance and chronicity, significant changes may be noted in plain films, in follow-through studies or small bowel enemata (Fisher *et al.*, 1975) (Fig. 3.12).

The bowel alterations are non-specific in character and similar patterns can be seen in other states of malabsorption and other parasitisms, such as by strongyloides. The duodenum and upper jejunum reveal coarsened thickened mucosal valvulae conniventes. This is associated with disturbed peristaltic activity, dilution of barium and flocculation from secretions (Fig. 3.13) (Marshak *et al.*, 1968). Generally one notes rapid transit, though Peterson (1957) emphasised delay in passage of barium. He also showed marked segmentation and other changes that may have been related to the barium preparation used. These disturbances disappear after therapy (Hoskins *et al.*, 1967).

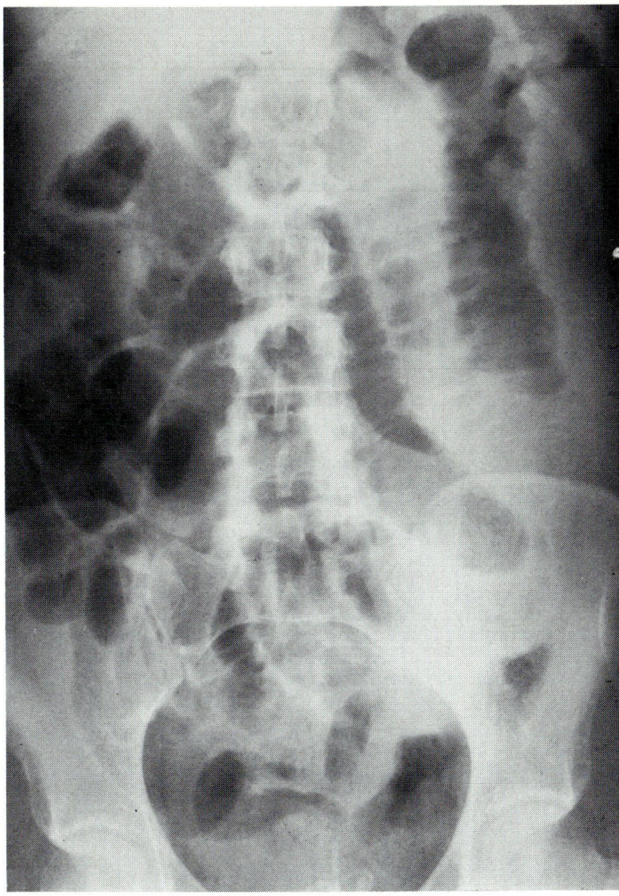

Fig. 3.12 Plain film abdomen of patient with giardiasis. Jejunal gaseous distension and prominent valvulae conniventes are revealed by luminal gas. (Courtesy of Prof. S. Siegelman, Baltimore; and *American Journal of Roentgenology*.)

The Johns Hopkins workers have commented on the presence of nodular lymphoid hyperplasia in small bowel and colon in patients with giardiasis in association with Ig A deficiency as well as in other forms of agammaglobulinaemia (Fisher *et al.*, 1973).

In a controlled study of Australian aboriginal children eradication of infestation led to a growth spurt. This vividly documents the malabsorptive consequences of giardiasis (Jose & Welch, 1970).

REFERENCES

Faust, E. C. & Gonzales-Mugaburu, L. (1965) Parasitological surveys in Cali, Departamento del Valle, Colombia, *American Journal of Tropical Medicine and Hygiene*, **14**, 276–289.

Fisher, G. M., Oh, K. S., Bayless, T. M. & Siegelman, S. S. (1975) Current perspectives in giardiasis, *American Journal of Roentgenology*, **125**, 207–217.

Hoskins, L. C., Winawer, S. J., Broitman, S. A., Gottlieb, L. S. & Zamcheck, N. (1967) Clinical giardiasis and intestinal malabsorption, Gastroenterology, **53**, 265–279.

Jose, D. G. & Welch, J. S. (1970) Growth retardation anaemia and infection with malabsorption and infestation of the bowel. The syndrome of protein calorie malnutrition in Australian aboriginal children, *Medical Journal of Australia*, **1**, 349–356.

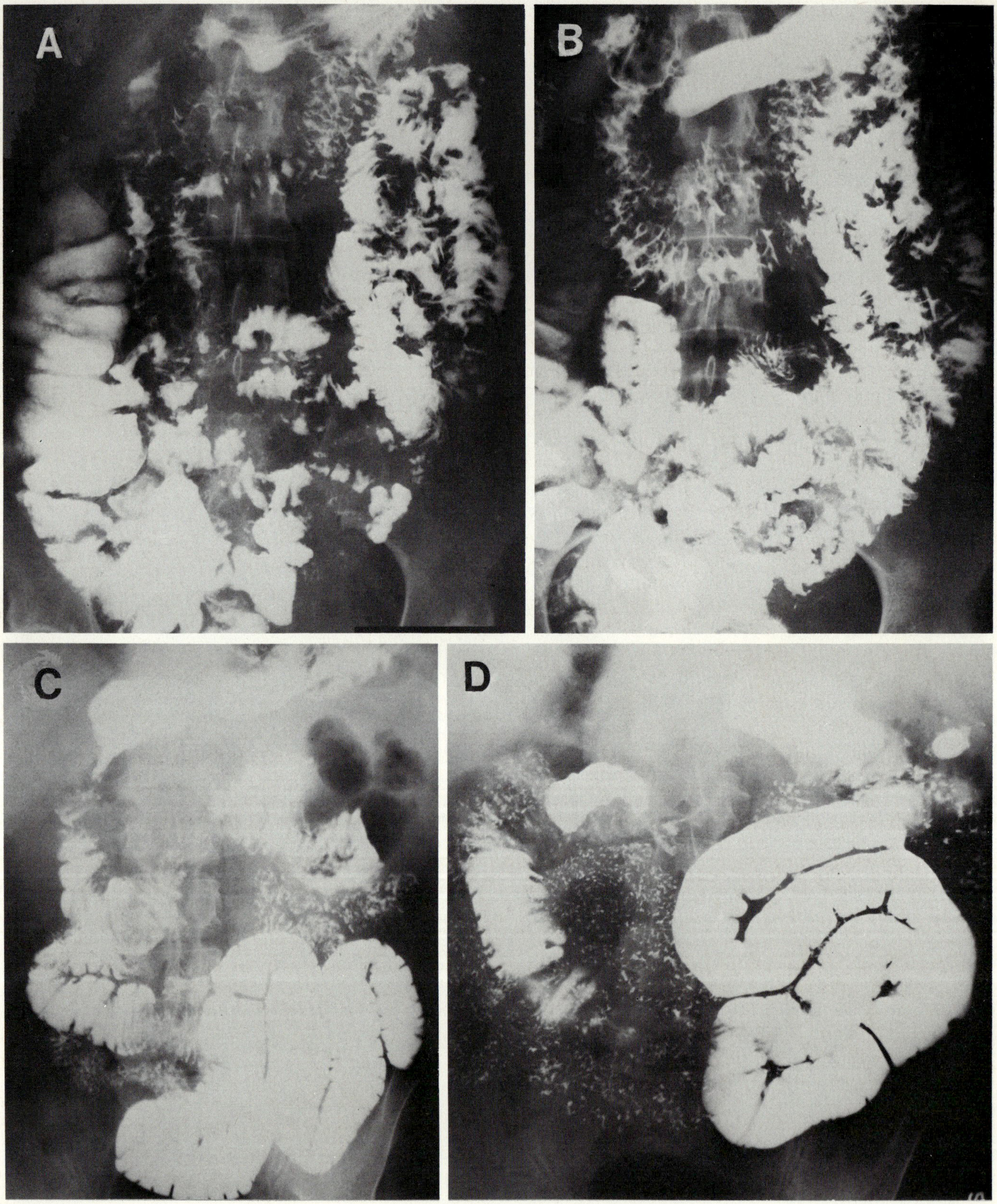

Fig. 3.13 Intestinal giardiasis. Series of films of barium follow-throughs indicates varying degrees of jejunal dilatation, exaggeration of mucosal circular folds, segmentation and moulage. (Courtesy of Prof. S. Siegelman, Baltimore; and *American Journal of Roentgenology*.)

Marshak, R. H., Ruoff, M. & Lindner, A. E. (1968) Roentgen manifestations of giardiasis, *American Journal of Roentgenology*, **104**, 557–560.
Peterson, G. M. (1957) Intestinal changes in Giardia Lamblia infestation, *American Journal of Roentgenology*, **77**, 670–677.
Wright, S. G., Tomkins, A. M. & Ridley, S. (1977) Giardiasis: clinical and therapeutic, *Gut*, **18**, 343–350.

INTESTINAL CAPILLARIASIS

Benjamin D. Cabrera

An intestinal parasitism that causes severe diarrhoea and malabsorption with a significant mortality (10 per cent) has been found with high prevalance in northern Luzon in the Philippines (Chitwood *et al.*, 1964; Whalen *et al.*, 1969). Two cases have been described from Thailand suggesting that other further foci of this disorder may exist (Pradatsundarasan *et al.*, 1973).

The disease is caused by a small hair-like nematode, Capillaria philippinensis. The females are 2·5 to 4·3 mm long and the males 2·3 to 3·1 mm long. The eggs measure 40 $\mu \times 20\ \mu$ with a fenestrated wall and flattened bipolar plugs and can be segmented or unsegmented (Cabrera *et al.*, 1967). The ova bear a resemblance to those of Trichuris trichiuria, and since the two organisms can be present in one patient distinction is important. All stages in the life cycle of the parasite: eggs, larval stages one to four, and adults can be found in the intestine (Fresh *et al.*, 1972). Adults can exist in the lumen or burrowed beneath epithelial mucosal wall of the distal jejunum and proximal ileum. Histologically the affected parasited mucosa does not show flattened villi in biopsies despite the marked malabsorption that may be present (Whalen *et al.*, 1969).

The presence of all stages in the bowel of man suggests that a self-propagating auto-infection can develop. To date no natural host reservoir is known despite extensive search. The diet of some of those afflicted includes raw or partially cooked fish, shrimps, dogs, goats and goat's intestine.

Diagnosis is established by stool examination with identification of the eggs, or less commonly larvae and adult worms, in direct faecal smears, or by acid ether concentration techniques (Cabrera *et al*, 1967). An intradermal test has been developed that may be a useful supplementary diagnostic tool (Cabrera & Silan, 1968).

The attack rate can be as high as a third of a localised population during an outbreak, and a mortality as high as 35 per cent has been recorded in males (Detels *et al.*, 1969). The disease is commoner as well as more severe in males.

Patients initially have vague abdominal pain and borborygmi, which after passing of two to six weeks is associated with profuse watery diarrhoea with bulky stools. The patients begin to lose weight, develop malaise and anorexia. As a result of a protein-losing enteropathy emaciation becomes marked with loss of fat and muscle bulk, and hypoproteinaemia results in oedema. Improvement can follow thiabendazole treatment.

Since there is a parasitism of the jejunum and proximal ileum associated with malabsorption and an exudative intraluminal process, it is not surprising that there are radiological abnormalities of the small bowel. These have been well described in 14 patients by Paulino and Wittenberg (1973) though previous workers had noted an abnormal small bowel pattern (Dauz *et al.*, 1967). These workers have noted increase in the size of the valvulae conniventes in the distal jejunum and proximal ileum of all cases. Dilatation of the small bowel beyond 3 cm was present in most instances in inconstant segments. Segmentation, flocculation and dilution were all seen in some cases but disturbances of transit times were not seen. The authors indicate that in comparison with sprue the dilatation in capillariasis is much less marked.

REFERENCES

Cabrera, B. D., Canlas, B. D. & Dauz, V. (1967) Human intestinal capillariasis. III Parasitological features and management, *Acta Medica Philippina*, **4**, 92–103.
Cabrera, B. D. & Silan, R. B. (1968) The intradermal test in the diagnosis of human intestinal capillariasis, *Acta Medica Philippina*, **4**, 175–180.
Chitwood, M. B., Valasquez, C. & Salazar, N. G. (1964) The physiological changes in a species of Capillaria causing a fatal case of human capillariasis, *Proceedings of the First International Congress of Parasitology*, Rome, **2**, 797–798.
Dauz, V., Cabrera, B. D. & Canlas, B. D. (1967) Human intestinal capillariasis. I Clinical features, *Acta Medica Philippina*, **4**, 72–83.
Detels, R., Gutman, L., Jaramillo, J., Zerrvdo, E., Banzon, T., Valera, J., Murrel, K. D., Cross, J. & Dizon, J. J. (1969) An epidemic of intestinal capillariasis in man, *American Journal of Tropical Medicine and Hygiene*, **18**, 676–682.
Fresh, J. W., Cross, J. H., Reyes, V., Whalen, G. E., Vylangeo, C. V. & Dizon, J. J. (1972) Necropsy findings in intestinal capillariasis, *American Journal of Tropical Medicine and Hygiene*, **21**, 169–173.
Paulino, G. N. & Wittenberg, J. (1973) Intestinal capillariasis—a new cause of a malabsorption pattern, *American Journal of Roentgenology*, **117**, 340–345.
Pradatsundarasan, A., Pecharamond, K., Chintanawongo, C. & Ungthavorn, P. (1973) The first case of intestinal capillariasis in Thailand, *South East Asia Journal of Tropical Medicine and Public Health*, **4**, 131–134.
*Whalen, G. E., Strickland, G. T., Cross, J. H., Vylangea, C., Rosenburg, E. B., Gutman, R. H. & Dizon, J. J. (1969) Intestinal capillariasis: a new disease in man, *Lancet*, **1**, 13–16.

TAENIA SAGINATA
BEEF TAPEWORM

Infection by this cestode comes from eating raw or inadequately cooked beef that contains the larval or cysticercal stage of T. saginata. Man is the only known definitive host of the adult parasite and does not acquire the cysticercal stage as happens with T. solium, the pork tapeworm.

The condition has been eliminated from most parts of the world as a result of beef carcass inspection. It is seen, however, where public health measures are lax or do not exist—particularly where people slaughter their own cattle and where local custom favours eating raw meat. It occurs in the Middle East, Central America and with nomadic groups in East Africa. Sporadic cases are discovered in travellers and field workers. The majority of cases are symptomless.

The life cycle is simple. The tapeworm inhabits the upper jejunum where its diminutive hookless head or scolex is attached to the mucous membrane. The 'body' consists of numerous segments, proglottids, that gradually enlarge in size caudally so that the sexually mature segments are about 7 mm by 20 mm. The more proximal proglottids are considerably smaller, measuring about a millimeter, and cannot be detected in films. According to Grahovac and colleagues (1970) the smallest segment that can be recognised radiologically lies 20 cm from the scolex, usually about half a metre beyond the duodeno-jejunal junction. The proglottids are flat, not greatly exceeding 2 mm in thickness. As the mature worm is usually between 5 and 10 metres in length and segments in continuity reaching the colon are rapidly broken off to accommodate the length, there is redundancy in the small bowel with the worm folded upon itself.

Mature segments and ova passed onto pasture may be ingested by cattle. Then an oncosphere is liberated into the herbivore's duodenum which passes through the intestinal wall to find the musculature to encyst and complete the life cycle.

Radiology has little role to play in diagnosis but since the features in barium studies are distinctive they should be recognised if seen (Hamilton, 1946; Monroe & Norton, 1962; Grahovac *et al.*, 1970).

The long cestode causes linear filling defects which increase in size distally (Fig. 3.14). The size depends not only on the distance from the scolex but also whether the flattened segments are seen *en face* or in profile. Barium is not taken up by the proglottids, unlike ascaris, but double linear defects with intervening barium may be seen because of the doubling up folds of the worm.

Individual segments have not been shown, though in veterinary practice like other tapeworms (Taenea pisiformis) they can be identified (Fig. 3.15).

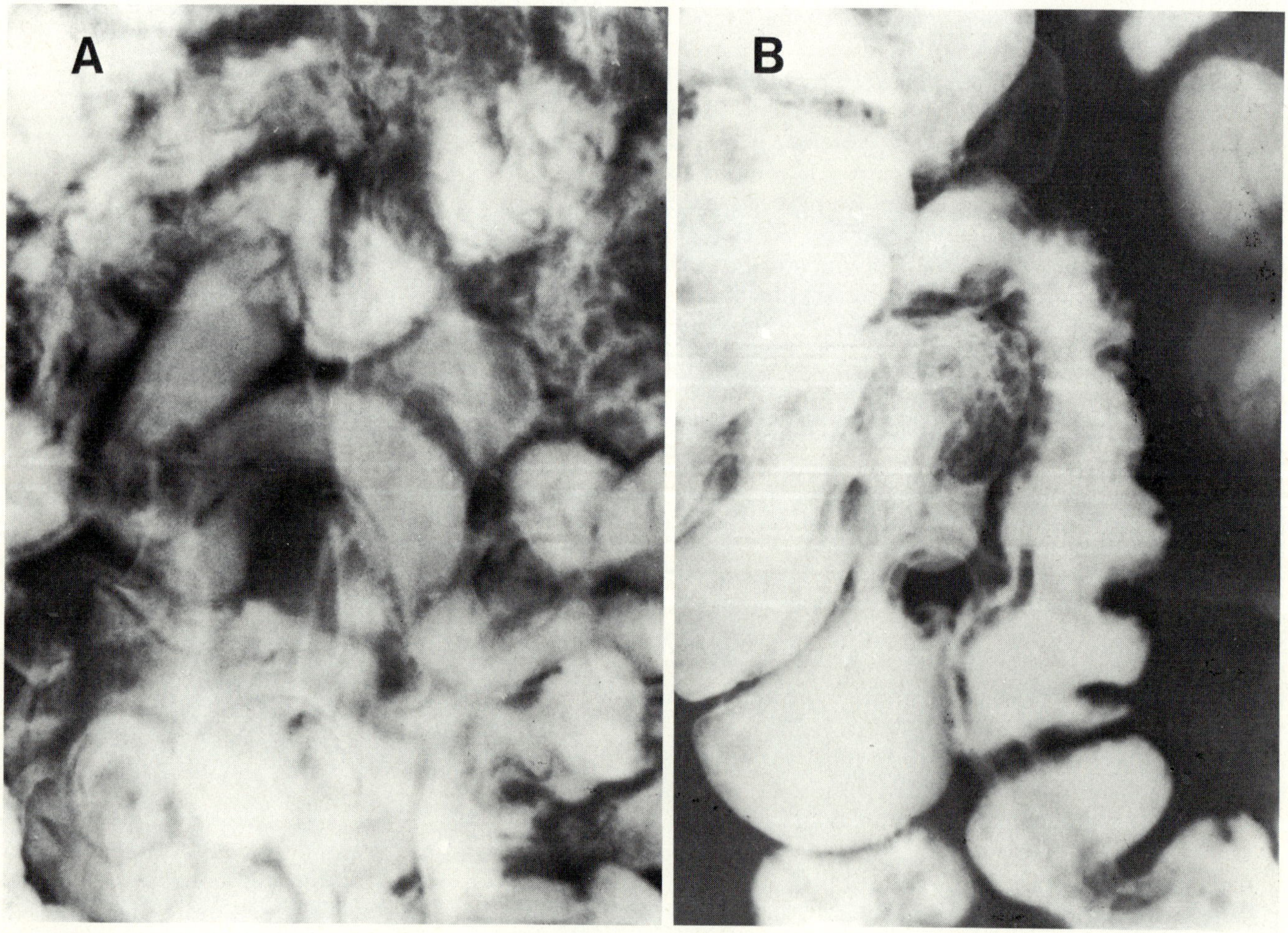

Fig. 3.14 Taenia saginata—**A.** The lower jejunum and ileum show a fine intraluminal curvilinear lucency due to a worm. In some loops it is bent upon itself to accommodate its length that is greater than that of the bowel. **B** is at the same magnification and indicates that the distal end of the worm is larger due to the greater size of the proglottid segments. (Courtesy of Dr. Z. Grahovac, Ottowa; and the *Journal of the Ca-adian Medical Association.*)

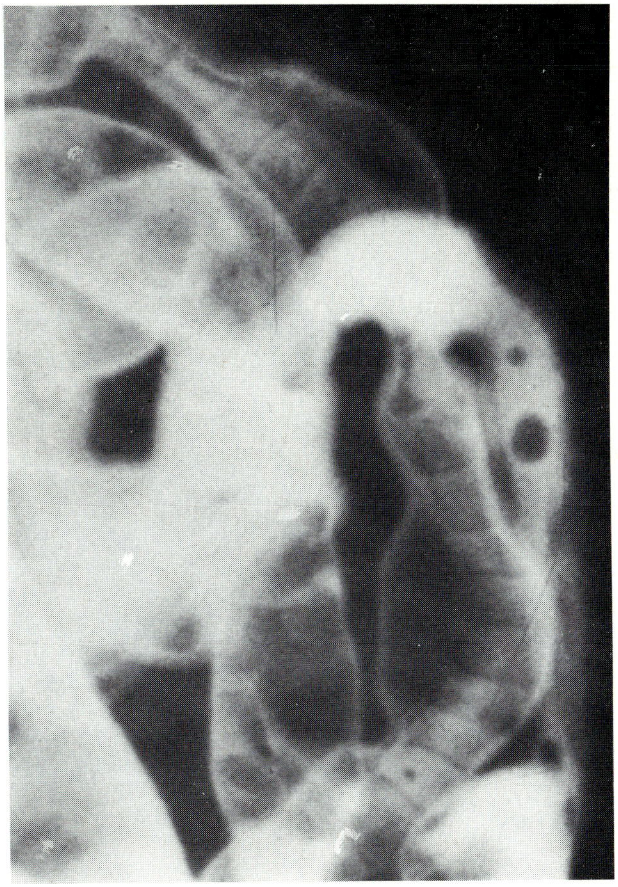

Fig. 3.15 Follow-through study in a cat harbouring Taenia pisiformis. This shows that proglottid segments are potentially visible. (Courtesy of Dr. V. Rendano, Guelph Veterinary College.)

Taenia saginata is usually noted incidentally during a follow-through examination. In an adequately prepared large bowel segments in the colon will have been removed by the cleansing process.

Precise identification of the tapeworm required stool examination for proglottids or ova or study of the passes scolex.

REFERENCES

Grahavoc, Z., Joanes, J. F. & Chew, F. M. (1970) The radiological diagnosis of tapeworms: two cases of Taenia saginata infestation, *Canadian Medical Association Journal*, **102,** 967–968.

Hamilton, J. B. (1946) Taenia saginata, *Radiology*, **47,** 64–66.

Monroe, L. S. & Norton, R. A. (1962) Roentgenographic signs produced by Taenia saginata, *American Journal of Digestive Diseases*, **7,** 519–522.

TAENIA SOLIUM PORK TAPEWORM

Taenia solium exists in man both as an intestinal tapeworm and as a cysticercus. The letter form is discussed in relation to muscle and the brain in the appropriate sections of the book. The condition is prevalent in Central and South America, the Middle East, Central and South Africa.

Generally intestinal infection is either symptomless or may cause mild diarrhoea. It is strange that to date we are not aware of a single account of the radiological appearances of this cestode in the alimentary tract.

Other cestodes

There are other less frequent tapeworms that may involve children in the tropics, such as the small H. nana. There are two, however, that are around 60 cm long and produce small proglottid segments about 3 mm long, shaped like rice grains, that should be visible in barium small bowel studies. Precise identification, as with all enteric parasites, depends on examination of ova and proglottids or the scolex if available.

Rallietina celebensis has been reported in children from Thailand, Indonesia, Formosa, the Philippines, Tahiti and Western Australia (Fain *et al.*, 1977; Margoni *et al.*, 1977). Inermicapsifer madagascarensis seems to be a tapeworm of Caucasian children in East and Central Africa and Malaysia (Bisseru & Smith, 1967; Hira, 1974; Goldsmid & Fleming, 1977). Both these parasites are believed to have as normal host rats and mice but the exact modes of transmission are not yet well understood.

REFERENCES

Bisseru, B. & Smith, G. (1967) Infection with Inermicapsifer madagascarensis in a child from Malaya, *Medical Journal of Malaya*, **21,** 374.

Fain, A., Limboo, P., Van Ros, G., de Mulder, P. & Herin, A. (1977) Presence du cestode Railletina celebensis (Janicki, 1902). Chez un infant originaire de Tahiti, *Annales de la Société Belge de Médecine Tropicale*, **57,** 137–142.

Goldsmid, J. M. & Fleming, F. (1977) Tapeworm infections of children in Rhodesia, *Central African Medical Journal*, **23,** 7–10.

Hira, P. A. (1974) Infestation of man by the cestode Inermicapsifer madagascarensis in Lusaka, Zambia, *Medical Journal of Zambia*, **8,** 35–38.

Margono, S., Handojo, I., Hadidjaja, P. & Mahfudin, H. (1977) Raillietina infections in children in Indonesia, *South East Asian Journal Tropical Medicine and Public Health*, **8,** 195–199.

TYPHOID—TYPHOID PERFORATION

Typhoid remains endemic in places where the water supply and food can become contaminated. The disease expresses itself in different fashions in various areas, but whether the modifications are due to differences in virulence of organisms, varying degrees of host resistance or other factors is not resolved. In this section only the abdominal manifestations will be discussed with emphasis on the diagnosis of perforation.

All age groups can be affected, though most clinical cases are in the second or third decades of life. The condition may be widespread in a community with S. typhi H agglutinin existing in 15 per cent of the population, as in Ghana.

Patients present with fever and often have diarrhoea and abdominal tenderness. By the end of the first week the lymphoid Peyer's patches in the distal ileum and the lymphoid follicles of the terminal ileum and colon have become swollen and hyperaemic. There may be intense inflammation by about the twelfth day which may resolve or progress to ulceration and later perforation. The latter complication generally develops at the end of the second or during the third week of the infection. Perforations are either transverse on the antimesenteric side of the distal ileum through a Peyer's patch or through a round slough in a lymphoid follicle. Haemorrhage may also occur at this stage. There can be multiple perforations.

Perforation has a varying incidence in different series, 3·5 per cent in 200 cases from Cairo; 0·5 per cent in 1088 cases from India; 0·7 per cent in 530 cases in Iraq and 18 per cent of 781 patients seen in Accra in a period of three years (Archampong, 1969).

Prior to perforation characteristic but non-specific changes may be evident in plain films of the abdomen. The inflamed terminal ileum interferes with the onward passage of intestinal gas which accumulates in the ileum, giving rise to some meteoric distension (Fig. 3.16) (Bohrer, 1966).

Kabakian and his colleagues (1975) in Beirut have performed barium studies on typhoid patients and shown a uniform dilatation of the distal ileum up to one and a half times its normal calibre. This begins abruptly in the last 10 to 15 cm of the ileum. Sometimes one can appreciate in the affected area a coarsely nodular and wavy linear

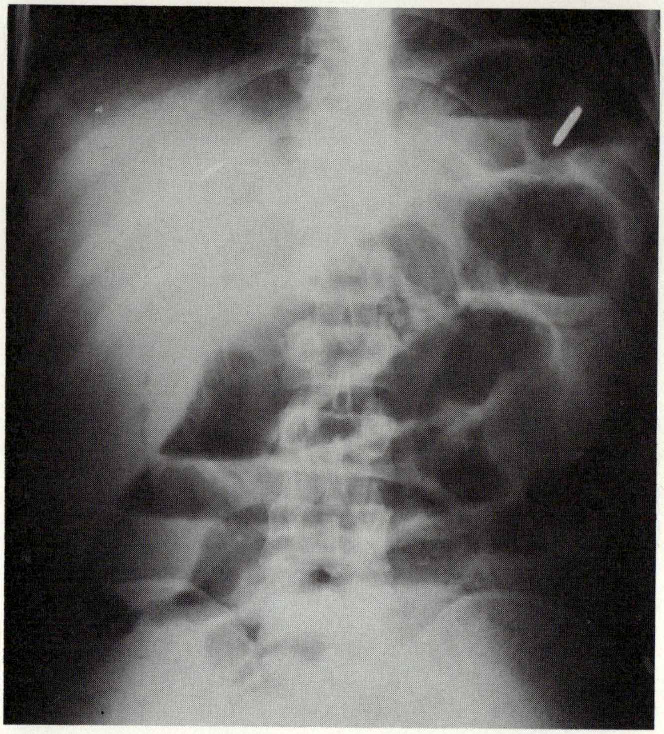

Fig. 3.16 Plain erect film of 'typhoid' abdomen. The ileus due to the inflamed Peyer's patches has produced proximal small bowel distension, fluid levels and an empty colon.

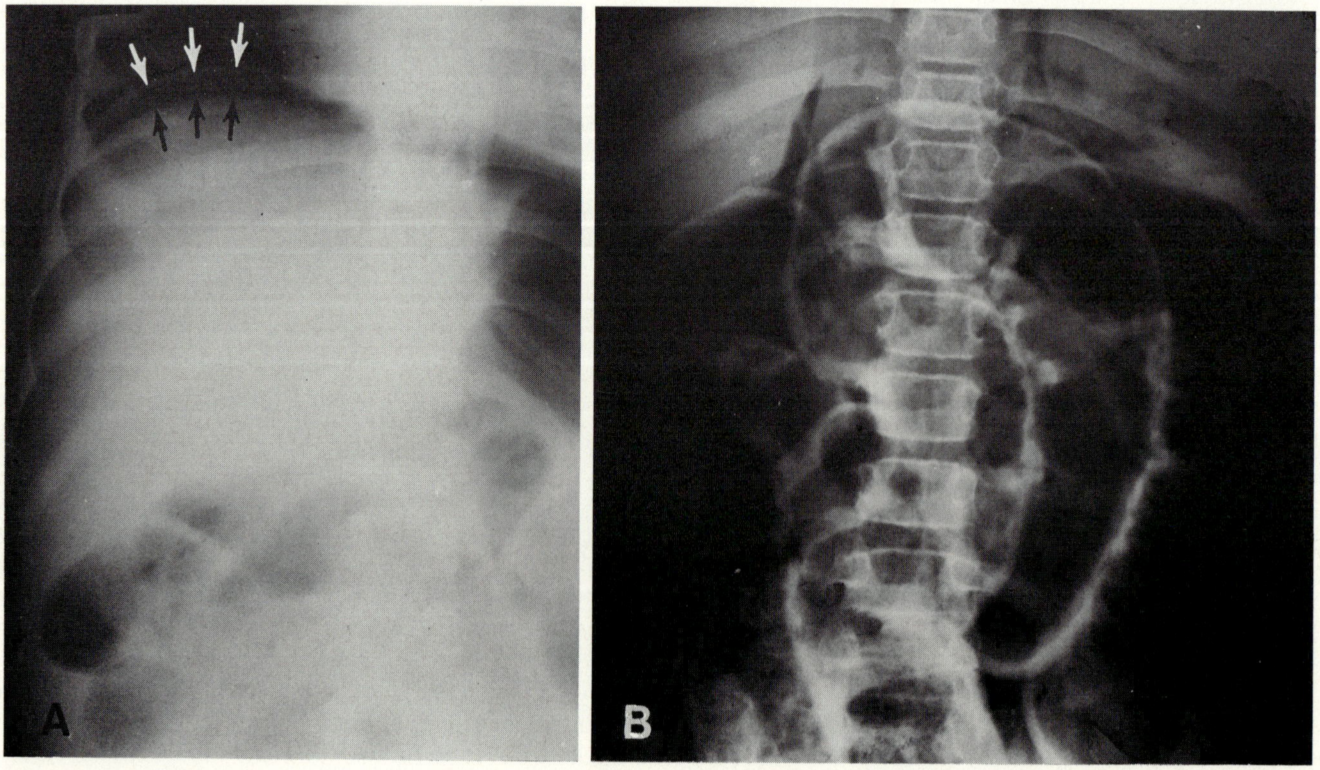

Fig. 3.17 **A.** Free gas between liver and diaphragm due to typhoid perforation. **B.** Extensive pneumoperitoneum with gas-distended small bowel from typhoid ileus. Note the 'double bowel wall' sign. (Courtesy of Prof. S. P. Bohrer and the *British Journal of Radiology*.)

mucosal pattern (Francis & Berk, 1974). At this stage there is no rigidity of the affected segment. It is claimed that a normal terminal ileum in a patient with a febrile illness virtually excludes typhoid as the cause (Kabakian *et al.*, 1975). In most circumstances laboratory facilities provide more specific diagnostic information and there is no need for barium studies.

When perforation occurs gas from the ileum is released into the peritoneal cavity and then the classic signs of gas under the diaphragm in an erect film, or against the upper flank in a decubitus lateral view, are seen (Fig. 3.17). A 'double contour' with gas outlining each side of the bowel is also common. Gas tends to remain in the ileum with a paucity of gas in the colon, in contrast to the normal ileus of peritonitis where there is often colonic gas as well (Bohrer, 1966). Erect films may show fluid levels when peritonitis develops. Disappearance of the normal fat flank stripe lucency can also be observed in late cases.

As the peritonitis progresses the features of generalised ileus become more obvious, but in most instances there is more small bowel accumulation of gas than one would anticipate. As surgical management of perforation shows a lower mortality than conservative medical management early diagnosis is of importance (Huckstep, 1960; Dickson & Cole, 1964; Archampong, 1969). Consequently radiology can offer considerable aid in cases of clinical uncertainty.

REFERENCES

Archampong, E. Q. (1969) Operative treatment of typhoid perforation of the bowel, *British Medical Journal*, **2**, 273–276.

Bohrer, S. P. (1966) Typhoid perforation of the ileum, *British Journal of Radiology*, **39**, 37–41.

Dickson, J. A. S. & Cole, G. T. (1964) Perforation of the terminal ileum, *British Journal of Surgery*, **51**, 893–897.

Francis, R. S. & Berk, R. N. (1974) Typhoid fever, *Radiology*, **112**, 583–585.

Huckstep, R. L. (1960) Recent advances in the surgery of typhoid fever, *Annals of the Royal College of Surgeons*, **26**, 207–230.

Kabakian, M. A., Nassar, N. T. & Nasrallah, S. M. (1975) Roentgenographic findings in typhoid fever, *American Journal of Roentgenology*, **125**, 198–206.

INTESTINAL TUBERCULOSIS

S. Chawla

In many parts of the tropical world where Crohn's disease is infrequent tuberculosis is by far the most common cause of granulomatous disease of the bowel.

Quantitatively it can pose a formidable problem, particularly in India (Vayda & Sodhi, 1978), where Chawla and her colleagues (1966) report that 15 per cent of all barium studies are on patients with tuberculous intestinal disease.

Since lesions are frequently multiple and may exist at several levels, tending to cause similar symptomatology, several segments of the gastro-intestinal tract are considered here together. It should be remembered that tuberculous ascites and mesenteric adenitis are frequently associated with the more focal intestinal lesions.

G.I. tuberculosis exists wherever human tuberculosis is widespread. It is more frequent in females than males. Nowadays reports invariably stress that it is due to the human form and not the bovine type of mycobacterium. Apart from isolated tuberculous peritonitis and adenitis, which is often a childhood disease, most adult patients present in the twenties or early thirties.

The symptoms vary somewhat, depending on the anatomic location and form of the lesion, but most reports emphasise the presence of weight loss and abdominal pain in about 90 per cent of patients (Werbeloff *et al.*, 1973; Kolawole & Lewis, 1975). Diarrhoea is present in a high proportion, though later as strictures form constipation becomes manifest. Palpable masses are not uncommon. In surgical series obstructive symptoms and perforations feature prominently (Bhansali, 1977).

Most writers on this topic have noted that pulmonary tuberculosis is often not detectable or apparently inactive in many cases of tuberculous enteritis, and they have further recorded that Mantoux and Heaf tests are sometimes negative.

When ascites is present microscopic and cultural examination of the fluid with high protein content can be of value. However, when fluid is absent or there is plastic peritonitis proof of the diagnosis has to be obtained in other fashions.

In plain films of patients with ascites a diffuse haziness may be noted, accompanied by a more central location of bowel gas which is not evident in the flanks. This can be confirmed by follow-through studies. With plastic or loculated peritonitis fixation of loops and retraction may be observed in barium studies.

Tuberculous mesenteric adenopathy may be associated with lymph gland enlargement elsewhere or may be isolated with or without ascites. The latter is known to follow rupture of a caseous gland into the peritoneal cavity.

Radiologically adenopathy becomes evident because of a mass lesion displacing structures such as the ureters or the duodenal loop; by compressing the lumen of the bowel as in duodenal ileus; or by interfering with the lymphatic absorption mechanism and producing a protein-losing enteropathy syndrome with characteristic small bowel mucosal changes (Fig. 3.18). Obviously such mass lesions of glands can on occasions be confused with lymphoma and Burkitt's disease.

Lymphangiography has been carried out in several centres (Werbeloff *et al.*, 1973; Beetlestone *et al.*, 1977) on patients with a mesenteric adenopathy (Fig. 3.19). As is to be expected caseous areas cause filling defects, glandular enlargement and obstructive features with collateral formation. The pattern of the involvement and flow indicates that the process is most marked in the proximal para-aortic nodes. Whether this is from the drainage of the gut

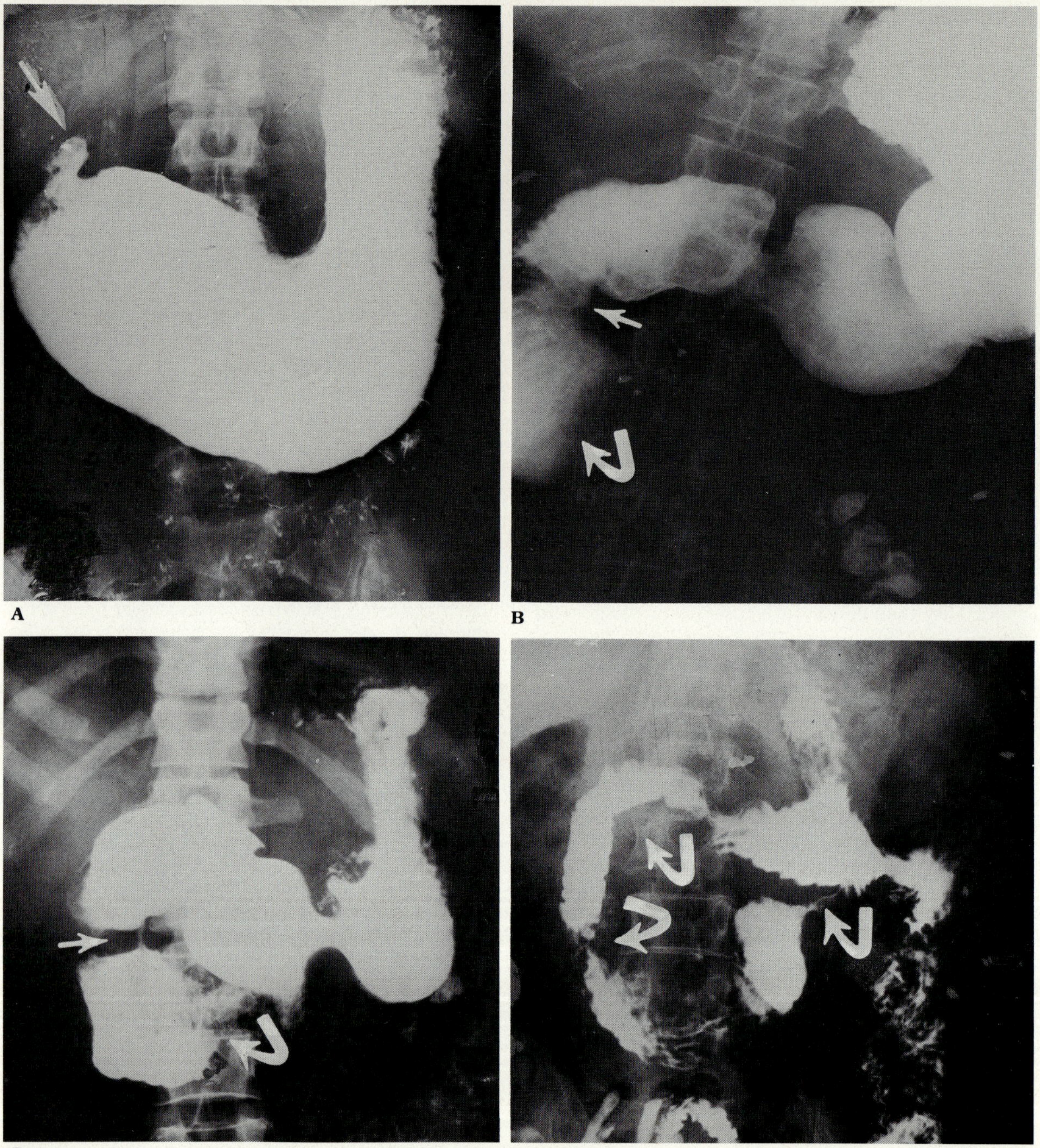

A B C D

Fig. 3.18 A–D. Gastric and duodenal tuberculosis composite. The straight arrows indicate intrinsic strictures of the gastric outlet and the second part of the duodenum. The curved arrows point to deformity consequent on tuberculous glandular masses.

is uncertain. Varicose draining channels emerge from lower nodes. This pattern differs from that seen in lymphoma.

Duodenal tuberculosis usually presents as a form of gastric outlet obstruction with vomiting and visible gastric peristalsis (Davey & Pearson, 1965; Chawla & Bery, 1969; Osime, 1977). This form is due to compression of the duodenum at the root of the mesentery by enlarged glands (Fig. 3.18). Retroperitoneal glands around the pancreas can also enlarge the duodenal loop and cause impressions on the medial aspect of the loop, or there may be frank mucosal tuberculous ulceration and hyperplastic infiltrating repair (Balikian *et al.*, 1967; Kolawole & Lewis, 1975). The pyloric glands and the antrum of the stomach may be affected in such cases. When this type of disease is present the patients have dyspeptic symptoms that simulate peptic ulcer disease or gastric carcinoma.

Lesions of the small bowel are usually said to be secondary even though the primary site may not be evident. Mucosal ulcers are well recognised at autopsy, but radio-

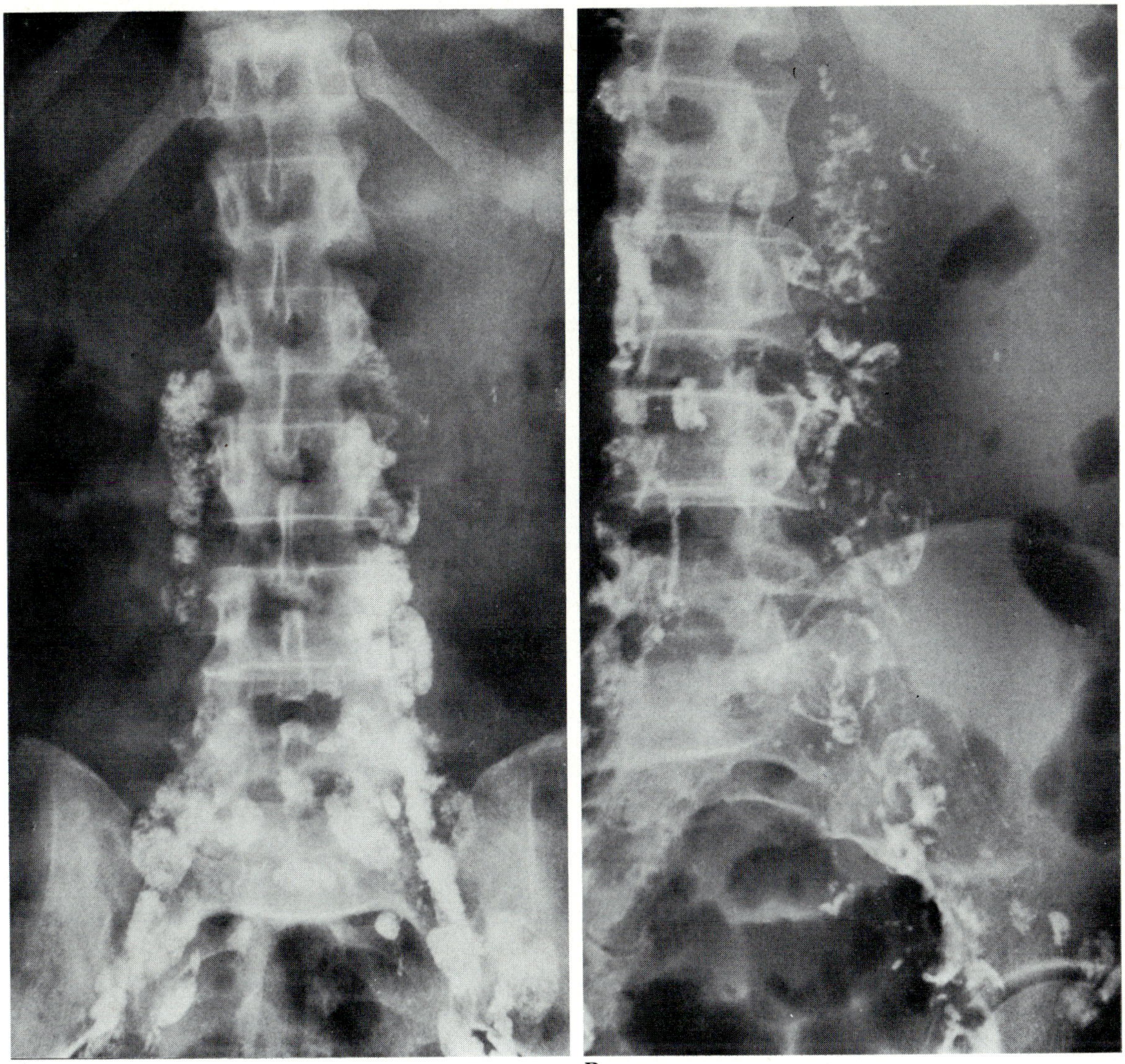

A B

Fig. 3.19 A, B. Lymphangiograms on two patients with proven tuberculous mesenteric adenopathy. Para-ortic nodes are enlarged and have filling defects. (Courtesy of Dr. Claire Beetlestone.)

logically these have not often been demonstrated. It is the later scarring or reactive phase involving the whole thickness of the bowel that is most often identified in patients investigated for obstructive symptoms.

Strictures in the small bowel are more frequent in the ileum than the jejunum and may be multiple at several levels with normal intervening bowel. Proximal to the narrowed area there may be small bowel distension and stasis (Fig. 3.20). The latter can lead to a striking but unusual radiographic feature—enteroliths. In India in a series of over 400 cases this developed in over 3 per cent of patients (Chawla *et al.*, 1966). The calculi are often multiple and form proximal to the stenosis. They may be totally radio-opaque or be evident as lamellated or ring densities. It should be remembered that enteroliths can develop in stagnant segments of small bowel such as diverticuli and Meckel's diverticulum (Brettner & Euphrat, 1970).

Perforation of bowel tuberculous ulcers with release of gas into the peritoneal cavity is a rare complication. So also is fistula formation through matted adherent loops. This complication features more in regional enteritis. Lesions of the distal ileum and the caecum frequently co-exist and produce a characteristic appearance (Fig. 3.21).

It is noteworthy that Anand (1956) found that there was no evidence of pulmonary tuberculosis in 78 per cent of his series of 50 patients with hypertrophic ileo-caecal tuberculosis (Fig. 3.22).

Ileo-caecal tuberculosis is the location of 85 per cent of tuberculous enterocolitis. Purely colonic lesions are infrequent and difficult to differentiate from stenosing malignant disease, though the young age of most cases would be unusual for colonic malignancy. Patients tend to present with subacute large bowel obstruction, and barium enema studies reveal one or more strictures which usually affect a short segment of bowel (Chawla *et al.*, 1971). Colonic mucosal ulcers can be diffuse. They are

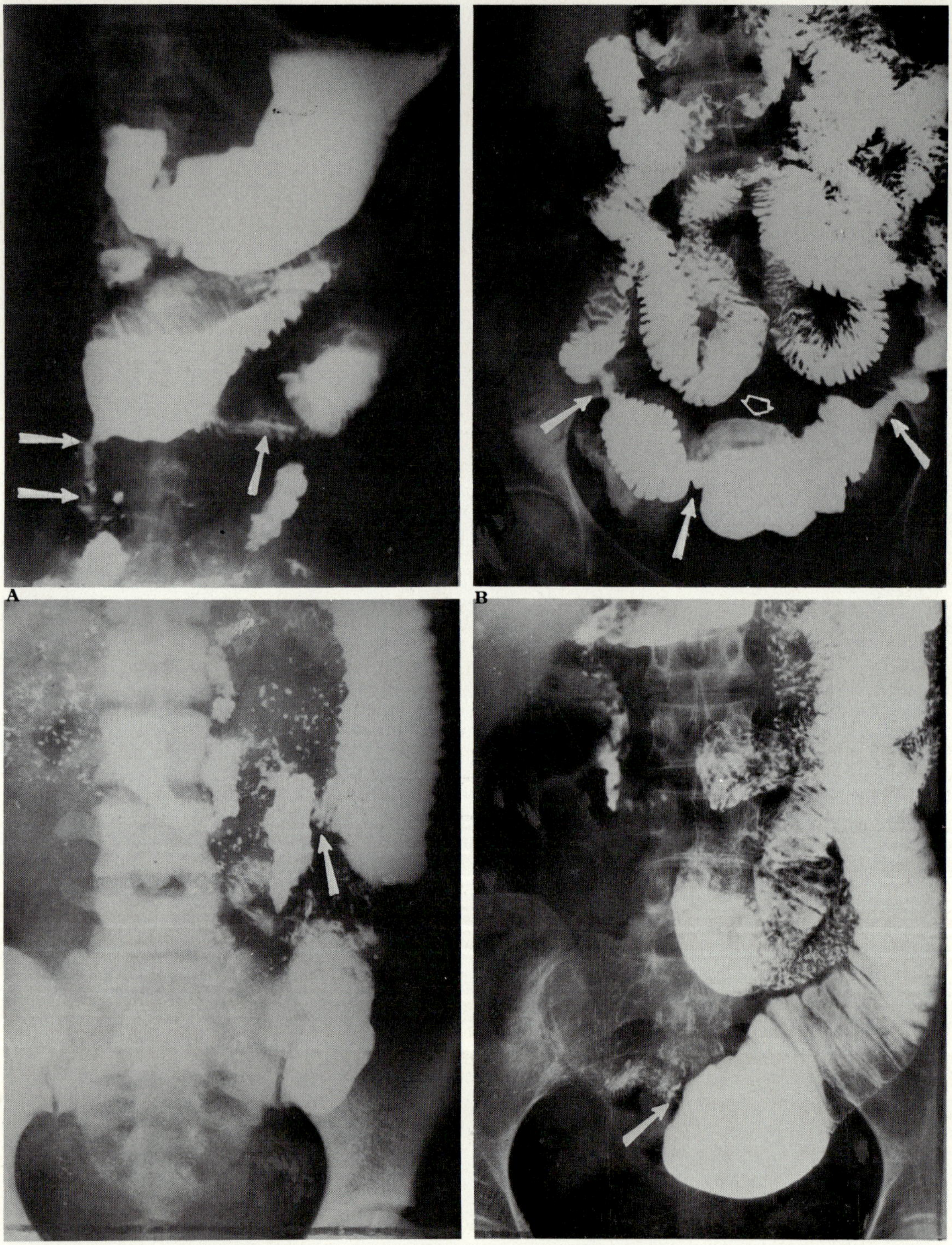

A B C D

Fig. 3.20 A–D. Appearances in four patients with tuberculous small bowel strictures shown by solid white arrows. In some cases these are multiple. In all proximal bowel dilatation is present. The small open arrow in top right view indicates an enterolith.

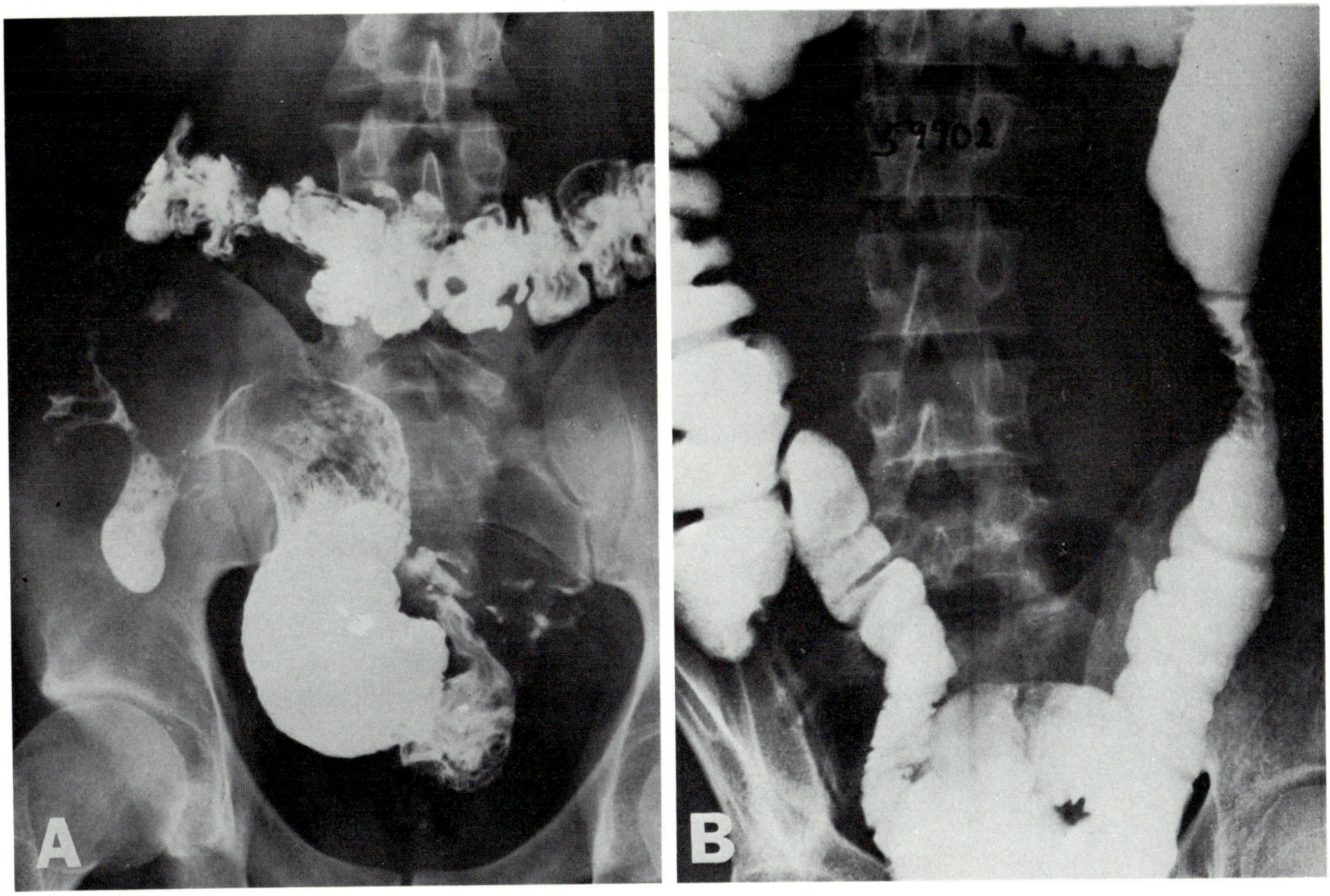

Fig. 3.21 **A.** Terminal ileal, caecal and ascending colon tuberculous strictures. **B.** Descending colon stricture.

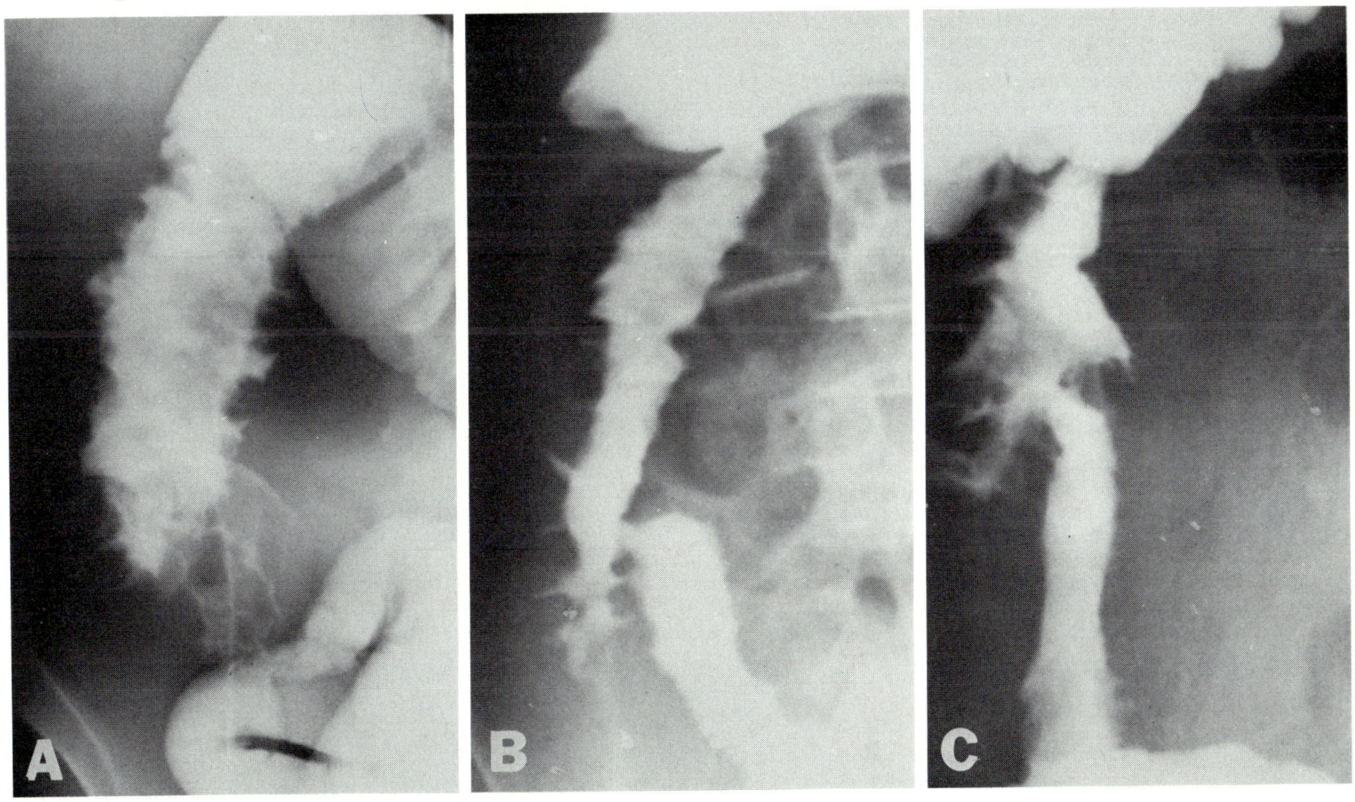

Fig. 3.22 **A, B, C.** Three Nigerian examples of hypertrophic ileo-caecal tuberculosis with characteristic cicatricial shortening of ascending colon and change in the ileal angle. The mucosa is totally destroyed and deep ulcers extend into the investing granuloma.

usually linear in an annular fashion and are often multiple (Fig. 3.23).

Rectal tuberculosis is distinctly rare, though the occurrence of tuberculous fistulae *in ano* suggests that the primary rectal lesion is not usually detected.

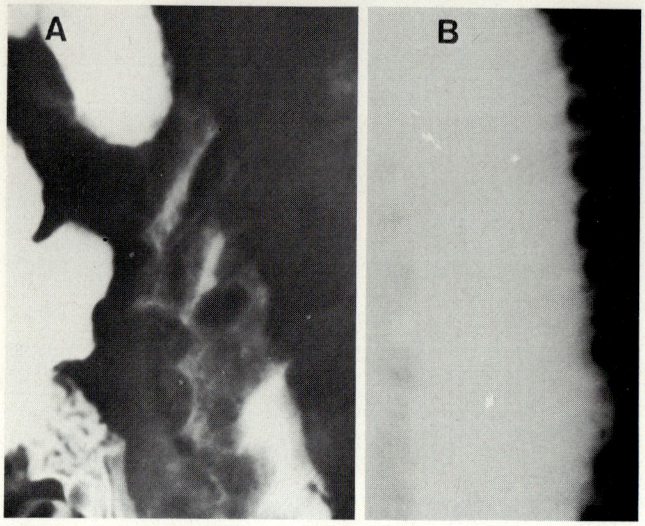

Fig. 3.23 **A.** Segment of transverse colon with long linear tuberculous ulcers and thumbprinting. **B.** Same case showing coarsely serrated tuberculous ulceration of the descending colon. These mucosal changes rapidly resolved with chemotherapy. (Courtesy of Dr. Giles Stephenson, Hamilton.)

REFERENCES

Anand, S. S. (1956) Hypertrophic ileo-caecal tuberculosis in India with a record of fifty hemicolectomies, *Annals of the Royal College of Surgeons*, **19**, 205–222.

Balikian, J. P., Yenikomshian, S. M. & Jidejian, Y. D. (1967) Tuberculosis of the pyloro-duodenal area, *American Journal of Roentgenology*, **101**, 414–420.

Beetlestone, C. A., Wieland, W., Lewis, E. A. & Itayemi, S. O. (1977) The lymphogram in abdominal tuberculosis, *Clinical Radiology*, **28**, 653–658.

Bhansali, S. K. (1977) Abdominal tuberculosis, *American Journal of Gastroenterology*, **67**, 324–337.

Brettner, A. & Euphrat, E. J. (1970) Radiological significance of enterolithiasis, *Radiology*, **94**, 238–288.

Chawla, S., Bery, K. & Indra, K. J. (1966) Enterolithiasis complicating intestinal tuberculosis, *Clinical Radiology*, **17**, 274–279.

Chawla, S. & Bery, K. (1969) Duodenal obstruction due to tuberculous lymphadenitis—a study of four cases, *Clinical Radiology*, **20**, 99–102.

Chawla, S., Mukerjee, P. & Bery, K. (1971) Segmental tuberculosis ot the colon (a report of ten cases), *Clinical Radiology*, **22**, 104–109.

Davey, W. W. & Pearson, J. B. (1965) Obstruction of the third part of the duodenum, *British Journal of Surgery*, **52**, 189–193.

Kolawole, T. M. & Lewis, E. A. (1975) A radiologic study of tuberculosis of the abdomen (gastrointestinal tract), *American Journal of Roentgenology*, **123**, 348–358.

Osime, U. (1977) Pyloric stenosis from tuberculosis, *Journal of the Royal College of Surgeons, Edinburgh*, **22**, 218–220.

Vaidya, M. G. & Sodhi, J. S. (1978) Gastro intestinal tuberculosis: a study of 102 cases including 55 colectomies, *Clinical Radiology*, **29**, 189–195.

Werbeloff, L., Novis, N. H., Bank, S. & Marks, I. N. (1973) The radiology of tuberculosis of the gastrointestinal tract, *British Journal of Radiology*, **46**, 329–336.

INTESTINAL SCHISTOSOMIASIS

Four species of schistosomal trematodes can cause intestinal lesions in man. S. japonicum occurs mainly in China, the Philippines and Japan; S. mansoni in Brazil, Venezuela, Puerto Rico and much of East, Central and West Africa, the Sudan, Nile delta, Mauritius and Malagasy; S. haematobium in Egypt, North Africa, West Africa, East and Central Africa, the eastern part of South Africa and parts of Iraq and Arabia; and S. intercalatum mainly in Zaire and the Cameroons (Van Wijk & Elias, 1975).

Mature eggs of all these parasites hatch on contact with water at an appropriate temperature to release motile miracidia. These seek out specific snail hosts where they undergo further maturation in the liver. After two sporocyst generations, ultimately cercariae are liberated into the water. Man contacting water with cercariae becomes infected when these penetrate unbroken skin. The cercariae lose their tail during this process and reach lymphatics or veins and are carried to the lungs, where most are filtered out and progress no further. The remainder reach the portal vein branches in the liver, to undergo further maturation and then descend against the flow of blood to find the veins of predilection: the vesical and uterine veins in the case of S. haematobium; the ileo-colic, colic, sigmoidal and haemorrhoidal veins with S. mansoni; the mesenteric veins with S. japonicum; and the rectal and sigmoidal veins with S. intercalatum. Naturally with such a complicated Odyssey many worms arrive in the wrong tributaries and so eggs from the 'wrong' source appear in the stools and urine of most infected persons. These four digenetic trematodes live in veins for many years in a state of permanent copulation producing ova. These are excreted in the faeces or urine to get to water and so maintain the cycle.

It is this oviposition that is responsible for the pathologic disturbances, as the flukes themselves cause relatively little trouble. Some eggs pass through the bowel lumen and are excreted. Others remain localised, unable to penetrate the wall, and die, exciting a localised inflammatory response around that causes thickening of the bowel wall. This fibrosis can progress to stricture formation (Chapman, 1966; and Francis & Wright, 1971). Lastly some eggs pass with a portal blood to embolise in the liver or, by portal systemic collaterals, to the lungs. Sequelae from these processes are discussed with the body systems involved.

The severity of symptoms is determined by the species, the worm burden, the intensity of ova deposition, the duration of the disease and host immunologic responses.

The initial passage of eggs is accompanied by bleeding. As the disease progresses bloody diarrhoea becomes manifest which sometimes, because of the exudation, produces loss of iron and a severe protein-losing enteropathy. Early in the disease colonoscopy or sigmoidoscopy reveals a swollen, congested mucosa with small punctuate haemorrhagic areas. Later oedema becomes more marked and mucosal ulceration occurs. The ulceration causes marked epithelial repair and inflammatory polyps develop which are usually multiple and can be large. Whether the polyps are due to redundant proliferative mucosa overlying disrupted cicatrised muscularis mucosa, or an epithelial covered schistosomal granuloma acted on by peristalais, is not agreed (Smith *et al.*, 1977). However, the epithelial activity gives rise to a higher incidence of bowel carcinoma than expected in association with S. japonicum and possibly S. mansoni infections. There appear to be significant differences in the schistosomal associated carcinomata compared with those in the general population in respect of age range, sex ratio and histopathology (Shindo, 1976).

The plain film of the abdomen is of little value, though radiographically visible colonic calcification in schistosomiasis has been recorded (Lehman *et al.*, 1971).

Barium studies are necessary to demonstrate bowel alterations. The small bowel is predominantly affected in S. japonicum infections and the later polypoid lesions should be detectable on a careful follow-through study or a small bowel enema. Coarsening and irregularity of mucosal folds with changes in motility have been recorded in 24 cases by Wang and Kuo (1958), and S. mansoni ileal stricture formation resembling Crohn's disease has been reported from the Sudan (Mynors, 1957).

In the large bowel polyps are the most striking lesions, which are best revealed by double contrast study so that the mucosal changes and extent of disease can be appreciated (Fig. 3.24). The polyps are usually rounded with no significant stalk and 1 to 2 cm in diameter. The rectum and sigmoid are most affected but lesions can be seen in the descending and transverse colon. Polyps are not seen as flagrantly in South America as in the Egyptian experience, where both S. haematobium and S. mansoni may often coexist (Cheever & Andrade, 1967). In a series from Egypt 20 per cent of patients with S. mansoni ultimately developed polyps in the colon. Follow-up by air contrast enemas revealed considerable improvement after Niridazole therapy (Farid *et al.*, 1973; Nebel *et al.*, 1974). Polyps, though infrequent, can be dramatic in New York City immigrant Puerto-Ricans (Chait, 1963).

A double contrast study can also demonstrate mucosal ulcers, and areas of mural fibrosis that cause localised narrowing. These can be almost obstructing in the rectosigmoid area. If narrowing is diffuse the appearance can be difficult to differentiate from lymphopathia.

Confirmation of the diagnosis can be obtained by microscopic examination of the stool or urine for ova, and by rectal biopsy.

Though angiography has been perfomed it has not proven to contribute to the diagnosis of polypoid disease (El-Sallab & Aboul-Enein, 1967).

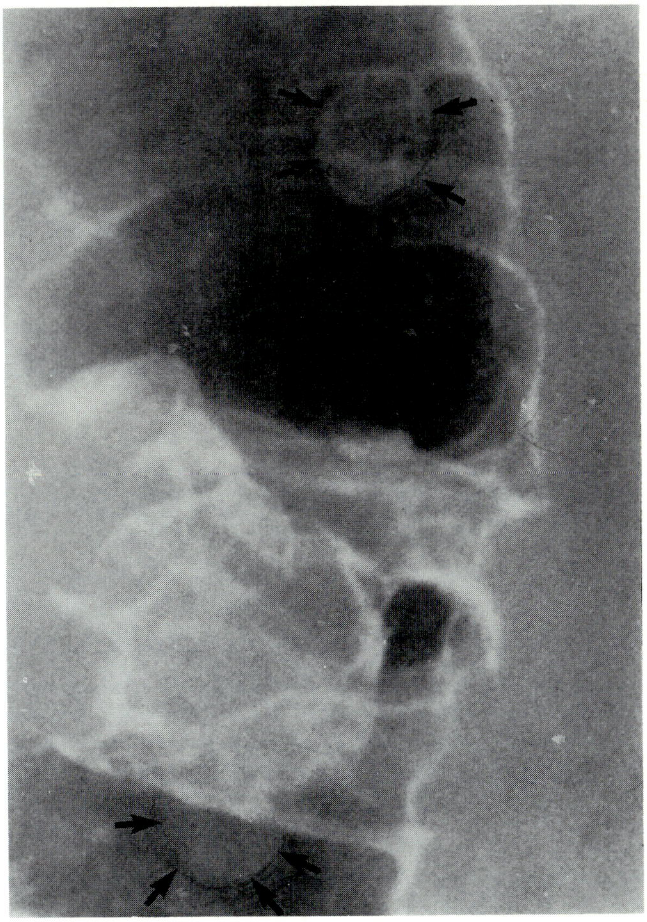

Fig. 3.24 Colonic segment with multiple S. mansoni polyps demonstrated by double contrast study. The black arrows indicate smaller inflammatory polyps.

REFERENCES

Chait, A. (1963) Schistosomiasis mansoni: roentgenologic observations in a non endemic area, *American Journal of Roentgenology*, **90,** 688–708.

Chapman, D. S. (1966) The surgical importance of bilharziasis in South Africa, *British Journal of Surgery*, **53,** 544–557.

Cheever, A. W. & Andrade, Z.A. (1967) Pathological lesions associated with schistomosa mansoni infection in man, *Transactions of the Royal Society of Tropical Medicine and Hygiene*, **61,** 626–639.

El-Sallab, R. A. & Aboul-Enein, A. A. (1967) Angiographic appearances of bilharzial mass of the colon. *British Journal of Radiology*, **40,** 151–153.

Farid, Z., Bassily, S., Sparks, H. A., El Masry, N. A., Young, S. W., Hassan, A. & Nebel, O. T. (1973) Reversibility of lesions in S. haematobium and S. mansoni infections, *Abstracts Ninth International Congress of Tropical Medicine and Malariology*, Athens, 84–85.

Francis, T. I. & Wright, S. G. (1971) Schistosoma mansoni infestation of the lower bowel in Nigerians, *Tropical and Geographical Medicine*, **23,** 84–88.

Lehman, J. S., Farid, Z., Bassily, S. & Kent, D. C. (1971) Colonic calcification and polyposis in schistosomiasis, *Radiology*, **93,** 379–380.

Mynors, J. M. (1957) Intestinal schistosomiasis resembling regional ileitis, *Transactions of the Royal Society of Tropical Medicine and Hygiene*, **51,** 45–47.

Nebel, O. T., El Masry, N. A., Castell, D. O., Farid, Z., Fornes, M. F. & Sparks, H. A. (1974) Schistosomal disease of the colon: a reversible form of polyposis, *Gastroenterology*, **67,** 939–943.

Shindo, K. (1976) Significance of Schistosomiasis japonica in the development of cancer of the large intestine, *Diseases of the Colon and Rectum*, **19,** 460–469.

Smith, J. H., Said, M. N. & Kelada, A. S. (1977) Studies on schistosomal rectal and colonic polyposis, *American Journal of Tropical Medicine and Hygiene*, **26**, 80–84.

Van Wijk, H. B. & Elias, E. A. (1975) Hepatic and rectal pathology in Schistosoma intercalatum infection, *Geographical Medicine*, 27, 237–248.

Wang, C. & Kuo, T. (1958) Roentgenologic changes of small intestine in Schistosomiasis japonica, *Chinese Journal of Radiology*, **6**, 247–253.

HELMINTHOMA

An inflammatory colonic mass related to parasitism by various Oesophagostomum species has been termed 'helminthoma'. The condition has been recorded over 35 times from Uganda, 10 times from Ghana and on occasions from Kenya, Sudan, Nigeria, the Ivory Coast, Brazil and Indonesia (Anthony & McAdam, 1972; Haaf & Van Soest, 1964).

The parasites, which are allied to hookworm, normally pass their life in pigs, sheep, cattle and monkeys. Man becomes an accidental host on consuming contaminated material containing rhabditoid larvae of O. apiostomum and O. stephanostomum. These encyst in the wall of the large bowel, usually around the caecum, exciting a considerable cellular reaction. The worm lies centrally in a small abscess-like cavity surrounded by a thick-walled eosinophilic granulomatous infiltrate that causes a mass. Since the tissue phase of the parasite is abnormal in man,

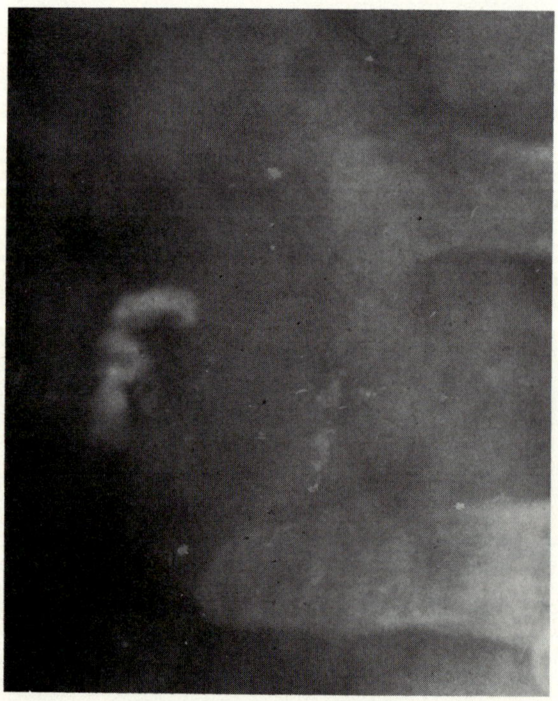

Fig. 3.25 Calcified parasite presumed to be O. apiostomum 10 years after surgery for helminthoma. (Courtesy of Dr. J. M. Welchman and *British Journal of Radiology*.)

the normal sequence of the mature worm returning to the lumen of the bowel to reproduce may not take place. The parasite may remain in an intramural position, it may enter the peritoneal cavity or it may lead to a cutaneous fistula through which it may be expelled.

Radiologically barium enema and follow-through studies can be useful. The characteristic lesion is an intramural filling defect of the caecum which has relatively smooth walls (Welchman, 1966). The mass can be pericaecal, displacing small bowel, as in a child who had lived in Uganda and became ill in Canada (Marshall & Deneka, 1969). This condition enters into the differential diagnosis of right iliac fossa masses. A presumptive diagnosis may be indicative of conservative management. In one patient followed up by Welchman a calcified parasite 2 cm long by 3 mm was noted in the right upper quadrant 10 years after an operated lesion in the transverse colon. Thus it would appear that the worm can calcify (Fig. 3.25 and 3.26).

There are other parasites that may cause bowel granulomata. Some forms of anisakiasis do not seek the stomach but localise in the ileum and caecum where they cause nodules, as with the larval stage of Contracaecum osculatum (Schaum & Mueller, 1967).

Angiostrongyliasis normally parasitises the vascular system of the rat but one species, A. costaricensis, can lead to adult worms in the distal branches of the superior mesenteric arteries of man, where it may cause thrombosis. The parasite, by depositing eggs in the caecal and ileal wall, produces nodular granulomas. Clinically the lesion can present as a subacute intestinal obstruction due to the mass, or as infarction of bowel following death of the intravascular parasite (Morera & Cespedes, 1971).

The condition has been seen in Costa Rica and Honduras. Children are mainly infected and complain of pain in the right iliac fossa. A mass can be palpated. On barium studies there is alteration to the bowel wall with rigidity and stretching of the mucosa (Morera, 1973).

In Australia a nematode, Spirurida physalopteridae, is reported to have caused infarcts and eosinophilic granulomata in the distal small bowel (Nicolaides *et al.*, 1977). As with A. costaricensis, parasitic embolism is the basic process that causes the lesions.

Various other parasites which may normally be in the abdomen, or where the abdomen represents an ectopic focus, can cause inflammatory intraperitoneal masses: ascaris, hookworm, sparganum, etc. These are discussed elsewhere.

There are a number of further parasites whose habitat in man is the bowel or bowel wall which are likely to cause radiologic abnormalities due to mucosal ulceration and granulomata, but we are not aware of any descriptions of the radiographic features.

Fasciolopsis buski is a common fluke infection of mainland South East Asia and parts of the south-west Pacific. Adult forms are attached to the duodenal and

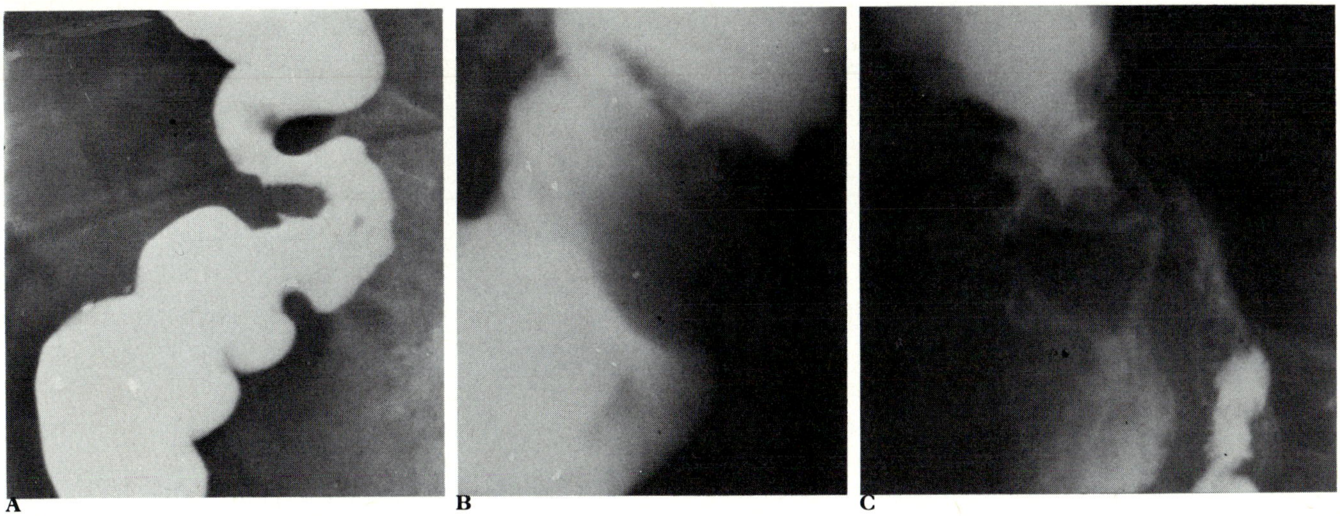

Fig. 3.26 A, B, C. Barium enemas from three patients with eosinophilic helminthoma granulomas showing mural filling defects from Tanzania. (Courtesy of Dr. M. Welchman.)

jejunal mucosa where they can cause severe diarrhoea, vomiting, intestinal obstruction and even death. Another fluke, Echinostoma ilocanum, parasitises the jejunal mucosa in the Philippines and parts of Indonesia. Jejunal mucosal ulcerations and even perforation can follow parasitism by Metagonimus yokogawai in the Far East and Heterophyes in Egypt. Gastrodiscoides hominis fluke attaches itself to the caecum and the proximal colon to cause mucosal ulceration and reaction in the bowel wall that can be associated with severe diarrhoea. Examination of the stools for ova should provide the diagnosis of these intestinal parasites that normally only affect the bowel in a superficial manner, yet on occasions can be more invasive (Spencer, 1973).

REFERENCES

Anthony, P. P. & McAdam, I. W. J. (1972) Helminthic pseudotumours of the bowel: thirty-four cases of helminthoma, *Gut*, **13**, 8–16.

Haaf, E. & van Soest, A. H. (1964) Oesophagostomiasis in man in North Ghana, *Tropical and Geographical Medicine*, **16**, 49–53.

Marshall, D. G. & Deneka, S. I. (1969) Abdominal abscess due to a helminthoma of the ascending colon, *Canadian Medical Association Journal*, **100**, 913–914.

Morera, P. (1973) Life history and redescription of Angio-strongylus constaricensis Morera and Cespedes 1971, *American Journal of Tropical Medicine and Hygiene*, **22**, 613–621.

Morera, P. & Cespedes, R. (1971) Angiostrongylus costaricencis n. sp. (Nematoda: Metastrongylcidea) a new lung worm occurring in man in Costa Rica, *Revista de Biologia Tropical*, Universidad de Costa Rica (San José), **18**, 173–185.

Nicolaides, N. J., Musgrave, J., McGuckin, D. & Moorhouse, D. E. (1977) Nematode larvae (Spirurida physalopteridae) causing infarction in the bowel in an infant, *Pathology*, **9**, 129–135.

Schaum, E. & Mueller, W. (1967) Die Heterocheilidiasis. Eine Infektion des Menschen mit Larven von Fisch-Ascariden, *Deutsche Medizinische Wochenschrift*, **92**, 2230–2233.

Spencer, H. (1973) In *Tropical Pathology* pp. 597–610. Heidelberg: Springer.

Welchman, J. M. (1966) Helminithic abscess of the bowel, *British Journal of Radiology*, **39**, 372–376.

AMOEBIASIS—AMOEBIC DYSENTERY

Amoebiasis is a worldwide problem with a high prevalence in areas of poverty associated with deficiencies in sanitation and water supplies. In Mexico City amoebiasis was found to be fourth in the causes of death—an indication of the magnitude that this problem can assume (Perez-Tamayo & Brandt, 1971).

It has been estimated that 20 per cent of the world's population may carry the parasite (Cardoso *et al.*, 1977), but only a small proportion develop clinical disease. Infection with Entomoeba histolytica exists in two forms: an asymptomatic carrier state in the colon characterised by the passage of infective cysts, and a symptomatic dysenteric disorder in which mobile trophozoites are passed. What determines the conversion of a tolerated parasite into an invasive pathogen is not well understood. It has been shown to be dependent on certain environmental alteration in the gut (e.g. pH and bacterial flora) as well as changes in the nutritional and immune status of the host. A further possibility is that strains of E. histolytica may vary in their virulence. Whatever the complex factors are that interact to determine the course of a particular infection, there is no doubt that analysis of series collected from various parts of the world reveals considerable differences in the incidence of the types of presentation, and the course and complications observed. What is seen in Mexico differs from the features noted in western Nigeria. The disease acquired by a visitor to an endemic area will have a different course from that expected in a local inhabitant.

Consequently amoebiasis can pose considerable difficulties in diagnosis. This is particularly so in areas where both ulcerative colitis and other forms of inflammatory bowel disease occur. Fortunately where Crohn's disease and ulcerative colitis are frequent amoebic dysentery is usually rare—and the converse applies.

Diagnosis is based on the identification of cysts and trophozoites of E. histolytica. Though examination of fresh stools may serve to establish the diagnosis, study of fresh mucus exudate obtained from the bowel lumen for haematophagous mobile trophozoites by proctoscopy, sigmoidoscopy or colonoscopy should not be neglected. Material should be obtained prior to washouts of the bowel (Pittman *et al.*, 1973). In non-endemic areas amoebic serologic tests, such as the indirect haemagglutination test or fluorescent antibody estimation, are useful in confirming both the diagnosis of colitis and invasive liver disease.

Systematic correlation of the endoscopic appearances of early lesions with their histologic basis has been carried out in a fine study on Malaysian aborigines (Prathrap & Gilman, 1970; Gilman & Prathrap, 1971). The earliest mucosal change was oedema of the folds, increased mucus production and some fine pinpoint depressions. This stage is characterised by glandular hyperplasia and stromal oedema and absence of tissue-penetrating amoebae. The next phase was termed 'lobular change', where in addition to the preceding alterations the mucosa was friable, had 1 mm superficial erosions and there were irregular raised lobules, each lobule of several millimetres, forming a reticular pattern. This appearance provides the background on which more severe ulcerative processes develop, such as necrotic ulcers 2 to 30 mm or more in size. These ulcers were of any shape and often irregular. Biopsies of the lobular change reveals that there are focal mucopenic depressions from localised loss of mucosal thickness due to disappearance of surface mucin and goblet cells, causing focal depressions or pseudo-ulcers. Large numbers of amoebae are present in the exudate. The ulcers initially contain sloughs and later have a red clean granular floor.

We have gone into some detail to describe the early lesions, as small areas of nodular oedematous mucosa can be detected as abnormal in double contrast studies (Fig. 3.27). Small ulcers may not fill with barium until the slough separates. They are then well defined. Larger lesions may show undermining.

Lesions may develop anywhere in the colon though, in addition to the rectum, the caecum has been said to be involved in 90 per cent of cases and the ileum remains free of the disease (Weinfeld, 1966). However, the appendix is not immune and can lead to symptoms suggestive of appendicitis. Appendiceal involvement is associated with a high incidence of liver abscess (Cardoso *et al.*, 1977).

Fulminating invasive amoebiasis can be diffuse and leads to an acute severe mucus bloody diarrhoea with extreme prostration, a high fatality rate, and features of toxic dilatation of the colon. This complication of panmural involvement is more frequent in children. We have seen it develop following the use of steroids in patients considered initially to have non-specific ulcerative colitis rather than amoebiasis (Case Records *N.E.J.M.*, 1977) (Fig. 3.28).

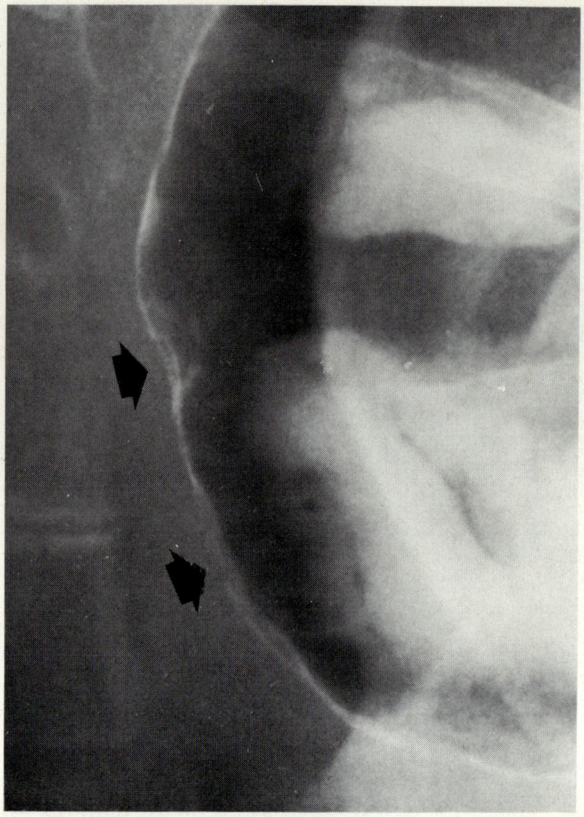

Fig. 3.27 Focal mucosal irregularities due to posterior rectal wall amoebic ulcers which are readily distinguishable from the thin white line of barium coating unaffected areas.

A more localised lesion is the amoeboma: an oedematous granuloma mass that intrudes into the lumen of the bowel and can lead to obstructive symptoms. About half amoeboma patients have a single focus, but multiple masses with skip lesion can be present. A striking characteristic of these masses is their potential for remarkably rapid resolution following treatment with emetine or metronidazole (Samuel, 1948; Balikian *et al.*, 1974).

The radiologic changes of intestinal amoebiasis may be confusing, difficult to interpret and are often not specific.

Though barium studies are generally the most informative, the value of plain abdominal films is not to be neglected, particularly in severe fulminating cases where toxic megacolon may develop. The appearance is then usually characteristic with gaseous distension of the colon most obvious in the transverse colon. The lumen of the bowel is devoid of solid material and the normal haustral configuration is abolished (Fig. 3.28). If the bowel wall thickness can be visualised anywhere it may show areas of thickening. The mucosal surface shows coarse wavy irregularities and perhaps 'thumbprinting' contour defects outlined by the gas (Fig. 3.28). The features are

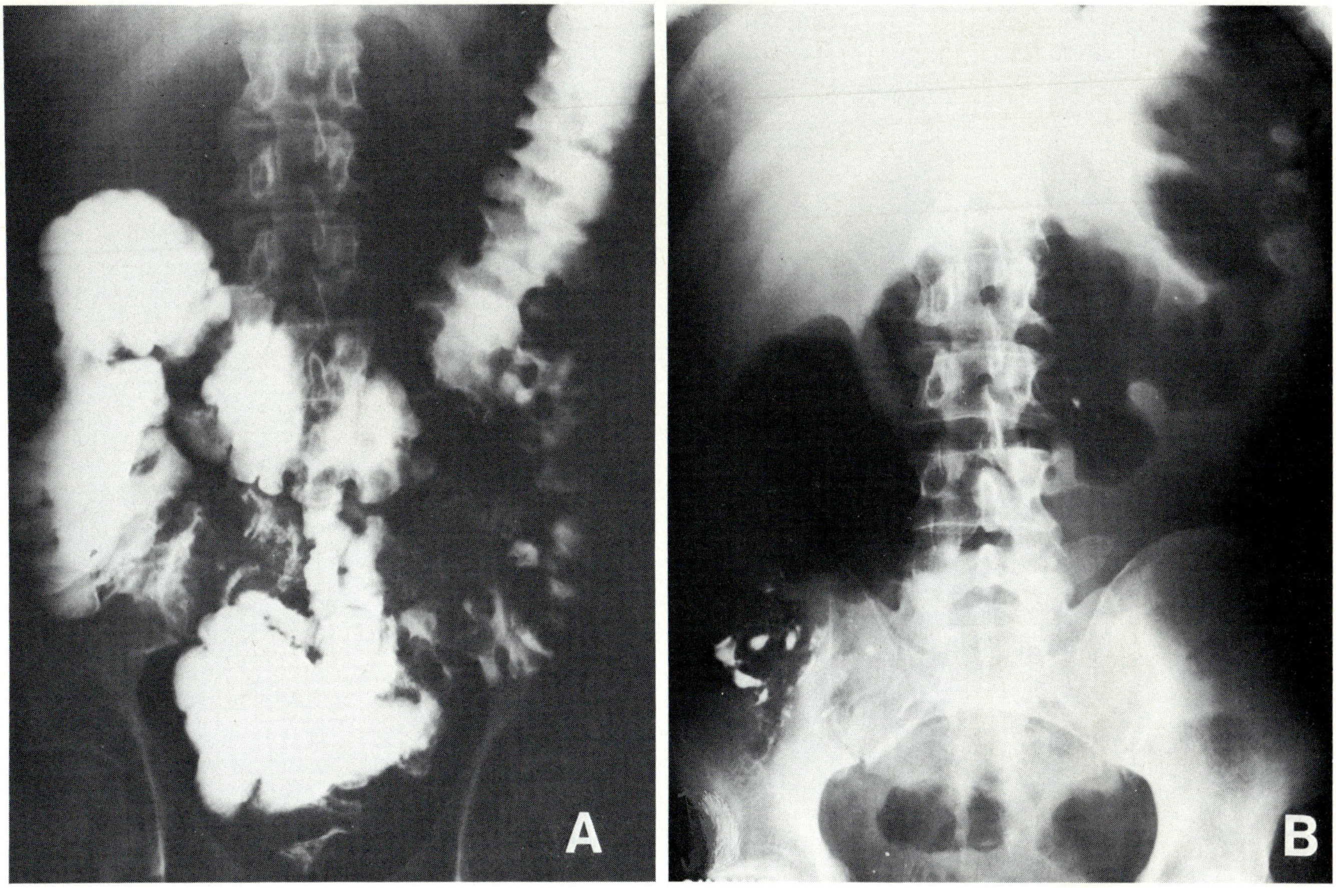

Fig. 3.28 Male aged 51 who developed 'toxic megacolon' during course of amoebiasis of six weeks duration after having been given steroids inadvertently. **A.** reveals multiple marginal thumbprinting mucosal irregularities. In the plain film a few days later there is gross distension of parts of large bowel.

due to oedema and swollen pseudopolyp tags. The features in amoebiasis can then be indistinguishable from those occurring in ulcerative colitis (Wruble *et al.*, 1966; Fargenburg *et al.*, 1967).

Plain abdominal films can reveal masses due to abscesses, hepatomegaly and perhaps constant rigid narrowed bowel segments outlined by gas when an amoeboma is present. Perforation of bowel is indicated by presence of free air in the peritoneal cavity.

Barium studies can be safely carried out except in severe fulminating cases where possible toxic dilatation is feared. Much of the descriptive literature on amoebic colonic disease is involved with careful detailed classification of haustral contour alterations. We believe that these are subjective findings that have no proven pathologic validity and, since they are not specific in any way, have little diagnostic value. The patients who clinically are problems do not yet have a diagnosis and suffer from chronic or mild diarrhoeal disease.

The radiologist must seek to identify the small mucosal lesions. For this purpose careful bowel preparation is necessary and a primary double contrast study is to be preferred to a conventional enema. The success of double contrast in showing the extent of disease and minute lesions of the mucosa in other inflammatory bowel disease has been established by many in recent years (Laufer, 1976), and this technique should be used in suspected amoebiasis unless there is toxic dilatation.

In a conventional enema the border of the lumen can show fine ulcers giving an irregular edge. Deep ulcers may undermine and be flask-shaped or even rarely track submucosally parallel to the lumen. In double contrast studies small ulcers and nodules are much easier to detect and the rectum should not be overlooked (Fig. 3.27). The lesions are patchy but larger than the apthous ulcers of Crohn's disease. The ileum is not involved though usually clearly shown, since the ileo-caecal valve is often patent in amoebiasis. The typical slightly conical caecum with a refluxing valve and a normal ileum is characteristic (Fig. 3.29).

If in addition ulcerative lesions are seen in the mucosa this provides reinforcement to a tentative diagnosis of amoebiasis and delineates areas for sigmoidoscopic or colonoscopic attention. The advantage of double contrast studies is that one is not restricted to visualising lesions tangentially on the borders of the lumen but can also display ulcers *en face*.

Ulcers often exist for a short segment and then intact

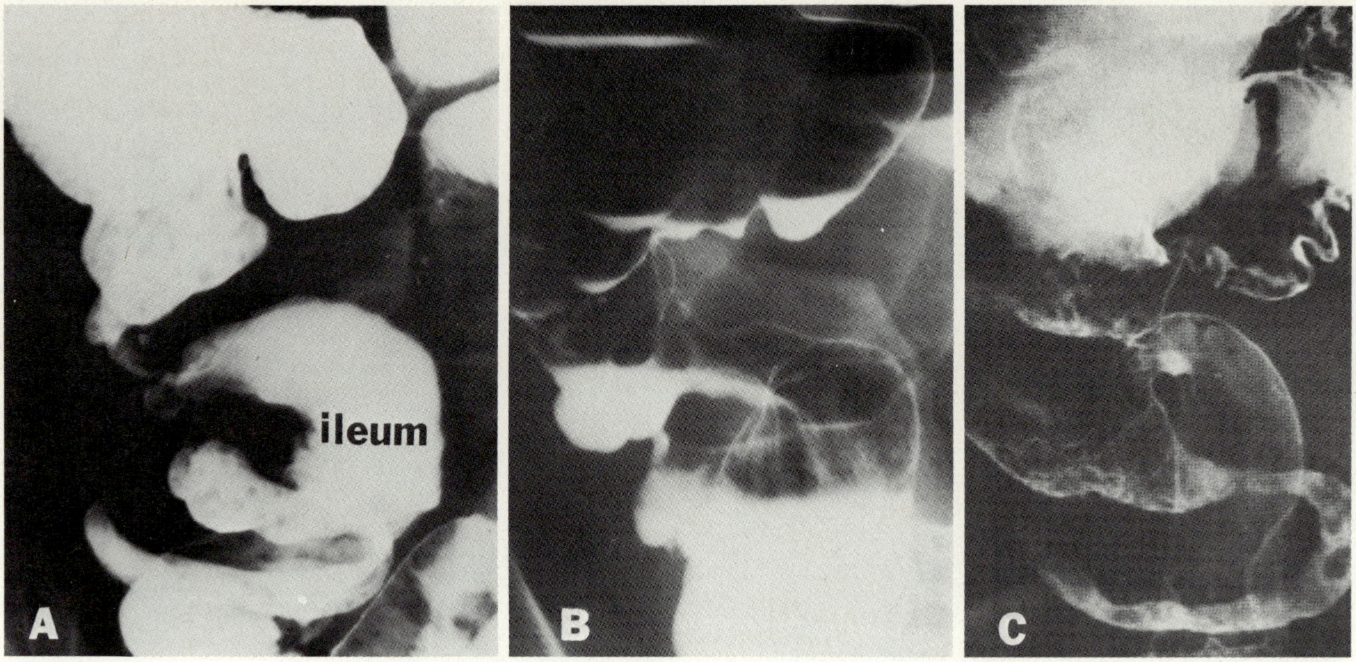

Fig. 3.29 Two patients with typical coned amoebic caecum. **A.** Single contrast with scarred caecum. **B** and **C.** Pointed caecum and widely patent terminal ileum.

mucosa is seen. Though postmortem and clinical studies indicate predominant involvement of caecum and ascending colon, ulcers *per se* are seen most often in the sigmoid and rectum in enema studies.

Amoebomas show as irregular segmental filling defects which do not expand. They may be multiple and are found with diminishing frequency in the caecum, ascending colon, rectosigmoid, transverse colon and descending colon (Delahaye *et al.*, 1964; Cardoso *et al.*, 1977) (Figs. 3.30 and 3.31). Re-examination after a week to ten days of adequate therapy will show remarkable resolution without stricture formation.

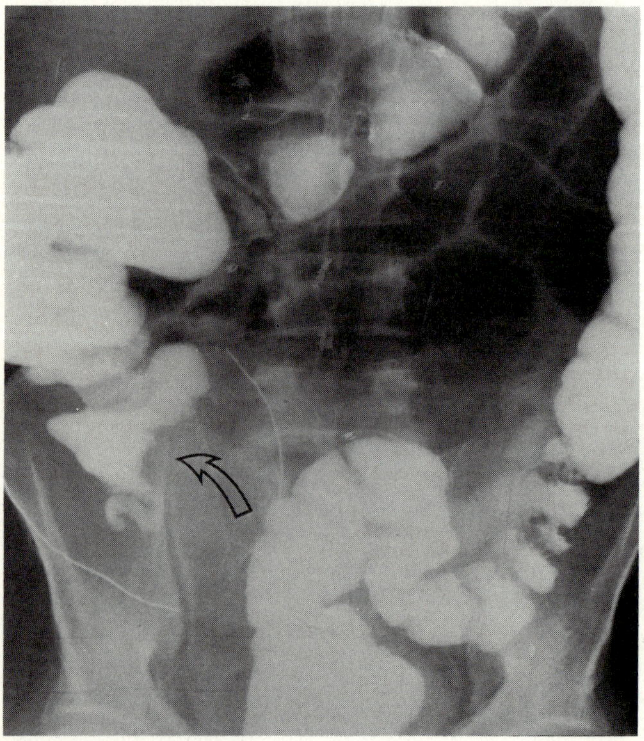

Fig. 3.30 Amoeboma extrinsic type filling defect marked by arrow. Wire indicates mass.

Stenosis following healing of inflammatory masses occasionally occurs and, as with amoebomas, several segments of bowel can be affected.

Perforation, abscesses, or tracking fistulae are occasionally seen.

In conclusion, barium studies can be useful as an aid to diagnosis but their value lies in providing morphologic information on the site of lesions for definitive diagnostic procedures as well as being helpful in follow-up studies.

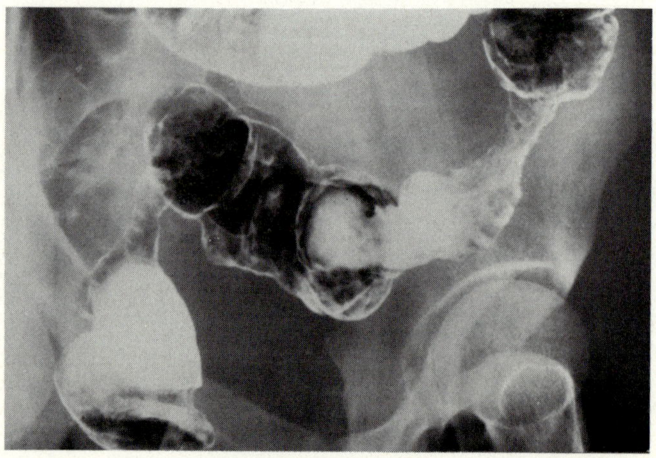

Fig. 3.31 Multiple amoeboma—until an adequate interval after therapy exclusion of permanent stricture is impossible.

The liver and lung complications are considered under their respective systems.

REFERENCES

Balikian, J. P., Uthman, S. M. and Khouri, N. F. (1974) Intestinal amoebiasis, *American Journal of Roentgenology*, **122**, 245–256.

Cardoso, J. M., Kimura, K., Stoopen, J., Cervantes, L. F., Elizondo, L., Churchill, R. & Moncada, R. (1977) Radiology of invasive amebiasis of the colon, *American Journal of Roentgenology*, **128**, 935–941.

Case records of the Massachusetts General Hospital (1977) *New England Journal of Medicine*, **297**, 322–330.

Delahaye, R. P., Jolly, R., Laaban, J. & Boursiquot, P. (1946) L'amibiase intestinale chronique (étude radiologique de 171 cas), *Journal de Radiologie et d'Electrologie*, **45**, 117–132.

Faegenburg, D., Chiat, M., Mandel, P. R. & Ross, S. T. (1967) Toxic megacolon in amebic colitis, *American Journal of Roentgenology*, **99**, 74–76.

Gilman, R. H. & Prathrap, K. (1971) Acute intestinal amoebiasis—proctoscopic appearances with histopathological correlation, *Annals of Tropical Medicine and Parasitology*, **65**, 359–365.

Laufer, I. (1976) The double contrast enema: myths and misconceptions, *Gastro-Intestinal Radiology*, **1**, 19–31.

Perez-Tamayo, R. and Brandt, M. (1971) In *Pathology of Protozoal and Helminthic Diseases*. p. 146. Ed. Marcial-Rojas, R. A. Baltimore: Williams & Wilkins.

Pittman, F. E., El-Hashimi, W. & Pittman, J. C. (1973) Studies on human amebiasis, *Gastro-Enterology*, **65**, 581–587.

Prathrap, K. & Gilman, R. (1970) The histopathology of acute intestinal amebiasis, *American Journal of Pathology*, **60**, 229–239.

Samuel, E. (1948) The radiological diagnosis of chronic amoebic colitis, *British Journal of Radiology*, **21**, 625–631.

Weinfeld, A. (1966) The roentgen appearance of intestinal amoebiasis, *American Journal of Roentgenology*, **96**, 311–322.

Wruble, L. D., Duckworth, J. K., Duke, D. D. & Rothschild, J. A. (1966) Toxic dilatation of the colon in a case of amoebiasis, *New England Journal of Medicine*, **275**, 926–928.

LYMPHOGRANULOMA VENEREUM

Lymphogranuloma, though worldwide in extent, is much more prevalent in the tropics than elsewhere. It is particularly frequent in the Caribbean and Central America, in tropical Africa, Southern India, Indonesia and New Guinea. This venereal disease is caused by Chlamydia trachomatis—organism classified between bacteria and viruses. The infective agent is closely related to that responsible for psittacosis.

The infection begins as a transient primary lesion, usually on the genitals, and is followed by suppurative inflammatory process of draining lymph nodes and adjacent tissues. The external evidence of the adenitis is usually inguinal gland swellings (buboes), particularly in males.

Proctitis, rectal fistulae and obstructing rectal fibrosis are later symptoms seen mostly in females. The pathogenesis of the rectal lesion is uncertain, but rectal intercourse is not necessary for its development.

The proctocolitis causes tenesmus and bloody diarrhoea. Symptoms can persist for long periods. The rectal mucosa ulcerates, the wall is infiltrated by plasma cell and lymphocyte granulomas so that the rectal wall and perirectal tissue gradually fibrose to cause short or long tubular strictures. These can be sufficiently narrow as to cause intestinal obstruction (Annamunthodo, 1961).

Diagnosis can be confirmed by the Frei skin test which remains forever positive in an infected patient. A complement fixation test has also been developed.

In clinical investigation changes can be observed sigmoidoscopically in the rectum and strictures can be palpated. Because of the infective nature of the disease care should be taken to avoid contamination. The disease has been transferred by an infected enema nozzle, so that disposable nozzles are an advantage and gloves should be worn when dealing with such patients (Annamunthodo, 1961).

Barium enemas document the site and length of the strictures, whether any communicating or blind fistulous tracks exist and can demonstrate mucosal ulceration (Annamunthodo & Marryatt, 1961) (Fig. 3.32).

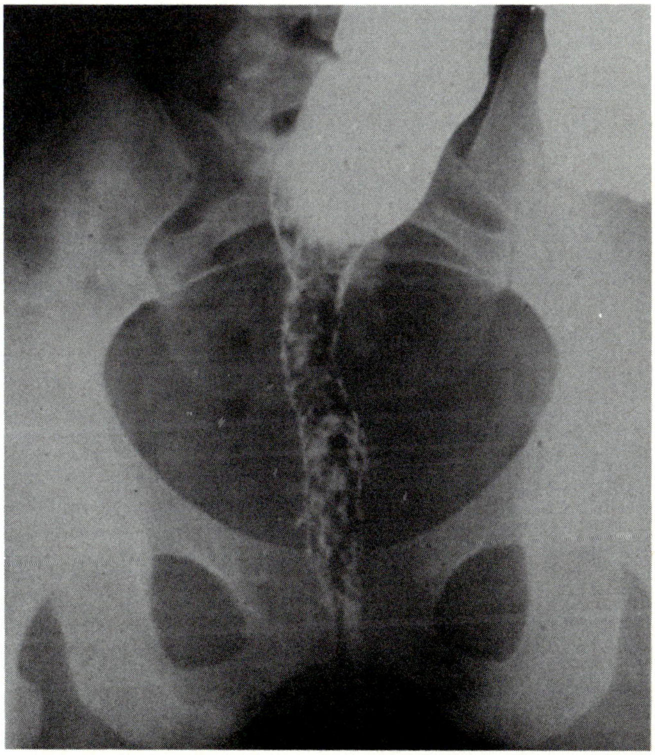

Fig. 3.32 Extensive mucosal ulceration with shortening and narrowing of rectum. The bowel proximal to the stricture can dilate in this Nigerian patient.

The strictures may be short, or a long tubular narrowing may occur with a markedly shortened cicatrised rectum that has a straightened course (Fig. 3.33). Proximal to the stricture the bowel may be dilated due to chronic obstruction. Abscesses and fistulae may be outlined.

REFERENCES

Annamunthodo, H. (1961) Rectal lymphogranuloma venereum in Jamaica, *Annals of the Royal College of Surgeons*, **29**, 141–159.

Annamunthodo, H. & Marryat, J. (1961) Barium studies in intestinal lymphogranuloma venereum, *British Journal of Radiology*, **34**, 53–57.

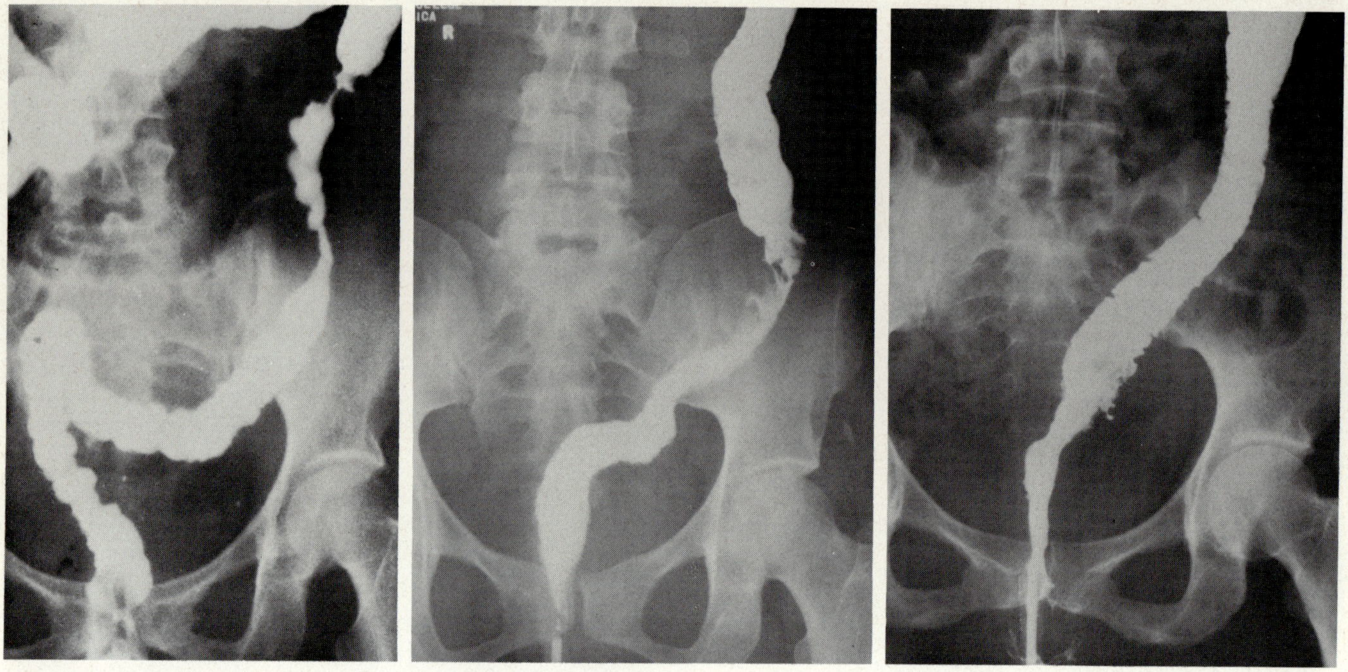

A B C

Fig. 3.33 A, B, C. Three Jamaican patients with lymphogranuloma of the colon and rectum. Cicatrisation has led to shortening and straightening of the bowel. Extensive mucosal ulceration is present as well as long strictures. (Courtesy of Dr. J. Marryat, Jamaica.)

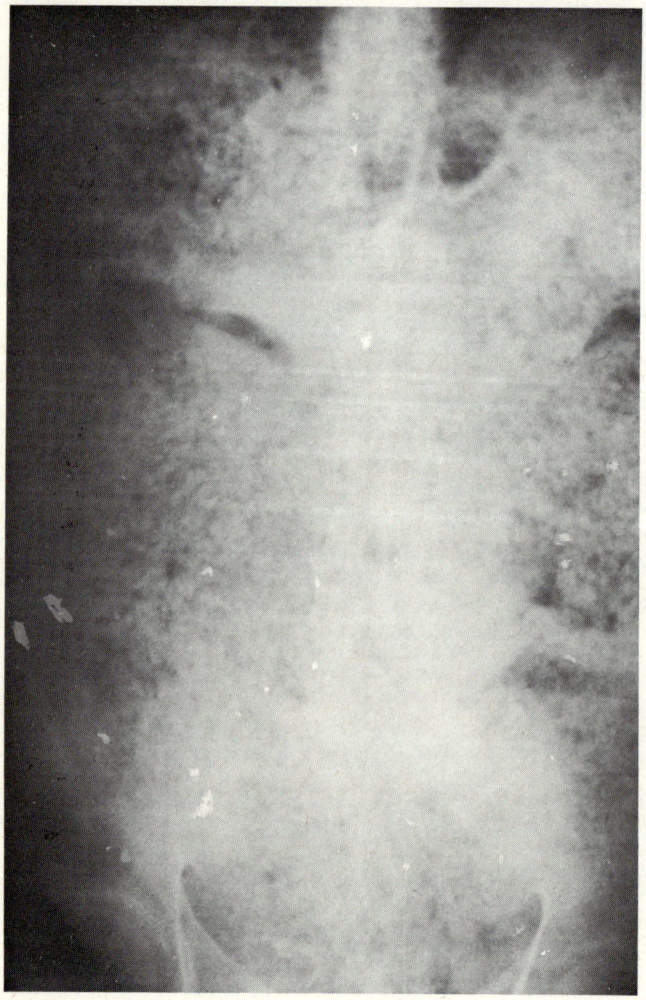

Fig. 3.34 Chagasic megacolon in plain film. The whole of the abdomen is obscured by opacity from enormous quantity of faecal contents in colon. (Courtesy of Dr. C. Simao, Ribirao-Preto.)

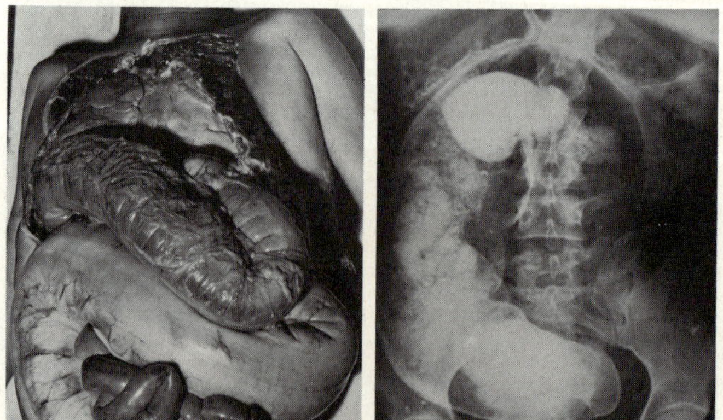

A B

Fig. 3.35 A, B. Autopsy to show gross dimension of sigmoid and of colon in an individual with chagasic megacolon. The enema outlines the dilated redundant sigmoid. (Courtesy of Prof. F. Koberle, Ribeirao-Preto.)

CHAGASIC MEGACOLON

In American trypanosomiasis megacolon develops in about a third of cases (Koberle, 1973). This occurs in the late chronic phase of T. cruzi infections when the autonomic tissues in the bowel wall have been severely depleted. The whole of the colon is involved and it may attain grotesque proportions with considerable stagnation of bowel contents (Figs. 3.34 and 3.35). There is no focal narrow zone as can occur in Hirschsprung's disease. A barium enema study, if required, should be done with considerable care and moderation, as the barium is likely to be retained and later harden. In this condition the colonic capacity can reach 20 litres so that enthusiasm to opacify the colon must be tempered by caution. Since the disease is, despite the stagnation, not precancerous, the need for enemas in this condition is probably limited.

Chagasic colonic disease predisposes to sigmoid volvulus in 10 per cent of cases (Ferreira-Santos & Carrill, 1964).

REFERENCES

Ferreira-Santos, R. & Carrill, C. F. (1964) Acquired megacolon in Chagas disease, *Diseases of the Colon and Rectum*, **7**, 353–364.

Koberle, F. (1963) Enteromegaly and cardiomegaly in Chagas disease, *Gut*, **4**, 399–405.

FUNGAL INFLAMMATORY BOWEL DISEASE

This type of bowel involvement is infrequent. Fungal lesions can cause mass lesions, ulcerative lesions and obstructing lesions.

Masses may be either intramural or extrinsic, often from enlarged lymph glands. Inflammatory masses of the bowel wall occur in Histoplasma capsulatum, H. duboisii infections, cryptococcosis and South American blastomycosis (Perez *et al.*, 1966; Unat *et al.*, 1960; De Moraes *et al.*, 1967). Involvement of lymph glands can lead to displacement of bowel or compression. Duodenal ileus may arise following adenopathy.

When mesenteric glands are involved marked swelling and prominence of valvulae conniventes may be seen (Bank *et al.*, 1965).

Mural involvement when it encircles bowel can cause narrowing that can simulate Crohn's disease.

Radiologically these dimorphic yeast infections are so variable in their appearance in the bowel that diagnosis can only be established by other means. Since the lesions are often not single, and the usual portal of entry is through the lungs, chest films may sometimes provide an aetiologic clue. Careful inspection of accessible skin lesions for biopsy can be very helpful.

REFERENCES

Bank, S., Trey, C., Gans, I., Marks, I. N. & Groll, A. (1965) Histoplasmosis of the small bowel with 'Giant' intestinal villi and secondary protein-losing enteropathy, *American Journal of Medicine*, **38**, 492–501.

De Moraes, C. R., Fiorillo, A. M. & Da Costa, J. C. (1967) Lesões Radiologicas intestinais na blastomicose sud-americana, *O Hospital*, **71**, 145–156.

Perez, C. A., Sturim, H. S., Kouchoukos, N. J. & Kamberg, S. (1966) Some clinical and radiographic features of gastrointestinal histoplasmosis, *Radiology*, **86**, 482–487.

Unat, E. K., Pars, B. & Kosyak, J. P. (1960) A case of cryptococcosis of the colon, *British Medical Journal*, **2**, 1501–1502.

TRICHURIS TRICHIURA
WHIPWORM, TRICHOCEPHALIASIS

Whipworm with a worldwide distribution is one of the most frequent intestinal helminthic infestations of man. It is most often seen in tropical and subtropical countries where both the worm burden and incidence may be high, particularly in children aged 3 to 9 living in conditions of overcrowding and poverty. Mentally defective children in institutions can have a high rate of infection in the U.S. and Europe.

Infection is acquired by ingesting mature eggs from the soil. Freshly passed ova in the stool take about three weeks to develop to a first stage larva within the egg. A suitable environment is necessary for this to take place. Warmth, dampness and shade are the optimal soil conditions.

The embryonated ova on ingestion releases the larva in the duodenum and upper small bowel, where they enter the crypts and grow. The larva migrate into the caecum and large bowel, where they gain attachment to the mucosa. The adult worms have a characteristic shape. The anterior portions of their bodies are thin and thread-like with the distal third, which contains the genital structures, being much wider. This is the portion that lies free in the lumen of the bowel, the thread-like segment lying in epithelial tunnels in the mucosa, where in most instances it seems to excite remarkably little reaction. The worms consume a slight amount of blood, far less than hookworms, but petechial haemorrhages and slight bleeding from the mucosa can occur in heavy infestations. The male worm is 3 to 4·5 cm long and the female is longer, 3·5 to 5 cm.

Most infections produce scant symptoms and diagnosis is only established through a stool examination where the characteristic eggs are evident. The quantity of ova can be used as rough determinant of the likely worm load. In moderate infestations vague abdominal pain, vomiting and diarrhoea have been attributed to the presence of the parasite. There is no doubt that with heavy worm loads mucous diarrhoea with blood streaking and abdominal cramps occur. Infection predisposes to rectal prolapse. Intussusception from a worm-laden caecum has been recorded by Reeder *et al.* (1968). Systemic disturbance such as weight loss, eosinophilia and anaemia may also be present in severe childhood infections (Kamath, 1973).

It is clear that radiology is not the means of establishing the diagnosis but, since children with blood-stained diarrhoea may be referred for barium enema studies, the characteristic appearance of the tail of the parasites as they lie in the bowel lumen should be recognised.

The paper by Fisher and Cremin (1970) illustrated the appearance of worms in double contrast studies. They cause curvilinear lucencies because of their barium coating. These are curled into complete rings or have an S-shaped configuration (Fig. 3.36). The outlined portion of the worms are usually just over 1 cm long, which is to be expected since the anterior thread-like two-thirds of the helminth are lying in the mucosa and submucosa and therefore inaccessible to coating. Worms may be identified in the caecum, transverse colon and even the sigmoid and the rectum.

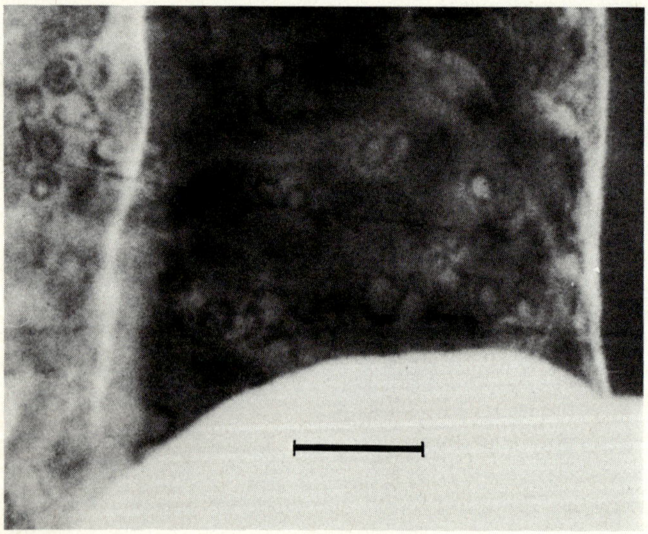

Fig. 3.36 Close up of double contrast enema of ascending colon in patient harbouring a heavy load of Trichuris trichiuria. Black bar marker is 1 cm long. (Courtesy of Dr. R. Fisher and Prof. B. Cremin, Capetown.)

REFERENCES

Fisher, R. M. & Cremin, B. J. (1970) Rectal bleeding due to Trichuris trichiura, *British Journal of Radiology*, **43**, 214–215.

Kamath, K. R. (1973) Severe infection with Trichuris trichiura in Malaysian children, *American Journal of Tropical Medicine and Hygiene*, **22**, 600–605.

Reeder, M., Astacio, J. & Theros, E. (1968) An exercise in radiologic pathologic correlation. *Radiology*, **90**, 382–387.

CROHN'S DISEASE AND ULCERATIVE COLITIS

These two conditions were once considered exceptional in the tropics but, though still uncommon, are being increasingly recognised. They do not yet numerically constitute a significant problem. Establishment of the diagnosis can be difficult, as specific infections such as amoebiasis, tuberculosis, yersinia, bacillary infections and other colonic conditions need to be excluded.

The presence of a mild form of ulcerative colitis has been established in India but the condition is rare in South East Asia, though seen occasionally in Sikh communities and in Sri Lanka (Tinckler, 1966; Chuttani *et al.*, 1967; De Silva *et al.*, 1976). Crohn's disease and ulcerative colitis occur infrequently in the Caribbean, Kenya and in the black population of South Africa (O'Donoghue & Clark, 1976; Whittaker, 1977; Giraud *et al.*, 1967).

We urge the use of the primary air double contrast enema in suspected cases to reveal the early mucosal changes, as the 'standard' enema only portrays mucosal features of the edges of the filled lumen (Fig. 3.37).

REFERENCES

Chuttani, H. K., Nigam, S. P., Sama, S. K., Dhanda, P. C. & Gupta, P. S. (1967) Ulcerative colitis in the tropics, *British Medical Journal*, **2**, 204–207.

De Silva, P. T., Talwatte, S. N. B., Burhan, M. N. & Wedisinghe, M. P. (1976) Ulcerative colitis in Sri Lanka, *Ceylon Medical Journal*, **21**, 232–238.

Giraud, R. M. A. & Luke, I. (1969) Crohn's disease in the Transvaal Bantu, *South African Medical Journal*, **43**, 610–612.

O'Donoghue, D. P. & Clark, M. L. (1976) Inflammatory bowel disease in West Indians, *British Medical Journal*, **2**, 796.

Tinckler, L. F. (1966) 'Non-incidence' of disease, *British Medical Journal*, **1**, 734.

Whittaker, L. (1977) Personal communication.

NON-SPECIFIC COLITIS

Patients who have had dysentery may develop a persistent diarrhoea even when no enteropathogens can be isolated. Similarly individuals who have suffered from traveller's acute colitis due to Escherichia coli may have continuing colonic symptoms. Barium studies are frequently requested in the work-up of these cases. Such investigations will exclude other underlying causes of diarrhoea not detectable by laboratory tests and can therefore be of value. Various haustral and motor changes have been described in barium studies and attributed to a 'post-dysen-

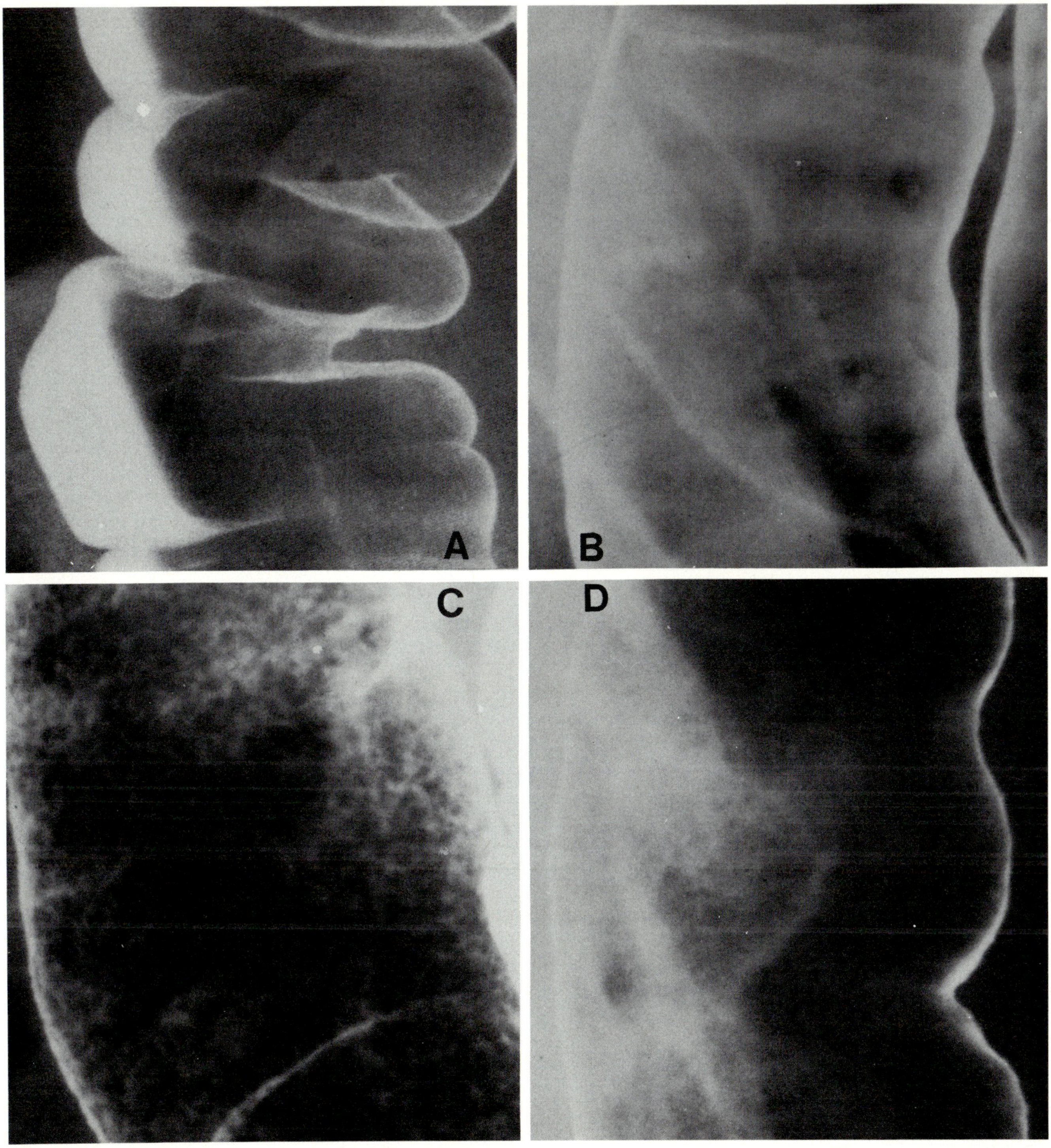

Fig. 3.37 Mucosal patterns in double contrast enemas in **A.** normal, **B.** apthous ulcers of Crohn's disease, **C.** ulcerative colitis, **D.** Yersinia enterocolitis. (Courtesy of Dr. Giles Stevenson, Hamilton.)

teric appearance'. We doubt the specificity and significance of such findings and believe that they are of slight diagnostic or management assistance.

There is no doubt that a post-dysenteric state exists clinically but it is at present poorly characterised endoscopically and radiologically. With acute or subacute salmonella enterocolitis the objective colonic changes disappear rapidly (Radšel-Medveščček *et al.*, 1977).

REFERENCE

Radšel-Medveščček, A., Žargi, R., Ačko, M. & Zajc-Satler, J. (1977) Colonic involvement in salmonellosis, *Lancet*, **1**, 601.

ACUTE INTESTINAL OBSTRUCTION

Though the causes of intestinal obstruction are manifold, local genetic, parasitic, dietary and unknown factors result in significant differences in the relative proportion of some entities in certain geographic locations. It is obviously impossible to give comprehensive coverage of this subject, but some conditions are discussed to indicate that differential diagnostic weighting must need alter in differing locations.

OBSTRUCTED HERNIA

In some temperate climate series of intestinal obstructions, herniae account for 25 to 50 per cent. In underdoctored areas there are many more individuals with untreated hernias, so it is to be expected that this condition is more common. Thus in Ghana at a large hospital hernias were responsible for 68·5 per cent of all obstructions, and in the Busoga district of Uganda strangulated hernias constituted 85 per cent of such abdominal emergencies (Badoe, 1970); Hancock, 1974). In the Busoga area most of the herniae are clinically direct type with specific anatomic features. This emphasises how pathology can be modified locally by genetic factors. Ischaemic strictures of small bowel attributed to the presence of chronic herniae have been described from Benin (Subbuswamyd & Iweze, 1977).

Since the diagnosis of the nature of the obstruction is usually clinically evident, radiology has little role in the diagnosis in most instances. The direct herniae have a high proportion of the Richter type.

INTUSSUSCEPTION

Obstruction due to intussusception is primarily an infant disease in Europe and North America. When seen in adults there is usually a cause such as a tumour or colonic anomaly at the apex of the lesion. The same conditions prevail in the East, but in a few areas of Africa extraordinarily high rates of intussusception occur in children and adults. These are considered idiopathic. Some patients have a long mesocaecum which may predispose to the condition. A seasonal incidence suggests that dietary intake or dietary excess may be a causative factor. High rates are known in Korea, Natal and in western Nigeria, where it is responsible for 27 per cent of all obstructions (Cole, 1965; Dietrick & Lee, 1965). In other areas such as Ghana, Senegal and Kenya it is a rare phenomenon.

Most intussusceptions are caeco-colic, and obstruction may be complete or incomplete depending on the duration and progression.

The plain film is usually helpful. The caecal area may appear 'empty'. A soft tissue mass may be evident somewhere in the line of the colon. The apex is sometimes outlined by a crescent of air (Fig. 3.38). The apex can be anywhere in the colon including the rectum and anus. Gas in a semicircular whorled pattern may be seen trapped in the intussuscipiens. Generally there is little small bowel gaseous distension. Barium enema studies will confirm the diagnosis in obscure cases (Fig. 3.39). Hydrostatic reduction for this type of intussusception has been found to be of little value.

SIGMOID VOLVULUS

The prevalence of sigmoid volvulus shows wide variations in different populations. It is alleged that it is commoner amongst those consuming a high residue diet which may cause a redundant colon. It is uncertain whether such an association is causal or due to genetic factors, since much of the world partakes of a fibre diet yet the frequency of volvulus varies. Genetic anatomic factors are probably important. In the U.S. volvulus is commoner in blacks than in whites.

In most of western Europe and Britain volvulus accounts for one to 4 per cent of intestinal obstructions. In Russia and India, by contrast, 30 per cent or more of obstruction are due to sigmoid volvulus (Ahsan & Rahman, 1967; Elmasri & Khalil, 1976). In Africa it represents 18 per cent of obstructions in the Sudan, 15 per cent in Uganda and the Bantus of the Transvaal, 12

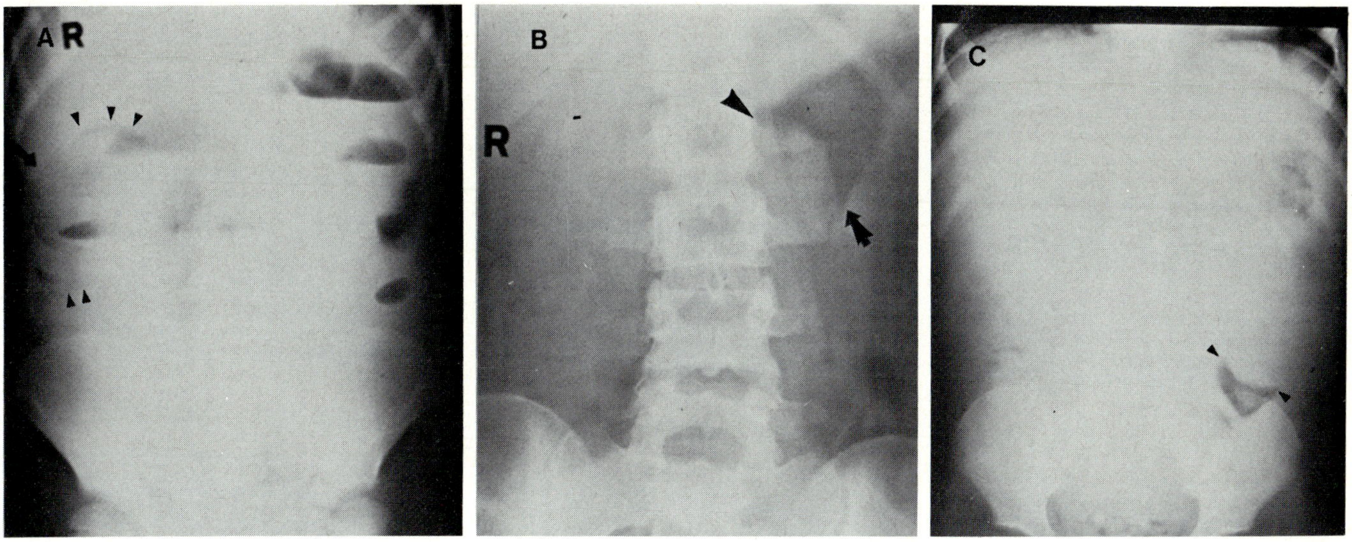

Fig. 3.38 Three patients with chronic intussusception. In **A** the apex is in ascending colon and gas (black arrows) is caught in curvilinear segments within the intussusception. In **B** the apex is outlined by gas in the transverse colon and in **C**, in the descending colon.

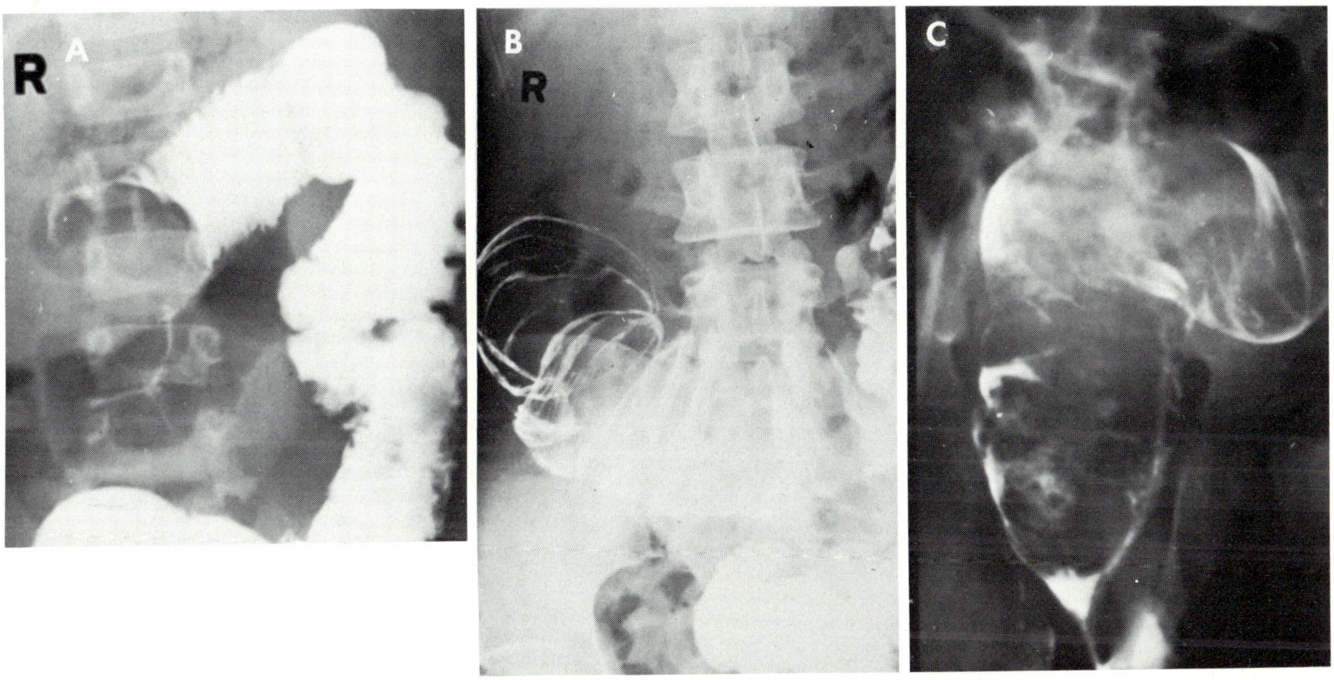

Fig. 3.39 Enema features of intussusception. In **A** the filling defect of the apex is outlined and in **B** and **C** barium has entered the sleeve space. In **C** the apex is presenting in the rectum.

per cent in Rhodesia, 9 per cent in the Ivory Coast (El Masiri & Khalil, 1976; White & Palmer, 1963; Skapinker, 1963; Cornet *et al.*, 1973). In one series 94 per cent were males (Hall-Craggs, 1960). By contrast it is infrequent in Nigeria, New Guinea and in Malaysia (Cole, 1965; Ti & Yong, 1976).

In Brazil the condition is frequent but there, and elsewhere in South America where Chagas' disease exists, chagasic megacolon is probably an important factor in aetiology (Oliveira *et al.*, 1963). Volvulus may develop in 10 per cent of cases (Ferreira-Santos & Carril, 1964).

In a plain abdominal film the typical case is readily evident. Arising out of the pelvis is a grossly gas-distended loop occupying much of the abdomen. There is an oblique line usually sloping towards the liver on the right, caused by the opposing walls of the twisted sigmoid obstructed loops (Fig. 3.40). The appearance has been likened to a kinked inner tube of a tyre. Small bowel gas does not accumulate greatly until late. If it is very obvious one should consider a complicated compound volvulus where the small bowel has also become implicated. This type is seen particularly in Rhodesia and Kenya (White & Palmer, 1963).

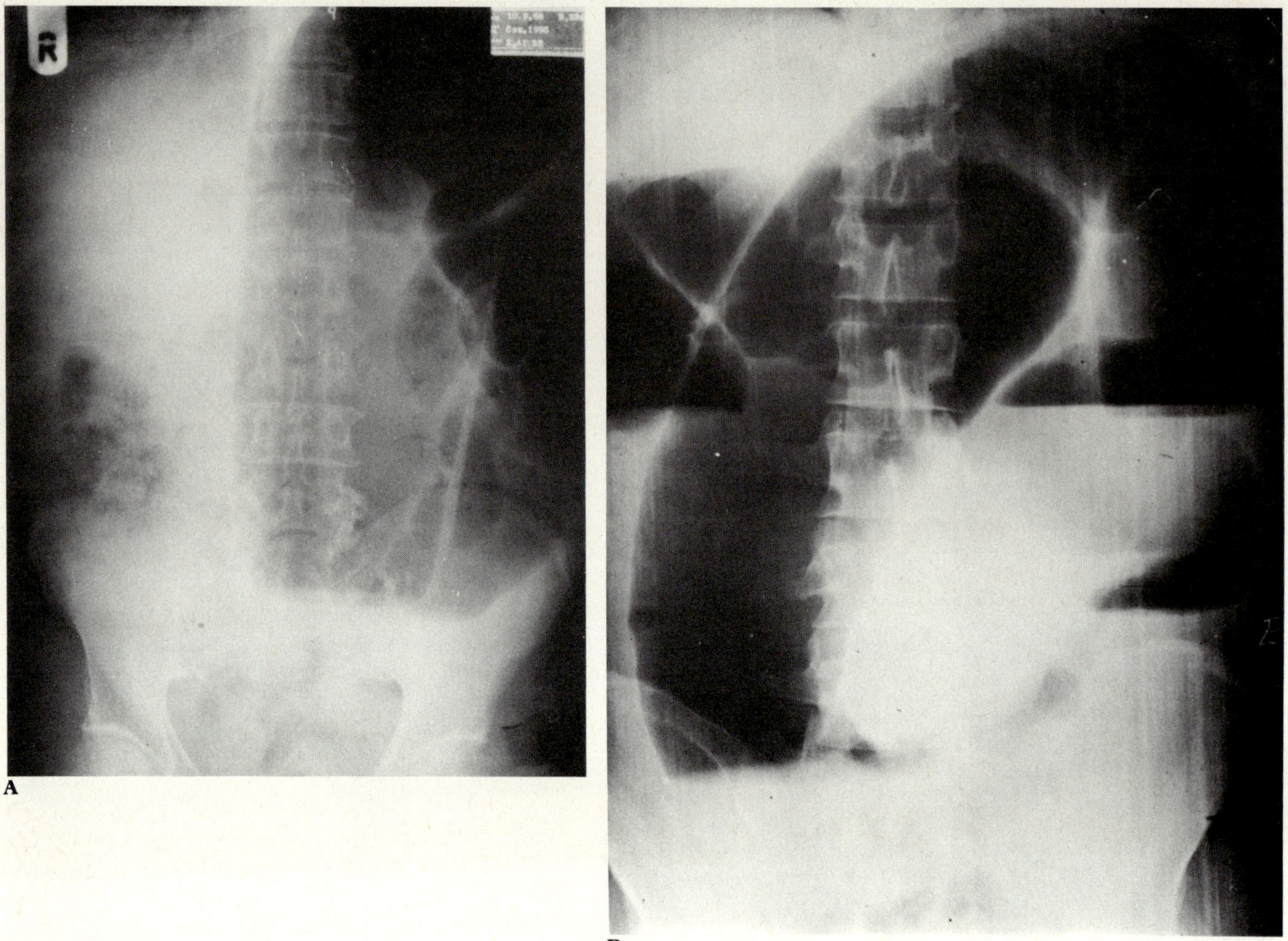
A

B

Fig. 3.40 A, B. Sigmoid volvulus. Classic gas-distended loop arising out of pelvis in two patients.

Barium studies are rarely indicated even though a characteristic appearance of a sharp-pointed bird beak obstruction may be evident. Enemas cause delay, add little information, and may make tube deflation more difficult. This manœuvre should not be attempted in late cases or those in whom a compound volvulus is suspected.

VOLVULUS OF THE SMALL BOWEL

In northern Uganda volvulus of the small bowel may account for nearly 20 per cent of intestinal obstructions not due to hernia (de Souza, 1976). The condition is also frequent in parts of Kenya.

Unlike most cases of small bowel volvulus, circulatory collapse prostration and systemic disturbances are not prominent unless bowel gangrene is present. The patients seen had drunk large amounts (several litres) of a local beer very rapidly during festivities. The beer was shown to contain considerable quantities of serotonin and it is considered that by its smooth muscle action the substance initiated the volvulus.

REFERENCES

Badoe, A. E. (1970) Acute intestinal obstruction Korle Bu Teaching Hospital, Accra 1965–69, *Ghana Medical Journal*, **9**, 283–287.

Cole, G. J. (1965) A review of 436 cases of intestinal obstruction in Ibadan, *Gut*, **6**, 151–162.

Cornet, L., Angate, Y., Breton, P., Coulibaly, A. O. & Benoit, G. (1973) 61 cas de volvulus du colon sigmoide, *Chirurgie*, **99**, 255–261.

De Souza, L. J. (1976) Volvulus of the small bowel, *British Medical Journal*, **1**, 1055–1056.

Dietrick, R. B. & Lee, M. H. (1965) Intussusception: a different clinical entity in Korea, *Surgery*, **57**, 651–654.

El Masri, S. H. & Khalil, T. (1976). Volvulus of the sigmoid in Khartoum, Sudan, *Tropical and Geographic Medicine*, **28**, 297–302.

Ferreira-Santos, R. & Carril, C. F. (1964) Acquired megacolon in Chagas disease, *Diseases of Colon and Rectum*, **7**, 353.

Hall-Craggs, E. C. B. (1960) Sigmoid volvulus in an African population, *British Medical Journal*, **1**, 1015–1017.

Hancock, B. D. (1974) Busoga hernia prevalence in abdominal emergencies in Busoga, Uganda, *Tropical and Geographical Medicine*, **26**, 15–25.

Oliveira, M. R. de, Cutait, D. E., Branco, P. D., Speranzini, M. B., Fujimura, I. & Campos, S. de M. (1963) Obstrucão Intestinal, I: Volvo

de sigmoide; estudo de 107 casos, *Revista Hospidale Clinicas Faculdade de Medicina Sao Paulo*, **18,** 469–479.
Skapinker, S. (1953) Acute mechanical obstruction in the Bantu, *South African Medical Journal*, **27,** 237–239.
Subbuswamy, S. G. & Iweze, F. I. (1977) Ischaemic strictures of the small intestine in Nigeria, *Gut*, **18,** 266–273.
Ti, T. K. & Yong, N. K. (1976) The pattern of intestinal obstruction in Malaysia, *British Journal of Surgery*, **63,** 963–965.
White, A. & Palmer, P. E. S. (1963) The radiology of intestinal obstruction in Rhodesia, *Clinical Radiology*, **14,** 211–218.

IDIOPATHIC TROPICAL SPRUE TROPICAL ENTEROPATHY

Tropical sprue can be difficult to diagnose since many of the clinical features can be simulated by other conditions so that exclusion of other enteropathies such as gluten sensitivity, tuberculous enteritis, Crohn's disease, coeliac disease, lymphoma blind loops, gut fistulae, strongyloidiasis and giardiasis is necessary. Recently the separate term tropical enteropathy has been popularised, but many workers believe that this represents a milder form of sprue rather than a distinct entity (Klipstein *et al.*, 1969).

Sprue can be described as a symptom complex but is best defined by nutritional and laboratory criteria.

The clinical features are those of malabsorption and diarrhoea with weakness, loss of weight, abdominal pain and distension, vitamin-deficient glossitis and stomatitis, and an anaemia that may be megaloblastic. The stools are bulky and steatorrhoea is generally present. Laboratory investigations disclose malabsorption of unrelated substances such as fat, xylose and vitamin B_{12}. A frequently used definition suggests that symptomatic malabsorption of at least two of these substances is required for the diagnosis of idiopathic tropical sprue if other causative factors can be eliminated.

Histologically the jejunum will show varying degrees of villous atrophy, round cell infiltration of the lamina propria, mucosal and epithelial cell thickening and goblet cell abnormalities (Floch *et al.*, 1962).

This condition occurs in the East in India, Ceylon, Singapore, Burma, Vietnam, Indonesia, the Philippines; in the Caribbean in Puerto-Rico and Haiti; in Africa in Rhodesia, Lagos and Durban (Jeejeebhoy *et al.*, 1968; Falaiye, 1970; Moshal *et al.*, 1975; Thomas & Clain, 1976). The geographical incidence is not defined precisely and it needs to be stated that the African reports are scant in comparison with the large number of cases from the Far East and India. Expatriates are liable to the disease after a stay in an endemic area, though no such cases have come to light from tropical Africa.

Therapy with tetracycline, folic acid and Vitamin B_{12} results in clinical improvement and regression of absorptive and jejunal changes. This therapeutic response also confirms the diagnosis of this idiopathic disorder.

The radiological manifestations are greatly dependent on the means used to study the small bowel (Laws *et al.*, 1963). A stabilised barium compound resistant to flocculation, though it may mask clumping changes, provides better delineation of the jejunal mucosa and calibre than standard barium and tap water. Probably better still is the administration of a good coating of a stabilised barium by a nasogastric tube whose tip has entered the duodenum.

The 'malabsorption pattern' shown in radiographs is of course not specific to sprue, but it is characteristic and the severity generally correlates well with the clinical and absorption defects (Caldwell *et al.*, 1965; Paterson *et al.*, 1965).

The lumen of the bowel is increased in calibre—this being defined as greater than 28 to 30 mm measured on the film. In addition the mucosal folds are prominent, being both deeper and thicker (Paterson & Baker, 1958) (Fig. 3.41). Flocculation, separating out of the barium and its clumping into segments, may be a feature if a standard barium is used.

Whenever investigating a patient with a possible diagnosis of sprue the study must proceed beyond the jejunum

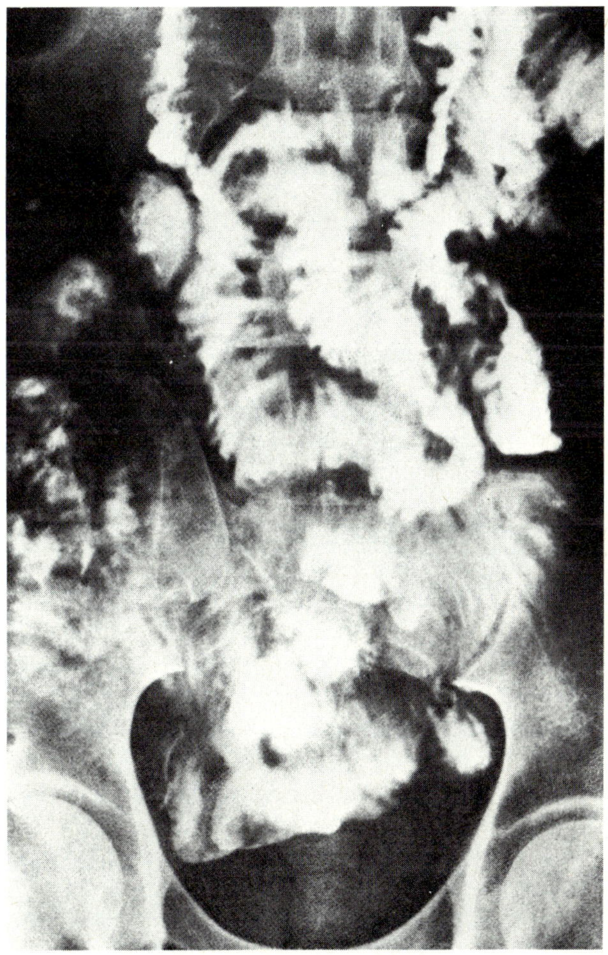

Fig. 3.41 Dilated small bowel, coarse exaggerated jejunal folds and segmentation in tropical sprue.

to exclude diverticuli, blind loops, enteric fistulae, Crohn's disease and tuberculosis in the ileum that could be present and be the cause of the patient's symptoms.

Other radiographic changes such as osteomalacia are exceptional.

REFERENCES

*Caldwell, W. L., Swanson, V. L. & Bayless, T. M. (1965) The importance and reliability of the roentgenographic examination of the small bowel in patients with tropical sprue, *Radiology*, **84**, 227–240.

Falaiye, J. M. (1970) Tropical sprue in Nigeria, *Journal of Tropical Medicine and Hygiene*, **73**, 119–125.

Floch, M. N., Caldwell, W. L. & Sleeny, T. W. (1962) Histopathologic basis for the interpretation of small bowel roentgenography in tropical sprue, *American Journal of Roentgenology*, **87**, 709–716.

Jeejeebhoy, K. N., Desai, H. G., Borkar, A. V., Deshpande, W. & Pathare, S. M. (1968) Tropical malabsorption syndrome in West India, *American Journal of Clinical Nutrition*, **21**, 994–1006.

Klipstein, F. A., Samloff, I. M., Smarth, G. & Schenk, E. A. (1969) Treatment of overt and subclinical malabsorption in Haiti, *Gut*, **10**, 315–332.

Laws, J. W., Booth, C. C., Shawdon, H. & Stewart, J. S. (1963) Correlation of radiological and histopathological findings in idiopathic steatorrhoea, *British Medical Journal*, **1**, 1311–1314.

Moshal, M. G., Hift, W., Kallichurun, S. & Pillay, K. (1975) Endemic tropical sprue in Africa, *Journal of Tropical Medicine and Hygiene*, **78**, 2–5.

Paterson, D. E. & Baker, S. J. (1958) The radiologic investigation of the small intestine in tropical idiopathic malabsorption, *Journal of the Faculty of Radiologists*, **9**, 183–194.

*Paterson, D. E., David, R. & Baker, S. J. (1965) Radiodiagnostic problems in malabsorption, *British Journal of Radiology*, **38**, 181–191.

Thomas, G. & Clain, D. J. (1976) Endemic tropical sprue in Rhodesia, *Gut*, **17**, 877–887.

DISACCHARIDE DEFICIENCY

Diarrhoea, cramps and abdominal distension can be due to lack of specific enzymes which stop hydrolysis of sucrose to glucose and fructose; and of lactose to glucose and galactose. Man is the only mammal that can produce lactase after weaning. However, much of the world's population, though producing lactase at birth and infancy, do not retain this enzyme in childhood and later life. Presence in adults of the enzyme appears to be an acquired genetic characteristic found amongst populations that traditionally consume milk and its products. Over many generations the large majority of Caucasian, Batutsi, Bahutu and Fulani can digest lactose, whereas most Bantu, Baganda, Yoruba, Ethiopians, Sudanese, some Indian groups, Eskimo, Australian aborigines, Chinese, Thai and Japanese are unable to do so (Davis & Bolin, 1967; Moodie, 1973; Elliot *et al.*, 1973; Varavithya *et al.*, 1976).

In those deficient in lactase, symptoms may begin at two to three years if challenged by food containing lactose. Abdominal distension, borborygmy, cramps and diarrhoea may then develop. These symptoms are due to the unhydrolysed sugar acting as an osmotic load which draws fluid into the lumen of the bowel. This distension induces increased peristaltic activity. The gas distension is considered to be due to bacterial fermentation of the unabsorbed sugar.

There are many ways of establishing the diagnosis, varying from a crude test for reducing substances in the stool, to administration of a test dose of lactase to establish whether the blood sugar level rises and the symptoms are reproduced. More elegantly and definitively enzyme histochemistry of Crosby capsule mucosal specimens may be carried out.

Changes can be readily demonstrated radiologically if 50 grams of lactose is added to a barium solution and swallowed (Laws & Neale, 1966; Prager & Amberg, 1967). Soon after, distension of the distal jejunum becomes apparent, combined with increased peristalsis. The transit time is markedly reduced with the head of barium in the transverse colon, perhaps in half an hour. The patient will usually experience symptoms.

Though this is a non-biochemical way of confirming lactase deficiency, it is only of value, pictorial curiosity apart, when blood chemistry may be difficult to obtain. Perhaps of greater importance is the danger of producing these appearances inadvertently. Sometimes sugars are added to barium to make them more palatable. Probably no proprietary bariums have such sugars, but the addition may occur at the local level during mixing. Sucrose produces similar changes in those who are sucrase deficient.

REFERENCES

Davis, A. E. & Bolin, T. (1967) Lactose intolerance in Asians, *Nature*, **216**, 1244–1245.

Elliott, F. G., Cox, J. & Nyomba, B. L. (1973) Intolerance au lactose chez l'adulte en Afrique Centrale, *Annales de la Société Belge de Médecine Tropicale*, **53**, 113–132.

Laws, J. W. & Neale, G. (1966) Radiological diagnosis of disaccharidase deficiency, *Lancet*, **2**, 139–143.

Moodie, P. M. (1973) *Aboriginal Health*. p. 222. Canberra: Australian National University Press.

Preger, L. & Amberg, J. R. (1967) Sweet diarrhoea. Roentgen diagnosis of disaccharidase deficiency, *American Journal of Roentgenology*, **101**, 287–295.

Varavithya, W., Valyasevi, A., Manu, P. & Kittikool, J. (1976) Lactose malabsorption in Thai infants and children: effects of prolonged milk feeding, *South East Asian Journal of Tropical Medicine and Public Health*, **7**, 591–595.

DIVERTICULAR DISEASE

Diverticular disease is now the most frequent morphologic abnormality of the colon in the Western world, though it was an almost unknown condition at the beginning of this century (Painter & Burkitt, 1971). The incidence of diverticula increases with age, reaching 42 per cent by the ninth decade in Utah (Smith & Christensen, 1959).

By contrast in many parts of the world diverticulosis of the sigmoid is a pathologic curiosity, though the incidence may now be rising in some large cities as the dietary pattern changes.

In series of barium enemas diverticula were found in Senegal in 0·5 per cent and in Nigeria 1·1 per cent (Cave *et al.*, 1963; Bohrer & Lewis, 1974). In a series of 2280 enemas carried out in Abidjan over 6 years, 28 cases of diverticulosis were observed. All but two were expatriates who constituted a small proportion of all the patients (Djedje & Lesquerre, 1974). Diverticular disease is rare in Malaysia (Ti & Yong, 1976), and also in Papua New Guinea as well as in Australian aborigines.

Generalised colonic diverticulae and predominantly right-sided colonic diverticula are probably genetically determined rather than acquired from a low fibre diet. Right-sided diverticula develop at a younger age than the sigmoid variety and are not accompanied by muscle hypertrophy. There are also racial differences in the right-sided form. They are rare in Caucasians but represent 60 per cent of diverticula in Japanese, 50 per cent in Hawaians and 33 per cent of Chinese with diverticula living in Hawaii (Peck *et al.*, 1969).

REFERENCES

Bohrer, S. P. & Lewis, E. A. (1974) Diverticula of the colon in Ibadan, Nigeria, *Tropical and Geographical Medicine*, **26**, 9–14.

Cave, L., Sankale, M., Bobo, J. & Serafino, G. (1963) Les differents aspects radiologiques de la pathologie Recto-colique à Dakar, *Bulletin de la Société Médicale d'Afrique Noire*, **8**, 397–402.

Djedje, A. T. & Lesquerre, C. L. (1974) Bilan statistique de 6 ans de radiologie digestive au C. H. U. Treichville, *Annales de l'Université d'Abidjan*, **8**, 116–121.

Painter, N. S. & Burkitt, D. P. (1971) Diverticular disease of the colon, a deficiency disease of Western civilisation, *British Medical Journal*, **2**, 450–454.

Peck, D. A., Labat, R. & Waite, V. C. (1968) Diverticular disease of the right colon, *Diseases of the Colon and Rectum*, **11**, 49–54.

Smith, C. C. & Christensen, W. R. (1959) The incidence of colonic diverticulosis, *American Journal of Roentgenology*, **82**, 996–999.

Ti, T. K. & Yong, N. K. (1976) The pattern of intestinal obstruction in Malaysia, *British Journal of Surgery*, **63**, 963–965.

MALIGNANCY OF THE GASTRO-INTESTINAL TRACT

Cancer of oesophagus

From the radiological aspect the radiographic features of oesophageal cancer in the tropics are little different from elsewhere, apart from the greater proportion of advanced tumours and lesions with complications such as fistulae. However, there are marked regional differences in incidence. Very high rates are known in the Transkei, the Nyanga region of Kenya, in Zambia, the Caspian shore of Iran, the Tachang area of Northern China and Curacao. In China the high incidence has long been known, but in some of the African areas it appears to have reached almost epidemic proportions in recent times. These very localised foci of oesophageal carcinomata are of considerable epidemiologic interest, though as yet no specific etiological factor has been found responsible.

There appears to be an association between the mega-oesophagus of Chagas' disease and oesophageal carcinoma, as the latter occurs in 10 per cent of cases (Hutt *et al.*, 1973).

Gastric cancer

Whereas gastric cancer is progressively becoming less frequent in parts of Europe and the United States, gastric carcinoma has unexpectedly high incidence in Japan, Finland, Iceland, parts of Russia, China, Chile, Costa Rica, Kivu province of the Congo, south-west Uganda and Rwanda-Burundi (Bijlsma, 1974). Though most of Africa has a low incidence of gastric cancer, negroes in U.S.A. have a rate similar to the white population. The etiological significance of these 'pockets' of relatively high incidence is important but no etiologic factor has emerged. In West Africa antral lesions are much more frequent proportionately than other gastric locations in comparison with experience elsewhere.

Burkitt's lymphoma of stomach

Gastric intramural and ulcerating mucosal masses are sometimes seen in children (Figs. 3.42 and 3.43). Often

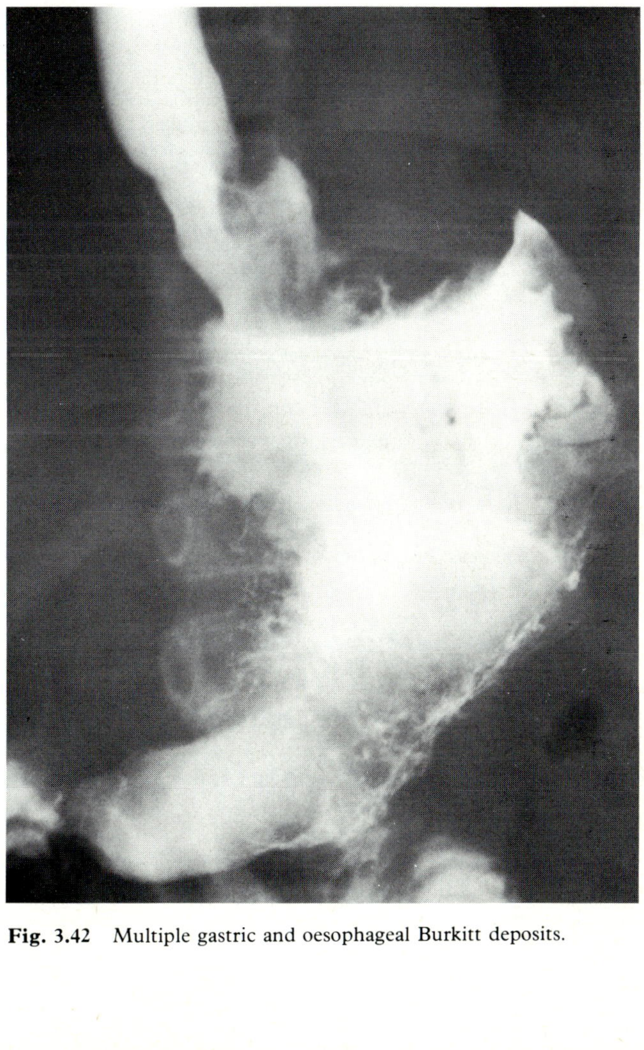

Fig. 3.42 Multiple gastric and oesophageal Burkitt deposits.

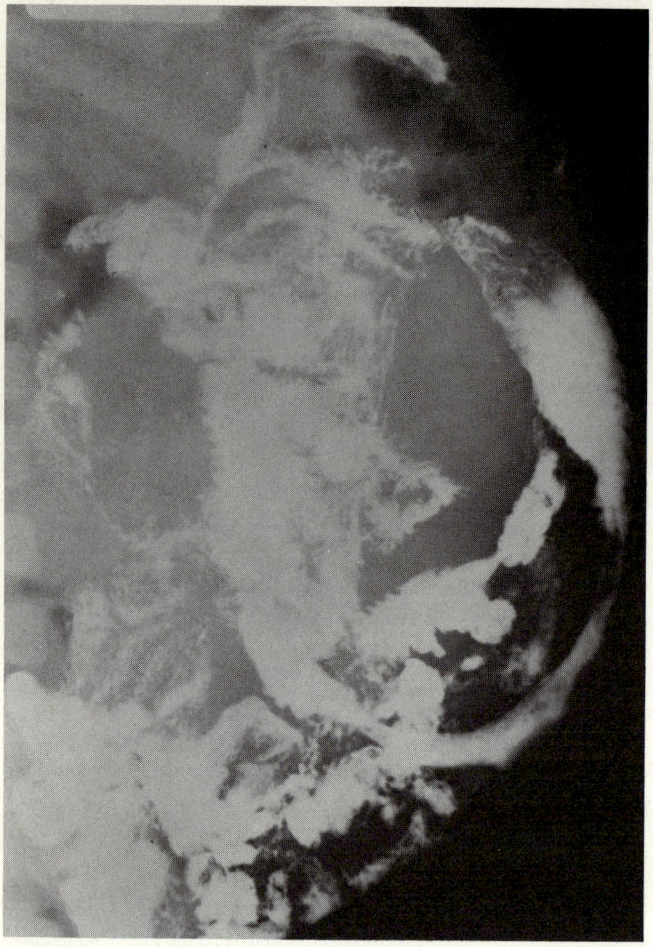

Fig. 3.43 Gross displacement of bowel by extrinsic masses and mural intestinal masses in Burkitt's lymphoma. Such patients show a protein-losing enteropathy.

such lesions are associated with mesenteric deposits and pancreatic masses so that the barium studies should include studies of the pancreas and small bowel. Ileal and jejunal lesions and intramural nodules may be present. Children with these lesions are often malnourished due to a protein-losing state. Marked improvement can follow chemotherapy with complete resolution of lesions.

Colonic cancer

Rectal and colonic cancer are discussed together even though etiologically there is evidence at times to suggest that they have differences, e.g. rectal cancer is commoner in males and colonic cancer in females.

Whilst rectal cancer is one of the most frequent malignancies of Europe and North America, it is not especially prevalent in tropical countries. Some workers have related this to high fibre diet allowing less time for degradation of cholesterol products into carcinogens—an attractive but unproven hypothesis, particularly as cancer occurrence is not increased in that supreme example of stasis: Chagasic megacolon.

Cancer of the large bowel is rare in Africa. This has been well documented for the Bantu. It is of interest that there is also a low adenomatous polyp rate. Thus no polyps were seen in 14 000 autopsies, and only six from surgical speciments, in the 2000-bed Baragwanath Hospital in South Africa over a 12-year period (Brenner & Ackerman, 1970).

Schistosomiasis due to S. japonicum has been shown to be precancerous where cancer occurs at an earlier age, with a different sex ratio and histopathology than large bowel cancers occurring in individuals without bilharzia (Shindo, 1976). The colo-rectal cancers of the Sudan occur at a young age and are often undifferentiated mucoid lesions (El Masri & Boulos, 1976). Perhaps these features may be related to high S. mansoni rates in the Sudan.

Visceral Kaposi deposits can simulate colonic neoplasia (Fig. 3.44).

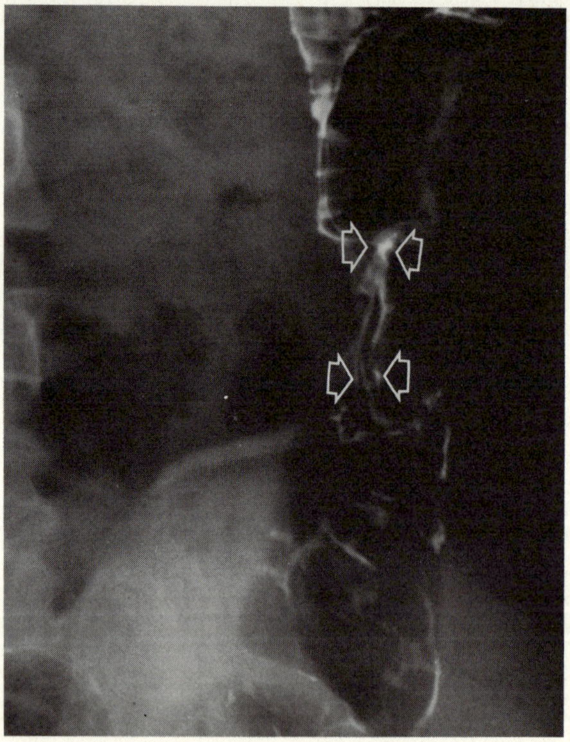

Fig. 3.44 Filling defect in double contrast enema due to a Kaposi sarcoma mural deposit in a Ugandan patient. (Courtesy of Dr. G. Davies.)

REFERENCES

Bijlsma, F. (1974) Gastric carcinoma in Uganda, *Tropical and Geographical Medicine*, **26**, 1–8.

Bremner, C. G. & Ackerman, L. V. (1970) Polyps and carcinoma of the large bowel in the South African Bantu, *Cancer*, **26**, 991–999.

Cockshott, W. P. (1965) Radiological aspects of Burkitt's tumour, *British Journal of Radiology*, **38**, 172–180.

El Masri, S. H. & Boulos, P. B. (1976). Prognosis of colo-rectal cancer in the Sudan, *Tropical and Geographical Medicine*, **28**, 187–190.

Hutt, M. S. R., Koberle, F. & Salfelder, K. (1973) In *Tropical Pathology*. p. 394, ed. Spencer, H. Heidelberg: Springer.

Shindo, K. (1976) Significance of Schistosomiasis japonica in the development of cancer of the large intestine, *Diseases of the Colon and Rectum*, **19**, 460–469.

MEDITERRANEAN LYMPHOMA AND ALPHA CHAIN DISEASE

J. S. Macdonald

Alpha Chain disease (Seligmann *et al.*, 1968) and Mediterranean lymphoma (Azar, 1962) are diseases of the young and early middle-aged, which present clinically with diarrhoea, weight loss, abdominal pain, malabsorption, finger clubbing and raised plasma alkaline phosphates (Doe, 1975). Mediterranean lymphoma appears to affect those of non-Caucasian origin, particularly Arabs and non-Ashkenazy Jewish populations in the Mediterranean area, while Alpha Chain disease is more widespread and has been reported in northern Europe, America and the Far East (Seligmann, 1975; Ramos *et al.*, 1978). There have been reported twelve patients of Spanish (? Arab admixtures) origin in Mexico (Ramos *et al.*, 1978). The sexes appear to be equally affected and in Alpha Chain disease there is a gammapathy with free alpha chain protein in the serum.

These are an interesting group of lymphomas since they display a premalignant phase which can be reversed by antibiotic therapy. It has been suggested by Seligmann *et al.* (1971) that the early changes of plasma cell infiltration could be attributed to continual intestinal infestation, so explaining the association of these diseases with those who live or have lived in the under-privileged areas. Yet many areas of high gut parasitism do not show evidence of the disease.

Pathologically the main feature is infiltration of the lamina propia of gut by plasma cells.

Radiological features

They have been discussed by Doe *et al.* (1976). The features seen on barium meal and follow-through examination consist of thickened mucosal folds, nodular mucosal pattern giving rise to a spiky contour (Fig. 3.45). Grossly enlarged mesenteric nodes may press on the gut, giving rise to a scalloped appearance, and narrowed rigid areas may be shown (Fig. 3.45). In Alpha Chain disease the whole length of the small gut may be involved, but Mediterranean lymphoma tends to involve the proximal small gut. Doe *et al.* (1976) described inconstant segmental dilatations and strictures. One of their patients also had hypertrophic osteo-arthropathy. At some stage of the disease the erect abdominal films may show fluid levels in the small bowel.

REFERENCES

Azar, H. A. (1962) Cancer in Lebanon and the Near East, *Cancer*, **15**, 66–78.

Doe, W. F. (1975) Alpha Chain disease: clinico pathological features and relationship to so-called Mediterranean lymphoma, *British Journal of Cancer*, **31**, Suppl. II, 350–355.

Doe, W. F., Henry, K. & Doyle, F. H. (1976) Radiological and histological findings in six patients with Alpha Chain disease, *British Journal of Radiology*, **49**, 3–11.

*Ramos, L., Marcos, J., Illanas, M., Hernandez-Mora, M., Perez-Paya, F., Picouto, J. L., Santana, P. & Chantar, C. (1978) Radiological characteristics of primary intestinal lymphoma of the 'Mediterranean' type: observations of twelve cases, *Radiology*, **126**, 379–385.

Seligmann, M. (1975) Alpha Chain disease: immunoglobulin abnormalities, pathogenesis and current concepts, *British Journal of Cancer*, **31**, Suppl. II, 356–361.

Seligmann, M., Danon, F., Hurez, D., Mihaesco, E. & Preud'Homme, J. L. (1968) Alpha Chain disease: a new immunological abnormality, *Science*, **162**, 1396–1397.

Seligmann, M., Mihaesco, E. & Frangione, B. (1971) Studies in Alpha Chain disease, *New York Academy of Science Annals*, **190**, 487–500.

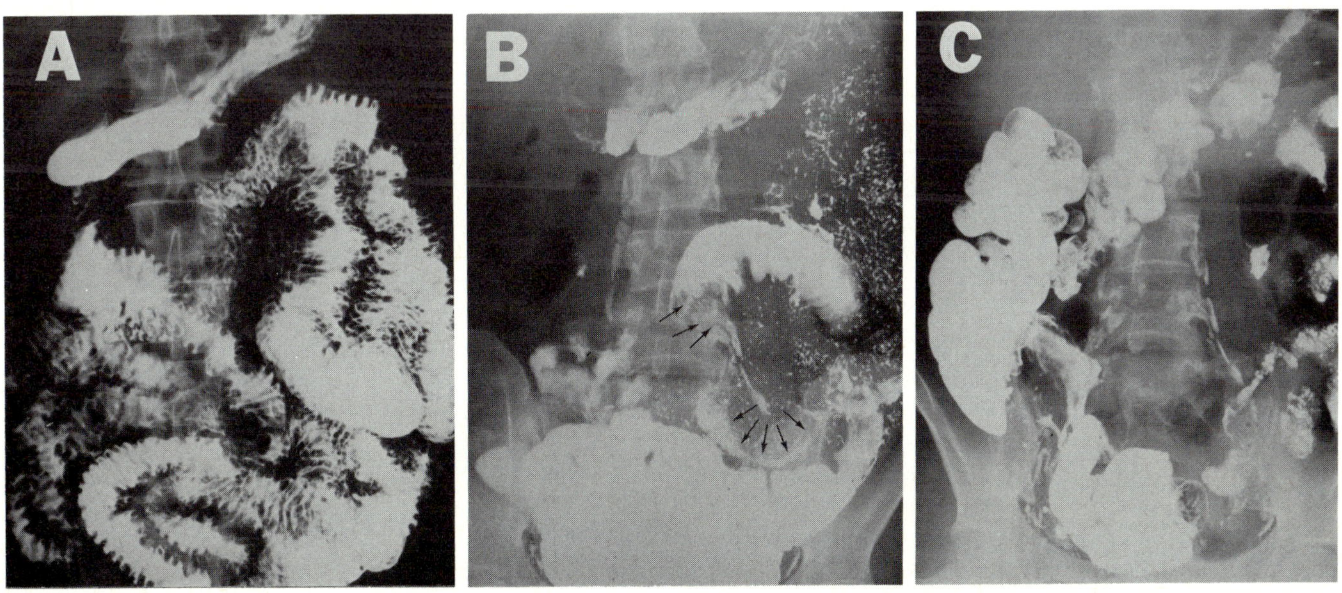

Fig. 3.45 **A.** Mediterranean lymphoma in 35-year-old Iraqi involving proximal small gut and showing exaggerated mucosal folds. **B.** 22-year-old female Filipino with Alpha Chain disease. Enlarged glands are extrinsically narrowing and compressing the bowel (black arrows). **C.** in the same patient there is also terminal ileal involvement.

BILIARY CALCULI

The radiological demonstration of biliary calculous disease probably does not pose any unique problems in any part of the world, but the indications, pattern and incidence of diseases is subject to considerable variations. Whether diet, hereditary factors or parasitic diseases mainly determine the differences is at present unresolved.

Gall-stones are uncommon in most of Africa and stones in the common duct are exceptional—though the prevalence is beginning to increase in the last decade in some centres. Burkitt, in a busy surgical practice in Uganda, encountered only one case of calculous disease in 17 years (Parnis, 1964). In a 3-year period out of 2375 general surgical cases (trauma excluded) seen in Kenyatta National Hospital in Nairobi, one common duct stone and seven patients with calculous cholecystitis were diagnosed (Miller, 1964). Similarly, reviewing 16 years' experience at the Kinshasa University clinics in Zaire, Ngala Kenda (1977) found only 32 cases of gall-stones. It is of interest to note that 38 per cent were under the age of 30 with a 4 to 1 female to male ratio. In the main University Hospital in Ghana only 0·4 per cent of surgical admissions were for biliary disease (Ampona, 1975). A combined radiographic, clinical and autopsy survey in Ibadan also disclosed a paucity of cases and a younger presenting age than that seen in Europe or North America (Parnis, 1964).

Autopsy series may be less clinically significant, since stones are often asymptomatic, but such statistics confirm the same trend. In Britain 15 to 20 per cent of the population harbour stones (Parnis, 1964), but out of 6773 autopsies in Uganda only 0·87 per cent had stones and 0·1 per cent in Kenya (Ower, 1964). In South Africa, Bantu women at autopsy have calculi four to six times less often than the Caucasian population (Trowell, 1960).

In many parts of the East, Indonesia and Thailand, gall-stones are rare (Stitnimankarn, 1960). Amongst the Japanese, Koreans and Singapore Chinese many biliary calculi lie in the intrahepatic bile ducts rather than in the gall bladder (Yessen, 1961; Maki, 1961; Hutt & Gibson, 1973). It has been suggested that ascariasis ova or flukes may determine this distribution but the evidence is not conclusive.

The low incidence of stones, and pigment stones in particular, in areas of East and West Africa where the S gene has a 20 per cent or even greater prevalence is surprising. In the U.S.A. the incidence of cholelithiasis in haemoglobin SS disease above the age of 10 years is increased and by the third decade 62 per cent can be affected. In haemoglobin SC disease the incidence is less (Phillips & Gerald, 1971). These American levels arre far higher than those seen by us in the West Indies and in East and West Africa.

A typhoid carrier state that proves difficult to eradicate by antibiotics is an indication for cholecystography. A proportion of such patients can be cured by removal of a calculous gall bladder.

REFERENCES

Ampona, A. A. D. (1975) Idiopathic intussusception in adult Ghanians, *Ghana Medical Journal*, **14,** 64–66.

Hutt, M. S. R. & Gibson, J. B. (1973) *Tropical Pathology*, ed. Spencer, H. p. 675. Heidelberg: Springer.

Jessen, C. (1961) Gallstones restricted to the biliary ducts: a review of 24 Korean cases, *Acta Chirurgica Scandinavica*, **283,** 242–248.

Miller, J. R. M. (1964) The pattern of general surgical disease in Nairobi, 1960–1963, *East African Medical Journal*, **41,** 419–429.

Ngala Kenda, J. F. (1977) Lithiase biliare chez l'africain, une revue de 16 ans aux cliniques Universitaire de Kinshasa, *Annales de la Société Belge de Médecine Tropicale*, **57,** 61–66.

Parnis, R. O. (1964) Gall bladder disease in Nigeria—a five year review, *Transactions of the Royal Society of Tropical Medicine and Hygiene*, **58,** 437–440.

Phillips, J. C. & Gerald, B. E. (1971) The incidence of cholelithiasis in sickle cell disease, *American Journal of Roentgeneology*, **113,** 27–28.

Stitnimankarn, T. (1960) The necropsy incidence of gallstones in Thailand, *American Journal of Medical Sciences*, **240,** 349–352.

Trowell, H. C. (1960) *Non-Infective Disease in Africa*. pp. 71–73. London: Edward Arnold.

AMOEBIC LIVER ABSCESS

Radiology and allied imaging techniques can be invaluable aids in the diagnosis of this complication of colonic amoebiasis. The incidence of amoebic liver abscess arising in clinical cases of colonic amoebiasis is not known, but it is certainly less than autopsy figures would suggest. This complication developed in 12 per cent of a series of 119 patients with amoebiasis (Radke, 1955), but in overall colonic disease a figure below 5 per cent seems more realistic.

Some years ago there was a prolonged controversy on whether amoebic hepatitis existed separately from liver abscess. The term was applied to a clinical syndrome popularised by Doxiades and his colleagues (1964) for patients with hepatomegaly, fever, amoebae in the stool and a good response to specific anti-amoebic therapy. These individuals were postulated as having a diffuse hepatic involvement causing hepatomegaly, but as no pathologic histologic basis has ever been established the concept is no longer accepted and such a symptom complex can be regarded as being due to the early stage of an undetected abscess.

A liver abscess presumably develops by portal venous dissemination from the colon. This route may partly account for the 80 per cent prevalence in the right lobe of the liver due to streaming of the portal venous blood from the more frequently and more heavily infected right side of the colon. The much greater volume of the right lobe compared with the left is also an obvious factor of importance. What is surprising is how often abscesses are solitary. Evidence from ultrasound and isotopic liver examinations support the frequency of isolated abscesses yet, in pathological terms of venous spread, one would expect multiple lesions. Occasionally abscesses coalesce to form a single lesion. In clinical cases probably three-quarters of abscesses are single.

This condition is seen most often in males, though the 89 per cent male preponderance recorded by Adi (1965) is exceptional. Those in the third and fourth decade appear most vulnerable, although the process can occur in childhood. The typical presentation is of abdominal pain, possibly referred shoulder pain, abdominal swelling and possibly diarrhoea. Anaemia and a raised E.S.R. are frequent. The alkaline phosphatase was raised in 71 per cent in the series of Lamont and Wicks (1976). Stool examination for trophozoites is usually unhelpful, but serological tests in invasave amoebiasis are frequently positive (Pittman *et al.*, 1973; Lamont and Wicks, 1976) and the procedure is particularly helpful in a non-endemic area where a previous infection is unlikely. Radiological changes are as frequent as any of the other features mentioned above and may be positive even in patients without clinical liver enlargement (Rowlands, 1963). Consequently it is an important task for the radiologist to detect liver enlargement, to show that it is due to an abscess and to determine whether extrahepatic spread has occurred.

Detection of liver enlargement is somewhat arbitrary and subjective in borderline cases. There are so many variables. Much depends on geometric technical factors and the stage of respiration when the film was obtained. Furthermore the patient's habitus and the normal range of variation are such that slight alterations can only be appreciated if serial films are obtained under similar conditions. Nevertheless, since enlargement is often in the superior part of the liver, radiographic evidence of enlargement often precedes clinical enlargement. Typically the diaphragm contour is more elevated than usual, with changes in contour anteriorly and medially (Fig. 4.24). This feature is often contrasted with the diaphragm alterations of subphrenic collections that tend to be most pronounced posteriorly and laterally. The degree of elevation may be dramatic (Fig. 4.24), but pleural fluid and lung consolidation may make it impossible to define the position of the diaphragm. A decubitus view of the left side up obtained with a horizontal beam is sometimes helpful if the fluid collection is mobile and shifts towards the mediastinum. Production of a pneumoperitoneum has also been used to resolve this difficulty and has the additional advantage that it can detect adhesions between the liver and the diaphragm. Thus it can help to separate primary changes in the thoracic cavity from those arising within the abdomen. Ellman and his colleagues (1965) found no false negatives by this procedure but its use is not generally recommended by us. The presence of a distended gall bladder detected in plain radiographs has been emphasised by Schmidt (1969).

Calcification rarely develops at the site of an amoebic liver abscess. Columbian workers have shown irregular amorphous calcification from this cause, and the phenomenon has also been seen on two occasions in Kenya (d'Alexandro, 1966; Whittaker, 1977).

Fluoroscopy can assess diaphragmatic movements but in our opinion a double exposure on the same film—one obtained in inspiration and the other in expiration—provides simple documentation of restriction of movement.

Basal linear subsegmental atelectases often accompany poor diaphragmatic excursions but the finding is non-specific, occurring also in pyogenic subphrenic collections and even with hepatomas.

The cause of the enlargement can be detected radiographically by contrast studies. Though arteriography has been used to show vessel displacement and the unperfused areas of the abscess, it is simpler and as effective to opacify the liver by a high dose of contrast medium by intravenous injection and perform tomography. Infusion can be used (De Morais & Medina, 1976; Palma *et al.*, 1977), but a large bolus of intravenous urography contrast medium (2 mg per kilogram of body weight) is usually effective (Fig. 3.46). Abscesses show as well-defined areas of translucency with sometimes some edge irregularities.

Ultrasound in B mode with and without grey scale clearly demonstrates most abscesses, giving indications of their size and depth (Fig. 3.46). Now that aspiration is seldom used for therapy or diagnosis, such information is not as important. It should be remembered that lymphoma deposits can also produce rounded trans-sonic areas. The lesions of hydatid cysts are usually better defined than abscesses and of course may show daughter cysts.

Obviously, when available, a computerised tomographic scan provides optimal morphological information (Fig. 3.46).

Opacification of abscesses following aspiration, with air or barium has been carried out. It clearly reveals the shaggy borders of the abscesses and can be used to follow resolution, since the sterile barium particles are phagocytosed by the Kupffer cells of the liver and so the area remains opaque (Harding *et al.*, 1970). However, as there are inherent risks in the procedure it is best avoided.

Extension of a liver abscess can be intraperitoneal or subphrenic, through the diaphragm into the thorax or from the left lobe into the pericardial cavity. Perforation into other viscera, pancreas, stomach and colon is rare, as is thrombosis and/or perforation into the vena cava.

The main problems in differential diagnosis lie with subphrenic suppuration from other causes and, in some parts of the tropics, exclusion of a hepatoma or Burkitt's lymphoma. The assistance of alkaline phosphatase determinations and serological studies in providing further evidence of an amoebic etiology is emphasised.

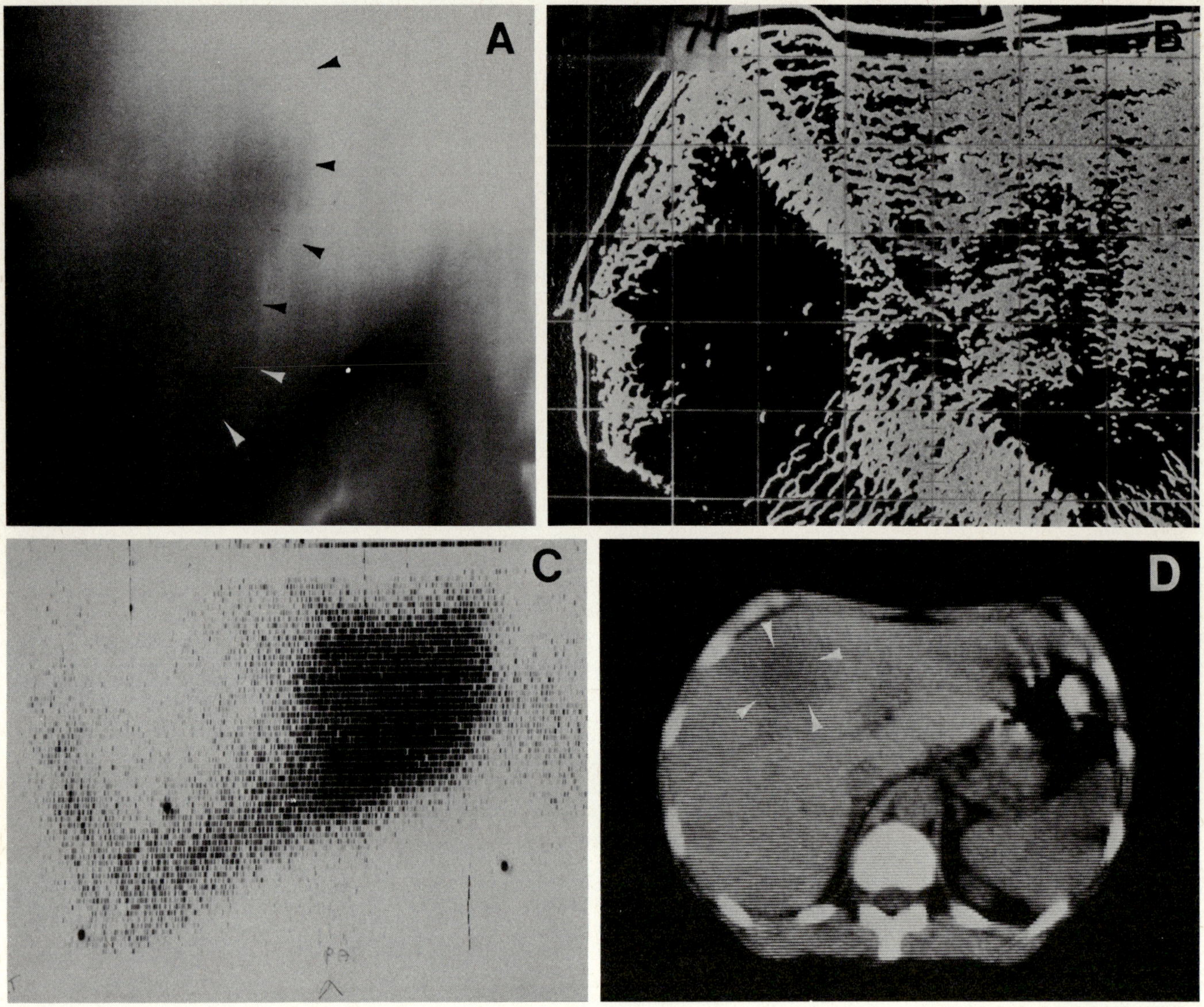

Fig. 3.46 Composite of amoebic abscesses. **A, B, C** same patient. **A.** Infusion hepato-tomogram reveals large, lobulated avascular area in liver. The mass is confirmed by the ultrasound and isotope studies. **D.** Shows a C.T. scan of an anterior abscess between white arrows. (A. Courtesy of Dr. Ants Toi, Hamilton. D. Courtesy of Dr. T. F. Meaney, Cleveland.)

REFERENCES

Adi, F. C. (1965) Clinical features of hepatic amoebiasis (a review of 120 cases, *West African Medical Journal*, **14,** 181–197.

d'Alexandro, A., Laga, J. & Vera, M. A. (1966) Cystic calcifications of liver in Colombia. Echinococcosis or calcified abscess, *American Journal of Tropical Medicine and Hygiene*, **15,** 908–913.

De Morais, J. A. D. & Medina, E. (1976) Essai sur la technique de visualisation des abscès amibiens hépatique, par coupes tomographique après perfusion de sels de l'acide triodobenzique, *Annales de la Société Belge de Médecine Tropicale*, **56,** 449–458.

Doxiades, T., Stergiou, L., Yiotsas, Z. & Tsitsanis, D. (1964) X-ray films in the diagnosis of chronic amoebic hepatitis, *British Medical Journal*, **1,** 343–346.

Ellman, B., McLeod, I. N. & Powell, S. J. (1965) Diagnostic pneumoperitoneum in amoebic liver abscess, *British Medical Journal*, **2,** 1406–1407.

Harding, T., Lewis, E. A. & Bohrer, S. P. (1970) Intra-cavity barium sulphate in the assessment of amoebic liver abscess, *Clinical Radiology*, **21,** 68–73.

Lamont, A. C. & Wicks, A. C. B. (1976) Amoebic liver abscess in Rhodesian Africans, *Transactions of the Royal Society of Tropical Medicine and Hygiene*, **70,** 302–305.

Palma, L. D., Bacarini, L. & Bazzochi, M. (1977) The use of abdominal contrast tomography in liver disease, *British Journal of Radiology*, **50,** 483–488.

Pittman, F. E., El-Hashimi, W. & Pittman, J. C. (1973) Studies on human amoebiasis, *Gastro-Enterology*, **65,** 581–587.

Radke, R. A. (1955) Amebomas of intestine: analysis of disease as presented in 78 collected and 41 unpublished cases, *Annals of Internal Medicine*, **43,** 1048–1066.

Rowlands, H. A. K. (1963) Radiological changes in amoebic liver abscess, *Journal of Tropical Medicine and Hygiene*, **66,** 113–123.

Schmidt, A. G. (1969) Plain film Roentgen diagnosis of amoebic hepatic abscess, *American Journal of Roentgenology*, **107,** 47–50.

Whittaker, L. R. (1977) Nairobi. Personal communication.

HYDATID LIVER DISEASE

Echinococcosis is a global problem caused by several species of echinocci: the worldwide E. granulosus that has a canine–ungulate cycle except in Alaska and Canada, where a moose–wolf dog passage is the rule, and in Australia where a dog–kangaroo cycle has been confirmed; E. multilocularis found in central and eastern Europe, Siberia, North Pacific Islands and Alaska, with a fox–rodent transmission that excludes herbivores; and E. oligarthrus of Central America and northern South America, with a feline–rodent cycle.

The large majority of infections acquired by man are due to E. granulosus. The specific prevalence in an area correlates with the state of development of the cattle industry. E. granulosus is a medical problem in parts of the Middle East: Lebanon, Syria, Iraq, Argentina, as well as Australia and Tasmania. In the Arctic and northern Canadian areas the disease appears to be milder and unrelated to cattle.

The sexually mature form of E. granulosus inhabits the intestinal tract of dogs. It is a small tapeworm of only a few segments, the last of which is gravid and discharges eggs. These are hardy, having a thick chitinous covering which envelops the oncosphere. The normal intermediate host acquires the eggs by eating contaminated pasture. In the duodenum of the intermediate host the embryo is freed, which then burrows into the gut mucosa, enters the circulation and is carried passively in the blood stream till it embolises. Then the cyst slowly grows, developing several layers: an outer adventitial derived from the host, an ectocyst laminated capsule, and a germinal layer which may show internal brood capsules. For the life cycle to be completed the definitive host, usually a dog, has to eat viscera containing a cyst with live embryo.

Cysts may be unilocular or form daughter cysts from the vacuolation of the germinal layer. Most cysts have a well-formed investing capsule, but with alveolar cysts spread by local infiltration or even more distal propagation can occur. This process is particularly associated with E. multilocularis, which is not a tropical parasite.

Since the embryos, having penetrated the gut, are carried by the portal blood stream to the liver, it is not surprising that in about half the patients with hydatidosis cysts are present there. It is said that embolisation usually occurs initially in the central veins of the hepatic nodules rather than portal tracts. Since the cyst develops at the rate of 1 mm a month, the precise site of lodgment is soon obliterated. A proportion of oncospheres pass unimpeded through the lung to arrest either in the pulmonary circulation, or survive that passage to traverse the heart and finally arrest systemically to embolise in various tissues. According to Poole and Marcial-Rojas (1971) approximately half the cysts develop in the liver, 20 per cent in the lungs, 4 per cent in the kidneys, 4 per cent in the muscle, 3 per cent in the spleen, 3 per cent in the central nervous system, 2 per cent in bone and the remainder with diminishing incidence in other tissues. These figures vary in different series, thus Little (1976) finds 30 per cent of cysts in the lungs. What is important is to stress the multiplicity of cysts in 41 per cent and that a quarter of patients with liver cysts also have lung lesions and 40 per cent with lung lesions have liver cysts (Little, 1976).

Though the radiological features can be highly suggestive precision in pre-operative diagnosis is aided by immunological tests. The time-tried intradermal Casoni test is positive in 90 per cent of patients, but has a 15 per cent false positive rate (Lass, 1973).

Perhaps more useful in management are the tests of greater sensitivity recently developed that may permit assessment of persistence of infection following surgery (*Lancet* editorial, 1976).

The radiological features in the liver may be a characteristic calcified cyst; the appearance of a non-specific space-consuming lesion; or, less commonly, due to communication between a cyst and the biliary passages. In the study of any suspected case simple chest, skull and abdominal radiography is obviously required.

Liver cysts are most often (80 per cent) in the right lobe of the liver. They are usually deep in the liver substance, but if superficially placed can then cause a localised distortion of the liver rather than general enlargement. As the cyst enlarges it produces compression of adjacent hepatic tissue and a host reaction characterised by a zone of reactivity and vascularity which is of help in angiographic diagnosis. In some patients calcification forms outside the laminated elastic membrane of the cyst, so that a calcified rim is not always necessarily indicative of a cyst with a dead sterile inner germinal layer. Viability of cysts diminishes with age, few being viable over the age of 60. Calcification was noted in 64 per cent of 149 cysts in Little's series (1976).

In a study from Colombia curvilinear irregular calcification similar to classic hydatid appearance was considered on the evidence to be due to remnants of amoebic abscesses. The likelihood of this cause of confusion must be rare (d'Alexandro *et al.*, 1966).

In plain films of the abdomen hepatomegaly of a localised bulge of the outline may be noted, which is most obvious when present on the diaphragmatic surface.

Calcification is the classical hallmark of hepatic cysts. The mineral may be deposited as a thin curvilinear rim (Figs. 3.47–3.49) or more diffusely in a denser amorphous pattern. Bonakdarpour (1967) has described a striking appearance attributable to calcification of daughter cysts, but this is very uncommon and must be due to a different process from the normal deposition of calcium in the false capsule formed from the host's tissues. This type of radiographic calcification is characteristic of the alveolar

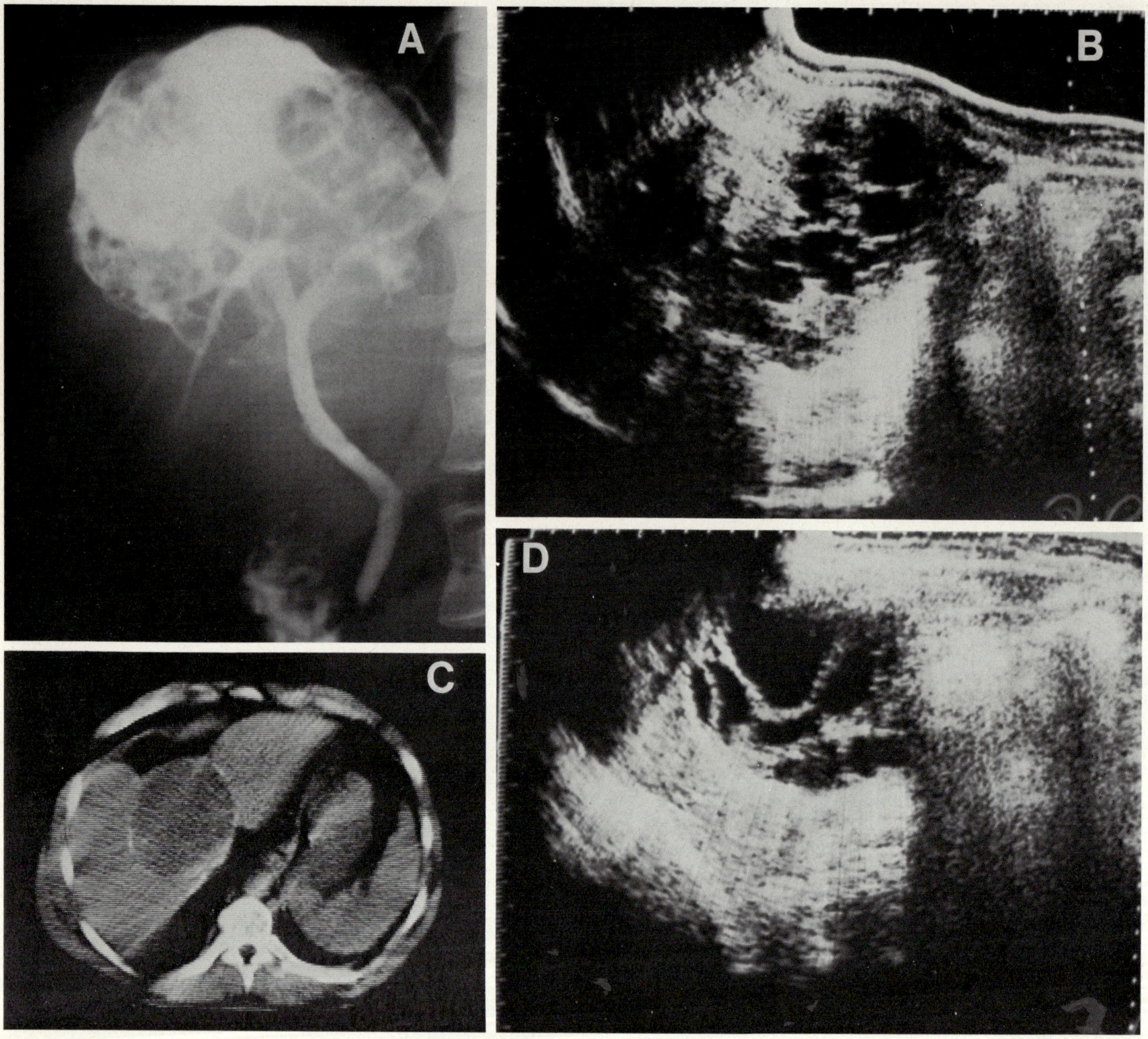

Fig. 3.47 Liver disease. **A.** Cyst with daughter cysts communicating with biliary tree opacified during percutaneous cholangiogram for jaundice. **B** and **D** show presence of multiple loculi due to daughter cysts in antero-inferior part of liver. **C.** Unilocular liver hydatid with traces of calcium in well-defined walls. (**A.** Courtesy of Dr. R. Tuttle, Hamilton. **B** and **D** Dr. Ants Toi, Hamilton. **C.** Dr. T. F. Meaney, Cleveland.)

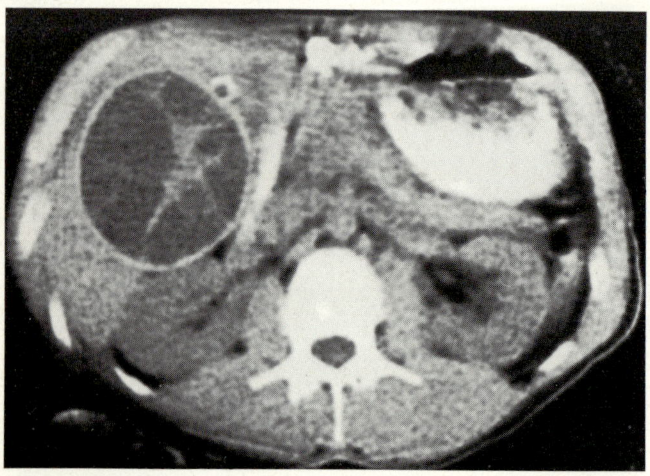

Fig. 3.48 Multilocular (daughter cysts) hydatid cyst of liver shown by C.T. scan. (Dr. W. Jeans, Bristol.)

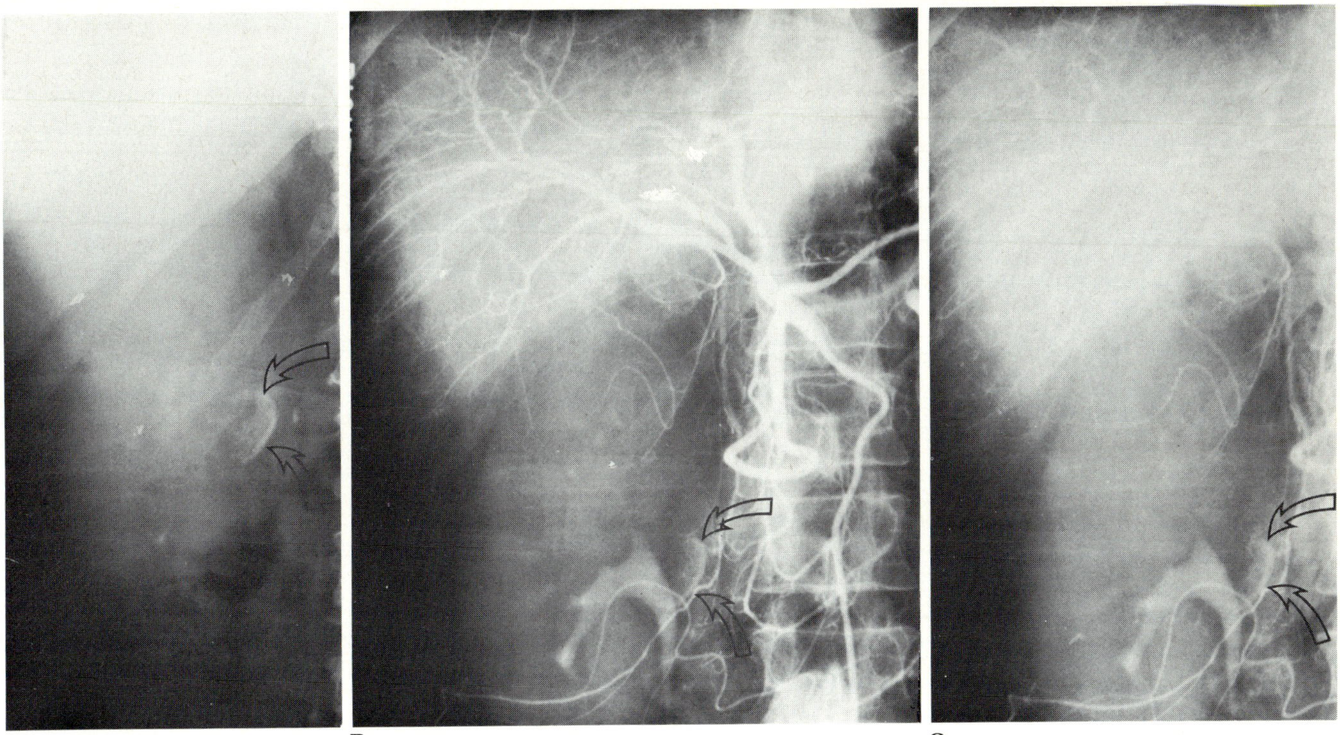

A B C

Fig. 3.49 A, B, C. Patient with enlarged liver and curvilinear calcification (arrowed). The coeliac angiogram reveals displacement of vessels around a large avascular area due to a hydatid cyst. (Courtesy of Dr. Prem Kapur, Hamilton.)

invasive disease due to E. multilocularis seen in Alaska (Thompson *et al.*, 1972).

When a cyst, by local pressure, compresses the common bile duct it can cause jaundice. More often jaundice is due to a growing cyst communicating with the biliary tree due to local pressure atrophy, as occurs in 16 per cent of liver hydatids (Kattan, 1977). The contents then drain and may plug the common bile duct. Recurrent jaundice, perhaps with cholangitis, can result from daughter cysts obstructing the bile ducts in an intermittent fashion during their passage. This may be shown by operative T tube cholangiography, or even during percutaneous cholangiography, which may be done when the ultimate diagnosis is unsuspected (Fig. 3.47) (Tuttle, 1970; Man *et al.*, 1977; Kattan, 1977.)

The cyst is a space-occupying lesion in the liver so that its presence can be detected by many methods. The first used technique was trans-splenic portovenography which could show distortion of the intrahepatic portal radicles and occasionally an avascular area in the hepatographic stage. Coeliac angiography has been used in many studies. Once again it shows distortion and displacement of the normal hepatic vasculature by the cyst and objectively reveals the avascular non-perfused cyst as a filling defect in the capillary phase (Fig. 3.49). In addition a denser hypervascular rim surrounds many cysts due to the capillary network in the adventitious cyst wall provided by the host. This rim can be half a millimetre to 4 millimetres with a sharper internal than external margin (Rizk *et al.*, 1971). Angiography by outlining the vasculature can provide useful morphologic information for the surgeon.

Isotopic techniques have proved reliable in demonstrating and locating mass lesions due to liver hydatids (Morris *et al.*, 1967).

More recently ultrasound has proven to be a very accurate means of displaying hydatid cysts with a 100 per cent reliability in some hands (Vicary *et al.*, 1977). The cysts are trans-sonic with a well-defined edge. Daughter cysts and loculi in a cyst are directly demonstrable (Fig. 3.47). The exact size and depth of a lesion is available from such studies.

Most recently whole body computerised scanning provides more elegantly and expensively similar and perhaps even more precise localisation and morphologic characteristics of a cyst. The well-defined margins are due to the different absorption characteristics of hydatid fluid and liver. A calcified rim is easily seen (Fig. 3.48).

Now that medical treatment of hepatic hydatid disease is available non-invasive methods of follow-up are going to assume greater importance (Bekhti *et al.*, 1977). Tomographic hepatography is the most generally available technique in the tropics, but ultrasound imaging and C.T. scanning when available have advantages.

REFERENCES

Bekhti, A., Schaaps, J-P., Capron, M., Dessaint, J-P., Santoro, F. & Capron, A. (1977) Treatment of hepatic hydatid disease with mebendazole: preliminary results in four cases, *British Medical Journal*, **2**, 1047–1051.

Bonakdarpour, A. (1967) Echinococcus disease—report of 112 cases from Iran and a review of 611 cases from the United States, *American Journal of Roentgenology*, **99**, 660–667.

d'Alexandro, A., Laga, J. & Vera, M. A. (1966) Cystic calcifications of liver in Colombia. Echinococcus or calcified abscess, *American Journal of Tropical Medicine and Hygiene*, **15**, 908–913.

Kattan, Y. B. (1977) Intrabiliary rupture of hydatid cyst of the liver, *Annals of the Royal College of Surgeons of England*, **59**, 108–114.

Lancet (1976) Editorial, **2**, 552–554.

Lass, N., Laver, Z. & Lengy, J. (1973) The immunologic diagnosis of hydatid disease—postoperative evaluation of the skin test and four serological tests, *Annals of Allergy*, **31**, 430–436.

Little, J. M. (1976) Hydatid disease at Royal Prince Alfred Hospital, 1964–1974, *Medical Journal of Australia*, **1**, 903–908.

Man, B., Kraus, L. & Motovic, A. (1977) Perforation of hydatid cyst into the common bile duct; report of four cases, *Tropical and Geographic Medicine*, **29**, 95–98.

Poole, J. B. & Marcial-Rojas, R. A. (1971) Echinococcosis in pathology. In *Protozoal and Helminthic Diseases*. pp. 635–657. Baltimore: Williams & Wilkins.

Rizk, G. K., Tayyarah, K. A. & Ghandur-Mnaymneh, L. (1971) The angiographic changes in hydatid cysts of the liver and spleen, *Radiology*, **99**, 303–309.

Thompson, W. H., Chisholm, D. P. & Tank, R. (1972) Plain film roentgenographic findings in alveolar hydatid disease—Echinococcus multilocularis, *American Journal of Roentgenology*, **116**, 345–358.

Tuttle, R. J. (1970) Cause of recurring obstructive jaundice revealed by percutaneous cholangiography—hydatid cyst, *New England Journal of Medicine*, **283**, 805–806.

Vicary, F. R., Cusick, G., Shirley, I. M. & Blackwell, R. (1977) Ultrasound and hydatid disease, *Transactions of the Royal Society of Tropical Medicine and Hygiene*, **71**, 29–31.

BILIARY INFECTIONS

Biliary ascariasis

The life cycle of Ascaris lumbricoides has already been described in the discussion of ascariasis of the intestinal tract.

Worms may migrate into the biliary passages. Sometimes multiple worms propel themselves head first through the papilla and have their tails lying free in the duodenum as they appear to have impacted. This process of forceful dilatation of the Sphincter of Oddi causes one of the severest pains known to man. Fortunately usually only a single worm at a time invades the biliary passages so that obstructive jaundice is inconstant unless multiple worms are present. In one clinical series a single worm was present in 83 per cent of cases of biliary tract invasion (Quant *et al.*, 1962). Some worms may enter the gall bladder or ascend into the hepatic ducts, where they eventually die. Organisms may be carried to the bile by the parasite so that cholangitis, suppurative intrahepatic cholangitis and even a subphrenic abscess can ensue (Reay *et al.*, 1964). When a worm dies in a duct and releases ova they cause a marked clinical reaction.

An ascarid entering the biliary system is one of the recognised causes of gas in the biliary tree in a plain film of the abdomen. The tail of the worm protruding into the duodenum after having entered the bile duct has been demonstrated in barium studies (Lieu, 1959). The impor-

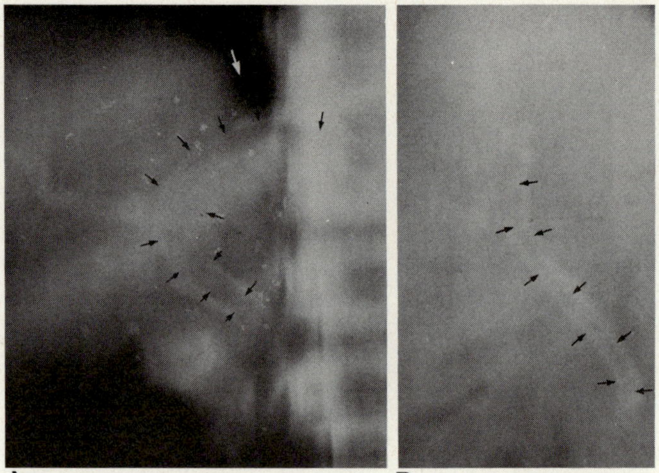

A B

Fig. 3.50 A, B. Ascariasis of biliary tree demonstrated by tomography during intravenous cholangiography. (Courtesy of Dr. Krige and Prof. Cremin.)

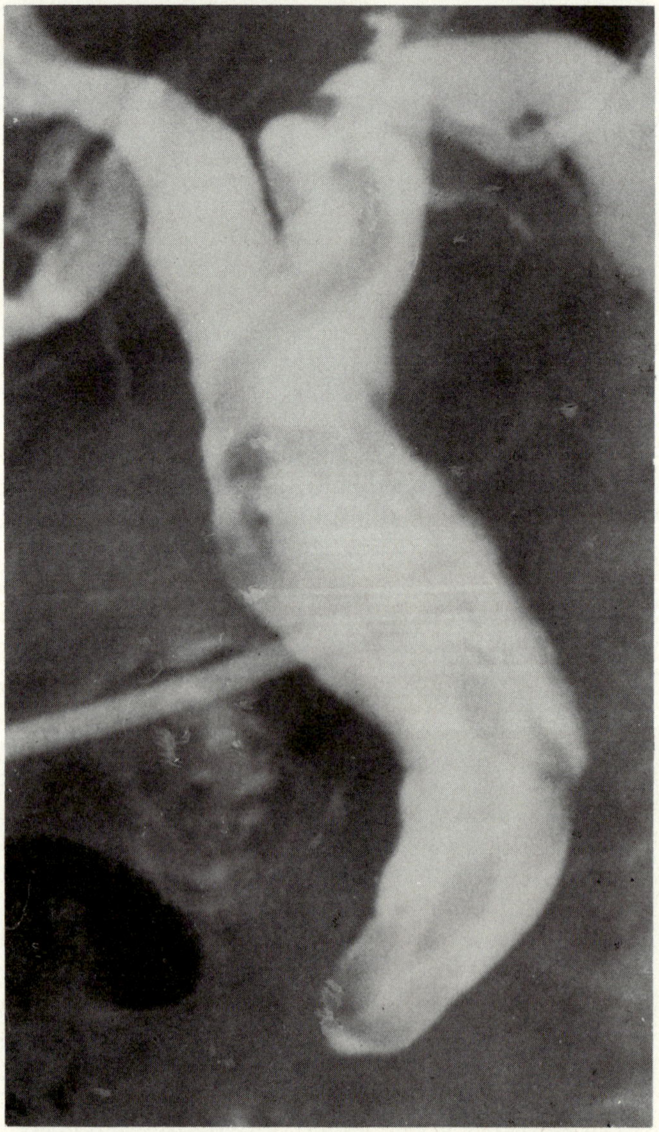

Fig. 3.51 Multiple filling defects due to ascaris in a dilated duct.

tance of intravenous cholangiography in the diagnosis is emphasised by the experience of Cremin (1969), who found ascarids in the bile passages in 40 out of 60 clinical cases. A normal cholangiogram or an obstructive process may also be demonstrated (Fig. 3.50). Generally an initial conservative approach to management is justified, as often the worms leave the bile passages spontaneously. If a repeat cholangiogram two weeks later reveals a worm, surgery is indicated (Fig. 3.51).

The condition is not rare in endemic areas and large series exist in the literature, such as the 600 cases of Schmauss and Tung (1959) and 110 of Hsu (1962).

REFERENCES

Cremin, B. J. (1969) Biliary parasites, *British Journal of Radiology*, **42**, 506–508.

Hsu, F. M. (1962) Clinical observations on 110 cases of ascaris invasion into the biliary tract, *Nagoya Journal of Medical Sciences*, **24**, 215–233.

Lien, S. H. (1959) Radiographic diagnosis of biliary ascariasis, *Chinese Medical Journal*, **78**, 545–555.

Quang, N. D., Schmauss, A. K. & Thu, N. X. (1962) Ascaridiasis der Gallenwege beim Kund, *Zeitschrift Troppenmedicine Parasitologie*, **13**, 318–331.

Reay, H. A. J., Dignon, A. P. & Maunder, C. (1964) Liver abscess caused by adult Ascaris lumbricoides, *British Medical Journal*, **2**, 553–554.

Schmauss, A. K. & Tung, T. T. (1959) Erfahrungen bei dem durch Parasitenbefall der tiefen Gallenwege ausgelosten abuten pankreasodem und der Pankreasnekrose nach Ulcusresektionen, *Langenbecks Archiv für Klirische Chirurgie*, **292**, 890–892.

DISTOMATA INFECTIONS CLONORCHIASIS OPISTHORCHIASIS

Clonorchiasis and opisthorchiasis are considered jointly, as they have many facets in common in their life cycle and in the consequences of their parasitism.

Clonorchis sinensis infection is a disease that occurs in parts of Korea, southern China, Taiwan, Hong Kong and Japan. In many of these areas the prevalence is on the wane due to control measures, improved drainage and industrial pollution which may inhibit the snail vectors.

Opisthorchiasis caused by O. felineus and O. viverini has a somewhat similar distribution as clonorchiasis, but in addition Thailand, Laos, western Malaysia and the Philippines are affected. In north-east Thailand prevalence rates over 80 per cent have been recorded in some districts.

As with many other forms of parasitic disease the symptoms are often related to the parasite load. A light infection may cause no obvious disturbance (Evans *et al.*, 1971). Evidence of this tolerance comes from a survey of Chinese living in New York City. Amongst immigrants from China, mainly Kwantung province, 26 per cent harboured the parasite as determined by stool tests, yet the majority had left their homeland over 20 years before (Kammerer *et al.*, 1977). Parasites have been known to persist for 50 years.

The life cycles are essentially similar, though the species of the intermediate hosts differ. The eggs are excreted in the stool already containing a miracidium. This hatches in a suitable snail first intermediate vector into sporocysts, rediae and subsequent cercariae. The latter penetrate the scale of certain cyprinoid fishes or carps, and encyst in tissues. If the fresh-water fish is then eaten raw by man, or other final hosts such as cats, pigs or dogs, the parasites excyst in the duodenum and ascend the common bile duct via the sphincter of Oddi. A small proportion may enter the pancreatic ducts. The parasites ascend against the bile flow into the more distal biliary radicles, and they seem to progress until they impact. Within about three weeks they mature, laying eggs and starting on a long hepatic career.

Clinically there may be no symptoms. Heavy infections produce certain host reactions and complications that ultimately bring the patient to medical attention.

The parasites in the biliary passages excite epithelial proliferation of the hepatic ductal tissue combined with a fibrosing mural and perimural process. The duct epithelium shows new mucin secreting glands and there is constant desquamation of the wall leading to debris in the duct system, in addition to the flukes. The latter vary in size according to species from 1 to 1·75 cm long and 0·2 to 1 mm in width, with a shape reminiscent of a broad leaf. Thousands of parasites may be recovered from ducts at autopsy. As a result of ductal changes, debris and parasites, mechanical obstruction develops and fusiform or saccular dilations form in multiple proximal tributaries of the hepatic biliary tree. These can be visualised by percutaneous cholangiography or by retrograde endoscopic techniques. (Ho, 1961; Okuda *et al.*, 1971; Evans *et al.*, 1971; Okuda *et al.*, 1973). Sometimes the obstruction becomes more severe with development of retention cysts in the biliary passages.

In cholangiograms the alteration in the lumen of a duct or ducts is readily apparent (Fig. 3.52) and small filling defects due to the flukes may be seen (Fig. 3.53). These have been likened in size and shape to dried tea leaves. The shape is obviously variable whether the flukes are seen in profile or *en face*. With clonorchiasis, gall-stones may develop in the hepatic duct and be another cause of filling defects. Such calculi are exceptional in opisthorchiasis (Wilde, 1973). In some instances examination of gall-bladder stones has revealed clonorchis parasitic fragments which may have acted as nuclei in an analogous manner to the ova of ascarids.

Acute suppurative cholangitis with E. coli is a complication that can further lead to distortion of the hepatic ducts from micro-abscess formation and later scarring. In an acute episode of infection, flukes may lose their hold and pass down the biliary tree and plug the common bile duct. The condition recurrent cholangitis can be associated with intrahepatic calculi but bears uncertain relationship to clonorchiasis (McFadzean & Ong, 1966). The same authors have shown a correlation between clonorchiasis

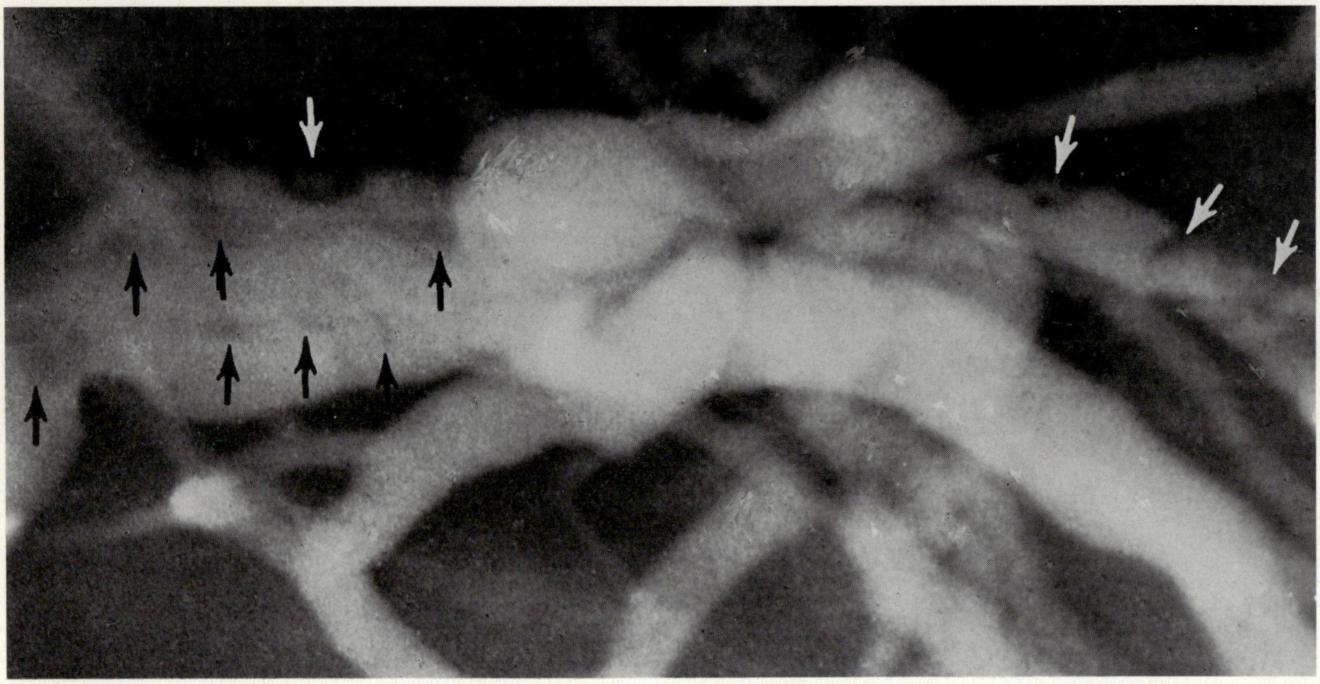

Fig. 3.52 Cholangiogram showing multiple small filling defect in large hepatic duct and branches due to clonorchis flukes. (Courtesy of Prof. J. Ho, Hong Kong.)

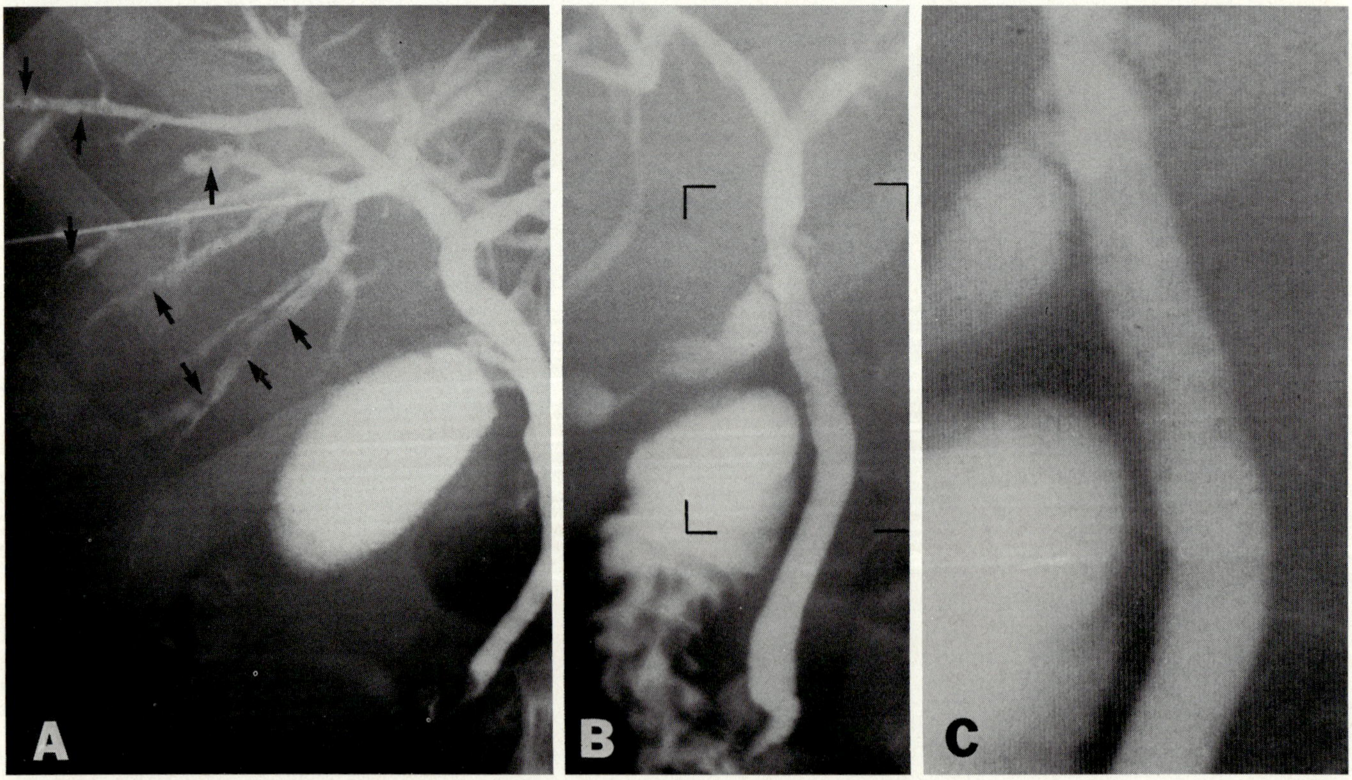

Fig. 3.53 Percutaneous cholangiogram with multiple filling defect in hepatic ducts and in a common bile of normal calibre. Clonarchis are best seen in close-up **C.** (Courtesy of Prof. Okuda.)

and a typhoid carrier state. Rarely in opisthorchiasis rupture of an infected abscess can occur into the lung with establishment of a fistula between the biliary and bronchial trees (Projyanonda and Tandhanand, 1961).

Cholangiocarcinoma, which can be multifocal, has a high incidence in opisthorchiasis, but whether this is so in clonorchiasis is not yet fully established (Fig. 3.54). Carcinoma of the cystic duct can also develop (Chainuvatti *et al.*, 1976).

A form of acute pancreatitis of low morbidity due to sinensis infection has been recorded in Hong Kong (McFadzean & Yeung, 1965).

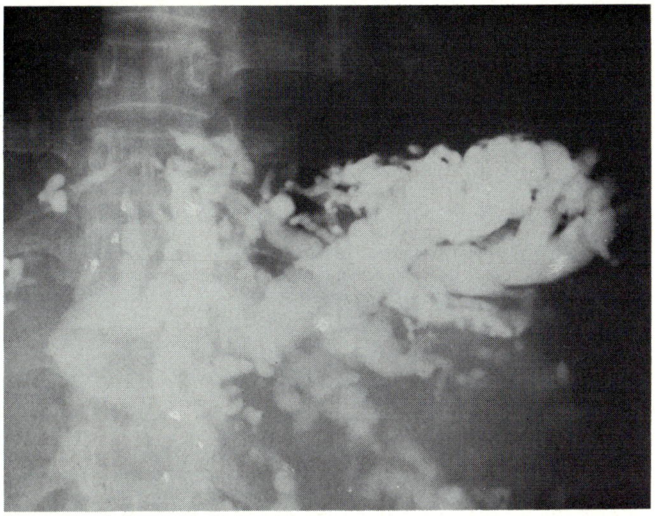

Fig. 3.54 Patient from Thailand with obstructed dilated intrahepatic ducts due to cholangiocarcinoma in a patient with opisthorchiasis. (Courtesy of Prof. Harold Jacobson, the Bronx, New York.)

REFERENCES

Chainuvati, T., Paosawadhi, A., Sripranoth, M., Manasatith, S. & Viranuvatti, V. (1976) Carcinoma of cystic duct associated with opisthorchiasis, *American Journal of Tropical Medicine and Hygiene*, 7, 482–486.

*Evans, H., Bourgeois, C. H., Comer, D. S. & Keschamras, N. (1971) Biliary tract changes in opisthorchiasis, *American Journal of Tropical Medicine and Hygiene*, **20**, 667–671.

Ho, H. C. (1961) *Tropical Radiology*, H. Middlemiss. pp. 140–141. London: Heinemann.

Kammerer, W. S., Van der Decker, J. A., Keith, T. B. & Mott, K. E. (1977) Clonorchiasis in New York City Chinese, *Tropical Doctor*, 7, 105–106.

*McFadzean, A. J. S. & Ong, G. B. (1966) Intrahepatic typhoid carriers, *British Medical Journal*, **1**, 1567–1571.

McFadzean, A. J. S. & Yeung, R. T. T. (1965) Acute pancreatitis due to Clinorchis sinensis, *Transactions of the Royal Society of Tropical Medicine and Hygiene*, **60**, 466.

Okuda, K., Shimokawa, Y. & Nakayama, Y. (1971) Roentgenologic visualisation of liver flukes, *Acta Hepato-Splenologica*, **18**, 46–50.

Okuda, K., Emura, T., Morokuma, K., Kokima, S. & Yokagawa, M. (1973) Clonorchiasis studies by percutaneous cholangiography and a therapeutic trial of toluene—2g4-diisothiocyanate, *Gastroenterology*, **65**, 457–461.

Prijyanonda, B. & Tandhanand, S. (1961) Opisthorchiasis with pulmonary involvement, *Annals of Internal Medicine*, **54**, 795–799.

Wilde, H., (1973) Biliary calculus associated with opisthorchiasis, *American Journal of Tropical Medicine and Hygiene*, **22**, 819–820.

LIVER FLUKES
FASCIOLIASIS

Liver flukes are flat, leaf-shaped hermaphrodites that in adult form parasitise the biliary tree. The main species is Fasciola hepatica, which occurs primarily in France, North Africa, South America, particularly Peru, the Caribbean, China and parts of Russia and Eastern Europe. A related species F. gigantica is endemic in parts of the Middle East, South East Asia, Hawaii and Africa. A larger digenetic trematode Fasciolopsis buski is widespread in South East Asia but affects the small bowel and colon rather than the liver.

The normal hosts for the adult flukes are sheep and cattle. The adult flukes, varying in size according to species, are approximately 25 to 15 mm. They produce operculated eggs when in the bile ducts which are voided in the faeces. The fertile ova liberate, after two weeks in water, a miracidium which is harboured in the liver of Lymnaea species of water snails. After passing through redial generations metacercariae are formed which attach themselves to various types of water vegetation, particularly watercress, and there encyst.

If the leaves are consumed by animals or man the larvae excyst in the upper small bowel in the presence of bile. The larvae actively penetrate the bowel wall, cross the peritoneal cavity to penetrate and burrow through the liver. Only a proportion reach the biliary passages, where they mature and proceed to lay eggs and so complete the cycle.

In man an acute phase characterised by epigastric and right upper quandrant pain, fever, and eosinophilia occurs several months after eating infected watercress. After a quiescent period non-specific symptoms and intermittent obstructive jaundice can occur.

Development of an inflammatory hepatic mass is uncommon (Kirk, 1961). Biliary cirrhosis is a rare but severe late complication. With Fasciolopsiasis of the Far East the adult flukes are attached to the mucosa of the small bowel and rarely the colon or stomach. They can cause diarrhoea, vomiting and facial edema with eosinophilia.

The radiological features of liver fluke infections have been described following cholangiography carried out during the course of cholecystectomies for obscure biliary symptoms or for known biliary calculi (Longo & Daraio 1953; Levrat *et al.*, 1963; Courbier *et al.*, 1966; Vayre & Robin, 1968). In such cases a narrow area of the common bile duct associated with a filling defect caused by the body of the adult fluke is seen. A small dot of contrast media may sometimes be seen, due to contrast within the sucker (Vayre & Robin, 1968).

Obviously operative cholangiography is not the only way to establish the diagnosis (Munro, 1965). If a liver fluke is suspected, stool examination for the presence of the characteristic ova is definitive. However, should the features just described be seen in an opacified common bile duct the liver flukes can be readily removed at surgery. Flukes in the more proximal portions of the biliary passages do not appear to have been described radiologically.

The filling defects in biliary passages due to opistorchiasis and clonorchiasis are considerably smaller, often multiple and may be associated with abnormalities of the hepatic ducts and intrahepatic calculi (Fung, 1961).

REFERENCES

Courbier, R., Villani, R. & Faini, M. (1966) Distomatose des voies biliares, *Marseille Chirurgical*, **16,** 638–645.

Fung, J. (1961) Liver fluke infestation and cholangio-hepatitis, *British Journal of Surgery*, **48,** 404–415.

Kirk, R. M. (1961) Fascioliasis presenting as a localised hepatic mass, *British Medical Journal*, **2,** 1333–1334.

Levrat, M., Tissot, A. & Pasquier, J. (1962) Distomatose hépato-biliare à forme d'ictère par retention guérie par le traitement médical, *Archives Françaises des maladies de l'appareil digestifs*, **52,** 351–355.

Longo, O. F. & Daraio, M. (1953) Distoma del coledoco-importancia de la colangiografia operatoria, La Prensa Medica Argentina, **40,** 2910–2911.

Munro, A. I. (1965) Liver fluke infestation and cholangio-hepatitis, *British Journal of Surgery*, **48,** 404–415.

*Vayre, P. & Robin, B. (1968) Distomatose choledocienne decouverte par cholangiographie per-operatoire lors d'une cholecystite lithiasique, *Journal de Chirurgie*, **96,** 553–556.

PORTAL HYPERTENSION

Portal hypertension can be the result of many processes, diverse both in aetiology and distribution. Below are briefly described a few entities that are either unique to specific areas in the tropics or have particularly high prevalence.

Umbilical sepsis

Infection of the cord acquired during cutting or following applications to the stump can lead to portal phlebitis via the umbilical vein. If the acute stage and the portal obliterative process are survived, portal hypertension frequently results with impaired liver function, splenomegaly and episodes of haematemesis. Detection of oesophageal varices and angiography are both technically difficult procedures in small infants. Portal venography is easier to perform and provides adequate information, revealing the degree of cavernous transformation of the portal vein from recanalisation as well as the collateral circulation (Fig. 3.55).

A similar process can arise from indwelling umbilical vein catheters in neo-natal intensive care units.

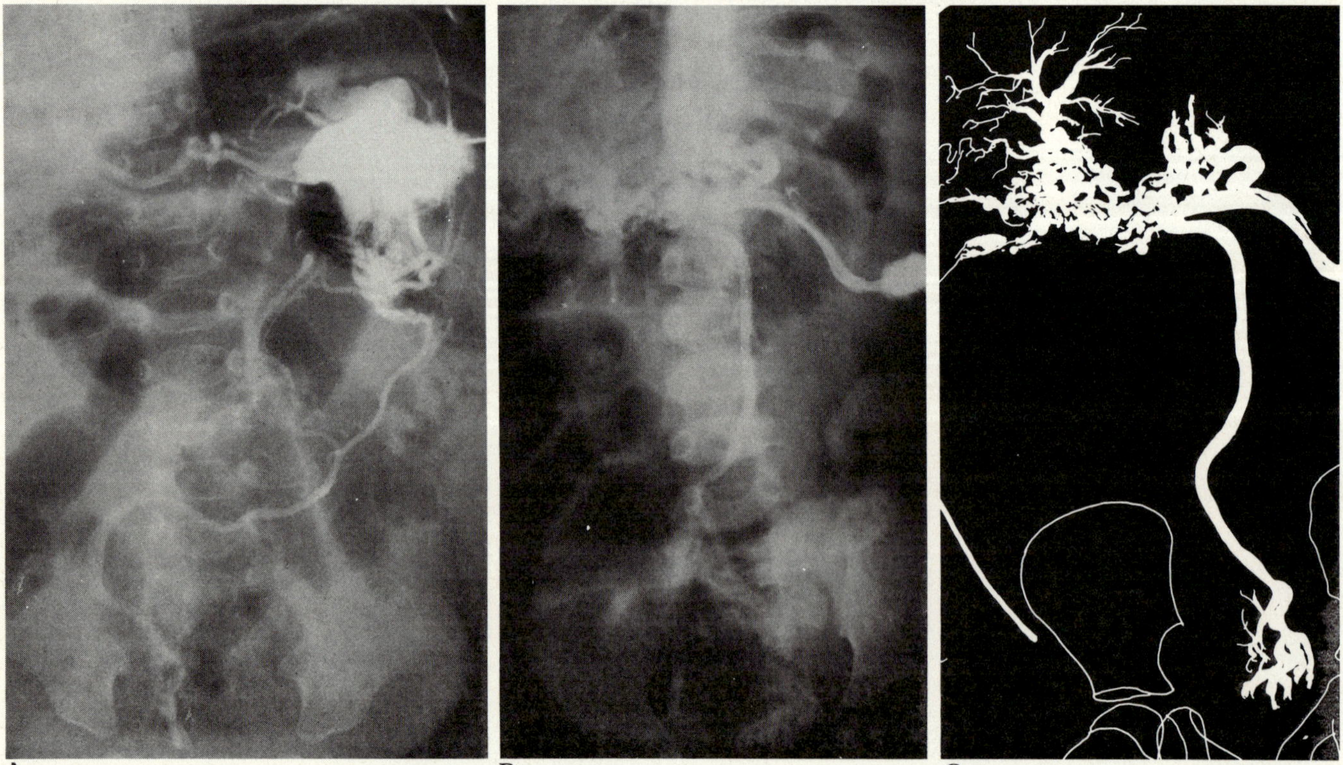

A B C

Fig. 3.55 A, B, C. Montage of trans-splenic portal venograms in 3-week and six-month-old infants who had had umbilical sepsis. In both there is porta hepatis obstruction and diversion of flow collaterals. The diagram and adjoining film indicate filling of the haemorrhoidal venous plexus.

Veno-occlusive disease

Alkaloids contained in 'medicinal' teas prepared from certain local plants can produce an obliterative endophlebitis of hepatic veins. This causes an intrahepatic obstruction with the development of a type of portal hypertension that simulates the Budd–Chiari syndrome (Brass *et al.*, 1954). We are not familiar with vascular radiology studies of these cases but percutaneous injection of contrast into the parenchyma of the liver should readily indicate whether hepatic venous flow obstruction is present (Ramsay & Britton, 1968).

In Japan there have been reports of a fibrous membranous obliteration of the vena cava at the level of the hepatic veins, causing hepatic venous obstruction (Kimura *et al.*, 1963).

Non-cirrhotic portal fibrosis of India

Portal tract fibrosis affecting medium-sized radicles of the portal vein has been described from India. There is no liver cell damage but the reduction in the lumen of branches of the portal vein causes portal hypertension. In the Delhi area this portal fibrotic process accounts for a quarter of all cases of portal hypertension (Sama *et al.*, 1971).

Bilharzial hepatic fibrosis

Embolising schistosomal ova produce a progressive obliterative process that impedes portal vein drainage, ultimately causing portal hypertension. The continuous arrival of ova from the mesenteric veins creates extensive fibrosis of the wall of the veins. Ova may penetrate there, causing further perivascular fibrotic thickening. The periportal venous fibrosis produces white rigid tubular pathways that have been likened to clay pipe stems. The role of immunologic factors and of embolising worms is less clear. The flukes are larger and presumably cause greater mechanical disturbances than ova. Considerable numbers of worms may become detached from distal veins and embolise to the liver following antimony and other forms of chemotherapy. With S. japonicum portal hypertension develops early, as the ovideposition occurs high up in the mesenteric veins. In S. haematobium infections the initial damage by eggs is primarily in pelvic veins, but with S. mansoni eggs reach distal branches of the portal venous system earlier. Once collaterals have formed to bypass the hepatic obstructive process, eggs may reach the lungs to damage the pulmonary arterial ramifications.

Opacification of the portal venous system by trans-splenic portal venography or consequent on coeliac and superior mesenteric arteriography does not usually demonstrate the distorted venous pattern characteristic of regenerative cirrhosis. A useful review of angiographic findings in S. mansoni cirrhosis is to be found in the paper by Sniderman & Sos (1978). Pruning of the portal tree and varying degrees of collateral formation are, however, evident. In Zambia bilharzial pipestem portal fibrosis is the most frequent cause of upper gastro-intestinal bleeding. Seventy per cent of ruptured oesophageal varices were from this cause (Carruthers & Sinha, 1978).

By creation of an extracorporeal circulation from the portal vein through a filter with return of blood to the femoral vein, it is possible to remove live worms as they are detached by the effects of antimony salts in the circulation.

Cirrhosis of the liver

Cirrhosis of the liver has a high incidence in much of Africa and in parts of the Far East, often in areas that also have a high prevalence of primary hepatocellular carcinoma. Though subnutrition and aflotoxins have been implicated in the aetiology, type B virus has assumed considerable aetiologic importance following Australia antigen studies. Owing to the post-necrotic scarring and the regenerating nodules, liver cirrhosis often causes considerable distortion of the portal venous and hepatic arterial architecture. Because of the association with neoplasia in many areas, care should be taken to determine whether any hypervascular areas seen in angiograms indicate a focus of liver carcinoma.

Other hepatic fibrotic processes

Hepatic fibrosis around the biliary tree, following suppurative cholangitis of the Far East, may occasionally obstruct portal flow, but even in endemic areas this is not a significant cause of portal hypertension. Bantu nutritional siderosis causes hepatic fibrosis but does not result in portal hypertension.

The congestive tropical splenomegaly syndrome does not normally produce a great elevation of the portal pressure, though this is a feature in some reports (Basu, 1958) of a form of the disorder from Bengal.

REFERENCES

Basu, A. K. (1958) Chronic 'Bengal' splenomegaly and allied states of portal hypertension, *Annals of the Royal College of Surgeons*, **8**, 137–158.

Brass, G., Jelliffe, D. B. & Stuart, K. L. (1954) Veno-occlusive disease of the liver with non-portal type of cirrhosis occurring in Jamaica, *Archives of Pathology*, 57, 285–300.

Carruthers, R. H. & Sinha, P. (1978) Bilharzial portal fibrosis: an important cause of portal hypertension, *Annals of the Royal College of Surgeons of England*, **60**, 49–52.

Kimura, C., Shirotani, H., Hirooka, M., Terada, M., Iwashaki, K. & Maetani, S. (1963) Membranous obliteration of the inferior vena cava in the hepatic portion (Review of 6 cases with 3 autopsies), *Journal of Cardiovascular Surgery*, **4**, 87–98.

Ramsay, C. G. & Britton, R. C. (1968) Intraparenchymal angiography in the diagnosis of hepatic veno-occlusive disease, *Radiology*, **90**, 716–726.

Sama, S. K., Bhargava, S., Gopi Nath, N., Talwar, J. R., Nayak, N. C., Tandon, B. N. & Wig, K. L. (1971) Noncirrhotic portal fibrosis, *American Journal of Medicine*, **51**, 160–169.

Sniderman, K. W. & Sos, T. A. (1978) Hepatic schistosomiasis: a case with intrahepatic shunting and extrahepatic portal vein occlusion, *American Journal of Roentgenology*, **130**, 565–567.

PYOGENIC CHOLANGITIS

A chronic suppurative disease of the liver has been well documented from Hong Kong and Singapore, but is also prevalent in adjacent parts of South East Asia (Harrison-Levy, 1962; Ong, 1962). A high proportion of patients have gall-bladder disease, but far more have intrahepatic biliary calculi or biliary mud. The alleged role of parasitic diseases such as clonorchiasis, opisthorciasis and ascariasis in the aetiology of such calculi is debatable. Whether the infection reaches the liver by ascent up the biliary passages or haematogenously through the portal vein is not known.

The condition gives rise to portal tract fibrosis arising from the repeated biliary infections. Small intrahepatic abscesses which communicate with the duct system may develop which are demonstrable by cholangiography (Fig. 3.56).

In a study by percutaneous cholangiography Yu and his colleagues (1973) emphasised the differentiating features in the appearances of pyogenic cholangitis from other causes of ductal dilatation. In other causes of obstruction the ducts not only dilate but become tortuous, whereas in pyogenic cholangitis the fibrosis of the wall renders the tube rigid, straight and pipe-like. Biliary mud and sludge may be seen distending portions of the ducts and in areas may produce cast-like filling defects as well as amorphous concrements. The common bile duct is usually around 20 mm in width. Small outpouchings and saccules due to abscesses related to the portal tracts are sometimes opacified.

REFERENCES

Harrison-Levy, A. (1962) The biliary obstruction syndrome of the Chinese, *British Journal of Surgery*, **49**, 674.

Ong, G. B. (1962) A study of recurrent pyogenic cholangitis, *Archives of Surgery*, **84**, 199.

Yu, S. F., Oon, C. L. & Kho, K. M. (1973) Local experience of percutaneous transhepatic cholangiography, *Singapore Medical Journal*, **14**, 13–18.

HEPATIC MALIGNANCY

S. B. Lagundoye

Primary liver cell carcinoma (hepatoma)

Primarily liver cell carcinoma is a common malignancy in much of the tropics, particularly affecting young men. It is seen in most of tropical Africa, in New Guinea, Formosa and the Chinese of Singapore. In parts of the Far East where clonorchiasis and opisthorchiasis are prevalent a cholangio carcinoma is seen.

To indicate the dimensions of the problem some statistics are revealing. In Mozambique this tumour occurs 500 times more often than in equivalent U.S. males aged 25 to 36 (Edington & Gilles, 1976). Lourenzo-Marques hepatoma represented 55 per cent of all malignancies; in the savanna of Nigeria 19 per cent and in Taiwan 15 per cent (Fakunle *et al.*, 1977; Yu, 1967).

A discussion of etiological factors would need to be discursive, as much is still speculative regarding the relationship of cirrhosis and viral hepatitis. Suffice to say that the alpha-foeto-protein is raised in 60 to 85 per cent of patients and that hepatitis B surface antigen can be detected in about half the patients (Abondo *et al.*, 1973; Fakunle *et al.*, 1977).

Clinically a hepatomegaly, which may be tender, is the obvious physical finding. A hepatic bruit due to the vascularity of the tumour can be heard in about a quarter to a third of cases—a useful differential point between hepatoma and amoebic abscess.

The tumour can be massive and localised, nodular or

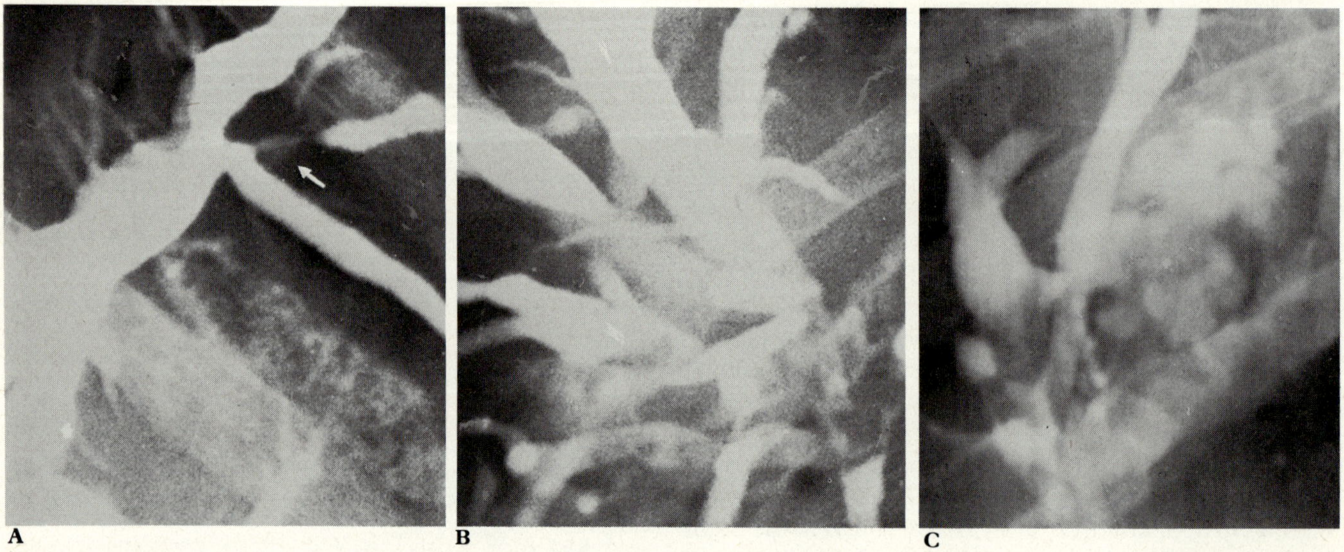

Fig. 3.56 A, B, C. Patients suffering from Far East cholangitis and clonorchiasis with strictures; dilatation of ducts from focal strictures; and irregular communicating abscess cavities. (Courtesy of Prof. Okuda and Prof. Ho.)

diffuse. It does not invade the diaphragm. Lung and bone secondaries are frequent. Ascites often develops but pleural collections are surprisingly infrequent. The liver is usually obviously enlarged in plain films unless ascites is present, when hepatomegaly may be difficult to detect radiologically. Elevation of the diaphragm is an early feature which can precede palpation of an enlarged liver edge (Payet *et al.*, 1956). The diaphragm does not often show a localised bulge, but rather a diffuse elevation which is much more frequent on the right side, though the left alone can be affected, or both domes together, particularly when ascites exists (Sanders, 1968).

If metastases are seen in the lungs the hepatic enlargement is readily differentiated from an amoebic abscess. Linear atelectasis of the overlying lung is often seen, but this interference with basal ventilation is non-specific and does not indicate the cause of the diaphragmatic elevation.

Calcification in hepatoma has been described but is extraordinarily rare (Allen & Holt, 1967).

Trans-splenic portal venography has been used to investigate these patients (Bovy, 1962). Since a proportion are cirrhotic the procedure documented the portal hypertension shunts. Often, unless encasement of a venous channel was clearly shown, the procedure did not truly differentiate hepatoma from other masses such as amoebic liver abscess. Selective angiography has now replaced venography, since the tumour is vascular and is supplied by the hepatic artery. Invariably the hepatic vessels have a wider lumen than normal. The branches are usually displaced by stretching around a mass to feed an area of increased vascularity which may show early venous shunting into portal vessels (Yu, 1967). There may be a marked capillary phase that serves to delineate more precisely the extent of the carcinoma deposits and whether the process is localised or diffuse (Fig. 3.57).

The significance of hepato-portal arteriovenous shunting in hepatoma has been investigated by Nagasue and colleagues (1977) on the basis of 80 cases studied in Japan. Such patients comprised 10 per cent of those in the series and all had oesophageal varices. Some other patients also had varices associated with venous obstruction by vessel encasement or thrombosis due to the tumour. Others have suggested that the combination of hepato-portal shunt with reversed flow associated with pressure defects in the portal vein is pathognomic for primary hepatoma (Rossi & Gould, 1970). Reversed flow and shunting is due to hepatic vein drainage obstruction and results in varices with haematemesis and splanchnic dissemination of secondary deposits.

In our view angiography is mainly worthwhile when the focus is considered localised and ablative surgery is being contemplated. Isotope studies are probably less sensitive in the detection of multiple foci. The role of ultrasound in management has not yet been assessed nor has the C.T. scan (Fig. 3.58). Since these last three modalities are not generally available we believe that if the diagnosis is diffi-

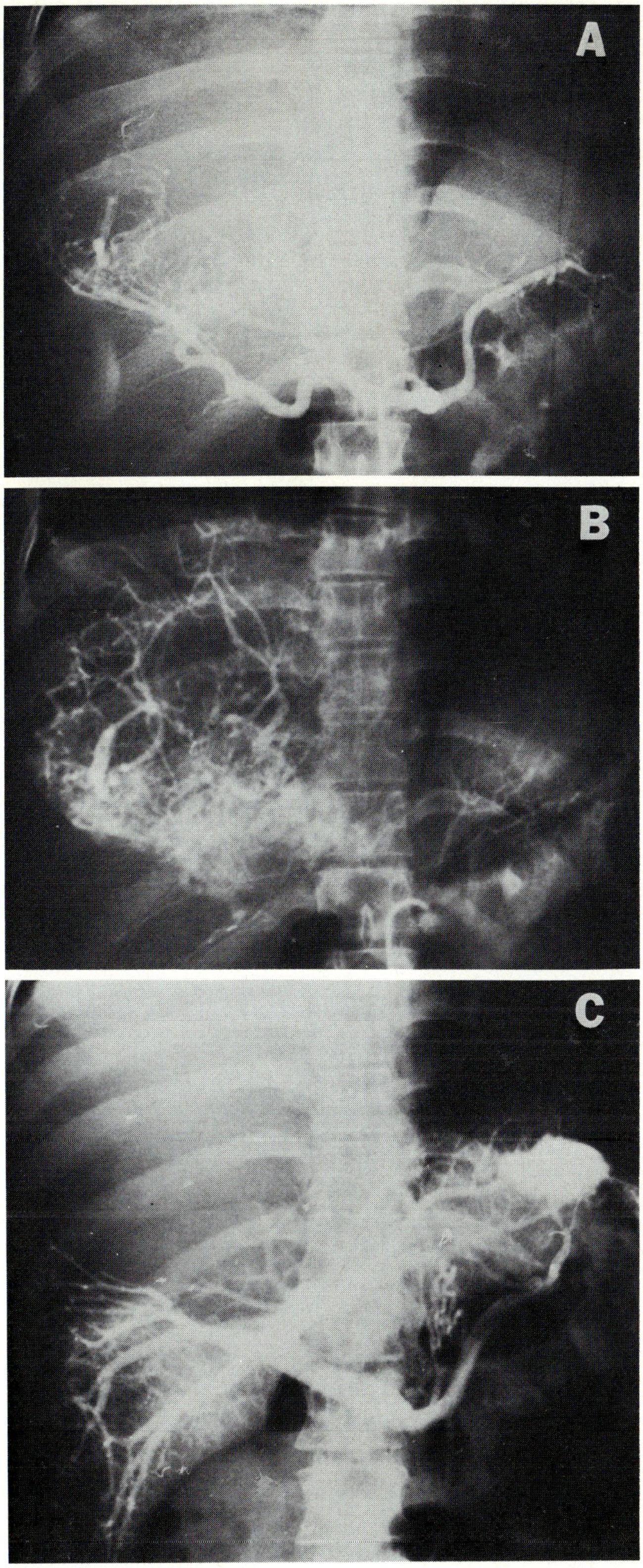

Fig. 3.57 **A** and **B** coeliac arteriogram and **C** trans-plenic phlebogram in patient with large superior hepatoma obstructing the hepatic vein outflow. Note that the neoplasm steals most of the arterial flow due to its low vascular resistance. There are no portal vein radicles in the area of neoplasia.

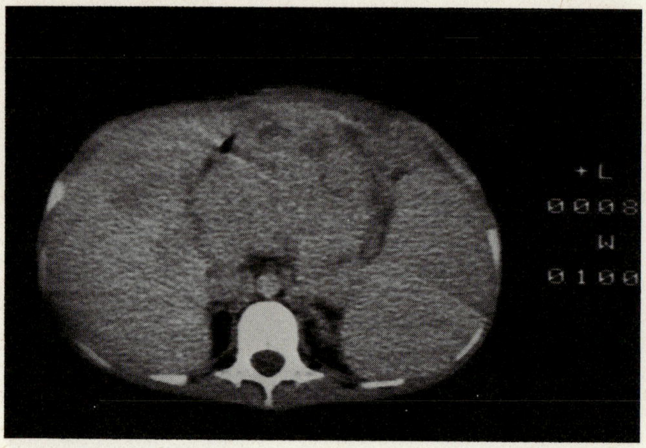

Fig. 3.58 Primary hepatoma. C.T. scan showing hepatoma in the right lobe of the liver with metastases within the left indicating inoperability. There are calcified foci in the tumour. Coeliac axis and superior mesenteric arteriography did not show the metastases in this patient. The pancreas appeared normal at arteriography, but could not be distinguished in the scan. (Courtesy of Dr. J. S. Macdonald.)

cult to establish, occasionally angiography may indicate the most rewarding area to approach for needle biopsy.

REFERENCES

Abondo, A., Quenum, C., N'Diaye, P. & Leger, H. (1973) Relations entre les caractères morphologiques et l'alpha-foeto-proteine au cours du cancer primitif du foie (à propos de 92 cas), *Bulletin Société Médicine d'Afrique Noire Langue Française*, **18**, 15–21.

Allen, R. W. & Holt, A. H. (1967) Calcification in primary liver carcinoma, *American Journal of Roentgenology*, **99**, 150–152.

Edington, G. M. & Gilles, H. M. (1976) *Pathology in the Tropics*. pp. 593–598. London: Edward Arnold.

Fakunle, Y. M., Ajdukiewicz, A. B., Greenwood, B. M. & Edington, G. M. (1977) Primary liver cell carcinoma in the Northern Guinea savanna of Nigeria, *Transactions of the Royal Society of Tropical Medicine and Hygiene*, **71**, 335–337.

Nagasue, M., Inokuchi, K. & Kobayashi, M. (1977) Hepatoportal arteriovenous fistula in primary carcinoma of the liver, *Surgery, Gynaecology and Obstetrics*, **145**, 504–508.

Payet, M., Pellegrino, A. & Pene, P. (1956) Etude clinique et radiologique des rapports Hépato-diaphragmatique et des poumons dans le cancer primitif du foie, *Journal de Radiologie et d'Electrologie*, **37**, 877–882.

Rossi, P. & Could, H. R. (1970) Angiography and scanning in liver disease, *Radiology*, **96**, 553–562.

Sanders, C. F. (1968) The plain chest radiograph in seventy five cases of primary carcinoma of the liver, *Clinical Radiology*, **19**, 341–346.

CARCINOMA OF THE BILIARY TRACT

Intrahepatic ductal carcinoma appears to be prevalent in areas where the flukes of clonorchiasis and opisthorciasis parasitise the biliary tree. Apparently they lead to epithelial proliferation and intraductal neoplasia which may be multifocal.

In much of Africa where gall-stones are rarely seen carcinoma of the gall bladder is rare. In South Africa the whites have nearly a 25 times greater incidence than the black population. The few gall-bladder neoplasms found in the black population are squamous cell carcinoma, whereas the tumour in whites is generally an adenocarcinoma (Becker & Chatgidakis, 1952).

REFERENCES

Becker, B. J. P. & Chatgidakis, C. B. (1952) Carcinoma of the gallbladder and cholelithiasis on the Witwatersrand; an autopsy survey of the racial incidence, *South Africa Journal of Clinical Science*, **3**, 13–22.

PANCREATIC LITHIASIS

A distinctive form of pancreatic calcification due to calculi in the pancreatic ducts has been noted in young people, particularly males, with diabetes in many parts of the tropics (Zuidema, 1959; Bourgoignie *et al.*, 1962; Kinnear, 1963; Shaper, 1964; Geevarghese & Pitchumoni, 1966). The initial reports came from Indonesia, but it is now realised to occur in Malaysia, India and other parts of the Far East, in Senegal, Ghana, Nigeria, the Congo, Uganda and elsewhere.

The condition is found in underweight individuals who have scanty scalp hair, atrophic skin reminiscent of kwashiorkor, and enlarged parotid glands. Most of the individuals have diabetes, which may be severe. Kinnear noted that 75 per cent of Nigerian diabetics under 20 years of age showed pancreatic calcification. Generally the external pancreatic secretions are not greatly disturbed, so that steatorrhoea and a malabsorption barium pattern are uncommon. Pain can be severe and necessitate pancreatic duct drainage procedures for relief. Following this type of surgery subsequent abdominal radiographs may show a slow disappearance of the calculi.

The etiology is considered to be related to chronic protein calorie malnutrition.

Radiologically the calcific densities are nodular of varying size and scattered throughout the gland (Fig. 3.59). The gland is often fibrotic and contracted, so that the calculi may be crowded together, but this is not constant.

Parenchymal calcification, as distinct from ductal calculi, can develop as a sequel to classical acute pancreatitis. Radiologically we do not know how this can be distinguished except that calculi may be larger than dystrophic foci.

Rarely calcification can be caused around dead schistosomal ova in the pancreas. In one such instance fine and diffuse opacities were clearly visible on a plain abdominal radiograph (Olurin, 1970).

REFERENCES

Bourgoignie, J., Sonet, J. & Dechef, G. (1962) Etude clinique du diabète sucre du Bantou de la région de Leopoldville, *Annales de la Société Belge de Médecine Tropicale*, **42**, 261–294.

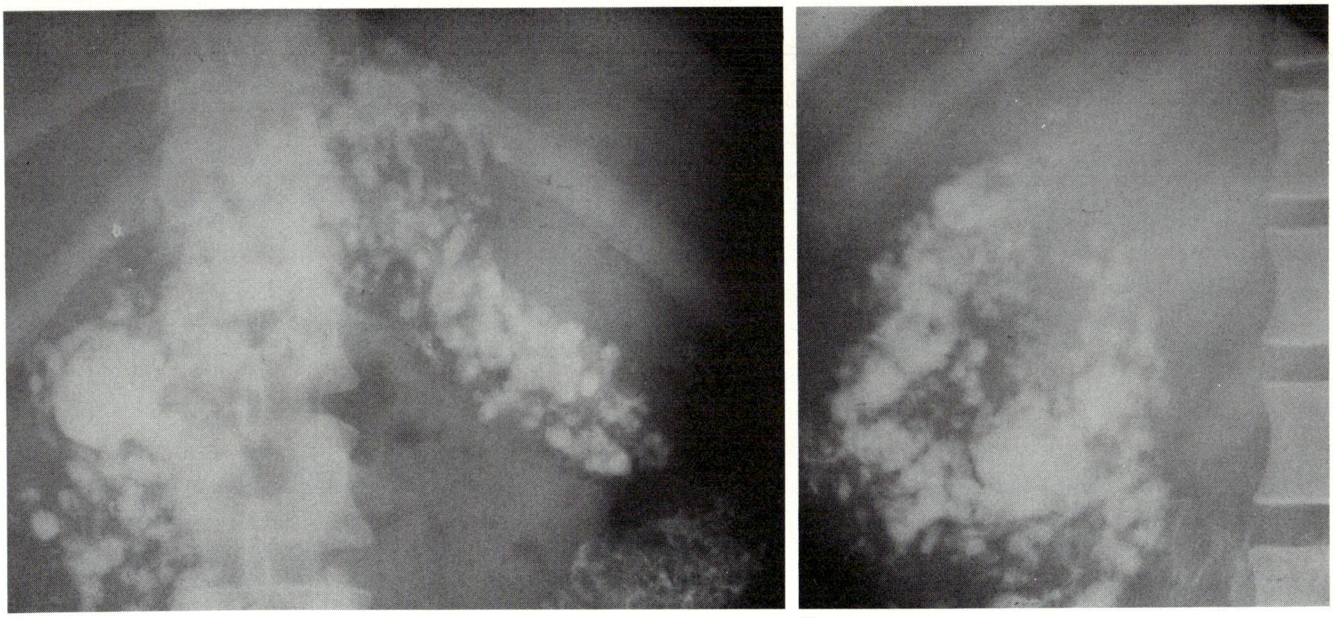

A B

Fig. 3.59 **A, B.** Gross pancreatic ductal lithiasis in a Nigerian diabetic. The concretions often appear more anteriorly than anticipated in the lateral view.

Geevarghese, P. J. & Pitchumoni, E. S. (1966) Pancreatic diabetes in Kerala, India, *Proceedings of the World Congress of Diabetes in the Tropics*, Bombay, 223.
Kinnear, T. W. G. (1963) The pattern of diabetes mellitus in a Nigerian teaching hospital, *East African Medical Journal*, **40,** 288–294.
Mahadevan, R. (1961) Pancreatic lithiasis—a follow-up of 21 cases, *British Medical Journal*, **1,** 626–629.
Olurin, E. O. (1970) Schistosomal pancreatic calcification, *Ghana Medical Journal*, **9,** 247–252.
Shaper, A. G. (1964) Aetiology of chronic pancreatic fibrosis with calcification seen in Uganda, *British Medical Journal*, **1,** 1607–1609.
Zuidema, P. J. (1959) Cirrhosis and disseminated calcification of the pancreas in patients with malnutrition, *Tropical and Geographical Medicine*, **11,** 70–74.

THE SPLEEN

Splenic enlargement is a feature of many tropical disorders. Clinical assessment of splenic size can be notoriously difficult. In radiographs assessment of a three-dimensional structure in two planes may be unreliable (Riemenschneider & Whalen, 1965), but a simple scheme can often provide an indication of spenomegaly. On a normal A.P. abdominal film taken at 100 cm anode–film distance the vertical distance between the tip and the diaphragm is measured. In an average adult 11·3 cm or more gives a 75 per cent probability that the weight is over 200 grams and so enlarged. The likelihood of enlargement is 98 per cent if the vertical distance is over 15 cm (Whitley *et al.*, 1966). Unfortunately splenic borders may be difficult to distinguish. If absolutely required isotopic evidence can provide useful size information. Splenic size can also be gauged by displacement of stomach, the splenic flexure and downward displacement of the left kidney (Forde *et al.*, 1960).

In plain films the spleen may cast a much greater diffuse density than normal if it carries a high iron burden, as in thalassaemic siderosis and in sickling disorders. In thalassaemia-S and in homozygous sickle cell disease fine speckled calcification or more amorphous patches may be noted (Fig. 3.60) (Lagundoye, 1971). The spleen in homozygous sickle cell disease is usually small (auto-splenectomy), but is large in most cases of haemoglobin S C disease.

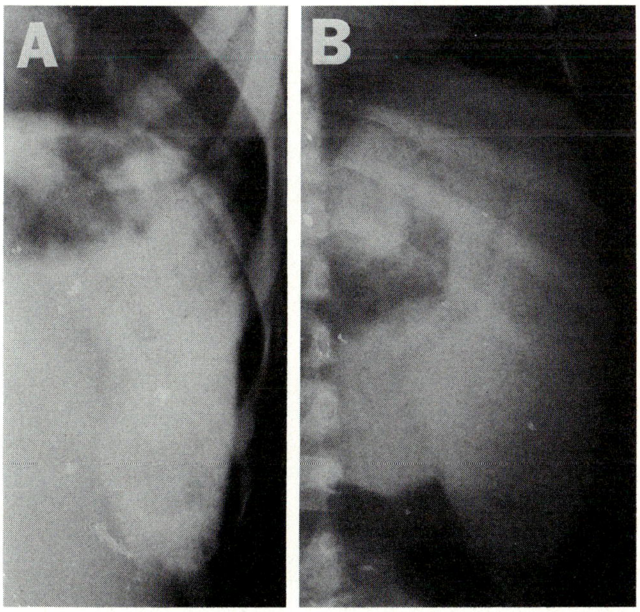

Fig. 3.60 **A.** Densely calcified small spleen of SS genotype. **B.** Large spleen with speckled calcification.

Calcification can occur in the spleen in certain granulomatous conditions such as tuberculosis and histoplasmosis. These foci are often multiple, irregular in shape and amorphous in character. Ring-shaped calcified hydatid cysts have a typical appearance.

Splenic abscess

Splenic abscesses of undetermined etiology have been reported from Zambia and Rhodesia for many years (Gelfand, 1950). Similar lesions have been noted in West Africa. It is likely that these are of multiple aetiologies. Splenic abscess can occur in the course of relapsing fever, develop in typhoid and with other salmonellae, and in amoebic infections. Rhodesian workers have also postulated tropical phlebitis of the splenic vein as an etiological entity. There is no doubt that in sickling areas a significant proportion of these abscesses are related to the S gene, in homozygous or heterozygous forms, including the carrier state (Cockshott & Weaver, 1962).

Such an abscess presents a characteristic appearance. The left diaphragm is raised and the stomach displaced medially by the bulk of the spleen. The spleen contains an irregular central cavity outlined by gas which will show a fluid level in the erect position (Figs. 3.61 and 3.62). Initially in the early stages when a patient has flank pain small bubbles can be appreciated over the spleen. These gradually coalesce as the centre of the spleen undergoes colliquative necrosis. At surgery the splenic vein is thrombosed. These cases in sicklers appear to represent massive infarcts. We have confirmed such infarction by angiography as have Yeung and Lessing (1976) and others by isotope studies in sickle cell C disease (Fishbone *et al.*, 1977).

These splenic abscesses can remain sterile but may become infected. The gas is at times endogenous and does not necessarily imply the presence of gas-forming organisms or fistulous communication with a viscus. Untreated the splenic contents may ultimately perforate the diaphragm to cause an effusion, or rupture into the lung to be expectorated. We have also seen pericardial communi-

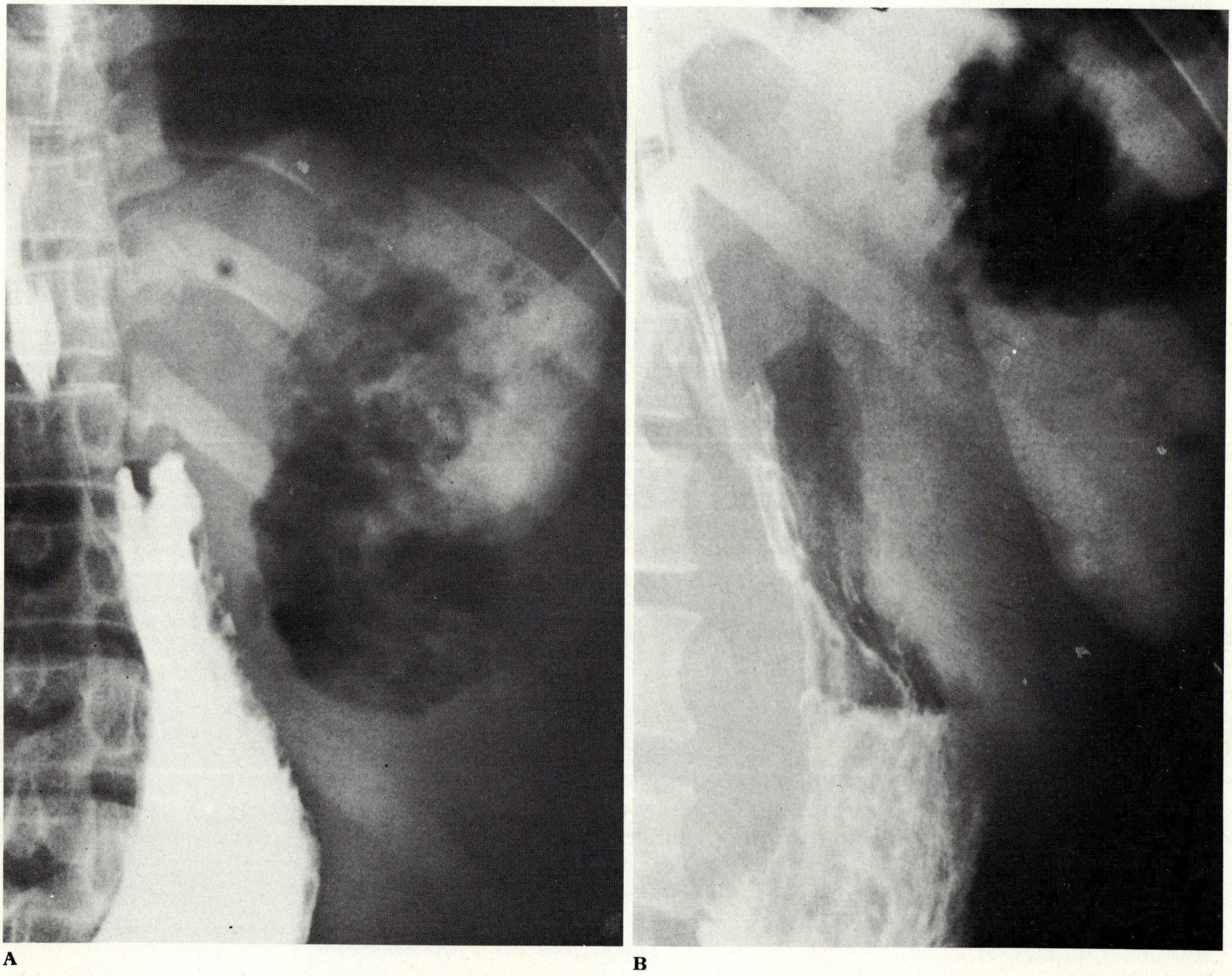

A B

Fig. 3.61 A, B. Gas-filled splenic abscess/infarct in a sickler. The spleen displaces the stomach. The abscess wall is irregular. Fluid levels develop in erect view.

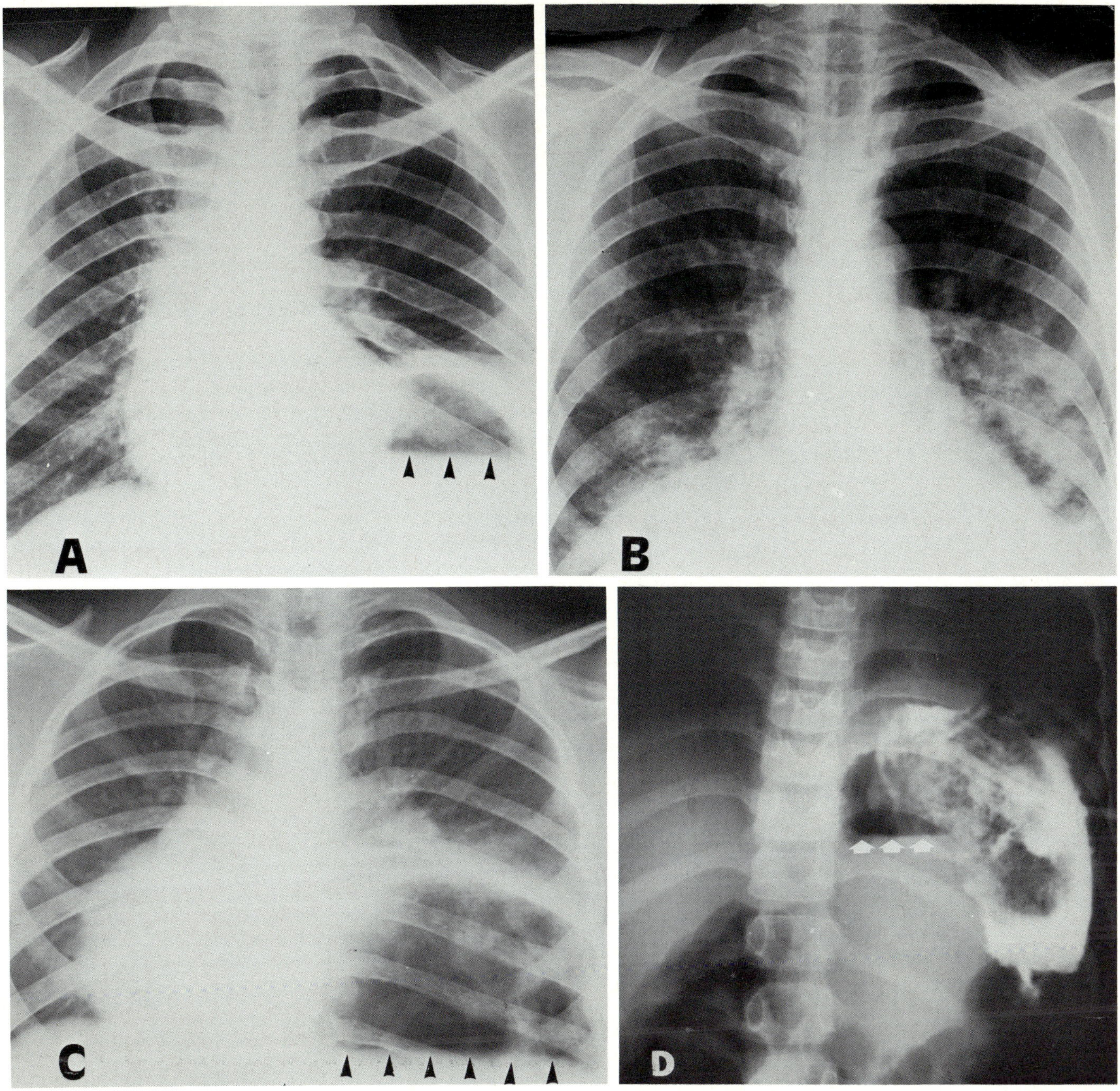

Fig. 3.62 Four sickling patients with 'splenic abscesses'. The elevated diaphragm and the thick-walled gas-filled cavities in **A** and **C** are splenic and not gastric. In **B** the abscess has ruptured through the diaphragm and aspiration of contents occurred. **D.** Another patient presented with a drain and the sinogram shows that the cavity occupies virtually all the splenic pulp and that infarcted material lies within.

cations with the development of pneumopericardium (Fig. 3.63).

It would seem likely that because of the frequency of splenomegaly due to malaria, kala-azar, brucellosis, schistosomiasis, etc., rupture of the spleen should be relatively more frequent in tropical areas compared with temperate zones. We know of no figures to support this contention. Indeed it has been asserted that the thickened capsule of the spleen in some conditions may contain subcapsular haematomas and so protect against rupture and secondary haemorrhage (Anand & Davey, 1965).

REFERENCES

Anand, S. U. & Davey, W. W. (1965) Surgery of the spleen in Nigeria, *British Journal of Surgery*, **52,** 335–344.

Cockshott, W. P. & Weaver, E. J. M. (1962) Primary tropical splenic abscess: a misnomer, *British Journal of Surgery*, **49,** 665–669.

Fishbone, G., Nunez, D., Leon, R., Paz, G., Isturiz, P. & McLoughlin, C. (1976) Massive splenic infarction in sickle cell hemoglobin C disease—angiographic findings, *American Journal of Roentgenology*, **129,** 927–928.

Forde, W. J., Ostrolenk, D. G. & Finby, N. (1960) Renal displacement associated with enlargement of the spleen, *American Journal of Roentgenology*, **84,** 889–897.

Gelfand, M. (1950) Tropical thromboangiitis of the splenic vessels and its relationship to primary splenic abscess, *Transactions of the Royal Society of Tropical Medicine and Hygiene*, **44,** 117–121.

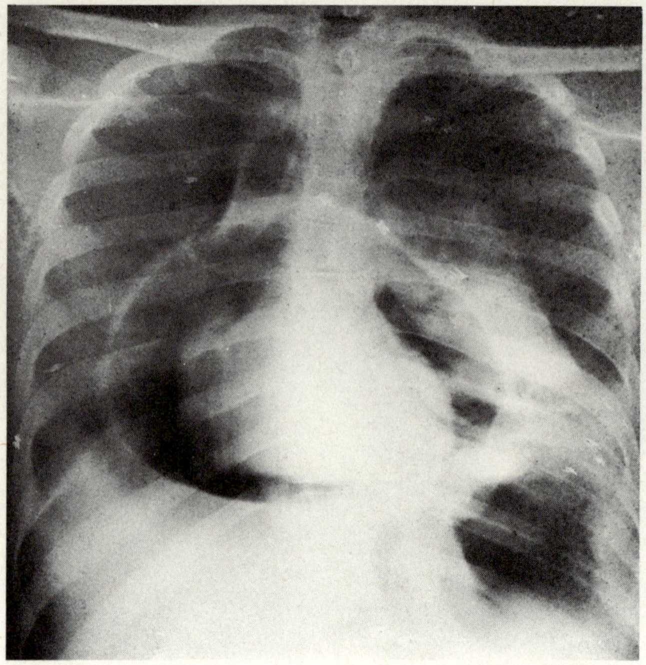

Fig. 3.63 Splenic abscess that has ruptured into pericardial sac, creating a pneumopericardium.

Lagundoye, S. B. (1971) Splenic calcification in sickle cell disease in Nigerians, *Tropical and Geographic Medicine*, **23**, 135–140.

Reinenschneider, P. A. & Whalen, J. P. (1965) The relative accuracy of estimation of enlargement of liver and spleen by radiologic and clinical methods, *American Journal of Roentgenology*, **94**, 462–468.

Whitley, J. E., Cooper, H. W., Hayes, D. M., Prichard, R. W. & Spurr, C. L. (1964) Radiodensities of the spleen associated with thalassemia-S disease, *American Journal of Roentgenology*, **91**, 900–902.

Whitley, J. E., Maynard, C. D. & Rhyne, L. (1966) A computer approach to the prediction of spleen weight from routine films, *Radiology*, **86**, 73–76.

Yeung, K. Y. & Lessing, L. S. (1976) Splenic infarction in sickle cell hemoglobin C disease, *Archives Internal Medicine*, **136**, 905–911.

TROPICAL SPLENOMEGALY SYNDROME

In malarial parts of the world splenomegaly is frequent. However, in some individuals an anomalous massive splenic enlargement develops associated with hypersplenism and high levels of IgM and malarial antibody production. The condition exists in Algeria and in Africa between the Sahara and Kalahari deserts, in Aden, New Guinea, Brazilian Indians and the subcontinent of India (Baruzzi *et al.*, 1971). In the latter area the disorder shows some differences in that the spleen is more fibrotic and portal hypertension is much more dominant (Basu, 1958). The more common form of the disease shows a large lymphoproliferative spleen (up to 2 kilograms) associated with neutropenia, anaemia and sometimes a 'leukaemoid' marrow. Prolonged anti-malarial therapy will show a good response in many cases.

The main role of radiology can be in certain instances the differentiation between this cause of portal hypertension and that due to other causes of Banti syndrome and veno-occlusive disease (Stein, 1958; Ramsay & Button, 1968). In most cases of the syndrome angiographic studies add little. Portal venography by splenic puncture documents the raised portal pressure in the splenic parenchyma (Williams *et al.*, 1966). The contrast when injected sometimes may remain stagnant and only slowly drain to show the splenic vein by diluted contrast. As a rule there is increase in the time taken to reach the liver and collateral pathways are not greatly evident. In the more fibrotic forms of the disease seen in Bengal and Hong Kong the degree of intrahepatic portal obstruction is greater but the condition may not be identical.

In the few cases where we have carried out splenic or coeliac axis angiography we have been disappointed in the degree of opacification of the splenic and portal veins, as the contrast was so diluted by the time it had traversed the massive spleen.

Thus radiology serves to exclude other causes of portal hypertension but is of limited value in management.

REFERENCES

Baruzzi, R. G., Camargo, M. E., Kameyama, I., Hoshino, S., Rabonato, C. & d'Andreth, C. (1971) Splenomegalia in Brazilian Indians from the Alto Xingu, *Annales de la Société Belge de Médecine Tropicale*, **51**, 205–214.

Basu, A. K. (1958) Chronic 'Bengal' splenomegaly and allied states of portal hypertension, *Annals of the Royal College of Surgeons*, **8**, 137–158.

Ramsay, C. G. & Britton, R. C. (1968) Intraparenchymal angiography in the diagnosis of hepatic veno-occlusive disease, *Radiology*, **90**, 716–726.

Stein, L. (1958) Portal venography with reference to veno-occlusive disease in Bantu children, *Medical Proceedings*, **4**, 31–37.

Williams, R., Parsonson, A., Somers, K. & Hamilton, P. J. S. (1966) Portal hypertension in idiopathic splenomegaly, *Lancet*, **1**, 329–333.

4. Chest

EOSINOPHILIA AND THE LUNG

There are a number of clinical forms of lung infiltrates associated with eosinophilia that occur in the tropics as well as in temperate zones. It is now evident that several clinical syndromes and aetiological agents can be defined. Certainly further developments and precision in aetiology will yet emerge but at the present time a descriptive radiological/clinical classification is convenient. We will consider 'tropical' eosinophilia, a respiratory syndrome associated with a filarial etiology; a Loeffler's type syndrome due to ascariasis; and a variety of pulmonary infiltrations associated with eosinophilia and related to diverse parasites as Toxocara canis (visceral larva migrans), Necator americanus, Capillaria aerophila and other nematodes. Furthermore, in the tropics other forms of cosmopolitan lung diseases with eosinophilia can occur such as allergic alveolitis and pulmonary infiltration with eosinophilia (P.I.E. syndrome of Reeder & Goodrich, 1952).

Patients undergoing chemotherapy for S. mansoni with trivalent antimonials consistently develop a clinico-radiological syndrome akin to that of larval ascariasis. It is believed that antigen released from the dissolution of adult worms reacts with lungs previously sensitised by schistosomes (Gelpi, 1973).

REFERENCES

Gelpi, A. P. (1973) Loeffler's syndrome and helminth infections: a reappraisal, *Abstracts, Ninth International Congress on Tropical Medicine and Malariology*, Athens, 173.

Reeder, W. M. & Goodrich, B. E. (1952) Pulmonary infiltration with eosinophilia (P.I.E. syndrome), *Annals of Internal Medicine*, **36**, 1217–1240.

PULMONARY FILARIAL DISEASE

The condition is found predominantly in children and young adults and there is an apparent increased male incidence. Racial differences in susceptibility have been recorded in some multiracial communities but no consistent pattern emerges. It is likely that such findings reflect social, economic and environmental differences between racial groups in a particular locality. Tropical eosinophilia (T.E.) has been recorded from India, Ceylon, Malaysia, Singapore, Thailand, Vietnam, Indonesia, Samoa, East, West and South Africa, Guyana, Curaçao and the Middle East.

The clinical onset is insidious with lassitude, slight fever and pyrexia and a cough worse at night. Wheezing and asthmatic symptoms follow. Lymphadenopathy is not usually present though slight splenomegaly and liver enlargement may become detectable. A massive eosinophilia is present associated with leucocytosis. A positive Dirofilaria immitis antigen reaction may be found. Response to therapy to diethylcarbamazine is usually prompt.

The cause appears to be filaria. Whether it is always a human pathogen or a vicariously acquired zoonotic strain, is not yet universally agreed. Webb and his colleagues (1960) showed microfilariae morphologically similar to Wuchereria bancrofti in the lungs, lymph nodes and livers of patients with T.E. in India. Joshi and his group (1969), also from India, found Brugia malayi microfilariae in the lung biopsies of T.E. patients. Dirofilaria have also been implicated (Wong, 1974). It is noteworthy that despite this suggestive evidence and the beneficial reaction to antifilarial carbamazine therapy, laboratory confirmation by the discovery of circulating microfilariae has proved to be extraordinarily difficult to obtain. However, circumstantial pathological, immunological and epidemiological evidence points to a filarial cause in many patients.

Despite the asthmatic clinical features the lung fields are not hyperlucent—indeed quite the contrary. A generalised loss of translucency has been emphasised by Herlinger. There may be slight hilar adenopathy with perihilar loss of definition and blurring of the vessel margins (Fig. 4.1). There is in addition a coarse interstitial pattern best seen peripherally where there is less overlapping. In some instances this may progress to the development of interstitial nodules 2 to 1 mm in size (Fig. 4.2). Small patches of consolidation can uncommonly occur.

The radiological changes following treatment by diethylcarbamazine are described by Herlinger (1963), who states that the loss of translucency resolves from the periphery towards the hilum and the process is usually complete in three days. In his experience the interstitial

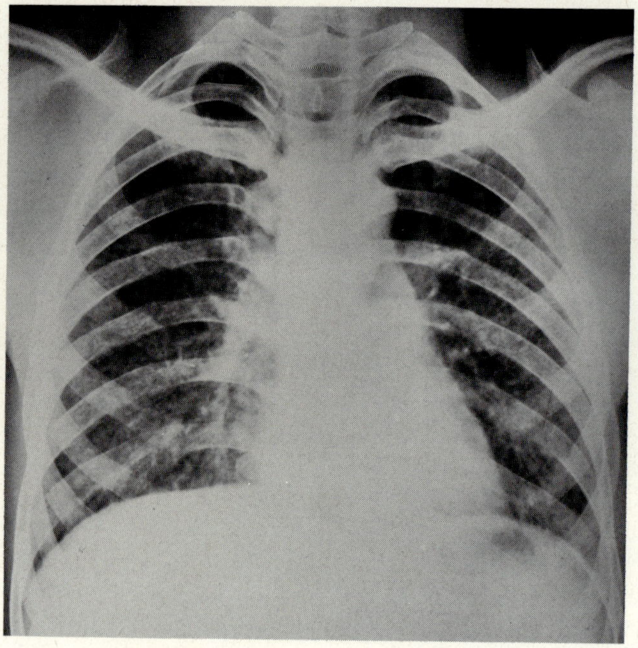

Fig. 4.1 Tropical filarial eosinophilia showing fine nodular opacities and increase in reticular pattern.

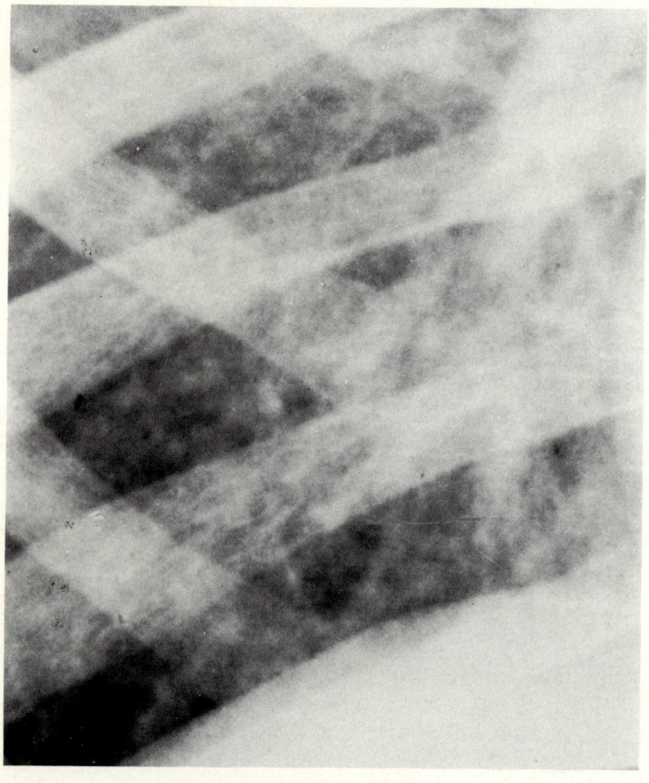

Fig. 4.2 Filarial tropical eosinophilia. Nodularity most marked at bases, loss of hilar definition.

changes disappeared within a week and the other changes took somewhat longer.

Evidence of obstructive airway disease is usually present and this feature takes longer to resolve.

Filarial lung disease associated with pulmonary hypertension has been described in Ceylon. This aspect is discussed with other pulmonary hypertension syndromes later in the next chapter. Filarial lung infarction is discussed later in this chapter.

REFERENCES

Herlinger, H. (1963) Pulmonary changes in tropical eosinophilia, *British Journal of Radiology*, **36,** 889–901.

Joshi, V. V., Udwadia, F. E. & Gadgil, R. K. (1969) Etiology of tropical eosinophilia, *American Journal of Tropical Medicine and Hygiene*, **18,** 231–240.

Webb, J. K. G., Job, C. K. & Gault, E. W. (1960) Tropical eosinophilia—demonstration of microfilariae in lung, liver and lymph nodes, *Lancet*, **1,** 835–842.

Wong, M. M. (1974) Experimental occult dirofilariasis in dogs with reference to immunological responses and its relationship to tropical eosinophilia in man, *Southeast Asian Journal of Tropical Medicine and Public Health*, **5,** 480–486.

LARVAL ASCARIASIS

The existence of a transient lung disorder in association with the migratory passage of ascarid larvae has been recognised for many years. Radiologically there may be fleeting changing infiltrates. Clinically the condition is characterised by minor or severe symptoms—the outcome being presumably determined by the size of the larval migratory load and the individual's immune state. A well-documented description of this disorder is provided by Phills and colleagues (1972). A high dose of embryonated larvae of Ascaris suum of the pig was maliciously given to four students. A lower respiratory tract illness developed with severe respiratory failure in some. Obstructive airway disease was present and associated with extensive alveolar non-segmental cloudy infiltrates that rapidly altered in appearance (Fig. 4.3). During this stage IgM and IgE globulins were raised. Gradually a severe eosinophilic leucocytosis formed.

The ascaris life cycle explains some of the pathological changes. Embryonated eggs are ingested and in the duodenum juvenile forms penetrate the bowel wall to enter mesenteric vessels or lymphatics and thence eventually reach the lung. There they undergo further developmental moults in the alveoli to migrate up the air passages over the epiglottis and back down the oesophagus till they finally reach the small bowel. It is thought that IgM is responsible for deposition of immune complexes around the larvae in the lungs, causing infiltrates, and that the level of IgE determines the asthmatic symptoms (Phills *et al.*, 1972).

The cases referred to were observed under virtual laboratory conditions and are not necessarily representative of the process that takes place in areas of high chronic infestation (Fig. 4.4). Spillmann (1975) in a rural survey searched for examples of this Loeffler's type of syndrome in a community of high ascariasis prevalence in Colombia,

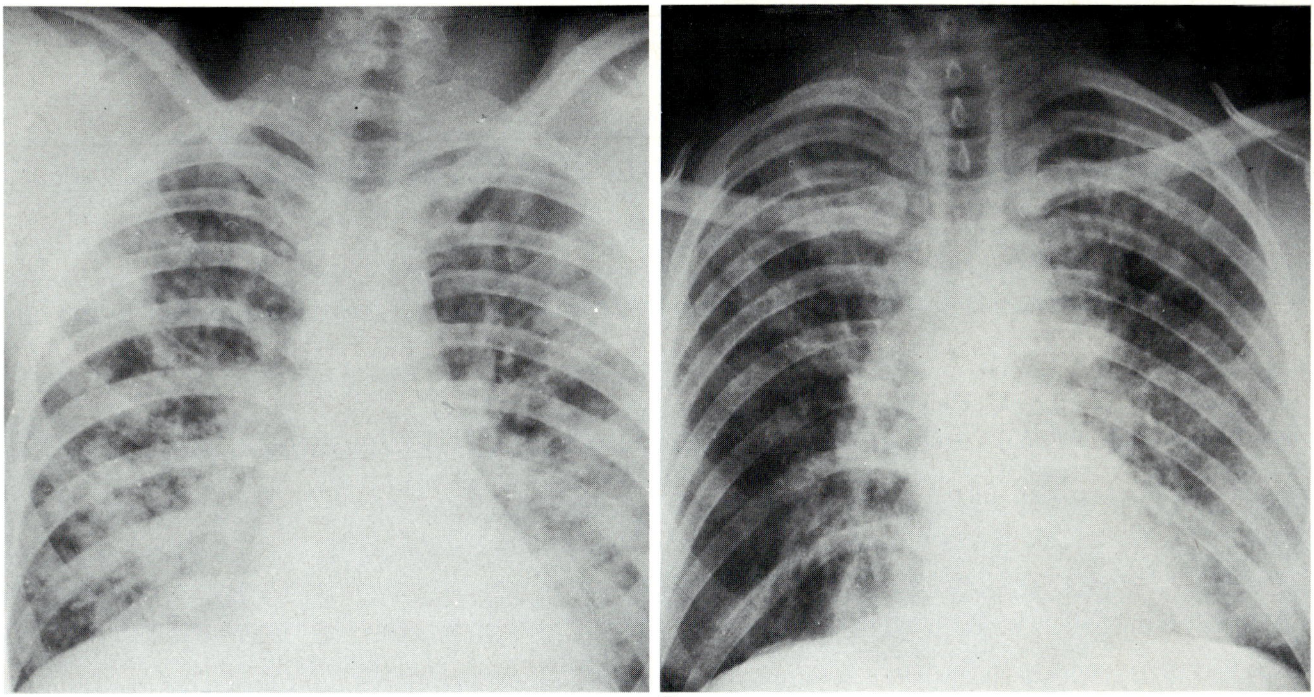

A B

Fig. 4.3 A, B. Ascaris suis—pulmonary infiltrates in students who had been malicously given ova of pork ascaris–see text. (Courtesy of Dr. G. Whiteman, Montreal, and *New England Journal of Medicine.*)

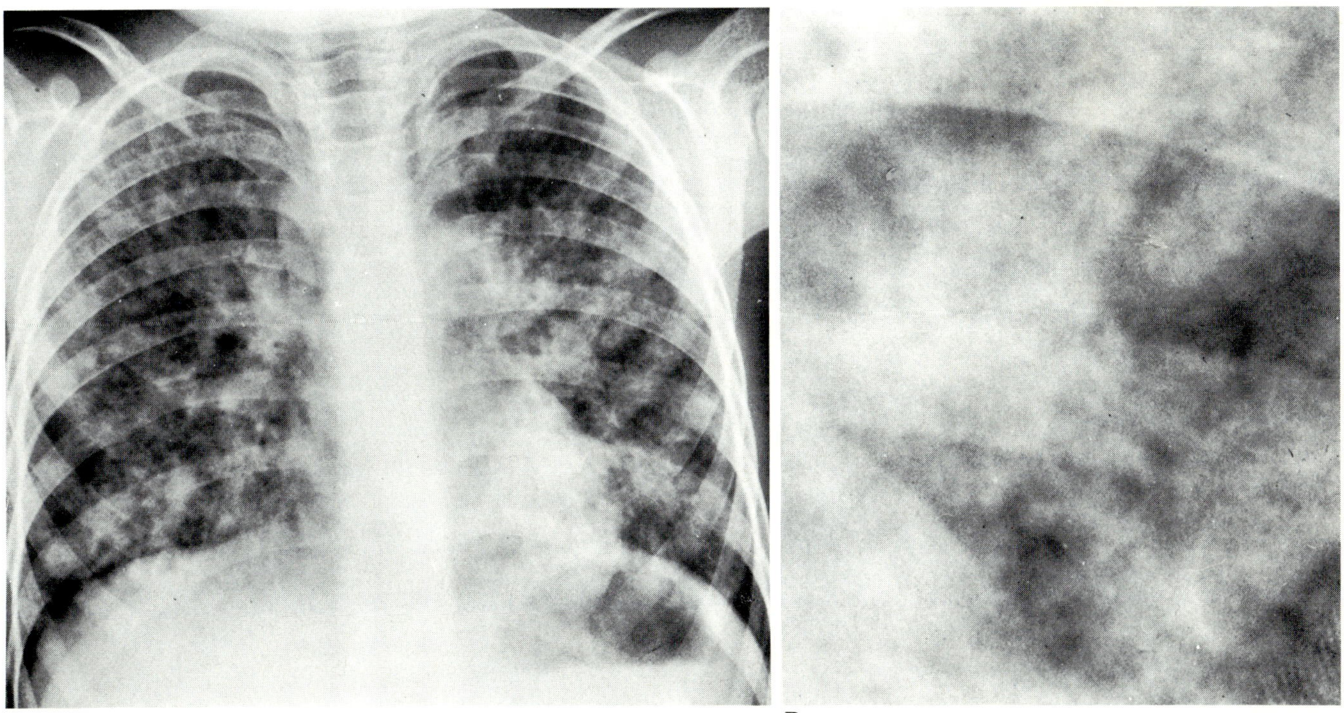

A B

Fig. 4.4 A, B. Extensive pulmonary infiltrates due to immature pulmonary ascaris forms in a Tamil child. Note alveolar infiltrate in the enlarged view. (Courtesy of Prof. J. Singh, Kuala Lumpur.)

and could discover only four cases out of over 13 000 individuals surveyed. Intermittent exposure to infection due to climatic factors that interrupt transmission leads to seasonal clinical pulmonary infiltrates with eosinophilia due to ascariasis in Saudi Arabia (Gelpin & Mustafa, 1969). The study of Vogel and Minning (1942), on larval pulmonary ascariasis in volunteers, emphasises the importance of immune factors in the development of the clinical disease.

In areas where ascariasis is common examples of pulmonary infiltrates may be seen in children of higher income groups, as well as occasionally in expatriates, who have been protected from previously acquiring the disease. Proof of the diagnosis in the acute pulmonary stage may be difficult, as ova may not yet be in the stools. Larvae are sometimes seen in the sputum or gastric washings.

A helpful feature is the dramatic change in the position of confluent infiltrates in radiographs obtained at intervals of a day or two, especially following specific therapy. The air space nature of the infiltrates and the hypervolaemia contrasts with the findings in filarial tropical eosinophilia.

REFERENCES

Gelpi, A. P. & Mustafa, A. (1967) Seasonal pneumonitis with eosinophilia—a study of larval ascariasis in Saudi Arabia, *American Journal of Tropical Medicine*, **16**, 646–657.

Phills, J. A., Harrold, A. J., Whiteman, G. V. & Perelmutter, L. (1972) Pulmonary infiltrates, asthma and eosinophilia due to Ascaris suum infestation in man, *New England Journal of Medicine*, **286**, 965–970.

Spillmann, R. K. (1975) Pulmonary ascariasis in tropical communities, *American Journal of Tropical Medicine and Hygiene*, **24**, 791–800.

Vogel, M. & Minning, W. (1942) Beitrage zur Klinick der Lungen Ascariasis und zur Frage, *Beitrage zur Klinik der Tuberkulose und Spezifischen*, **98**, 620–654.

PULMONARY CAPILLARIASIS

At present there is but scant information on human parasitism due to Capillaria aerophila. This is an ubiquitous nematode of dogs and cats but human infestation is rare. The parasite inhabits the air passages of dogs and transmission is through contaminated soil. The majority of case reports have come from the Soviet Union but examples have been recorded from Morocco and Iran (Condert *et al.*, 1972; Aftandelians *et al.*, 1977).

Patients have episodes of asthma and may show a minor degree of eosinophilia. The parasites deposit eggs in mucosal tunnels in the trachea and bronchi. These are subsequently coughed up and swallowed. Diagnosis by search for the eggs in the sputum or in the stool is worth carrying out in suspected cases.

Chest radiographs show hyperventilated lungs from an obstructive airway process and a diffuse reticular nodular perihilar infiltrate. Some hilar lymphadenopathy may be present (Fig. 4.5). These features can resemble those encountered in tropical eosinophilia.

REFERENCES

Aftandelians, R., Raafat, F., Taffazoli, M. & Beaver, P. C. (1977) Pulmonary capillariasis in a child in Iran, *American Journal of Tropical Medicine and Hygiene*, **26**, 64–71.

Condert, J., Despeignes, J. & Battesti, R. (1972) A propos d'un cas de capillariose pulmonaire, *Bulletin de la Société de Pathologie Exotique*, **65**, 841–848.

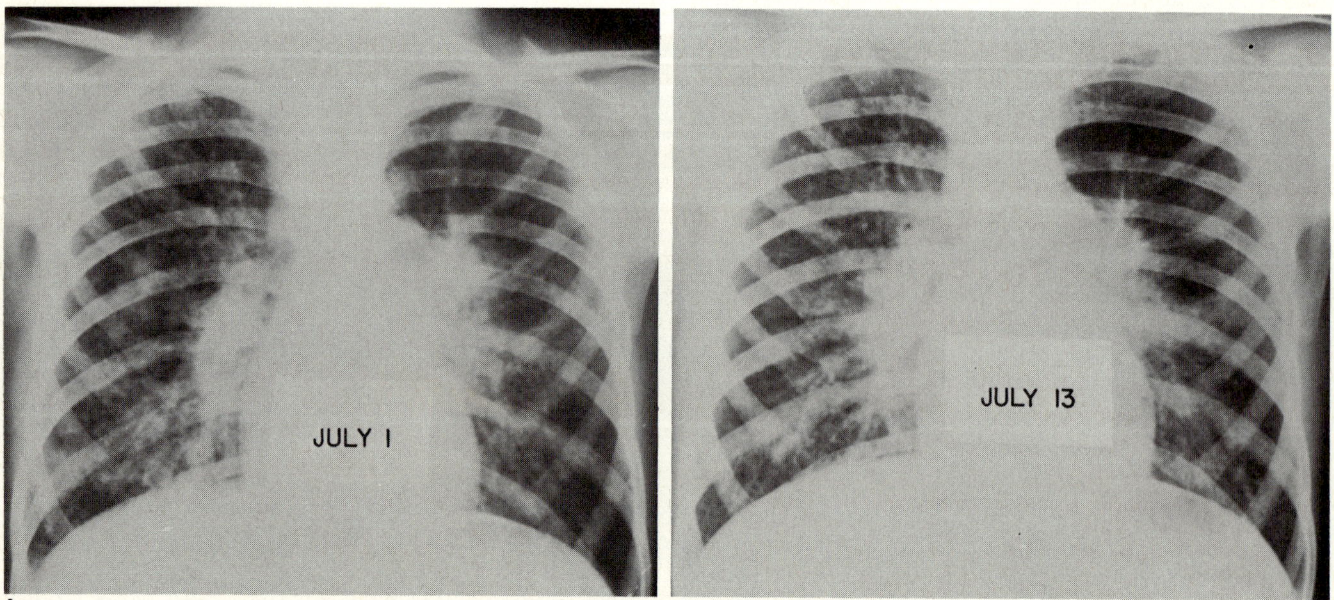

A B

Fig. 4.5 A, B. Capillaria aerophilia infection showing changes over two weeks. Extensive perihilar infiltrates and diffuse nodular air space and interstitial densities. (Courtesy of Dr. R. Aftandelians, Tehran.)

STRONGYLOIDES STERCORALIS LUNG

Strongyloides are frequent parasites of the human gastrointestinal tract. They have an obligatory passage through the respiratory tract during their parasitic life cycle but despite this, the pulmonary features are usually subclinical or insignificant, consisting of a transient dry cough and vague chest pain, as described in an experimental self-infection by Desportes (1944). At other times the parasitic pulmonary passage can lead to more severe symptoms with asthma, haemoptysis and severe eosinophilia (Jones, 1950; Nwokolo & Imohiosen, 1973).

Recently several authors have emphasised the importance of debilitating states; conditions of altered immune response as in leukaemia and lepromatous leprosy; and the exhibition of steroid drugs leading to the development of increased virulence and pathogenicity of this parasite (Rivera, 1970; Seabury *et al.*, 1971). Nwokolo and Willis 1966) have warned against the use of steroids in an endemic area without first excluding strongyloidiasis infection.

The lung can be involved in several fashions. In the normal course of development the filariform infective larvae penetrate the skin from soil that has been contaminated with rhabditiform larvae. The filariform larvae pass into blood vessels and reach the pulmonary interstitial space and enter the alveoli. This process may cause slight reaction and exudate formation but a Loeffler type syndrome can develop with transient pulmonary exudates. In the lung, partial maturation occurs with the adolescent male and female worms entering the air passages and ascending the trachea to pass down the oesophagus. The females burrow in the duodenal and jejunal mucosa and the males are expelled.

If for any reason the worms in the lungs are impeded in their passage, or there is a heavy infestation, some worms mature in the bronchiolar mucosa and lead to a chronic granulomatous process with rhabditiform larvae in the sputum. The worms may cause the formation of cavities in the lung with surrounding consolidation readily detected in radiographs (Seabury *et al.*, 1971).

In hyperinfections due to rhabditiform larvae developing into infective filariform larvae and autogenous reinfection occurring, an interstitial pattern and confluent infiltrations 2 to 6 cm in diameter may be seen in radiographs in association with slight hilar adenopathy (Petterson *et al.*, 1974).

In conclusion, strongyloidiasis under certain adverse circumstances can produce clinical, haematological and radiological features indistinguishable from Loeffler's syndrome; and at other times even cavitation.

REFERENCES

Desportes, C. (1944) Sur strongyloides stercoralis (Bavay 1876) et sur les strongyloides de primates, *Annales de Parasitologie*, **20,** 160–190.

Jones, C. A. (1950) Clinical studies in human strongyloidiasis. I. Semeiology, *Gastroenterology*, **16,** 743–756.

Nwokolo, C. & Imohiosen, E. A. E. (1973) Strongyloidiasis of respiratory tract presenting as asthma, *British Medical Journal*, **2,** 153–154.

Petterson, T., Stenstrom, R. & Kyronseppa, H. (1974) Disseminated lung opacities and cavitation associated with strongyloides stercoralis and schistosoma mansoni infection, *American Journal of Tropical Medicine and Hygiene*, **23,** 158–162.

Rivera, E., Maldonado, N., Velez-Garcia, E., Grillo, A. J. & Malaret, G. (1970) Hyperinfection syndrome with strongyloides stercoralis. *Annals of Internal Medicine*, **72,** 199–204.

Seabury, J. H., Abadie, S. & Savoy, F. (1971) Pulmonary strongyloidiasis with lung abscess, *American Journal of Tropical Medicine and Hygiene*, **20,** 209–211.

Willis, A. J. P. & Nwokolo (1966) Strongyloidiasis, *Lancet*, **1,** 1396–1400.

GNATHOSTOMIASIS

Thailand and Japan are the main sites for human infection by Gnathostoma spinigerum because of the popularity of the consumption of uncooked fish. The adult parasite is found in the stomach of dogs, cats and wild felines. Ova are passed in the faeces where they form larvae that undergo further maturation in cyclops in water. Subsequently certain fishes, frogs and snakes that ingest infected cyclops become intermediate hosts and harbour the parasite encysted in muscle. If the animal is then consumed by the definitive host the cyst-wall is digested and a complicated migration ensues, beginning and ending in the stomach.

Man becomes infected by eating raw fish or poorly cooked chickens. In man the gnathostomes migrate primarily in the subcutaneous tissues, and subcutaneous nodules form when the parasite is no longer migratory. Ectopic localisation in the abdomen and chest can give rise to tumour-like masses. The parasite may cause bronchial obstruction and consolidation with eosinophilia (Pryyananda *et al.*, 1955; Nitidandhaprabhas *et al.*, 1975a, b), and therefore can cause the pulmonary eosinophilia syndrome. Clinically the behaviour often resembles larva migrans.

REFERENCES

Nitidandhaprabhas, P., Sirikarna, A., Harsomburama, K. & Thepsithar, P. (1975a) Human urinary gnathostomiasis, *American Journal of Tropical Medicine and Hygiene*, **24,** 49–51.

Nitidandhaprabhas, P., Hanchansin, S. & Vongsloesvidhaya, Y. (1975b) A case of expectoration of Gnasthostoma spinigerum in Thailand, *American Journal of Tropical Medicine and Hygiene*, **24,** 547–548.

Pryyananda, B., Pradatsundarasar, A. & Viranuvatti, V. (1955) Pulmonary gnathostomiasis—a case report, *Annals of Tropical Medicine and Parasitology*, **49,** 121–122.

'MEASLES' PNEUMONIA

Measles is one of the most important causes of childhood mortality in much of the tropics. In Africa over half of all children will have developed measles by the age of one and a half (Morley *et al.*, 1967). The severity of the disease is influenced by age and state of nutrition—the outcome being more favourable in older children of normal weight range (O'Donovan & Barua, 1973).

It is frequently said that the pneumonia associated with measles has no distinctive features and that a direct viral aetiology is more often responsible for respiratory symptoms than the presence of bacterial superinfection. This is certainly true for older children and those who are well nourished, but in busy hospital practice where many children are underweight, bacterial infections become significant.

The changes in chest radiographs are not specific, consisting of infiltrates that are usually poorly defined, patchy, and combine features of air space diffuse clouding and interstitial opacities (Fig. 4.6). The extent of lung involved correlates well with the clinical severity of the disease (O'Donovan & Barua, 1973).

A complication that in measles is often attributed to Gram negative organisms, though staphylococci are not unusual, is the extension of disease to the pleura and mediastinum. This is usually heralded by the development of interstial air in the lungs, pneumomediastinum and pneumothorax. Surgical emphysema of the neck and flanks, pyopneumothorax and tension pneumothorax are common outcomes (Fig. 4.7). It is increasingly recognised that poor nutrition leads to a greater likelihood of these complications (Serres *et al.*, 1970; Familusi & Bohrer, 1972; O'Donovan & Barua, 1973).

The radiological features of pneumomediastinum, pneumothorax and pyopneumothorax are those to be anticipated (Fig. 4.8). The soft tissues of the lateral chest wall will often be deficient due to the malnutrition (Lagundoye, 1974).

REFERENCES

Familusi, J. B. & Bohrer, S. P. (1972) Pneumomediastinum and pneumothorax in childhood, *Zeitschrift für Tropenmedizin und Parasitologie*, **23**, 211–220.

Lagundoye, S. B. (1974) Subcutaneous fat and muscle layer in chest x-rays of children with kwashiorkor, *Environmental Child Health*, **1**, 287–290.

Morley, D. C., Martin, W. H. & Allen, I. (1967) Measles in East and Central Africa, *East African Medical Journal*, **44**, 497–508.

O'Donovan, C. & Barua, K. N. (1973) Measles pneumonia, *American Journal of Tropical Medicine and Hygiene*, **22**, 73–77.

Serres, J. J., Pene, P., Bourgeade, A. & Lesquerre, C. (1970) Etude radiologique du pneumomediastin spontané chez l'enfant rougeoleux en milieu tropical, *Journal de Radiologie et de Médecine Nucléaire*, **5**, 369–372.

PLAGUE

Plague, the medieval 'Black Death', due to Yersinia pestis, still occurs in outbreaks in many parts of the world. The

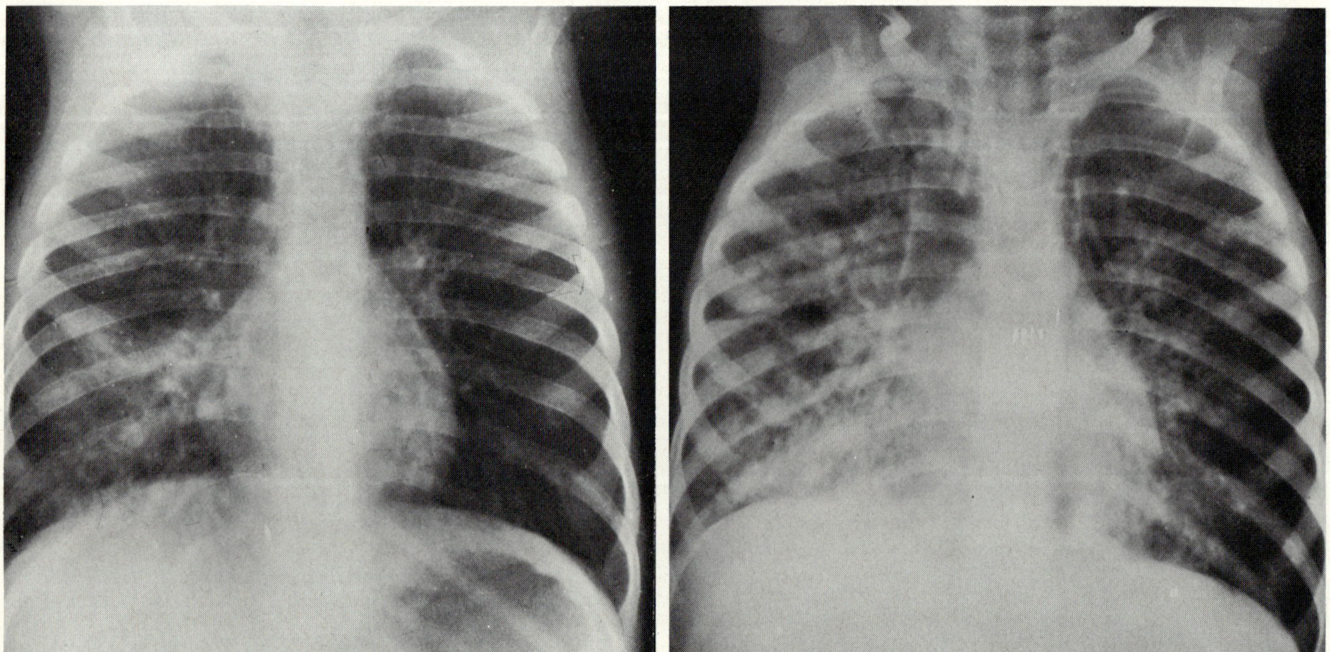

A B

Fig. 4.6 A, B. Two examples of 'measles' pneumonia to indicate the non-specificity of the infiltrates. Note the paucity of flank soft tissues indicative of malnutrition. (Courtesy of Prof. S. P. Bohrer, Ibadan.)

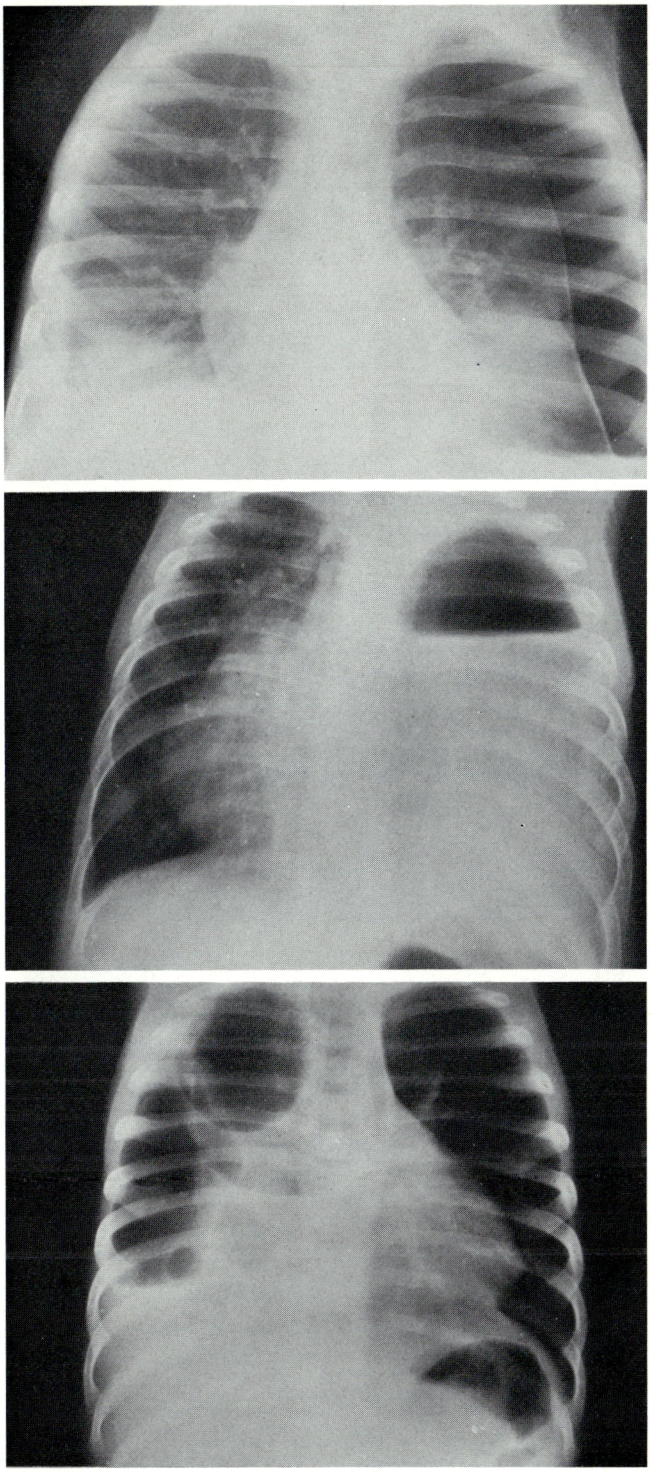

A

B

C

Fig. 4.7 **A, B, C.** Complications of 'measles' pneumonia—pneumothorax, pyopneumothorax and pyopneumothorax with loculation. Note the tissue wasting in these malnourished children. (Courtesy of Prof. S. P. Bohrer, Ibadan.)

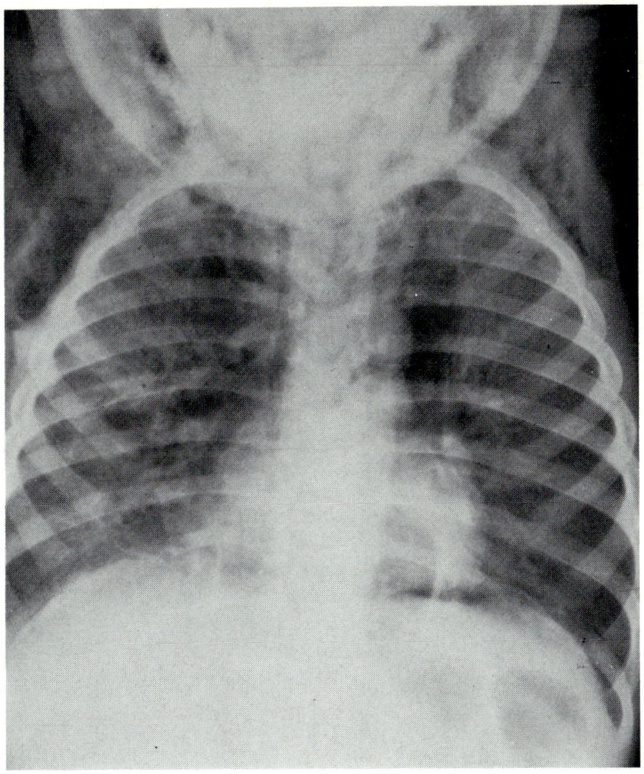

Fig. 4.8 Pneumomediastinum, surgical emphysema and small pneumothorax complicating measles.

infection is present in different varieties of rodents and transmitted by flea bites. Human infections can be from flea bites derived from wild rodents, as in hunters, or more commonly after transmission of the infection to rats and their fleas. Man-to-man transmission by droplet infection from patients where the lungs are implicated is particularly serious.

In 1975, 1478 cases of plague were reported worldwide with 99 fatalities. (There were incomplete returns from Vietnam.) In Africa cases were reported from Angola, Malagasy and Lesotho and Rhodesia (Namibia and Libya had recent outbreaks); in Asia, Vietnam and Burma Shan states had outbreaks; in the Americas there were 496 cases in Brazil, 20 in the U.S.A. and isolated cases in Peru and Bolivia (W.H.O., 1976).

Following a flea bite the organism localises to the regional lymph glands which become swollen, haemorrhagic and may suppurate, causing the buboe. Systemic infection ensues with prostration, rigors, peripheral vascular failure and endotoxin damage that leads to widespread haemorrhages. There may be involvement of the lungs with infected, haemorrhagic oedematous fluid infiltrates, giving rise to bronchopneumonic ill-defined consolidation, possibly associated with pleural effusions. This is a late, usually terminal stage not often documented radiologically. However, what is important is that such a patient, coughing and disseminating highly infective droplets, can be responsible for a primary pneumonic plague where the lungs, rather than flea bites, are the portal of entry. In such circumstances the 'buboe' forms in the hilar and mediastinal glands, which rapidly enlarge due to haemorrhagic oedematous infiltration. There is probably no other condition that leads so rapidly to hilar adenopathy (Fig. 4.9). In plague the lung fields can become the site of bronchopneumonic haemorrhagic consolidation which can rapidly become massive and confluent (Fig. 4.10). The use of specific antibiotic therapy has greatly changed the prognosis of this severe disease.

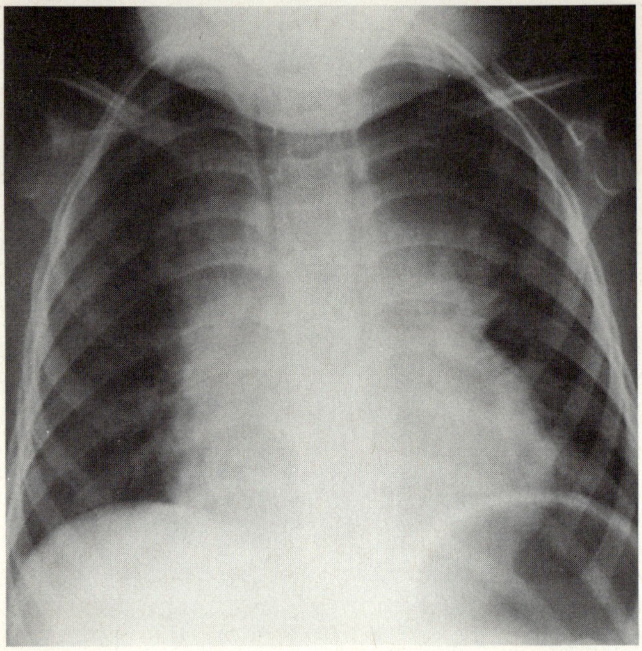

Fig. 4.9 Three-and-a-half-year-old Navajo Indian boy with proven plague and pericardial effusion and massive bilateral hilar adenopathy. (Courtesy of Prof. R. Moseley, New Mexico.)

The majority of patients are never radiographed. In theory the endotoxin effects and disseminated intravascular coagulation noted at autopsy could produce a 'shock lung' appearance in radiographs, as is documented in the illustrated case of Dr. Robert Moseley (Fig. 4.10).

In all suspected cases search for inguinal or axillary buboes should be made and, if found, they should be aspirated and examined by methylene blue staining and by culture (Butler, 1972).

REFERENCES

Butler, T. (1972) A clinical study of bubonic plague, *American Journal of Medicine*, **53,** 268–276.

World Health Organisation (1976) *Weekly Epidemiological Record*, **51,** 237–238.

LEPTOSPIROSIS

T. M. Walker

Leptospirosis is a multisystem disease caused by any of a large number of serotypes of the Leptospira spirochete. It is found in all parts of the world, although it is commoner in tropical than temperate climates. Infection may

A

B

C

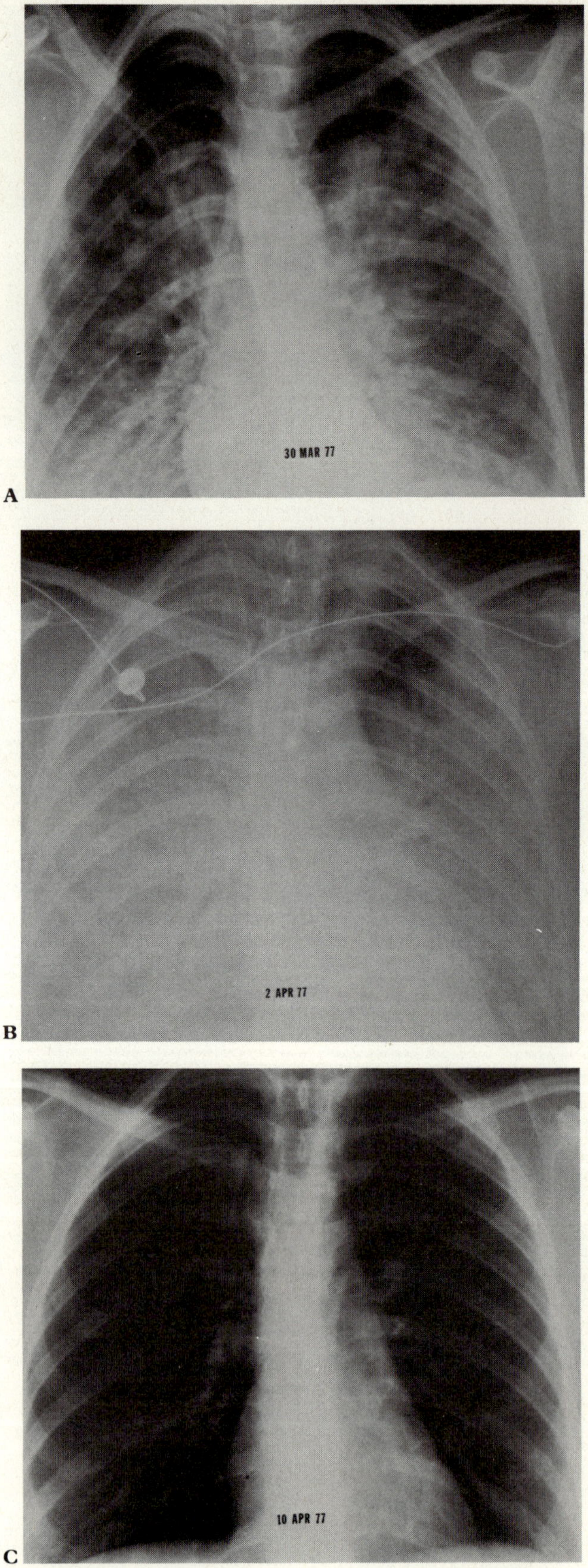

Fig. 4.10 **A.** Thirty-five-year-old Spanish-American female who developed acute chest symptoms on March 30. **B.** The disease developed rapidly with complete consolidation by April 2 and **C.** complete clearing by April 10. Proven case of plague pneumonia. (Courtesy of Prof. R. Moseley, New Mexico.)

cause a wide variety of symptoms, including hepatitis, renal failure, meningitis and a large number of less severe symptoms. Diagnosis is usually made either by serology, or by isolation of the organism from blood, urine or sputum.

Pulmonary changes detectable by radiology are found in up to a half of patients with leptospirosis. These have been associated with haemoptysis, which can be life-threatening (Burke *et al.*, 1976). Many of the lung lesions consist of basal linear collapse, with or without small areas of consolidation, and are entirely non-specific; however, they occur with sufficient frequency to suggest that they are part of the leptospiral infection. Pleural and pericardial effusions have also been described (Feigin *et al.*, 1973); Ghosh & Stevenson, 1977).

Intrapulmonary haemorrhage and oedema are responsible for more extensive lung involvement. Several different patterns may be found: small uniformly distributed discrete infiltrations; diffuse patchy infiltrations; and large areas of consolidation, often involving both lungs (Havens *et al.*, 1941; Silverstein, 1953; Wang *et al.*, 1965; Poh & Soh, 1970; Feigin *et al.*, 1973; Berman *et al.*, 1973; Burke *et al.*, 1976) (Fig. 4.11). These changes may all be different stages of the same pathological process. If treatment is successful, there is full resolution of the opacities, often within a few days.

Renal failure only occurs in a small number of patients with leptospirosis, and is not associated with any specific appearances on excretion urography. The renal size is usually normal, and there is reduced or absent excretion of contrast medium, without gross structural change. Decrease in renal size with calyceal distortion and clubbing has been reported after several months (Bain *et al.*, 1973).

Leptospirosis frequently produces generalised lymphadenopathy, and this is reflected in the appearances at lymphography. The para-aortic nodes are slightly enlarged and foamy, as may be found in other causes of diffuse inflammatory disease.

REFERENCES

Bain, B. J., Ribush, N. T., Nicoll, P., Whitsed, H. & Morgan, T. C. (1973) Renal failure and transient paraproteinaemia due to Leptospira pomona, *Archives of Internal Medicine*, **131**, 740–745.

Berman, S. J., Tsai, C., Holmes, K., Fresh, J. & Wratten, R. (1973) Sporadic anicteric leptospirosis in South Vietnam, *Annals of Internal Medicine*, **79**, 167–173.

Burke, B. J., Searle, J. F. & Mattingly, D. (1976) Leptospirosis presenting with profuse haemoptysis, *British Medical Journal*, **2**, 982.

Feigin, R. D., Lobes, L. A., Anderson, D. & Pickering, L. (1973) Human leptospirosis from immunised dogs, *Annals of Internal Medicine*, **79**, 777–785.

Ghosh, S. K. & Stevenson, J. (1977) Leptospirosis, *Practitioner*, **218**, 376–382.

Havens, W. P., Bucher, C. J. & Reimann, H. A. (1941) Leptospirosis—a public health hazard, *Journal of the American Medical Association*, **116**, 289–291.

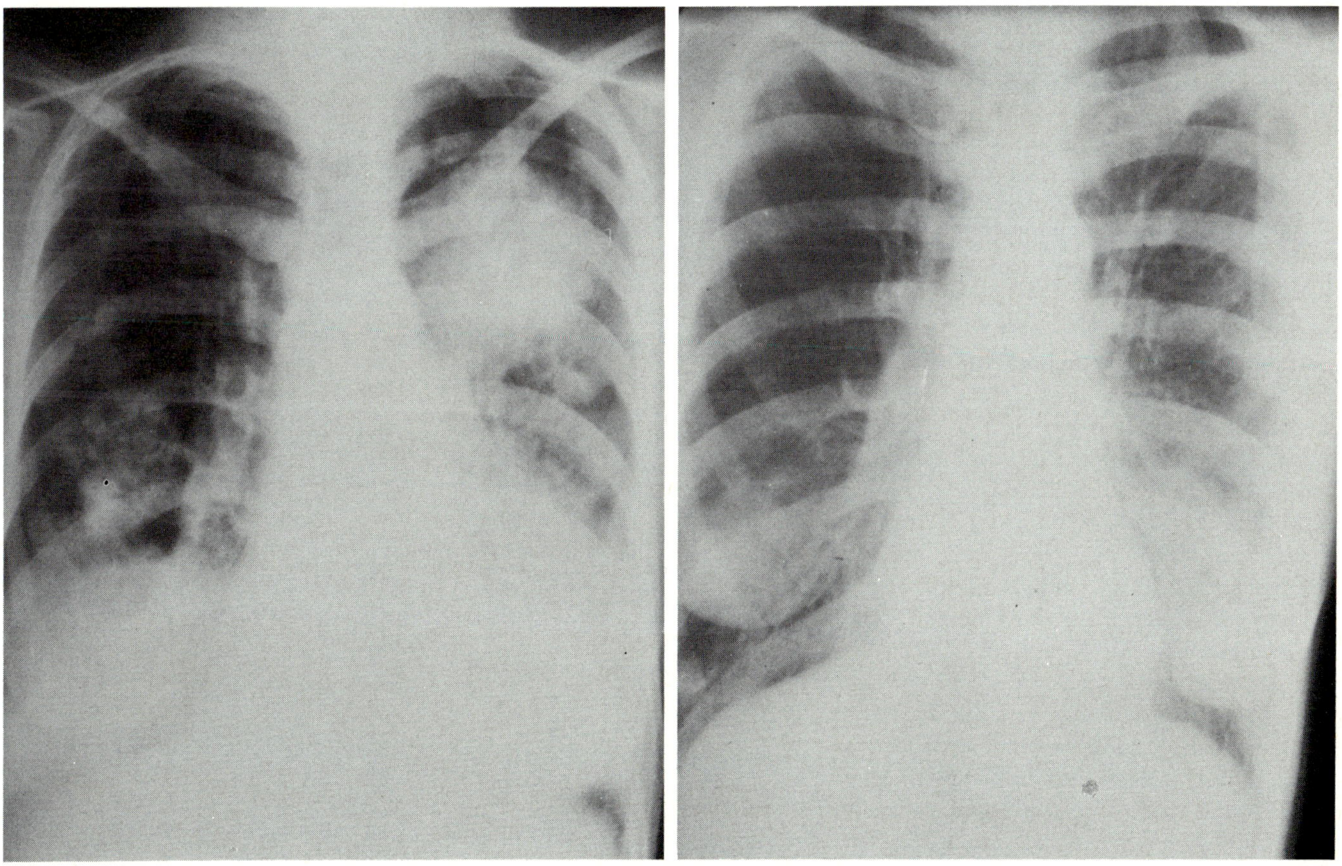

A B

Fig. 4.11 A, B. Multiple areas of pulmonary consolidation in a patient with leptospirosis. Resolution has occurred six weeks later.

Poh, S. C. & Soh, C. S. (1970) Lung manifestations in leptospirosis, *Thorax*, **25**, 751–755.
Silverstein, C. M. (1953) Pulmonary manifestations of leptospirosis, *Radiology*, **61**, 327–334.
Wang, C-P., Ch'i, C-W. & Lu, F-L. (1965) Studies on anicteric leptospirosis: III. Roentgenologic observations of pulmonary changes, *Chinese Medical Journal*, **84**, 298–306.

PULMONARY MELIOIDOSIS

James T. Lambeth

Melioidosis is a disease caused by infection with the organism Pseudomonas pseudomallei. It is apparently of uncommon occurrence, but most frequently acquired in South East Asia, extending through New Guinea to Queensland. Endemic regions, possible sources of infection, clinical manifestations and pathology are discussed in the section on Pseudomonas pseudomallei osteomyelitis.

Melioidosis has a wide clinical spectrum conveniently separated into acute, less acute, chronic and subclinical varieties (Thin *et al.*, 1970). The acute form of the disease may be fulminating and fatal. Onset of symptoms is usually sudden, although it may be preceded by a brief period of malaise. The signs and symptoms most frequently noted in acute pulmonary melioidosis are fever, productive cough, weight loss, pleuritic pain, haemoptysis and rales (Everett & Nelson, 1975). Progressive dyspnoea, pulmonary consolidation and hepatosplenomegaly associated with bacterial dissemination may lead rapidly to death in a few days. A less acute form of pulmonary involvement has been increasingly recognised with a milder symptom complex (Spotnitz *et al.*, 1967; Weber *et al.*, 1969; Everett & Nelson, 1975). In the chronic indolent form of the disease the clinical picture closely mimics chronic pulmonary tuberculosis (Sheehy *et al.*, 1967). Serologic surveys (Nigg, 1963) suggest that there is significant subclinical disease in some endemic pockets and that the true incidence of human experience with this infection may be much higher than the relatively few fulminating cases emphasised in the medical literature prior to recent French and American military adventures in South East Asia. Such studies suggest that as much as 7 to 10 per cent of populations in some endemic regions survive unrecognised or asymptomatic infections with Ps. pseudomallei. Therefore it seems likely that melioidosis, instead of being rare, is one of the more common diseases of South East Asia, if not of other endemic regions, but only occasionally causes diagnosed illness (Spotnitz *et al.*, 1967). A positive diagnosis can only be made by recovery of the organism on culture from sputum, blood or infected purulent material. In difficult cases serial indirect haemaglutination titres may be useful if available. Melioidosis should be borne in mind in the differential diagnosis of septicaemia, chest infection, or other febrile illness in any patient who is in, or who has visited, an endemic area (*Lancet*, 1975).

Radiographic features

The chest roentgenogram is useful to characterise the appearance of the lung disease and to follow the course of the illness. Acute fulminant disease is characterised by a pattern of irregular, vaguely nodular infiltrates, 5 to 10 mm in diameter, disseminated throughout both lungs. As the suppurative pneumonic disease progresses these enlarge, coalesce and cavitate (Fig. 4.12). A pattern of rapidly progressing bronchopneumonia with consolidation of single or multiple lobes may also occur acutely (James *et al.*, 1967). In the less acute form of the disease in which the patient is only mildly ill the roentgen pattern may be that of a mild bronchopneumonia or pneumonitis, frequently involving the upper lobes. With appropriate antibiotic therapy in diagnosed cases the chest radiograph may return to a normal appearance or show only some minor fibrotic residual (Spotnitz *et al.*, 1967). In chronic disease the roentgenographic pattern, as with the clinical

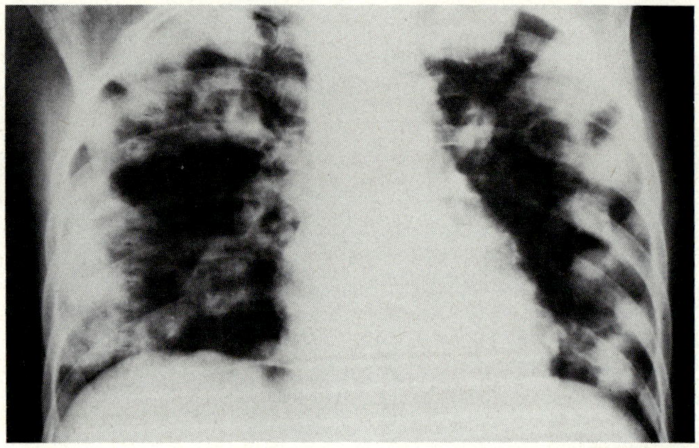

Fig. 4.12 Vietnamese female febrile and toxic three weeks post-partum. Blood culture positive for Ps. pseudomallei. Cavitating septic emboli present.

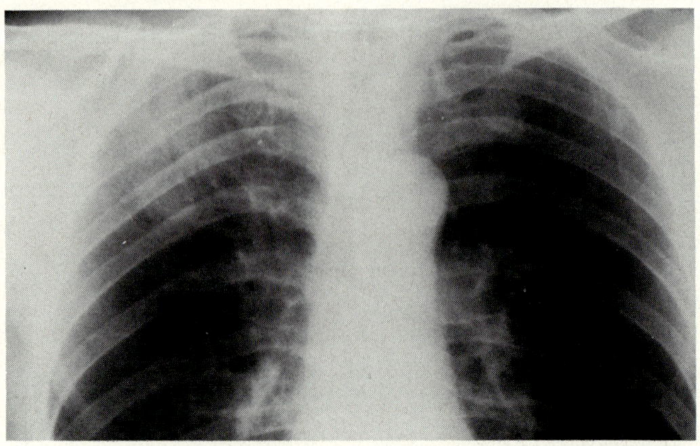

Fig. 4.13 Philippine male with chronic cough and right upper lobe infiltrate. Ps. pseudomallei obtained from culture of sputum.

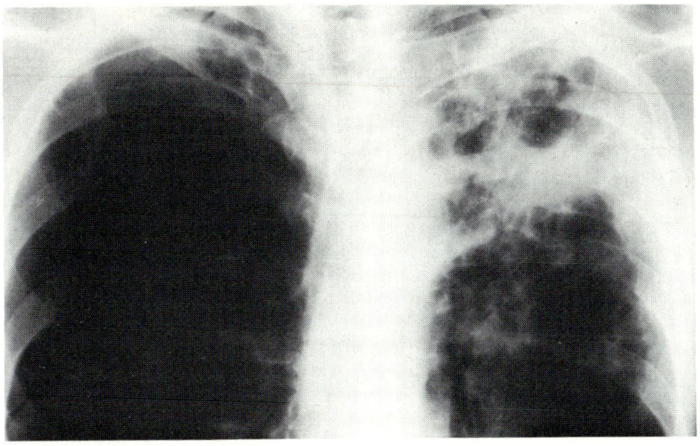

Fig. 4.14 Left upper lobe cavitary disease with negative tuberculosis cultures and skin test. Indirect haemaglutination titres for Ps. pseudomallei positive. Presumptive melioidosis.

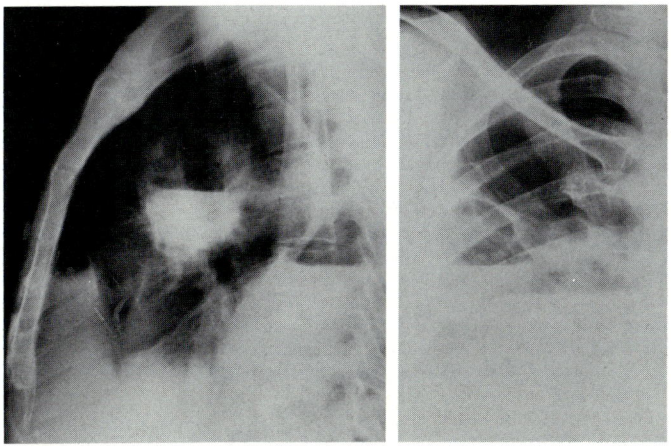

Fig. 4.15 Melioidosis—lateral and frontal views of a 46-year-old male with right upper lobe abscess, pneumothorax and loculated pyopneumothorax. (Courtesy of Dr. W. B. Young, London.)

picture, closely mimics pulmonary tuberculosis. It may appear as an unresolved pneumonia, a pulmonary infiltrate without associated hilar lymphadenopathy, a cavitary lesion or a lung abscess (Sheehy *et al.*, 1967). The upper lobes are the most frequent site of involvement (Figs. 4.13–4.15).

REFERENCES

Everett, E. D. & Nelson, R. A. (1955) Pulmonary melioidosis. Observation in thirty-nine cases, *American Review of Respiratory Diseases*, **112**, 331–340.

James, A. E., Dixon, G. D. & Johnson, H. F. (1967) Melioidosis. A correlation of the radiologic and pathologic findings, *Radiology*, **89**, 230–235.

Lancet (1975) **ii**, 962.

Nigg, C. (1963) Serological studies on subclinical melioidosis, *Journal of Immunology*, **91**, 18–28.

Sheehy, T. W., Deller, J. J. & Weber, D. R. (1967) Melioidosis, *Annals of Internal Medicine*, **67**, 897–900.

Spotnitz, M., Rudnitzky, J. & Rambaud, J. J. (1967) Melioidosis pneumonitis. Analysis of nine cases of a benign form of melioidosis, *Journal of the American Medical Association*, **202**, 950–954.

Thin, R. N., Brown, M., Stewart, J. B. & Garret, C. J. (1970) Melioidosis, a report of ten cases, *Quarterly Journal of Medicine*, N.S. **39**, 115–127.

Weber, D. R., Douglass, L. E., Brundage, W. G. & Stallkamp, T. C. (1969) Acute varieties of melioidosis occurring in U.S. soldiers in Vietnam, *American Journal of Medicine*, **46**, 234–244.

PULMONARY NOCARDIOSIS

The Nocardia are ubiquitous saprophytes in nature that invade man by a puncture wound of the skin or by inhalation. The organisms are related to the actinomycetes but are aerobic and usually semiacid fast. They resemble some fungi in having a propensity to form grains of clumped colonies and 'balls' in lung cavities. Two species are mainly responsible for clinical cases, N. asteroides and N. brasiliensis. The latter is more liable to give rise to a local spreading granuloma at the portal of entry, as discussed in the section on Mycetoma.

In many countries the disease is seen in a debilitated host with deficient immunological status due to underlying disease or iatrogenic causes. However, cases occur spontaneously from time to time and it is our impression that it is more frequent in the tropics. The disease has occurred spontaneously in chimpanzees. Diagnosis is important, as therapy is effective. Since the disease can cause either a miliary pattern or a chronic destructive suppurative lesion of the lung it can be confused with tuberculosis, klebsiella infections and actinomycosis.

The classic onset of high fever, rigors and prostration following a penetrating thorn wound is not often seen. The explosive onset is probably during haematogenous spread, and miliary lesions in the lungs can occur at this stage. The patient has more acute systemic disturbances

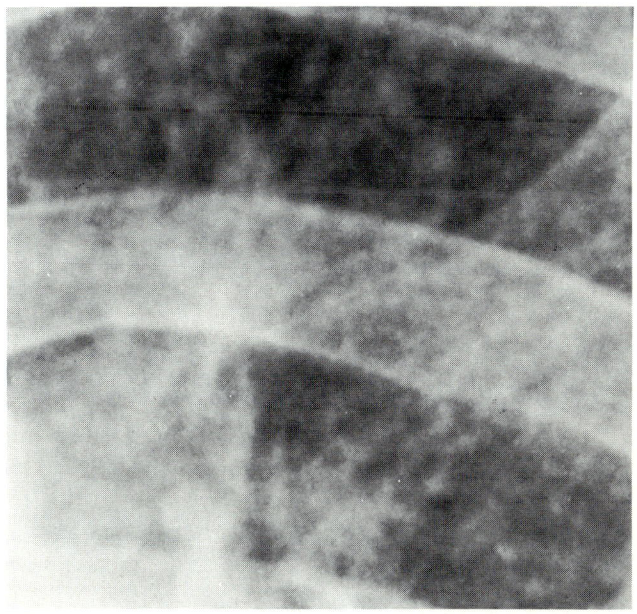

Fig. 4.16 Generalised systemic nocardiosis. Interstitial nodular densities of 1 to 2 mm in size.

than one expects in tuberculosis. The appearance fits the classical miliary picture (Fig. 4.16). Few such cases have been described (Hunter *et al.*, 1954).

More commonly there is a more focal lobar suppurative pneumonia that can involve any part of the lungs, though the bases are most frequently affected. The process does not resolve and cavitation ensues. Several parts of the lung can be affected but usually the infection is restricted to a lobe. The lesion may break down, leading to a cavity system that is colonised by other secondary invaders. Empyema and draining sinuses may develop late in the disease. Without therapy there is a significant mortality (Webster, 1956; Holdaway *et al.*, 1967; Grossman *et al.*, 1970). In a suspicious case request for cultural confirmation is urgent. We have seen several cases when the nature of the disease was only recognised after examination of the resected specimen.

REFERENCES

Grossman, C. B., Bragg, D. C. & Armstrong, D. (1970) Roentgen manifestations of pulmonary nocardiosis, *Radiology*, **96,** 325–330.

Holdaway, M. D., Kennedy, J., Ashcroft, T. & Kay-Butler, J. J. (1967) Pulmonary nocardiosis in a three year old child, *Thorax*, **23,** 375–381.

Hunter, R. A., Willcox, D. R. C. & Woolf, A. L. (1954) Aerobic actinomycosis with a report of a case resembling miliary tuberculosis, *Guy's Hospital Report*, **103,** 196–206.

Webster, B. H. (1956) Pulmonary nocardiosis, *American Review of Tuberculosis and Pulmonary Disease*, 73, 485–500.

PULMONARY MYCOSES

A full discussion of this complicated topic is beyond the scope of this section. As most of the mycoses, apart from the blastomycoses and African histoplasmosis, are not mainly tropical pathogens there is considerable documentation of this topic in conventional reference texts.

The main problem that mycoses pose to both clinicians and radiologists is differentiation from tuberculosis and chronic processes as melioidosis. Since dual infections can occur complex diagnostic problems can arise (Sarosi *et al.*, 1970). As both tuberculosis and the mycoses have a similar portal of entry; are influenced in their course by the development of host hypersensitivity; can involve lymph nodes, pleura and ribs; and can produce pulmonary exudation, fibrosis, cavitation and calcification; differentiation can be difficult. Purely radiological distinction is impossible, though lack of therapeutic response may sound the alert to use other diagnostic tools. Clinical or radiologic evidence of other inflammatory foci in the skin, bone or viscera may help, but ultimately laboratory resources are required for specific diagnostic categorisation.

Histoplasma duboisii is worth a comment since it behaves so differently from its cosmopolitan kin H. capsulatum. The latter usually involves the lungs, whereas the former preferentially invades the marrow and bones, the skin and the liver and only exceptionally the lung. Consequently experience with pulmonary histoplasmosis is limited. Histologically the lesions are predominantly interstitial granulomata present diffusely in the distal airways, and alveolar involvement is not marked. These features may suggest a haematogenous dissemination rather than extension of inhaled spores. The nodular disseminate densities and reticular pattern conform to the histological picture (Cockshott, 1968) (Fig. 4.17). More confluent opacities have also been observed.

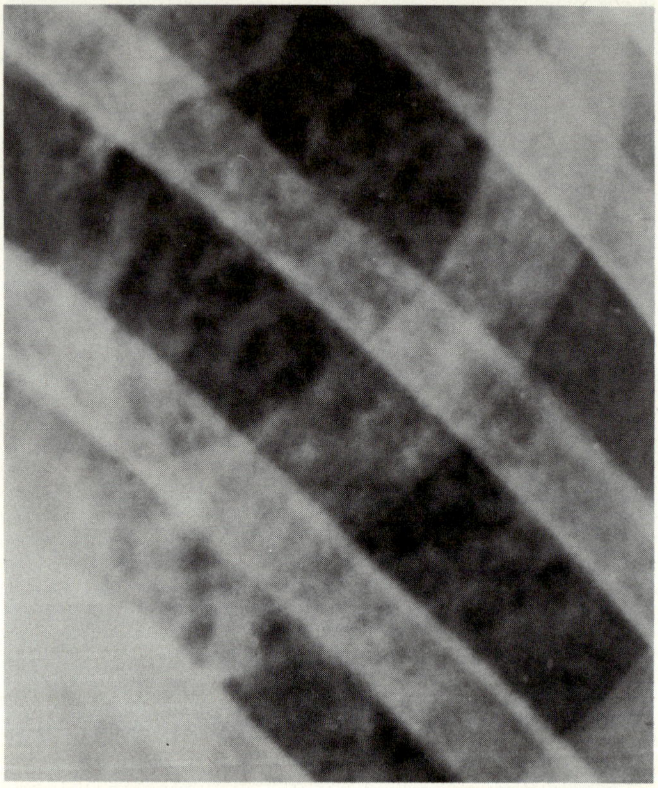

Fig. 4.17 Histoplasmosis duboisii with multiple interstitial nodular densities of a miliary type.

REFERENCES

Cockshott, W. P. (1968) *Systemic Mycoses*. pp. 118–122. London: J. & A. Churchill.

Sarosi, G. A., Parker, J. D., Doto, I. L. & Tosh, F. E. (1970) Chronic pulmonary coccidioidomycosis, *New England Journal of Medicine*, **283,** 325–329.

PULMONARY TUBERCULOSIS

Taiwo M. Kolawole

Pulmonary tuberculosis remains a major public health problem in developing areas of the world a quarter of a century after the introduction of specific chemotherapy.

Prevalence remains high in Asia in Japan, Malaysia, Singapore, Vietnam, Sarawak, Korea and India; in much of Africa, particularly Somalia, Algeria and Swaziland; in Oceania, Polynesia and Papua New Guinea; and in the urban peripheries of large Brazilian cities (Allan, 1973; Fukushima, 1974; Stradling *et al.*, 1975; Thestrup, 1975; Weg, 1976; Bulla, 1977; W.H.O., 1977). In some of these areas between 40 and 80 per cent of the children have evidence of having been infected by the age of 14. In Europe and the Americas the highest prevalence is under 20 per cent conversion by the age of 14, and generally the incidence of infection is well below that figure.

It has been estimated that there are approximately seven million cases of infectious tuberculosis in the world, with three-quarters of these in developing countries. Three and a half million new infectious cases are added each year. Tuberculosis still ranks as an important cause of death, with about half a million fatalities worldwide accounting for 10 per cent of all deaths in some areas (Weg, 1976). In parts of Asia 60 deaths per 100 000 population have been attributed to tuberculosis.

Immigrants from Asia and Africa to Europe have high notification rates: thus Indian immigrants have 27 times the rate of tuberculosis compared with Indians born in Britain, and for those from Pakistan the rate is 54 times greater (Stead *et al.*, 1968); Smythe *et al.*, 1971).

Mycobacterium tuberculosis is responsible for nearly all pulmonary mycobacterial infections. M. bovis, which is now insignificant in human disease due to pasteurisation and diary hygiene, rarely causes lung manifestations beyond adenopathy. The 'atypical', 'anonymous' or 'chromogenic' mycobacteria do cause pulmonary disease and can present diagnostic difficulties but numerically constitute a negligible problem in the tropics compared with M. tuberculosis.

B.C.G. vaccination programmes have been used in certain communities to modify the immune state of the childhood population.

Infection is acquired by inhalation of organisms from aerosols or contamination from the sputum of open cases. The response is partly dependent on the load of organisms and the state of resistance. The initial lesion is exudative and involves the alveoli. With the development of hypersensitivity after a few weeks caseation develops. This focal lesion and the associated regional adenopathy constitute the primary focus. Secondary tuberculosis results from exposure to a further exogenous source or reactivation due to altered immunological factors of a previously inactive focus that contains viable organisms. The primary infection is usually self-limiting and may be subclinical in the tropics (Onadeko & Sofowora, 1975), but it may progress with haematogenous dissemination causing miliary disease; extend to adjacent structures as the pleura and pericardium, or remote sites such as bone.

Radiological features of childhood T.B.

In radiological practice in the tropics patients often present at a late stage and are usually markedly underweight and may show signs of frank kwashiorkor (Bohrer & Sinette, 1968; Kolawole *et al.*, 1975).

A minority of children may show a primary complex or initially an area of consolidation with later adenopathy. More often adenopathy is seen without any parenchymal lesion. However, the majority of cases show both a segmental opacity and adenopathy. Glandular enlargement is not restricted to the draining area but often involves the paratracheal, para-aortic, carinal and hilar glands. Supraclavicular and cervical adenopathy and even axillary node enlargement may also be detectable clinically. Naturally the adenopathy may compress the airway, widen the carinal angle and lead to obstructive symptoms with collapse or focal obstructive emphysema (Fig. 4.18).

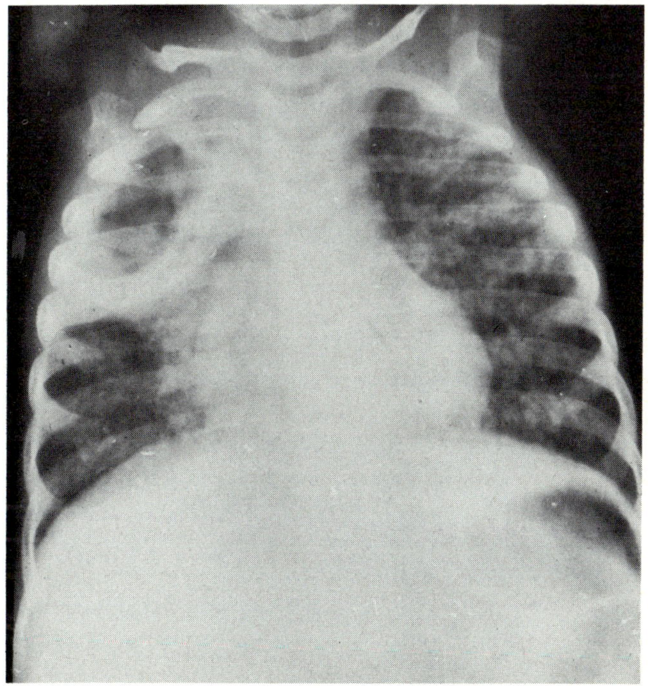

Fig. 4.18 Child with primary tuberculosis. Adenopathy present, obstructive right upper lobe lesion, middle lobe infiltrate and bronchopneumonic air space lesions of left lung.

The classical European right middle lobe syndrome is not often encountered, but compression of the left stem or left upper lobe bronchus is well recognised in Africa, New Guinea and in Asia. It is believed that the enlarged carinal glands and para-aortic glands mechanically compress the bronchus. This can progress to destruction of left upper lobe or left lung from mechanical obstructive factors rather than due to tuberculosis *per se*. This produces a severe type of bronchiectatic excavating destruction of the left lung that may require pneumonectomy (Fig. 4.19) (Palmer & Rothman, 1963; Grillo, 1970). A few cases of primary infection progress to miliary dissemination or

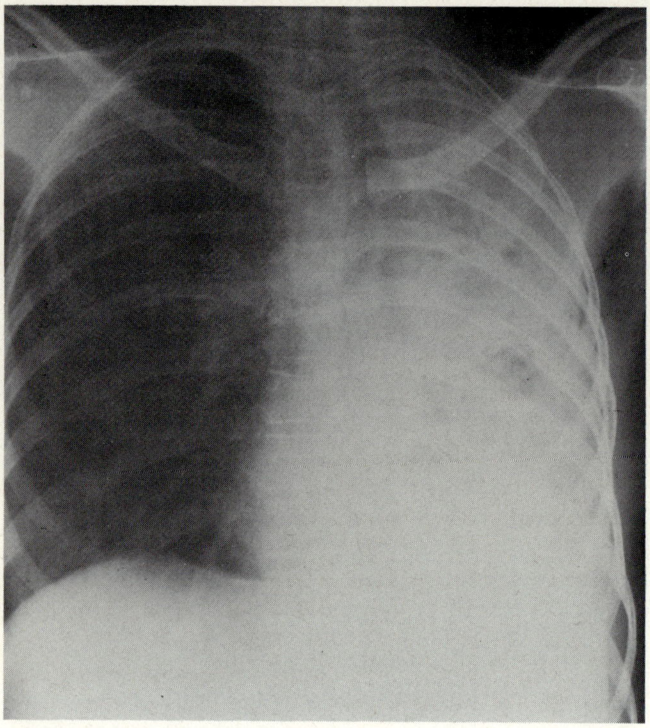

Fig. 4.19 Adult with typical left bronchus syndrome with pleural thickening, fibrosis and bronchiectasis. This is considered to be the end result of childhood primary tuberculosis.

pleural collections which generally resolve with appropriate therapy.

True miliary foci are pinhead in size, situated interstitially. In the early stages individual foci are not clearly distinguishable in radiographs and what is observed are summation densities of foci in different planes. By the time the mottling is 1 mm in size recognition presents no problem.

Adenopathy and segmental lesions resolve in between six months to a year after therapy.

Calcification of affected lymph nodes can develop as rapidly as three months, though it usually is noted between six months and a year after therapy (Bohrer & Sinette, 1968). Calcification may be noted in supraclavicular, cervical and axillary nodes. Parenchymal calcification is less frequent than that in nodes.

Thin-walled cavities of an obstructive type sometimes develop during therapy. These pneumatoceles from a focal ball valve obstruction can grow alarmingly. Such 'cysts' rarely rupture and most eventually regress.

Adult patterns

The apical and posterior segments of the upper lobes are the site of predilection with about equal incidence on each side (Kolawole *et al.*, 1975). Lower lobe bronchopulmonary segment lesions tend to occur in women, younger patients and diabetics (Doost & Vessal, 1975). In a Rhodesian survey the frequency of diametric lesions (e.g. right upper lobe and left lower lobe) in females was noted (Palmer & Rothman, 1963).

The main difference between adult tuberculosis in the tropics and the Western world is the severity of cavitation, pleural thickening and fibrosis with consequent deformation of trachea and contraction of lung segments.

The destroyed left lung syndrome has been discussed under the childhood manifestations (Fig. 4.19). In adult life it can lead to severe episodes of haemoptysis that can be exsanguinating. Dr. Jacque Kerfelec (1977), at Abidjan in the Ivory Coast, has shown by angiography that the bronchial artery vasculature is greatly hypertrophied with rich branching in the cavitating scarred bronchiectatic segments. Bronchial artery embolisation with autologous clot has been successfully used to control haemorrhage.

The differential diagnosis in adults includes chorion carcinoma secondaries which can mimic bronchopneumonic tuberculosis; histoplasmosis duboisii that may simulate miliary tuberculosis; and certain chronic destructive or suppurative processes such as blastomycosis or melioidosis that can closely resemble chronic tuberculous disease.

REFERENCES

Allan, W. G. L. (1973) Tuberculosis in Hong Kong ten years later, *Tubercle*, **54**, 234–246.

Bohrer, S. P. & Sinnette, C. H. (1968) Primary pulmonary tuberculosis in children seen at University College Hospital, Ibadan, *West African Medical Journal*, **17**, 54–60.

Bulla, A. (1977) Tuberculosis patients—how many now, *WHO Chronicle*, **31**, 279–286.

Doost, J. Y. & Vessal, K. (1975) Pulmonary tuberculosis in diabetes mellitus, *Tropical and Geographical Medicine*, **27**, 351–353.

Fukushima, K. (1974) Recent status of tuberculosis in children in Japan, *Bulletin International Union Tubercle*, **49**, Suppl. 1, 78–79.

Kerfelec, Jacques (1977) Personal communication to editors.

Kolawole, T. M., Onadeko, B. O., Sofowora, E. O. & Esan G. F. (1975) Radiological patterns of pulmonary tuberculosis in Nigeria, *Tropical and Geographical Medicine*, **27**, 339–350.

Onadeko, B. O. & Sofowora, E. O. (1975) Miliary tuberculosis of the lung in Nigerian adults, *East African Medical Journal*, **52**, 390–395.

Palmer, P. E. S. & Rothman, W. T. (1963) The incidence and pattern of chest disease in an African hospital, *Clinical Radiology*, **14**, 178–192.

Smythe, P. M., Schonland, M., Brereton-Stiles, G. G., Cooradra, N. M., Grace, H. J., Leoning, W. E. A., Hofayane, A., Parent, M. A. & Vox, G. A. (1971) Thymolymphatic deficiency and depression of cell mediated immunity in protein-calorie malnutrition, *Lancet*, **2**, 939–943.

Stead, W. W., Kerby, G. R., Schlueter, D. P. & Jodahl, C. W. (1968) The clinical spectrum of primary tuberculosis in adults: confusion with re-infection of the pathogenesis of chronic tuberculosis, *Annals of Internal Medicine*, **68**, 731–745.

Stradling, P., Newell, D. J., Pines, A., Ridehalgh, F., Somner, A. R., Springett, V. H. & Stevenson, D. K. (1975) Tuberculosis among immigrants related to length of residence in England and Wales, *British Medical Journal*, **3**, 698–699.

Weg, J. G. (1976) Diagnostic standards of tuberculosis (revised), *Journal of the American Medical Association*, **235**, **13**, 1329–1330.

World Health Statistic Report (1977) **30**, 9–10.

PARAGONIMIASIS EPIDEMIC/ENDEMIC HAEMOPTYSIS PULMONARY DISTOMIASIS

Paragonimiasis is a disorder due to trematodes of various

Paragonimus species. There are three main foci of the disease: the Far East with the chief affected areas being Korea, China, Thailand, Taiwan, the Philippines and Japan; Africa in the eastern parts of Nigeria, the Cameroons, Gambia and the Congo valley; and finally South America. The disorder is most prevalent in Asia, but the West African foci have received prominence in recent years (Kerfelec *et al.*, 1968; Ogakwu & Nwokolo, 1973; Voelker & Sachs, 1977). In the past P. westermani was considered the sole species pathogenic to man, but on the basis of morphologic differences P. africanus, P. uterobilateralis and P. tuanshanensis, P. szechuanensis, P. caliensis and P. peruvianus have emerged as pathogens in the Cameroons, eastern Nigeria, China, Colombia and Peru (Miyazaki, 1973; Voelker & Sachs, 1977).

The definitive hosts of the Paragonimus lung flukes are man and various carnivores such as cats, tigers, lions and leopards and domesticated pigs and dogs. There are two intermediate hosts: firstly snails of several genera and subsequently various crabs and crayfish.

From the adult worm in the lung the ova are released in the sputum, or if swallowed, in the patient's stools. The eggs have a characteristic morphology with an operculum and are readily identifiable microscopically. The eggs require water for continuation of the life cycle but can remain dormant for a period till circumstances are suitable. The free-swimming miracidia are released after three weeks in optimal circumstances. These invade the soft head of certain snails and develop into a sporocyst, which in turn produces two rediae generations before liberating cercariae. This snail cycle takes about three months. The free-swimming cercariae then either penetrate the crustacean hosts' articulations or the gills to form the metacercariae that are infective to man when ingested. Some crabs can also acquire cercariae by eating infected snails.

The cycle so far is complex but so is the subsequent migration and maturation in the definitive host. On eating inadequately cooked infected crustaceans or contaminated food, the encysted metacercariae are released in the small bowel, which they penetrate to enter the peritoneal cavity and then leave it to enter the abdominal wall musculature where they mature for a week. They then re-enter the peritoneum and penetrate the diaphragm to get into the pleural cavity and cross the visceral pleura to mature in the lungs within cystic lesions. In experimental animals it has been noted that a haematoma develops in the lung in the area of penetration with the fluke lying in the haemorrhagic space. Gradually a cyst-wall forms around the 'cavity' (Chung, 1971). The flukes within measure 0·8 to 1·6 cm by 0·4 to 0·8 cm.

From the foregoing it is not surprising that the migration pathway is not completed to the lung by all the metacercariae. Some get lost in the peritoneum where they can give rise to symptoms, others arrive in ectopic localisations where they form abscesses or even cause cerebral lesions. For the extrapulmonary radiological features see section on Cerebral Parasitism.

The radiological appearances have been well documented in four studies. Miller and Walker (1955) investigated 227 released Korean prisoners of war with the disease; Ogakwu and Nwokolo (1973) analysed the features in 100 Nigerian patients; Kerfelec *et al.* (1968) described 24 cases from the Cameroons; and Yokogawa *et al.* (1963) described the changes after chemotherapy in Japanese patients.

Precise diagnosis is important, since patients with cough and haemoptysis can readily enter a tuberculosis therapy programme if not recognised. Diagnosis obviously depends on identification of operculated eggs in the sputum or, less frequently, stools. Often the radiological features are reasonably suggestive and differ from those encountered in tuberculosis. However, as 14 to 21 per cent of proven cases with pulmonary symptoms have normal radiographs at some stage it is important to realise the need for sputum studies for parasitic ova, even in patients with normal chest films.

The exact appearance in a chest radiograph appears to be determined by the stage of the disease. Most of the lesions are closely related to but separate from the pleura. The fluke, after penetrating the visceral pleura, creates a haemorrhagic reaction which causes a localised opacity with indefinite borders. If the fluke is migrating these may resolve, only to develop again in an adjacent area. Should the worms remain *in situ* an elongated, sometimes multilocular cavern forms which develops thickened walls of compressed lung and reactive fibrous tissue. Usually a single fluke is in such a space (they are hermaphrodites) but two can exist together.

There is no site of predilection for involvement, though the midzones may show a greater prevalence. Multiple foci exist in two-third of patients, but generally less than three foci are seen in an individual.

Three main radiographic forms can be recognised. A poorly defined clouding with an alveolar pattern of density is noted in about a third of cases, but it is our belief that if radiographs were taken at an earlier stage this proportion would be higher. These lesions become better defined (Fig. 4.20) and linear fibrotic streaking may be evident. Eventually after establishing communication with the bronchial tree the most characteristic cystic lesion or 'cavern' can be recognised. These ring lesions are usually 1 to 2 cm in size but can vary from 0·5 to 4 cm (Miller & Walker, 1955). No fluid levels are detectable in these lesions.

Cystic lesions are often obvious on plain films but tomography delineates their ramifications (Fig. 4.21). The frequency of this finding may depend, once again, on the stage of disease. Miller and Walker noted cysts in nearly two-thirds of their patients and ring shadows were found in 82 per cent of Suwanik and Harinsuta (1959) in Thai patients. Even though the lesions are located in the sub-

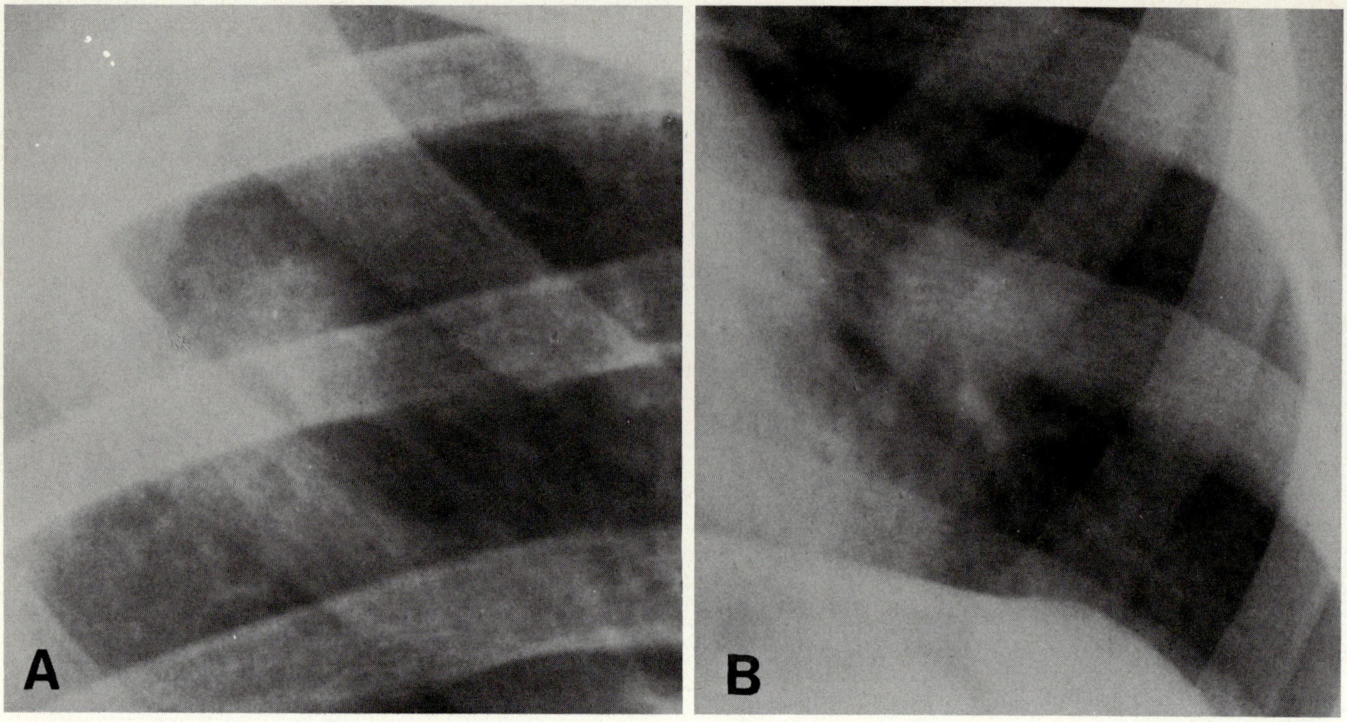

Fig. 4.20 Paragonomiasis. Early upper lobe module **A** and layer lower lobe poorly defined opacity. Both lesions resolved with menichlopholan therapy. (Courtesy of Prof. C. Nwokolo, Enugu, Nigeria.)

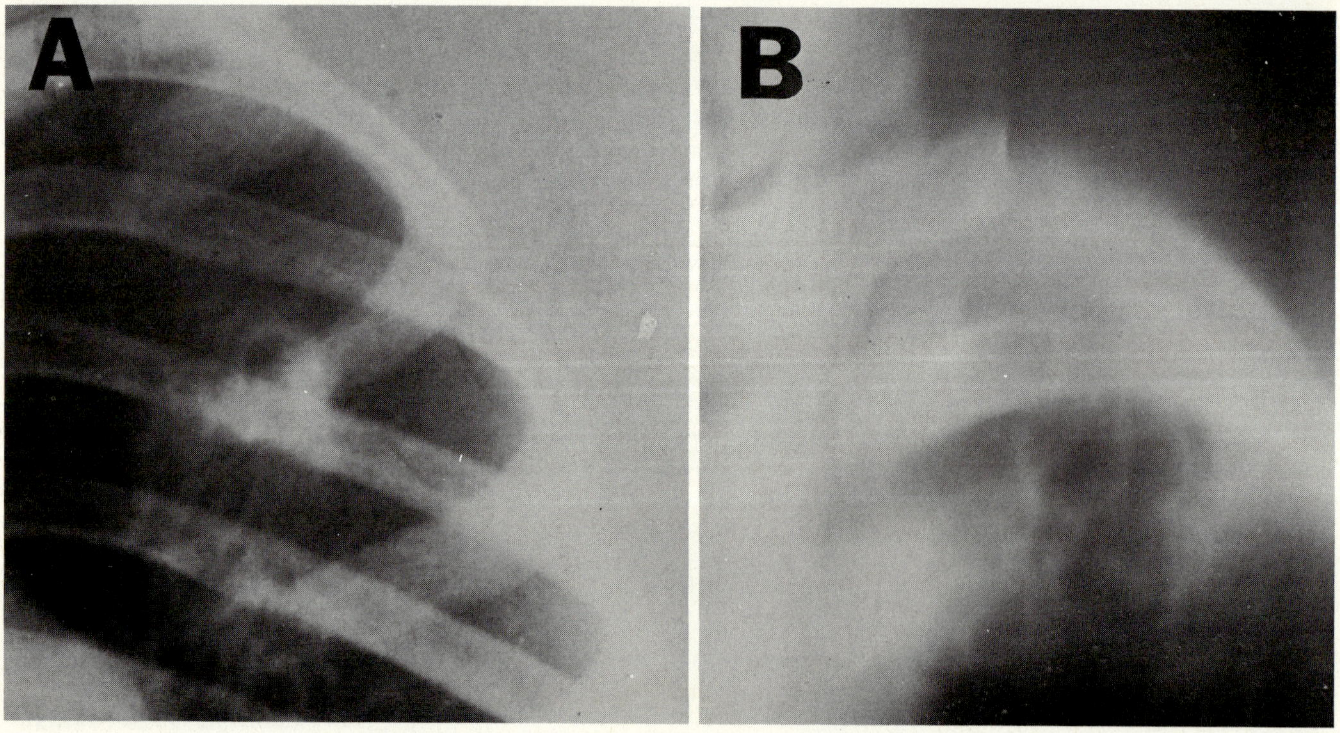

Fig. 4.21 Paragonomiasis. **A.** Parasitic cavern lesion. **B.** Multilocular apical small cavities with thin walls in patient from Cameroons. (Film A, courtesy of Prof. C. Nwokolo, Enugu, Nigeria.)

pleural areas, Chung (1971) has shown in experimental animals that the bronchial arteries supplying the area hypertrophy, thus explaining the haemoptysis.

Various workers have noted the rapid resolution of lesions after chemotherapy. The ill-defined opacities may leave no trace and other foci shrink and fibrose. Calcification is reported but the eventual incidence in treated patients is not known.

Despite the complicated migration route with a period in the pleural cavity, pleural effusions and empyemata are rare—under 3 per cent. Pleural fibrosis is, not surprisingly, much more frequent.

In this description a chronology of the x-ray features has been implied. These views are based on the animal studies of Chung (1971) and appear to fit the clinical pattern. Whether the temporal speculations are entirely correct or not, it is important to emphasise the changeability of the early lesions and the equally dramatic improvement after chemotherapy.

REFERENCES

Chung, C. H. (1971) Human Paragonimiasis, *Pathology of Protozoal and Helminthic Diseases.* Marcial-Rojas. pp. 504–535. Baltimore: Williams & Wilkins.

Kerfelec, J., Pappinuto, J. P., Garreta, L. & Ducloux, J. M. (1968) Aspects radiocliniques de la distomatose pulmonaire à propos de 24 cas observes au Cameroun occidental, *Annales de Radiologie*, **11**, 515–524.

Miller, M. F. & Walker, R. (1955) The Roentgen characteristics of pulmonary paragonimiasis, *Radiology*, **65**, 231–235.

Miyazaki, I. (1973) Recent advance in Paragonimus research with special reference to taxonomy, *Ninth International Congress on Tropical Medicine and Malaria*, Athens, 151.

Ogakwu, M. & Nwokolo, C. (1973) Radiological findings in pulmonary paragonimiasis as seen in Nigeria based on one hundred cases, *British Journal of Radiology*, **46**, 699–705.

Suwanik, R. & Harinsuta, C. (1959) Pulmonary paragonimiasis, an evaluation of roentgen findings in 38 positive sputum patients in an endemic area in Thailand, *American Journal of Roentgenology*, **81**, 236–244.

Voelker, J. & Sachs, R. (1977) Uber die Verbreitung von Lungenelgen (Paragonimus africanus and P. uterobilateralis) in West Kamerun and Ost Nigeria auf Grund von untersuchungen an Subwasserkrabben auf Befall mit Metacercarien, *Tropen Medizin und Parasitologie*, **28**, 120–133.

Yokogawa, M., Iwasaki, M., Shigeyasu, M., Hirose, H., Okura, R. & Tsuji, M. (1963) Chemotherapy of Paragonimus with Bithionol Studies on the minimum effective dose and changes in abnormal x-ray shadows in the chest after treatment, *American Journal of Tropical Medicine and Hygiene*, **12**, 859–869.

PULMONARY HYDATID DISEASE ECHINOCOCCOSIS OF LUNG

Hydatid disease in the lung is next in frequency to that occurring in the liver. Hexacanth embryos that have not been filtered out by the hepatic sinusoids pass through the right side of the heart, where most then lodge in the pulmonary vascular bed.

In different series the relative incidence of lung and liver hydatids shows considerable variation, with a preponderance of liver disease in most reports. Whether the varying frequencies are due merely to referral pattern anomalies or diagnostic accuracy, or are real and represent species variation, is not known. The disease is most often acquired by children but can be seen in all ages. It should be remembered that there is a high incidence of liver cysts in those with lung cysts (40 per cent, Little, 1976), so that routinely it should be determined whether there are any liver foci in any suspected or confirmed case of pulmonary hydatid disease.

In the lungs a hydatid cyst develops more rapidly than in the liver, presumably as lung tissue is more compressible. Rates of up to 6 cm a year occur (McPhail & Arora, 1967). Further, since expansion towards the hilum meets greater resistance due to vascular and cartilagenous structures, the cysts tend to expand peripherally so that most, if they attain a large size, grow towards the pleura and so have an edge close to or even adherent to the pleura. Spontaneous external rupture into the pleural space is a rare but most serious complication.

Many hydatids are initially symptomless and their discovery must await an incidental chest radiograph. When a cyst communicates with the bronchial tree or becomes infected definite symptoms of cough, expectoration, fever, etc. arise, and the radiographic manifestations differ from those of the uncomplicated cyst.

Lung hydatids, as in the liver, have three layers: an outer adventitial layer formed by the reactive tissues of the host and compressed lung; a laminated parasitic ectocyst; and an internal germinal layer. The cyst contains fluid, scolices and perhaps daughter cysts if it has been stimulated by a hostile environment.

In the uncomplicated cyst the borders are well defined (Fig. 4.22). The shape is usually spherical but if large, due to the effect of gravity on the fluid contents, the most dependent portion may change shape with posture. Since a horizontal beam is needed to show this sign, erect and decubitus views are required. This feature has no specific diagnostic implication beyond suggesting the presence of a fluid-containing lesion. If a single lesion is detected a search should be made to find a further lesion, as this occurs in nearly a third of cases. If serial films of a focus are available a change in diameter of up to 7 mm per month may be noted when a cyst is in a growing stage.

Cysts can occur anywhere in the lungs. The lower lobes are more involved than the upper.

The well-defined margin is lost if the pericyst becomes infected with the development of an adjacent pneumonitis. Leakage or aspiration of the contents of a cyst also leads to areas of consolidation.

If air enters around the cyst, or into the cyst, the well-known crescent sign and its variants is seen (Fig. 4.22). When air has penetrated the laminated membrane an air fluid level may form in the cyst which can become obscured if the upper cyst wall collapses and floats on the

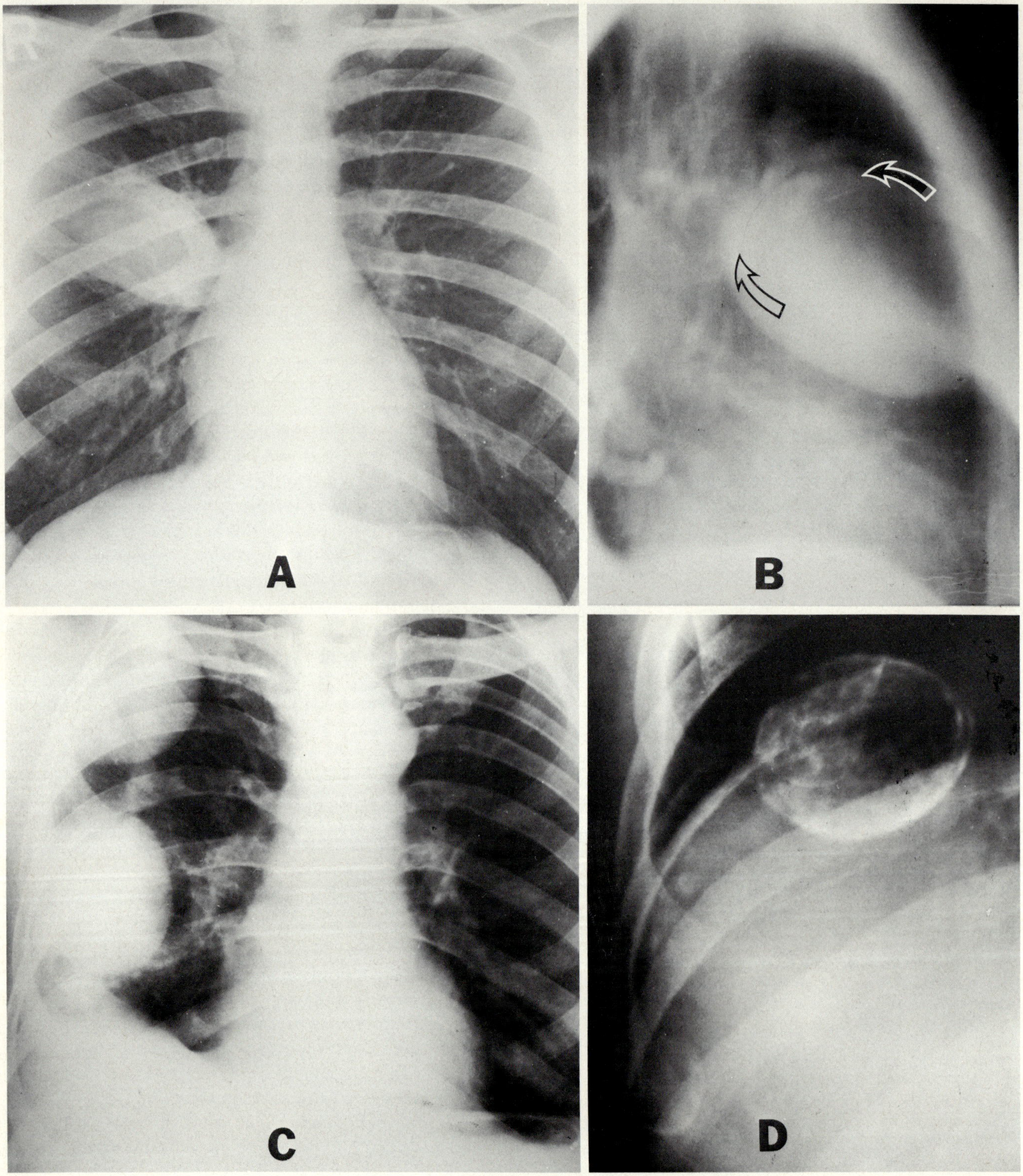

Fig. 4.22 Pulmonary hydatid disease. **A.** Right upper lobe cyst. **B.** Communicating cyst with crescent of air (arrowed) between adventitia and ectocyst. **C.** Multiple pulmonary hydatids with liver and pleural involvement. **D.** Multiple calcified hepatic hydatids. The larger focus has penetrated the diaphragm.

fluid, or if daughter cysts are present (Cuthbert, 1975).

Secondary pulmonary hydatids can form from rupture of lesions through the diaphragm by extension of hepatic or splenic foci.

A particular type of lung hydatid disease carries a severe prognosis due to pulmonary embolism and pulmonary hypertension.

This form develops from recurrent pulmonary embolism of intracardiac hydatids (Gilsanz, 1977). About 50 cases have been recorded of such embolic dissemination. In such cases conventional hydatid cysts may be present in the lungs and sometimes contour deformity of the cardiac silhouette due to cardiac hydatids. Clinically the course is one of repeated pulmonary embolism with the development of pulmonary hypertension.

The Casoni and complement fixation test are positive in about half the cases but the likelihood of a positive result, particularly of the latter test, is higher after cyst rupture (Nicks, 1967).

REFERENCES

Cuthbert, R. (1975) Sylvatic pulmonary hydatid disease—a radiologic survey, *Journal of the Canadian Association of Radiologists*, **26**, 132–138.

Gilsanz, V., Campo, C., Cue, R., Estella, J., Estrada, R. V., Perez-Oteiza, C., Rabago, G., Rebollar, J. L. & Zarco, P. I. (1977) Recurrent pulmonary embolism due to hydatid disease of the heart, *British Heart Journal*, **39**, 553–558.

Little, J. M. (1976) Hydatid disease at Royal Prince Alfred Hospital 1964–1974, *Medical Journal of Australia*, **1**, 903–908.

McPhail, J. I. & Arora, J. S. (1967) Intrathoracic hydatid disease, *Diseases of the chest*, **52**, 772–781.

Nicks, R. (1967) Thoracic hydatid cysts, *Medical Journal of Australia*, **1**, 999–1004.

PULMONARY AMOEBIC DISEASE

L. R. Whittaker

Intrathoracic manifestations of amoebiasis are not as rare as the literature might suggest. A difficulty has been to establish clear-cut pathological proof of the disease, as confirmation by identification of amoebae from lung material is difficult to achieve (Herrera-Llerandi, 1966; Wilson, 1971). This poses problems in assessing the frequency of amoebic pulmonary disease. The usual figure quoted is a 20 per cent incidence of lung foci in patients who have hepatic amoebic abscesses. Modern therapy is changing this.

A classic paper published by Oschner and DeBakey (1935) has influenced thinking on this subject for many years. They considered five routes of invasion which have, in our belief, unnecessarily complicated understanding of the pathogenesis. Their haematogenous route is theoretically possible but must indeed be rare. Similarly the presence of separate lung and liver lesions is distinctly unusual. For practical purposes we consider that almost all lesions represent direct extension of a liver focus.

Radiologically the initial lesion simulates any other subphrenic mass, with restriction of movement and possibly elevation of the right dome of the diaphragm. This can be confirmed by fluoroscopy, or if this is not available by inspiration and expiration exposures taken on the same film without the patient moving. Pleural blurring may be evident.

Classically most abscesses appear to track through the bare area of the liver and cause some pleural reaction, possibly with fluid, which serves to wall off the pleural cavity. The slow pace of progression permits this, so that initial free perforation into the pleural cavity is rare. Then the inflammatory mass most often dissects, because of anatomical relationships, along the oblique fissure (Whittaker, 1963). The lungs remain clear at this stage but a widening and bulging of the right oblique fissure becomes clearly evident (Fig. 4.23).

The subsequent course depends largely on management. Bursting into the pleural cavity with the formation of an amoebic empyema with a bronchopleural fistula can ensue (Fig. 4.24); or the loculated mass in the oblique fissure may penetrate the lung parenchyma. Then a lung abscess develops which soon establishes communication with the bronchial tree. An irregular thick-walled cavity,

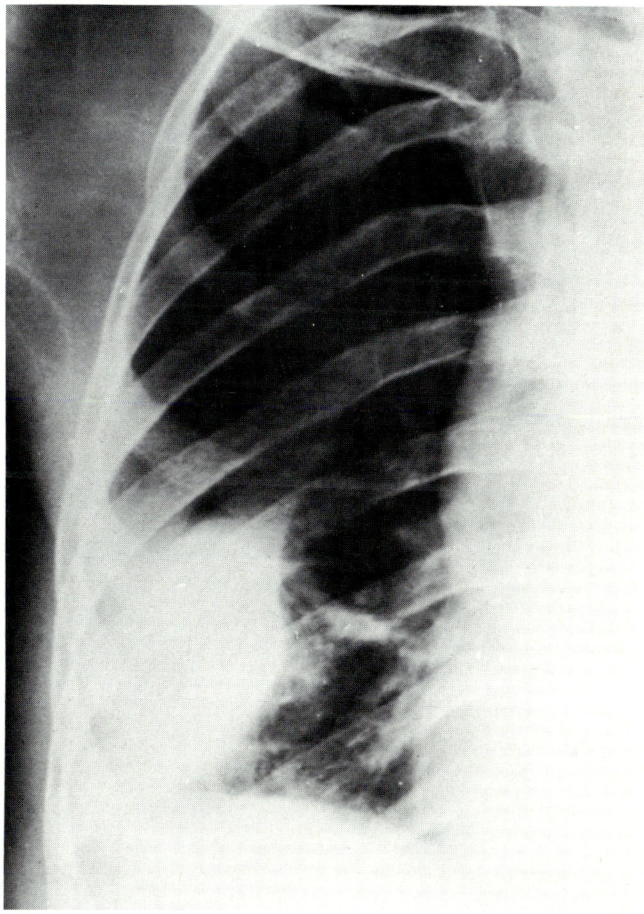

Fig. 4.23 Amoebic liver abscess tracking in the right oblique fissure. There is also some plate atelectasis.

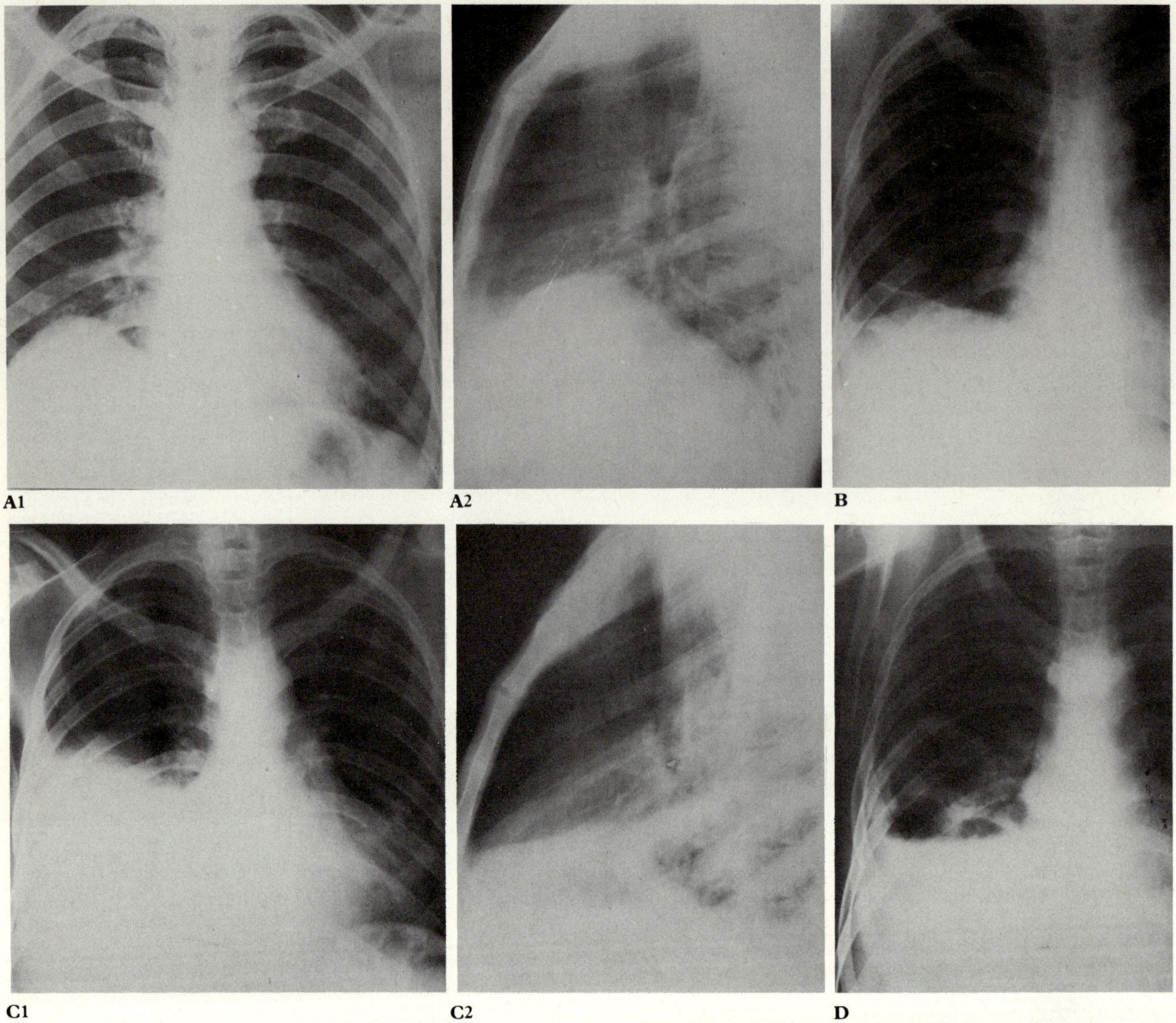

Fig. 4.24 A–D. Progression of an amoebic liver abscess extending to pleura. A bronchopleural fistula develops (see text).

possibly with a fluid level, may subsequently be seen in radiographs. In the initial stages following perforation into the lung temporary spill aspiration changes may be noted elsewhere in the lungs.

As an additional diagnostic manœuvre bronchography may occasionally be useful in delineating the precise morphology if surgery is being contemplated, but this procedure is of limited management value in the acute stage.

Most reported series strongly emphasise the right-sided nature of amoebic thoracic disease, though in some series only about three-quarters of cases involve the right side (Milroy-Paul, 1960; Herrera-Llerandi, 1966). It must not be forgotten that left lobe disease of the liver can cause amoebic pericarditis.

Since, without therapy, lung complications have serious sequelae and high mortality, early diagnosis is of great importance (Ducloux *et al.*, 1967).

REFERENCES

Ducloux, J. M., Duclous, M., Calvez, F., Astruc, R. & Fournier, H. (1966) Les pleuro-pneumopathies amibiennes, *Annales de Radiologie*, **10,** 341–360.

Herera-Llerandi, R. (1966) Thoracic repercussions of amoebiasis, *Journal of Thoracic and Cardiovascular Surgery*, **52,** 361–375.

Oschner, A. & DeBakey, M. (1935) Liver abscess. I. Amoebic abscess, *American Journal of Surgery*, **29,** 173–194.

Oschner, A. & DeBakey, M. (1936) Pleuropulmonary complications of amebiasis, *Thoracic Surgery*, **5,** 225–258.

Paul, M. (1960) New concepts on amoebic abscess of the liver, *British Journal of Surgery*, **47,** 502–514.

Whittaker, L. R. (1963) Intrathoracic complications of ruptured amoebic liver abscess, *East African Medical Journal*, **40,** 95–104.

Wilson, E. S. (1971) Pleuropulmonary amebiasis, *American Journal of Roentgenology*, **111,** 518–524.

MALARIA—'SHOCK LUNG' MALARIAL RESPIRATORY INSUFFICIENCY

The Vietnam war brought to light a rare form of acute respiratory distress syndrome associated with P. falciparum malaria in patients who usually did not come from an area of 'stable' malaria but were newcomers to a malarial zone. The condition has a high fatality rate but intensive therapy can bring about survival (Godard, 1971; Punyagupta, 1974; Marks, 1977).

The condition starts suddenly around the fourth day of the disease, is progressive and is often fatal within a day. All patients show a heavy parasitaemia and most exhibit mental and neurological evidence of cerebral malaria. The cause of the process is uncertain, but it is similar to other types of 'shock lung' with profound alterations to the microcirculation and increase in interstitial fluid in the lung and later pulmonary oedema (Brooks, 1968). This occurs in the absence of cardiovascular, renal or electrolyte disturbances that could lead to pulmonary oedema. Brain hypoxia, cerebral oedema, disseminated intravascular coagulation have all been implicated as the pathophysiological basis.

Radiologically the chest radiographs initially show perihilar increase in interstitial fluid with a reticular pattern which merges with areas of gross pulmonary oedema.

The pulmonary vasculature shows no significant plethora or redistribution, and indeed its relatively normal features contrast with the fluid accumulation in the lungs. Obviously the central interstitial fluid and oedema extending to the lung periphery is not pathognomic of 'malarial' lungs, as these features can occur in other conditions where the microcirculation of the lung is altered, such as in Gram negative septicaemia, fat embolism, etc.

REFERENCES

Brooks, M. H., Kiel, F. W., Sheehy, T. W. & Barry, K. G. (1968) Acute pulmonary edema in falciparum malaria. A clinicopathological correlation, *New England Journal of Medicine*, **279**, 732–737.

Godard, J. E. & Hansen, R. A. (1971) Interstitial pulmonary oedema in acute malaria, *Radiology*, **101**, 523–524.

Marks, S. M., Holland, S. & Gelfand, M. (1977) Malarial lung: report of a case from Africa successfully treated with intermittent positive pressure ventilation, *American Journal of Tropical Medicine and Hygiene*, **26**, 179–180.

Punyagupta, S., Srichaikul, T., Nitiyanant, P. & Petchclai, B. (1974) Acute pulmonary insufficiency in falciparum malaria: summary of 12 cases with evidence of disseminated intravascular coagulation, *American Journal of Tropical Medicine and Hygiene*, **23**, 551–559.

FILARIAL PARASITIC LUNG INFARCTION

Several parasites have been recorded as embolising via the pulmonary artery system to cause lung infarcts. Infarcts may be due to the presence of adult worms or parasitic elements such as hydatids in the circulation, which lead to obstruction by mechanical blockage and inflammatory tissue reaction around the parasite.

Such a process is often subclinical and only detected following the incidental discovery of a peripherally situated opaque 'coin lesion' in the lung (Beskin, 1966; Spear *et al.*, 1968; Yoshimura & Yokagawa, 1970). This form of clinically silent lesion can be due to Dirofilaria immitis, a parasite of some mammals, particularly the dog. Man acquires infection through the bite of a mosquito vector that has had a blood meal from an infected dog two weeks earlier. Microfilariae then mature in the right heart and from there enter the pulmonary vessels and embolise.

The radiographic appearances described are non-specific, small, 2 to 4 cm rounded peripheral opacities that do not calcify (Leonardi *et al.*, 1977). Diagnosis has invariably been made following histological examination of the surgical specimen. The adult D. immitis skin antigen intradermal test has been positive in some cases but this lacks specificity. The paucity of case reports (18 from U.S.A., mainly the Southern States) and from Japan and Australia probably does not reflect the true incidence of this process (Moorhouse *et al.*, 1971, 1976).

In experimentally infected dogs adult worms are visible as filling defects in pulmonary angiograms (Wong, 1974).

In contrast to the apparently symptomless emboli due to Dirofilaria those attributed to Wuchereria bancrofti and Brugia malayi cause symptoms of chest pain and haemoptysis. Eosinophilia is not necessarily a feature. The pulmonary opacities recorded are larger and segmental or subsegmental. Surgical exploration to exclude malignancy leads to discovery of the embolic worm, the specific species diagnosis being inferred from histological criteria (Beaver *et al.*, 1971; Beaver & Cran, 1974).

Despite the presence of adult filarial worms in the lungs these patients have not shown the radiological features of pulmonary eosinophilia that are thought to be due to microfilariae.

REFERENCES

Beaver, P. C., Fallon, M. & Smith, G. H. (1971) Pulmonary nodule caused by a living Brugia Malayi-like filaria in an artery, *American Journal of Tropical Medicine and Hygiene*, **20**, 661–666.

Beaver, P. C & Cran, I. R. (1974) Wuchereria-like filaria in an artery associated with pulmonary infarction, *American Journal of Tropical Medicine and Hygiene*, **23**, 869–876.

Beskin, C. A., Colvin, H. & Beaver, P. C. (1966) Pulmonary dirofilariasis cause of pulmonary nodular disease, *Journal of the American Medical Association*, **198**, 665–667.

Leonardi, H. K., Lapey, J. D. & Ellis, F. H. (1977) Pulmonary dirofilariasis: report of a human case, *Thorax*, **32**, 612–615.

Moorhouse, D. E., Abrahams, E. W. & Stephens, B. J. (1971) Human pulmonary dirofilariasis in Queensland, *Medical Journal of Australia*, **2**, 1230–1233.

Moorhouse, D. E., Abrahams, E. W. & Stephens, B. J. (1976) Human pulmonary dirofilariasis associated with pleural effusion, *Medical Journal of Australia, Journal of Australia*, **2**, 902–903.

Sear, H. C., Daughtry, D. C., Chesney, J. O., Gentsch, T. O. & Larsen,

P. B. (1968) Solitary pulmonary lesion due to dirofilaria, *New England Journal of Medicine*, **278,** 832–833.

Wong, M. M. (1974) Experimental occult dirofilariasis in dogs with reference to immunological responses and its relationship to tropical eosinophilia in man, *Southeast Asian Journal of Tropical Medicine and Public Health*, **5,** 480–486.

Yoshimura, M. & Yokogawa, M. (1970) Dirofilaria causing infarct in human lung, *American Journal of Tropical Medicine and Hygiene*, **19,** 63–67.

NEO-NATAL RESPIRATORY DISTRESS SYNDROME

In many tropical areas there are large numbers of low birth-weight babies that are 'small' for the gestational age. Yet paradoxically the mortality of equivalent gestation age groups is initially lower than in North America because of the low incidence of the various respiratory distress syndromes (Effiong & Dawodu, 1977). This is due to the fact that these low weight children are not premature, so that pulmonary dysmaturity is not to be expected.

REFERENCES

Effiong, C. E. & Dawodu, A. H. (1977) Neo natal morbidity and mortality in a special care baby unit in Nigeria: preliminary report and prospective study, *East African Journal of Medical Research*, **4,** 25–29.

'BLACK FAT' LIPID PNEUMONIA

For many years in Kentucky a type of tobacco has been prepared for export to Central America (Panama, Honduras); South America (Guyana); the Caribbean (Bahamas, Dominica, Virgin Islands); and West Africa. This tobacco has mineral oil and Vaseline added to keep it moist and to give flavour. The tobacco leaf is smoked and the lipid subsequently condenses in the lungs to produce a diffuse interstitial pneumonia and vasculitis (Miller *et al.*, 1971). In Guyana, where the condition has been intensively studied, one-fifth of the Indian population over the age of 55 were smokers of this product. Patients after many years of using black fat become increasingly breathless, develop a cough, lose weight, may show central cyanosis, and a few go on to develop cor pulmonale as a result of the pulmonary fibrosis (Miller *et al.*, 1971).

Radiologically the initial changes are those of a fine reticular pattern of interstitial fibrosis. Gradually this becomes more nodular (Fig. 4.25). Massive coalescent fibrosis is a late stage when diability is severe (Fig. 4.26). Fortunately the popularity of this type of smoke is now declining, so that the dimensions of this public health problem are being reduced. Also see page 191.

REFERENCE

Miller *et al.* (1971) The lipoid pneumonia of Blackfat tobacco smokers in Guyana, *Quarterly Journal of Medicine*, NS. **40,** 457–470.

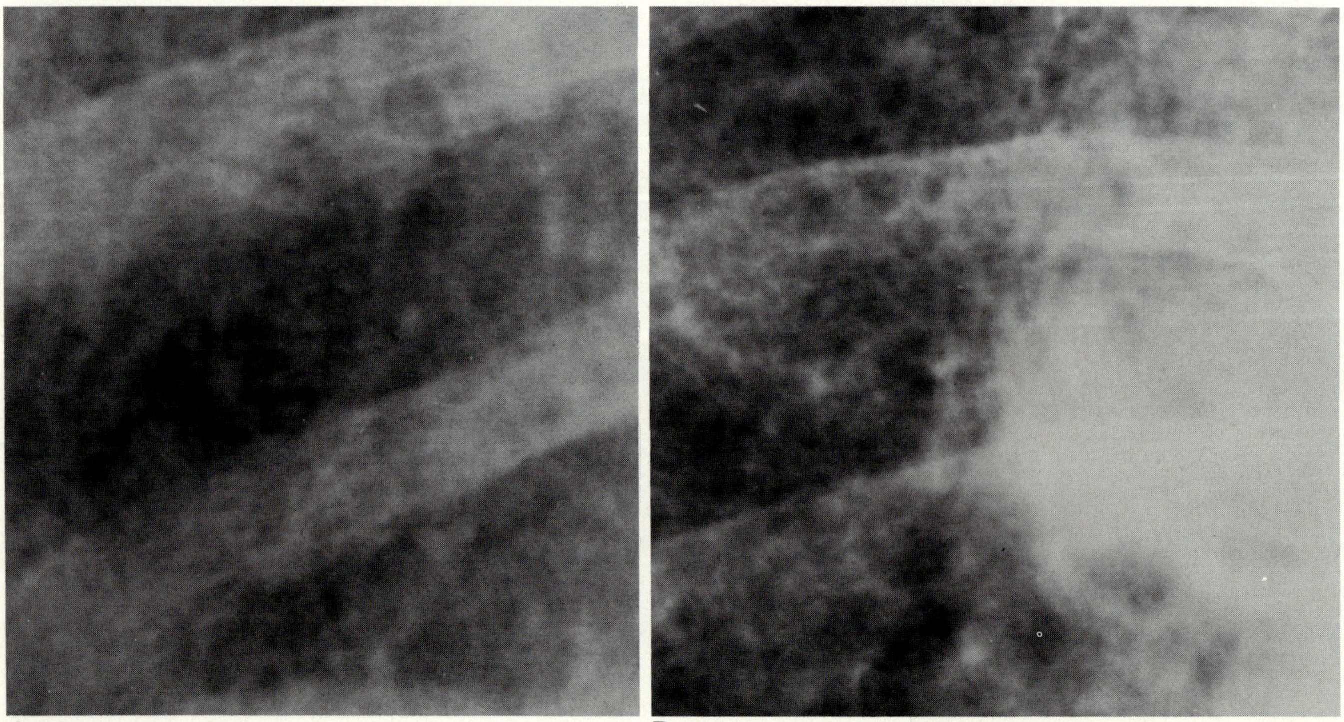

A B

Fig. 4.25 A, B. Blackfat lipoid pneumonia and interstitial fibrosis. Confluent areas are present in the more advanced case on right. (Courtesy of Dr. G. J. Miller, Trinidad.)

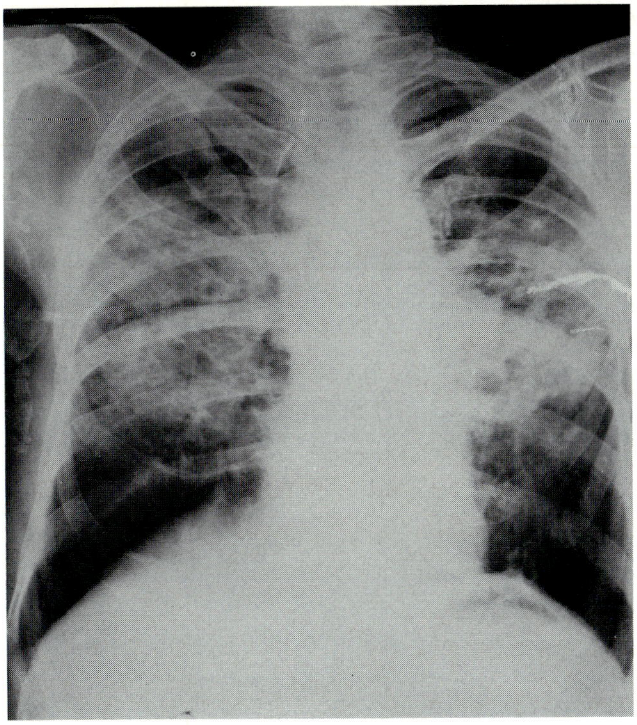

Fig. 4.26 Extensive pulmonary fibrosis in blackfat tobacco pneumonia. (Courtesy of Dr. G. J. Miller, Trinidad.)

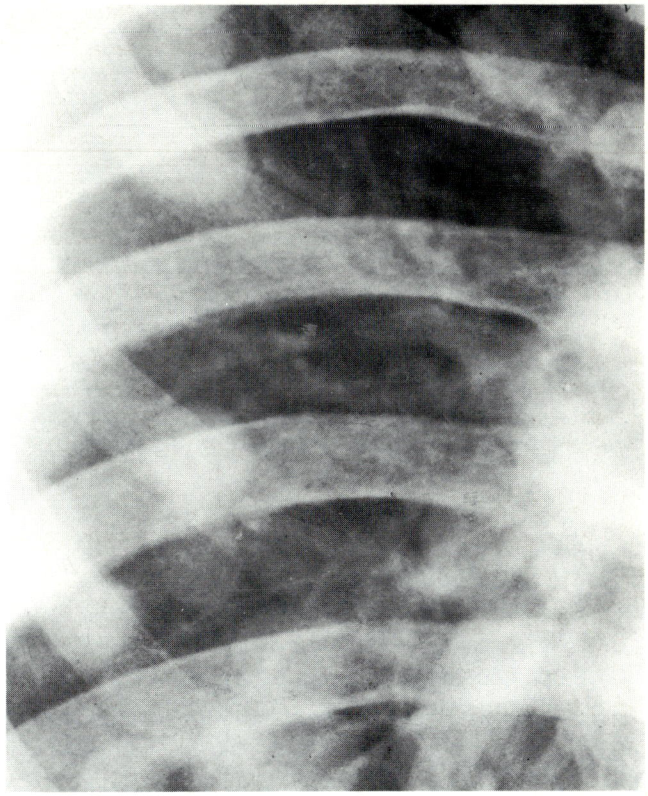

Fig. 4.27 Typical multiple rounded metastases of varying size due to chorion cancer.

MALIGNANT TROPHOBLASTIC DISEASE

Malignant trophoblastic disease (M.T.D.) is a frequent neoplasm in the Philippines, Indonesia, South East Asia and West Africa. The lungs are the most common site of metastases. Even normal pregnancy trophoblast embolises to the lungs but does not develop further. The same applies to vesicles and molar tissue from hydatidiform mole, but once again the tissue rarely proliferates. With the more invasive moles and chorion cancer pulmonary deposits grow. Thus it can be seen that trophoblastic tissue has a propensity for venous dissemination and may cause significant lung lesions which can bring the patient to medical attention, rather than the pelvic lesion producing the presenting symptom.

There are several forms of pulmonary metastases. In one series 68 per cent of patients with M.T.D. had lung deposits (Evans *et al.*, 1965). Deposits classically are multiple well-defined rounded opacities of varying size (Fig. 4.27). Such a variety does not pose a significant diagnostic problem though one feature may be perplexing. Some metastases may slowly regress and involute even without therapy, whilst others are enlarging. This type of concentric reduction in size contrasts with large foci that may cavitate following the establishment of a communication with the bronchial tree (Fig. 4.28). Regression of lung

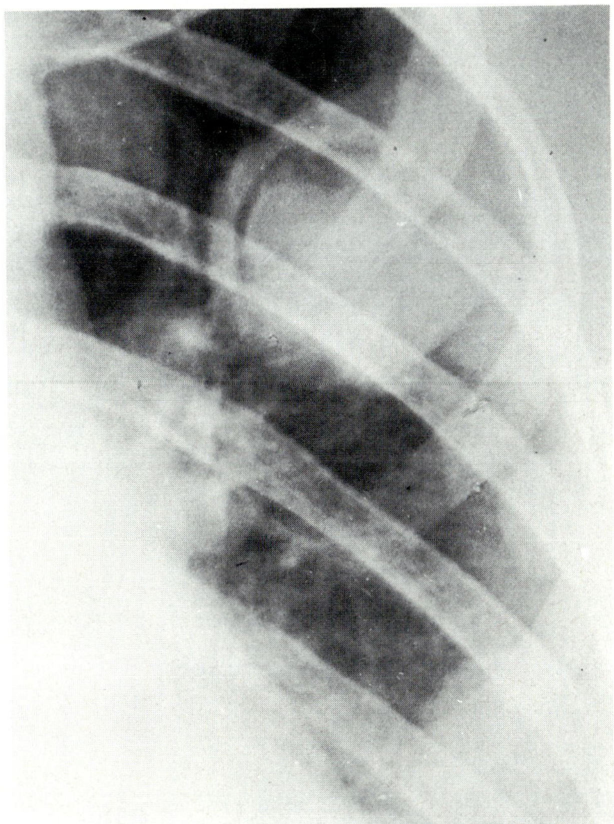

Fig. 4.28 Large cavitating necrotic secondary deposit of malignant trophoblastic disease that has established bronchial communication.

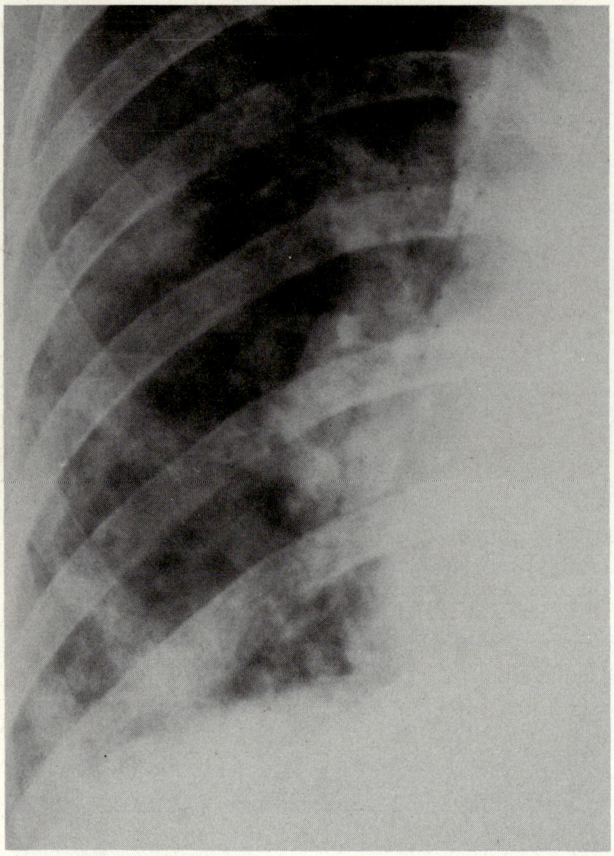

Fig. 4.29 Diffuse ill-defined metastases of malignant trophoblastic disease simulating an air space inflammatory process.

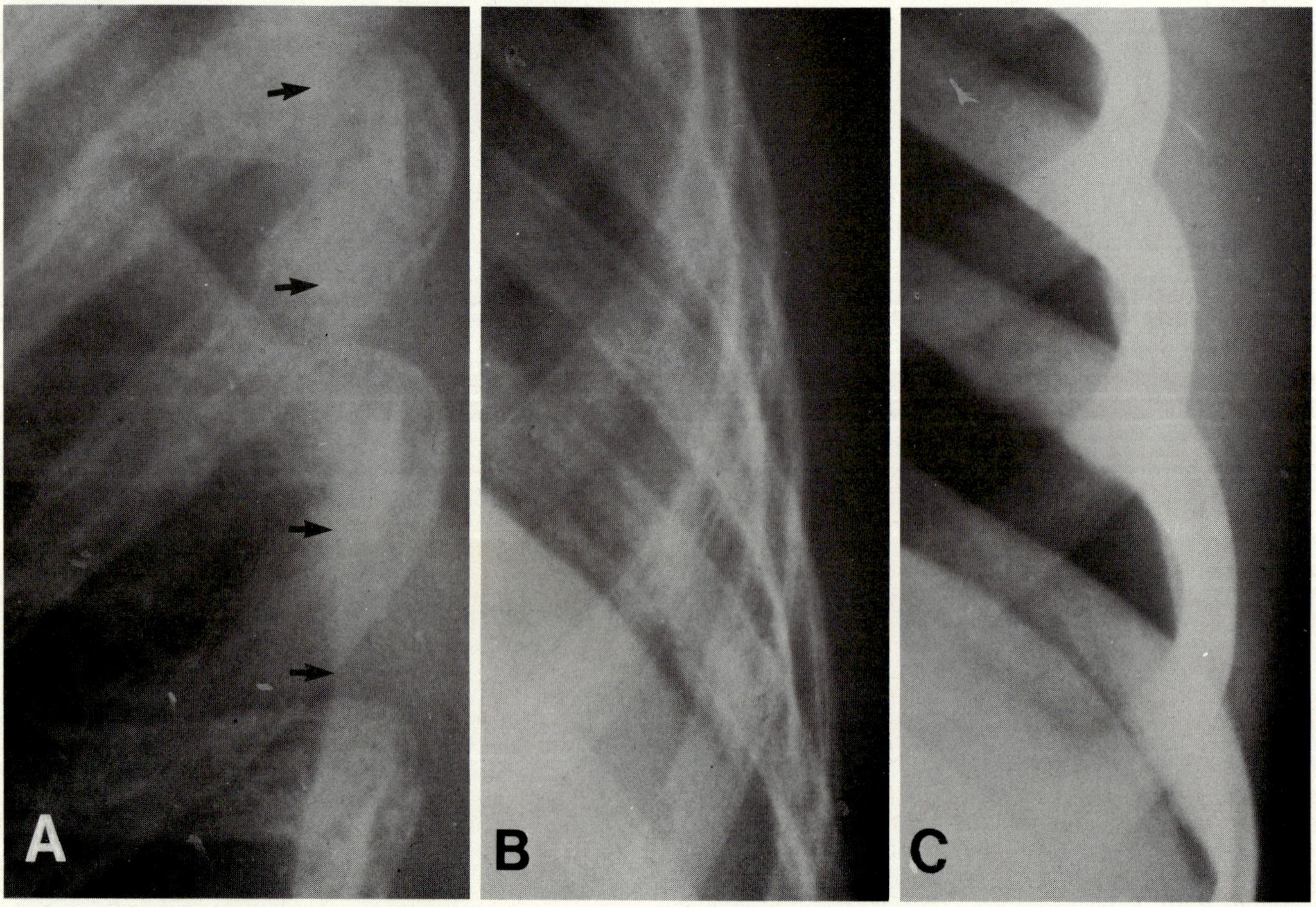

Fig. 4.30 Series of rib films obatined over eighteen months in a patient with sickle cell anaemia with rib infarcts infected by Salmonella. In acute phase **A.** note the extrapleural reaction. **B.** Multiple ribs showing destruction and early periosteal reaction. **C.** Ultimately ribs are sclerotic and there is persistent pleural thickening.

metastases after chemotherapy is to be expected. Calcification may develop at the site of deposits (Cockshott & Hendrickse, 1969).

More confusing are deposits that are multiple, small and ill-defined and simulate an inflammatory process (Fig. 4.29). This is due to the trophoblast deposits having an invasive haemorrhagic border that fills adjacent alveoli and gives rise to a fine patchy alveolar pattern. We have seen such patients diagnosed initially as tuberculosis. Pleural effusions due to haemorrhage from a subpleural deposit or as a result of infarction are not uncommon.

Dyspnoea may be an acute symptom from pelvic tumour emboli (Bagshawe & Garnett, 1963). These can cause pulmonary infarction if large enough to plug a segmental vessel, or lead to severe pulmonary hypertension if numerous enough to cause restriction of the pulmonary vascular bed (Hendrickse *et al.*, 1965).

REFERENCES

Bagshawe, K. D. & Garnett, E. S. (1963) Radiological changes in the lungs of patients with trophoblastic tumours, *British Journal of Radiology*, **36,** 673–679.

Cockshott, W. P. & Hendrickse, J. P. deV. (1969) Pulmonary calcification at the site of trophoblastic metastases, *British Journal of Radiology*, **42,** 17–20.

Evans, K. T., Cockshott, W. P. & Hendrickse, P. deV. (1965) Pulmonary changes in malignant trophoblastic disease, *British Journal of Radiology*, **38,** 161–171.

Hendrickse, J. P. deV., Willis, A. J. P. & Evans, K. T. (1965) Acute dyspnoea with trophoblastic tumours, *Journal of Obstetrics and Gynaecology of the British Commonwealth*, **72,** 376–383.

RIB AND EXTRAPLEURAL LESIONS

In chest films the ribs are inevitably studied. There are inflammatory and neoplastic rib lesions that may produce puzzling appearances.

Infarcts and salmonella infections of ribs in individuals with HbS disease are usually bilateral, not absolutely symmetrical and affect a number of ribs, usually between the fourth and the ninth. Why the bilateral multilevel distribution is a puzzle. Presumably there is impairment of venous drainage through the azygos intercostal system which leads to lowering of oxygen tension in the medullary cavity of several ribs and subsequent infarction. At this initial stage there may be considerable rib pain. Rapidly hyperaemia develops and repair with central rarefaction and investing periosteal new bone takes place. Should secondary infection supervene the inflammatory process is much more marked and the extrapleural reaction may cause considerable displacement of the pleura (Fig. 4.30). This should not be confused with a pleural effusion. Subsequently a period of repair with sclerosis takes place. The eventual outcome may be dense confluent sclerosis (Fig. 4.30) or this may be patchy.

Tuberculosis of ribs is usually closely related to the costochondral junction and can be difficult to detect because of the variable appearances in this region. The posterior neck of the rib can become involved by contiguity. In the chest penetrated films will reveal a vertebral focus and a paravertebral mass. Oesteolytic lesions developing elsewhere in the rib can be difficult to detect and may require tangential oblique views for their display. Abscesses form and spread under the muscle layers and may point at a considerable distance from the focus. There are no pathognomic appearances, since the lesions cause localised destruction arising in the marrow (Fig. 4.31). The chief dif-

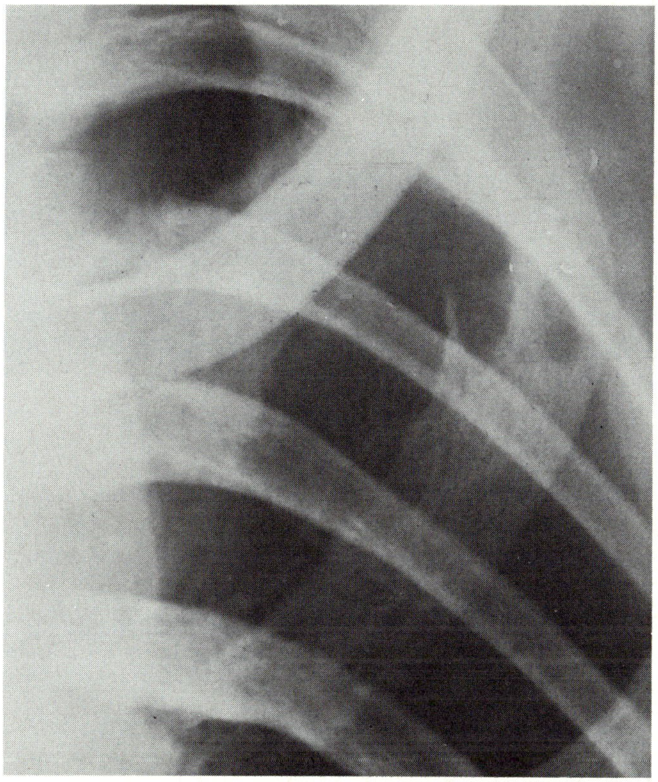

Fig. 4.31 Multiple rounded destructive foci of second rib due to tuberculosis.

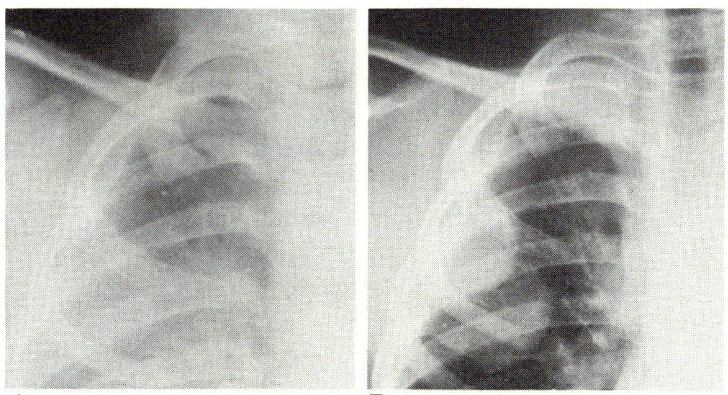

A B

Fig. 4.32 A, B. Burkitt's lymphoma of ribs with extrapleural extension taken five weeks apart. The later film shows extrapleural extension.

ferential considerations are a dimorphic yeast infection or histiocytosis.

Burkitt's lymphoma deposits in ribs cause permeative destruction, beginning in the marrow space and eventually breaching the cortex to spread extrapleurally. This can readily simulate a pleural effusion but evidence of bone destruction and extrapleural rounded masses should prevent diagnostic confusion (Fig. 4.32).

5. Cardiovascular System

MALNUTRITION, KWASHIORKOR AND THE HEART

The heart becomes small after prolonged protein calorie deficiency. Cardiac failure and sudden death may follow. There is no doubt of the reduced heart weight at autopsy but weight *per se* is only one, albeit important, variable that contributes to the radiographic size of the heart in a chest film. Apart from geometric factors that can be standardised (A.P. or P.A.; anode–film distance), the blood volume, the heart rate, the phase of the respiratory and cardiac cycles and the peripheral resistance are important factors that can alter the transverse diameter and the cardiothoracic ratio. The level of the diaphragm can be assessed visually so that subjective correction for expired or overinflated lungs is possible. Though blood volume estimations are rarely available in tropical clinical practice, it is known that rapid compartment shifts of fluid from electrolyte changes can follow initiation of kwashiorkor treatment. These effects are in turn reflected by cardiac enlargement, and increased pulmonary vasculature. Such findings in patients with treated kawashiorkor are not unusual.

In a series of 56 children with kwashiorkor only seven had a transverse diameter of the heart that fell within two standard deviations of aged matched controls (Smythe *et al.*, 1962). In a study of adults with malnutrition microcardia was also noted (Altemus Reed, 1967).

Lagundoye (1974) has suggested that the lateral chest wall in radiographs mirrors the nutritional state. He has shown that in children the subcutaneous fat layer of the soft tissue is depleted in malnutrition more rapidly than the muscle 'water density'. Indeed the fat layer could not be measured in 45 per cent of children with kwashiorkor and a layer of 1 mm or under was seen in 79 per cent of such patients. A muscle layer between 1·5 and 3 mm was observed in 79 per cent of well-nourished controls but only in 19 per cent of those with kwashiorkor and marasmus.

Children with kwashiorkor show initially a small heart that enlarges rapidly in transverse diameter under therapy, due largely to blood volume changes, so that serial study of the fat layer of the lateral chest wall at the level of the 9th and 10th ribs provides a useful additional indicator of nutritional change.

In malnourished children the lung fields are often very clear with oligaemia (Lagundoye & Reddy, 1970). This is again probably a reflection of a low cardiac output and hypovolaemia. The rapid change in lung appearance and heart enlargement is most readily explicable in this manner.

In adults with malnutrition associated with alcoholism, beri beri can develop, but the typical high output (up to 17 litres/minute) hyperkinetic Wenckebach phenomenon described from Java in the early days of this century is not often seen, though it still occurs in South East Asia (Thailand, Burma, Vietnam, the Philippines). These hearts are large in radiographs. Enlargement is generalised and the pulmonary vasculature is plethoric. With specific vitamin supplements there can be striking reduction in heart size within a month or so (Byrne-Quinn & Fessas, 1969).

In the urban African of Johannesburg a form of congestive cardiomegaly due to a dilated hypertrophied heart that often had endocardial mural thrombi was attributed to subnutrition (Higginson *et al.*, 1952). If this is indeed the aetiology the cardiac findings differ markedly from those due to other forms of qualitative/quantitative malnourishment.

REFERENCES

Altemus Reed, L. (1967) Malnutrition with microcardia, *American Journal of Roentgenology*, **99**, 674–680.

Byrne-Quinn, E. & Fessas, C. H. (1969) Beri beri heart disease in London, *British Medical Journal*, **2**, 25–28.

Higginson, J., Gillanders, A. D. & Murray, J. F. (1952) *The Heart in Chronic Malnutrition*, **14**, 213–224.

Lagundoye, S. B. (1974) Subcutaneous fat and muscle layers in chest x-rays of children with Kwashiorkor, *Environmental Child Health*, **20**, 287–290.

Lagundoye, S. B. & Reddy, S. (1970) Chest x-ray changes in Kwashiorkor, *Journal of Tropical Paediatrics*, **16**, 124–126.

Smythe, P. M., Swanpoel, A. & Campbell, J. A. H. (1962) The heart in Kwashiorkor, *British Medical Journal*, **1**, 67–73.

ANAEMIA AND THE HEART

Anaemia is a common problem in many tropical areas. Though the aetiology can be multifactorial (malaria, lack of dietary iron or folate, haemaglobinopathies, etc.), there is no doubt that the most frequent cause is hookworm infestation followed by association with pregnancy. In Kampala 47 per cent of the male and 69 per cent of female hospital admissions for anaemia could be attributed to hookworm (Knight, 1973).

If the drop in haemoglobin is gradual few symptoms develop until the level of Hb reaches 6 or so grams per 100 ml, though the additional burdens of pregnancy or exercise may precipitate failure at that or even higher levels. The haemodynamic responses of anaemia are well known. Because of tissue hypoxia there is a drop in peripheral resistance due to vasodilatation. The cardiac output increases and the circulation time is lessened. Such patients, at rest at any rate, can compensate for the anaemia.

Radiologically there is increase in the cardiac transverse diameter of the heart. Enlargement appears to be generalised and it is difficult to identify the size of individual chambers. The silhouette is usually globular. The pulmonary outflow tract may bulge. The pulmonary arteries and veins are prominent and there is greater perfusion of the upper lobes in the erect position than is normally seen.

The plethoric lung fields are the result of the high output state and the hypervolaemia. Pulmonary oedema is rarely seen, but small pleural collections may occur due to the haemodynamic state and the hypoproteinaemia that accompanies hookworm disease. Changes in children are much more marked radiographically than is the case with adults, as is the reversion to normal appearance as the haemaglobin rises with treatment (Figs. 5.1 and 5.2).

The hyperkinetic hypervolaemic circulation of anaemic patients can readily be overloaded by transfusion so that packed cells or replacement transfusions are used rather than whole blood. In other situations over-transfusion can produce radiologically detectable pulmonary oedema, but in anaemic hearts right-sided failure dominates and the lung fields remain free of oedema, though small pleural effusions may be noted.

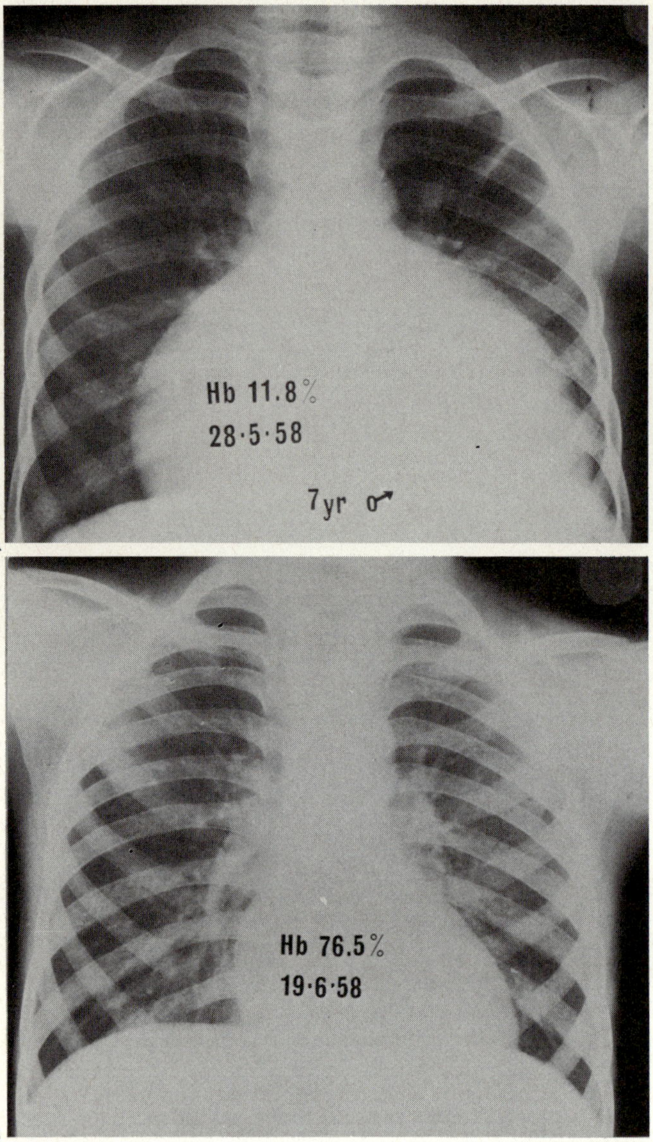

A

B

Fig. 5.1 A, B. Seven-year-old Nigerian child with hookworm anaemia. The change in the shape and size of the heart over a three week interval during which the haemoglobin rose 64 per cent is remarkable.

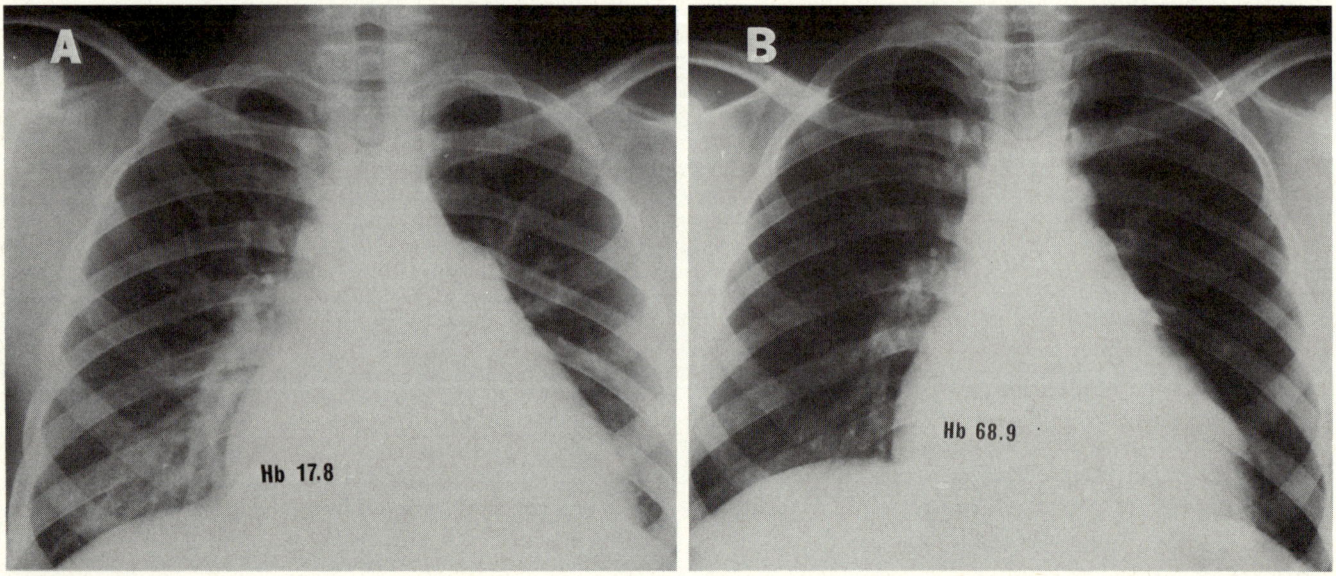

Fig. 5.2 A, B. Chest films of adult with severe anaemia obtained before and after elevation of the haemoglobin level. Initally **A.** There is cardiomegaly and pulmonary artery prominence. After treatment **B.** A considerable improvement is noted.

Though the cardiac contours may simulate pericardial collections, the typical oligaemic low output state of the latter differs from the plethoric pulmonary vasculature of the high output hyperkinetic anaemic state.

REFERENCES
Knight, R. (1973) In *Cardiovascular Disease in the Tropics*, pp. 232–242. London: British Medical Association.

SICKLE CELL ANAEMIA

Patients with sickle cell anaemia in the tropics invariably have cardiomegaly, though this feature is reported in fewer patients with the disease (75 per cent or less) in the United States (Riggs & Rockett, 1968). Cardiac enlargement is generalised and the features differ little from those encountered in anaemia due to other causes, except possibly being at times more severe than expected from the level of haemaglobin present. Disproportionate cardiac enlargement in relation to the level of anaemia is seen in older children and youths. Perhaps the chronicity of the process and episodes of sickling and thrombosis in small myocardial vessels may contribute to the cardiomegaly. Some patients develop elevation of the pulmonary arterial pressure. This can be acute in onset following embolism of marrow fragments after 'bone crisis', or develop slowly due to repeated episodes of intravascular sickling and thrombosis in lung vessels. This state is manifest in radiographs by the development of increasing prominence of the pulmonary outflow tract and main hilar arterial vessels (Fig. 5.3).

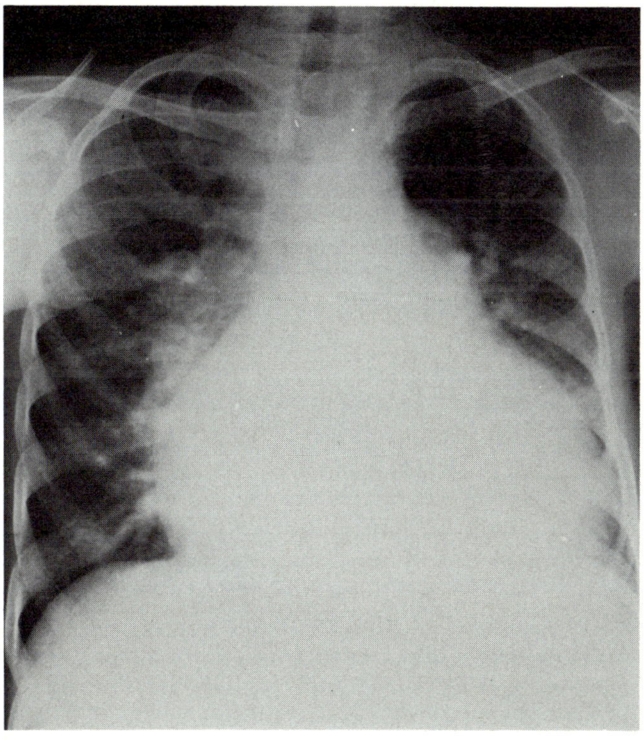

Fig. 5.3 Chest of adult with homozygous sickle cell anaemia. Pulmonary hypertension was present. There is cardiomegaly, a large pulmonary artery and obvious hila.

In heterozygotes cor pulmonale can develop acutely from showers of marrow emboli from infarcted lumbar spine bodies at the time of delivery or during exercise and can be fatal (Shelley & Curtis, 1958; Jones *et al.*, 1970).

Heterozygote sicklers without anaemia can develop cardiomegaly with cardiac failure, but it is uncertain whether this is directly due to the genetic abnormality, or is a consequence of an alcoholic form of cardiomyopathy, since some such individuals are alcoholics (Fleischer & Rubler, 1968).

REFERENCES
Fleischer, R. A. & Rubler, S. (1968) Primary cardiomypopathy in non anaemic patients. Association with sickle cell trait, *American Journal of Cardiology*, **22**, 532–537.
Jones, S. R., Binder, R. A. & Donowho, E. M. (1970) Sudden death in sickle cell trait, *New England Journal of Medicine*, **282**, 323–325.
Riggs, W. & Rockett, J. F. (1968) Roentgen chest findings in childhood sickle cell anaemia, *American Journal of Roentgenology*, **104**, 838–845.
Shelley, W. M. & Curtis, E. M. (1958) Bone marrow and fat embolism in sickle cell anaemia and sickle cell haemoglobin disease, *Bulletin of the Johns Hopkins Hospital*, **103**, 8–18.

HYPERTENSION

In tropical countries there are some isolated communities where the blood pressure does not rise with age. The Chinese of Szechwan, urban Delhi Indians, the Orang Asli of Malaysia, Polynesians and Melanesians, New Guinea highlanders, Brazilian Indians, Australian aborigines, Bushmen of the Kalahari and a number of African nomadic groups such as the Masai (Shaper, 1974). However, there is evidence to indicate that as the process of acculturation proceeds the pressure comes to the same level and relates to age, as in more sophisticated populations.

Essential hypertension is, apart from the rare societies just mentioned, a global problem. In Jamaica in a mass miniature radiographic survey of a rural hillside community aortic dilatation was present in the chest films of 8 per cent of men and 8·4 per cent of women, and was consistently related to higher blood pressure levels than those with a normal aorta. Furthermore there was also an association with aortic regurgitation that did not correlate with treponemal serology (Stuart *et al.*, 1962). In Nigeria an association between hypertension and radiographic aortic dilatation has been confirmed (Ikeme *et al.*, 1975).

In the aetiology of hypertension in the tropics renal disease is now considered to be less important than formerly. Glomerulonephritis is more significant than pyelonephritis. We have seen endemic areas of schistosomiasis where the incidence of pyelonephritis scarcely differed from a control group. However, gonococcal strictures can be causally related to hypertension (Somers, 1964).

Renal vascular disease due to primary aortitis assumes a much greater importance aetiologically in those communities where atheroma is rare. There primary aortitis is a frequent cause of hypertension in children.

The role of hypertension in the development of idiopathic cardiomegaly is not yet understood.

REFERENCES

Ikeme, A. C., D'Arbela, P. G. & Somers, K. (1975) The role of hypertension in the pathogenesis of idiopathic cardomegaly in the tropics, *Cardiologie Tropicale*, **1**, 135–141.

Shaper, A. G. (1974) In *Cardio Vascular Disease in the Tropics*, pp. 77–83. London: British Medical Association.

Somers, K. (1964) Gonococcal urethral strictures and hypertension, *British Journal of Venereal Diseases*, **40**, 194–195.

Stuart, K. L., Miall, W. E., Tulloch, J. A. & Christian, D. E. (1962) Dilatation and unfolding of the aorta in a Jamaican population, *British Heart Journal*, **24**, 455–463.

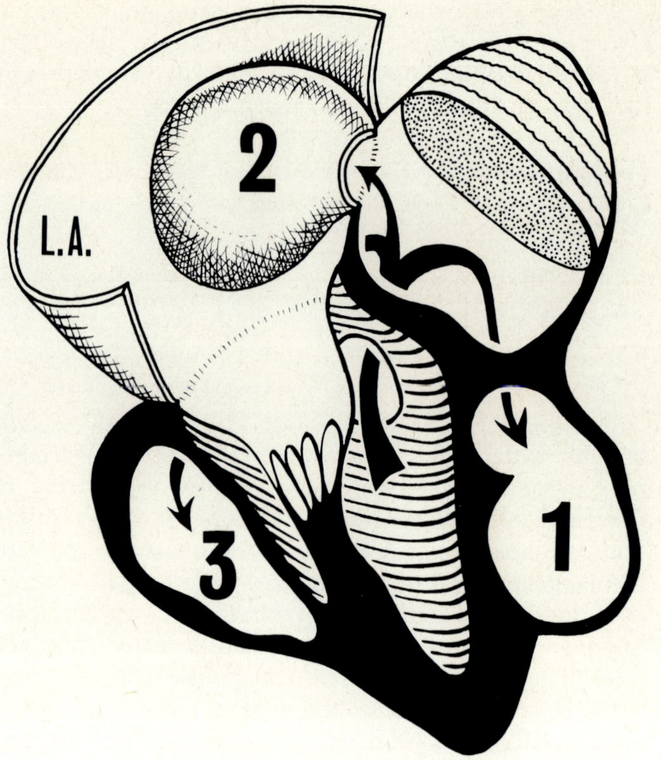

Fig. 5.4 Diagrammatic expression of paths of extension of an L.V. aneurysm from the ostium and initial loculus that contains lamellated clot. Spread can occur into the myocardial wall (1); by bulging into the left atrium (2); and by dissecting around the annulus fibrosus (3). (Courtesy of *British Journal of Radiology*.)

ANNULAR SUBVALVAR LEFT VENTRICULAR ANEURYSMS

An unusual form of aneurysm of the left ventricle has been reported from Equatorial Africa, Central and South Africa; also from the West Indies, Brazil and the United States, as well as sporadically elsewhere. Virtually all the patients have been of African ancestry. The first example was recorded by Corvisart in 1813 in a negro from Martinique living in Paris. The condition is not unduly rare, as 46 cases were seen in one institution over a span of eight years (Cockshott *et al.*, 1967).

The entity is seen most often in males with a peak incidence in the third decade. Many patients are asymptomatic when the aneurysm is discovered incidentally in a chest radiograph or during fluoroscopy for a barium study. Others present with a degree of left-sided failure which may be of acute onset or chronic in nature. Embolic phenomena from displaced intracardiac thrombi may also provide the initial symptoms (Abrahams *et al.*, 1962).

The aneurysm system is a complex three-dimensional structure. The most frequent type originates from an opening behind the posterior leaflet of the mitral valve. From there extension may take place in several directions (Fig. 5.4). It generally burrows in the upper part of the myocardium. Where this extension is close to the pericardial surface a 'blow-out' bulge develops, deforming the cardiac contour. The aneurysm not infrequently has a loculus extending around the annulus fibrosus of the mitral ring, rendering that valve incompetent. Much less often a component of the aneurysm can bulge into the left atrial cavity posteriorly above the mitral valve. Thrombus formation occurs spontaneously in loculi which have relatively stagnant flow. This leads to lamellated clots which later may calcify. Some of the thrombotic process can occlude a loculus at the same time that extension is taking place elsewhere. The coronary vasculature is universally normal apart from displacement when a large aneurysm causes extrinsic pressure and deviates a vessel from its usual course. Patients with calcified aneurysms are often asymptomatic. These aneurysms do not rupture spontaneously.

Little is known as to the aetiology. The marked racial predilection in negroes living in differing environments is suggestive of a genetic factor; but the ethnic genetic diversity (Bantu and non-Bantu) is difficult to reconcile. Infective mycotic aneurysms have been suggested. Whether the frequent coexistence of active or old tuberculous infection is casual or causal is not settled but this seems an unlikely aetiology (Abrahams *et al.*, 1962; Beheyt & Joris, 1963; Lintermans, 1976). Several analogous cases have followed trauma with the development of a pseudo-aneurysm, but this possibility is not applicable in most instances (Hertzeanu *et al.*, 1976). We believe that a congenital weakness at the junction of the mitral annulus and the wall of the left ventricle is the cause of

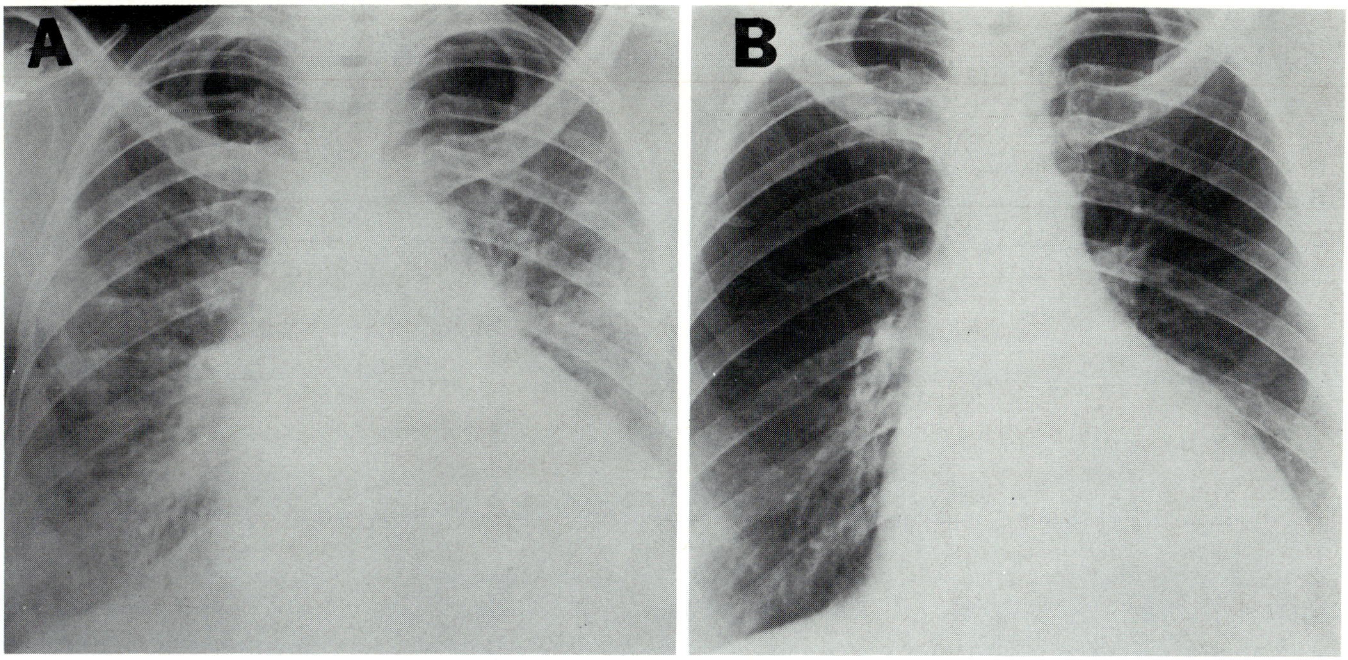

Fig. 5.5 Adult with left ventricular aneurysm presented initially with a greatly enlarged heart and evidence of marked left ventricular failure **A.** Several weeks later after symptomatic treatment the lungs have cleared, the heart is smaller **B.** Note in this case absence of left-sided contour deformity.

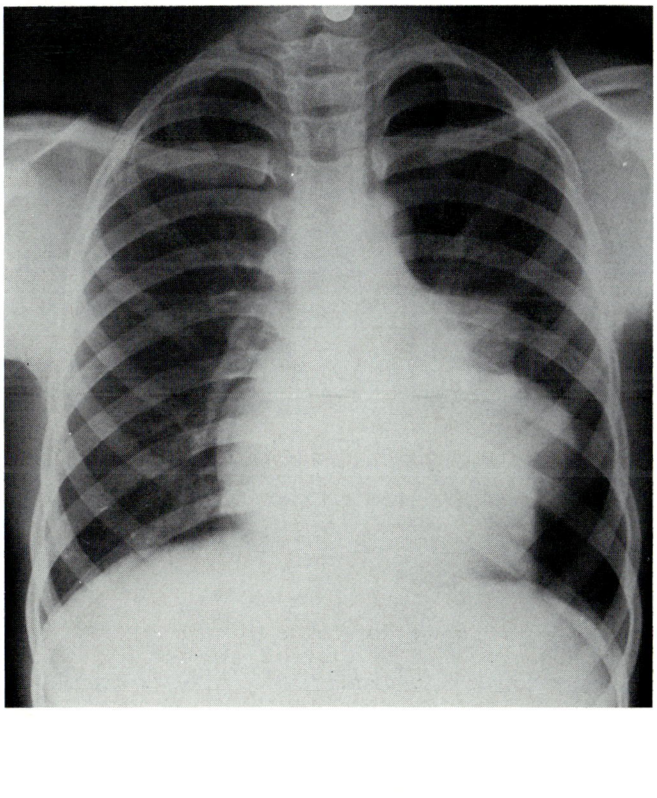

Fig. 5.6 Typical contour of L.V. aneurysm with two bulges projecting from left border. No evidence of left-sided failure.

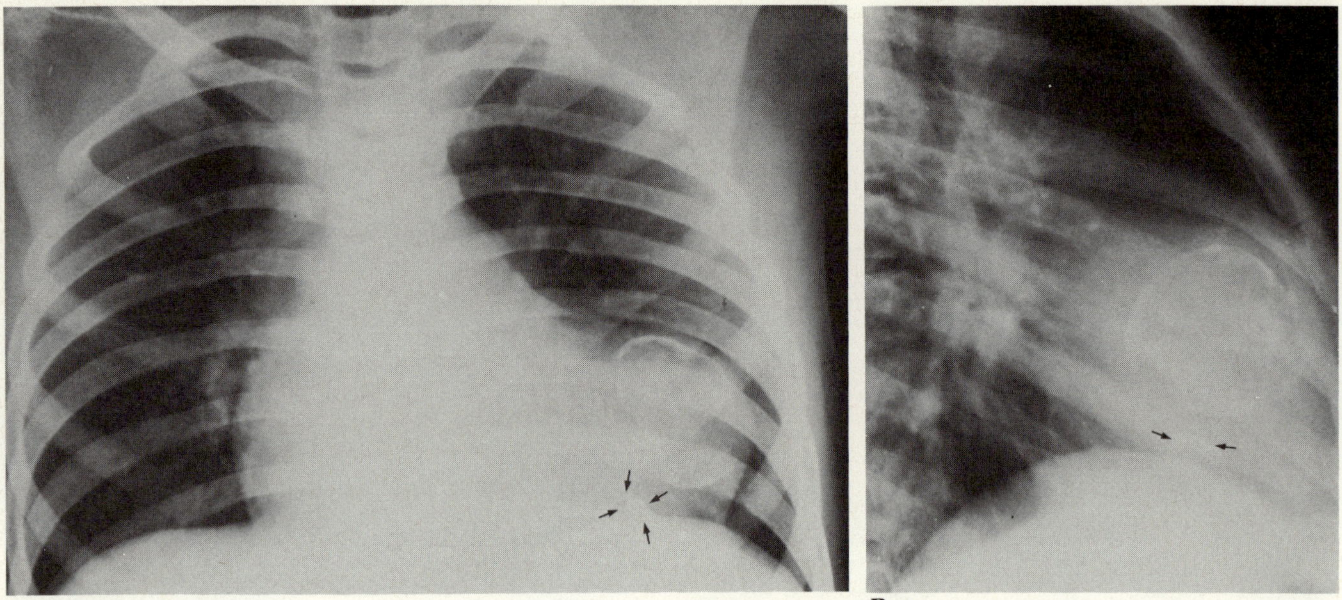

A B

Fig. 5.7 **A, B.** Heart with prominent large left-sided bulge. Within this a large calcified loculus and a smaller calcified area (arrowed) is seen. At angiography the larger loculus was obliterated.

the 'herniation' of the high pressure left ventricular cavity.

The heart is enlarged radiographically in most instances. It may be greatly so in those presenting with acute pulmonary oedema of sudden onset, or those in more chronic failure. With treatment and time, hearts may diminish in size (Fig. 5.5). The more obvious anomalies relate to deformation of the cardiac outline (Fig. 5.6). These may be appreciated as a silhouette anomaly or an internal 'double contour' due to a loculus projecting from the heart *en face* with air-filled lung tissue providing contrast. In loculi that extend inferiorly there may be displacement of the air-filled gastric fundus. Calcification of one or more loculi is seen in about 30 per cent of patients (Fig. 5.7). In those with acute onset it can be observed to develop within three years. Such marginal curvilinear calcification associated with cardiac bulges are only seen apart from aneurysms, in cardiac hydatids.

Angiography confirms the diagnosis. If a loculus is not obliterated by clot its size and communications will be delineated. It is best to avoid introducing a catheter initially into a loculus until a left ventricular injection has established that it does not contain clot that could embolise. Multilocular extensions can be difficult to elucidate and there may be need for injections and films in multiple oriventations (Fig. 5.8). In these cases mitral incompetence with reflux of contrast medium is common. The cases that present surprises are those where the basic heart shape in the P.A. projection is not specific and yet angiography clearly reveals an inferior loculus that may be more capacious than the left ventricular chamber (Fig. 5.9).

Systolic expansion is not a feature of these aneurysms. The therapy of these aneurysms is not settled; several patients with the simple type with a small opening have had surgical repair of the ostium with obliteration of the aneurysm.

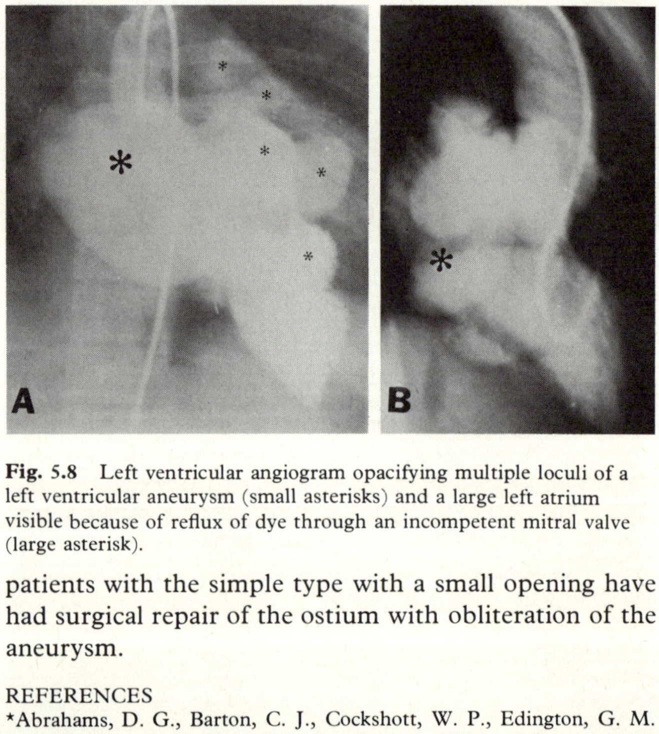

Fig. 5.8 Left ventricular angiogram opacifying multiple loculi of a left ventricular aneurysm (small asterisks) and a large left atrium visible because of reflux of dye through an incompetent mitral valve (large asterisk).

REFERENCES

*Abrahams, D. G., Barton, C. J., Cockshott, W. P., Edington, G. M. & Weaver, E. J. H. (1962) Annular subvalvular left ventricular aneurysms, *Quarterly Journal of Medicine*, **31**, 345–360.

Beheyt, P. & Joris, H. (1963) L'aneurisme ventriculaire gauche chez le jeune Africain; à propos de 9 nouveaux cas, *Acta Cardiologica*, **18**, 113–142.

Cockshott, W. P., Antia, A., Ikeme, A. & Uzodike, V. O. (1967) Annular subvalvar left ventricular aneurysms, *British Journal of Radiology*, **40**, 424–435.

Hertzeanu, H., Veutsch, V., Yahini, J. H., Lieberman, Y. & Neufeld, H. N. (1976) Left ventricular aneurysm of unusual aetiology: a report of two cases, *Thorax*, **31**, 220–225.

Lintermans, J. P. (1976) L'aneurisme ventriculaire gauche chez le jeune Africain, *Cardiologie Tropicale*, **2**, 13–25.

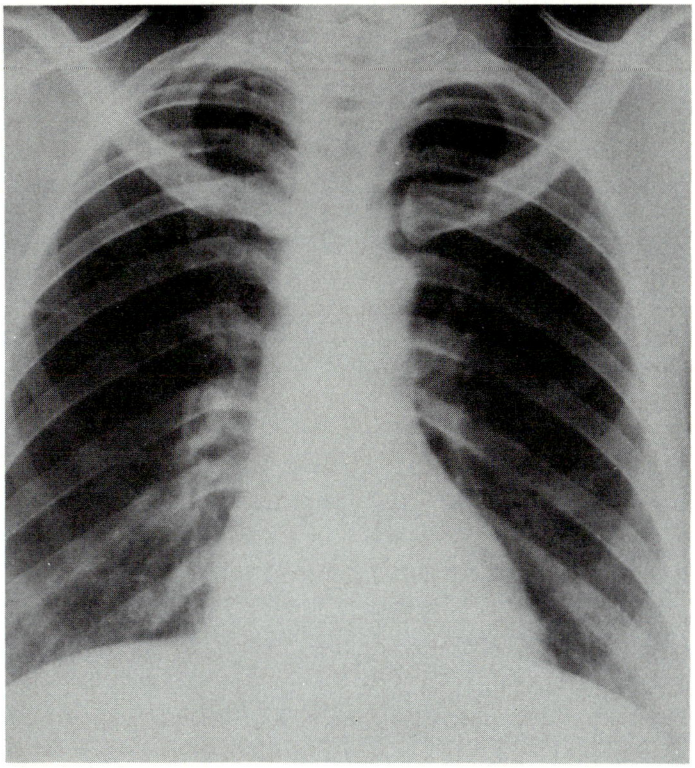

A

Fig. 5.9 Chest film with no gross heart enlargement or silhouette abnormality **A.** The left ventricular angiogram with A.P. view **B** and lateral **C** reveals an aneurysm larger than the ventricular cavity which is elevating the left atrium, which is visible due to mitral incompetence.

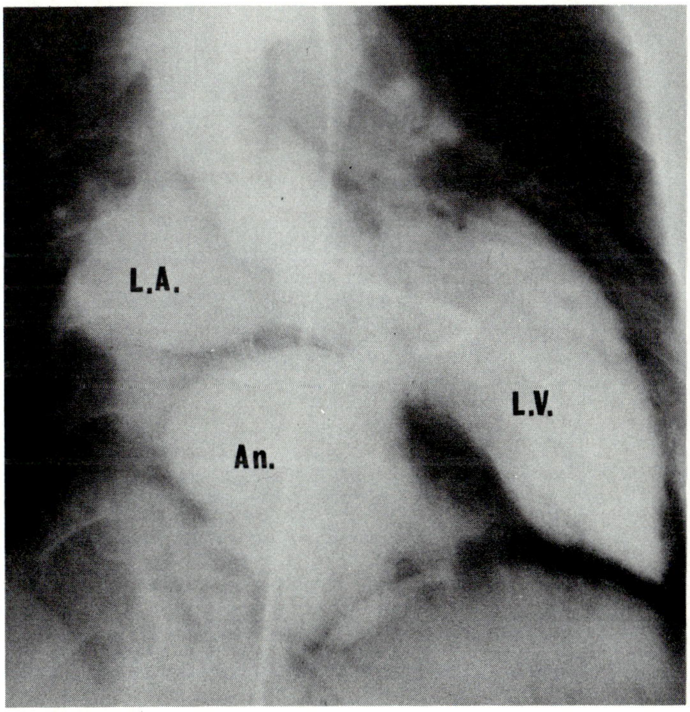

B

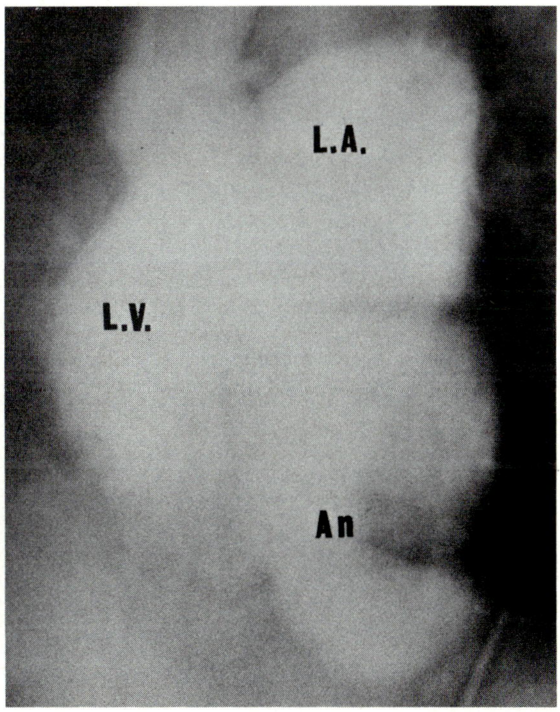

C

IDIOPATHIC CARDIOMEGALY

A type of heart failure associated with cardiac enlargement with intact valves and coronary circulation is seen in much of the tropical and subtropical world. Though obscure cardiomyopathies exist throughout the world, they assume proportionately greater significance in those communities where ischaemic heart disease is rare.

Idiopathic cardiomegaly is difficult to define in either pathological or clinical terms. There are no clearly recognised agreed or specific morbid anatomic features. In clinical practice the term seems to be employed as a scrap heap for those cases where conventional labels are inappropriate. In using this designation there is tacit understanding that probably a multitude of undefined entities are nosologically included which only have in common unexplained heart muscle malfunction.

The natural history of this group of disorders is variable. The consequences in children who recover from the acute phase are benign; the post-partum variety is somewhat more severe, and episodic; adult types may resolve or be rapidly progressive with or without hypertension (Ikeme, 1976). Indeed the whole role of essential hypertension in the pathogenesis of some obscure cardiopathies is at present under consideration in several studies (Falase, 1977).

Since the clinical presentations of these disorders is banal and unspecific at this stage of disease identification, a description of the distribution must necessarily be imprecise. Forms of idiopathic cardiomegaly are common in many areas: sub-saharan Africa, the West Indies, Central and Latin America, India and Japan, etc. In Ibadan idiopathic cardiomegaly represented 30 per cent of all patients seen in an adult cardiac clinic and was the second cause of death from cardiac causes (Cockshott *et al.*, 1967; Brockington & Bohrer, 1970).

At necropsy the hearts are heavy with dilated chambers and a flabby myocardium. Sometimes there is thinning of the left ventricular apex so that this area may be only 2 to 3 mm thick. The histological changes are surprisingly unremarkable.

In chest radiographs the heart is invariably enlarged with a mean C.T. ratio in one series of 0·67 (Cockshott *et al.*, 1967). The shape suggests generalised enlargement and in a proportion of cases it may be possible to conclude that the left side is mainly affected. The aorta is often dilated and unfolded (Brockington & Bohrer, 1970). The cardiac borders, particularly the left, are frequently well defined as though etched. It is hard to believe that this is merely due to the low amplitude of the cardiac contractions, but we have no better explanation. There is no cardiac calcification.

In an episodic disorder such as idiopathic cardiomegaly the heart dimensions tend to wax and wane with the clinical state. Similarly the lung fields may show normal

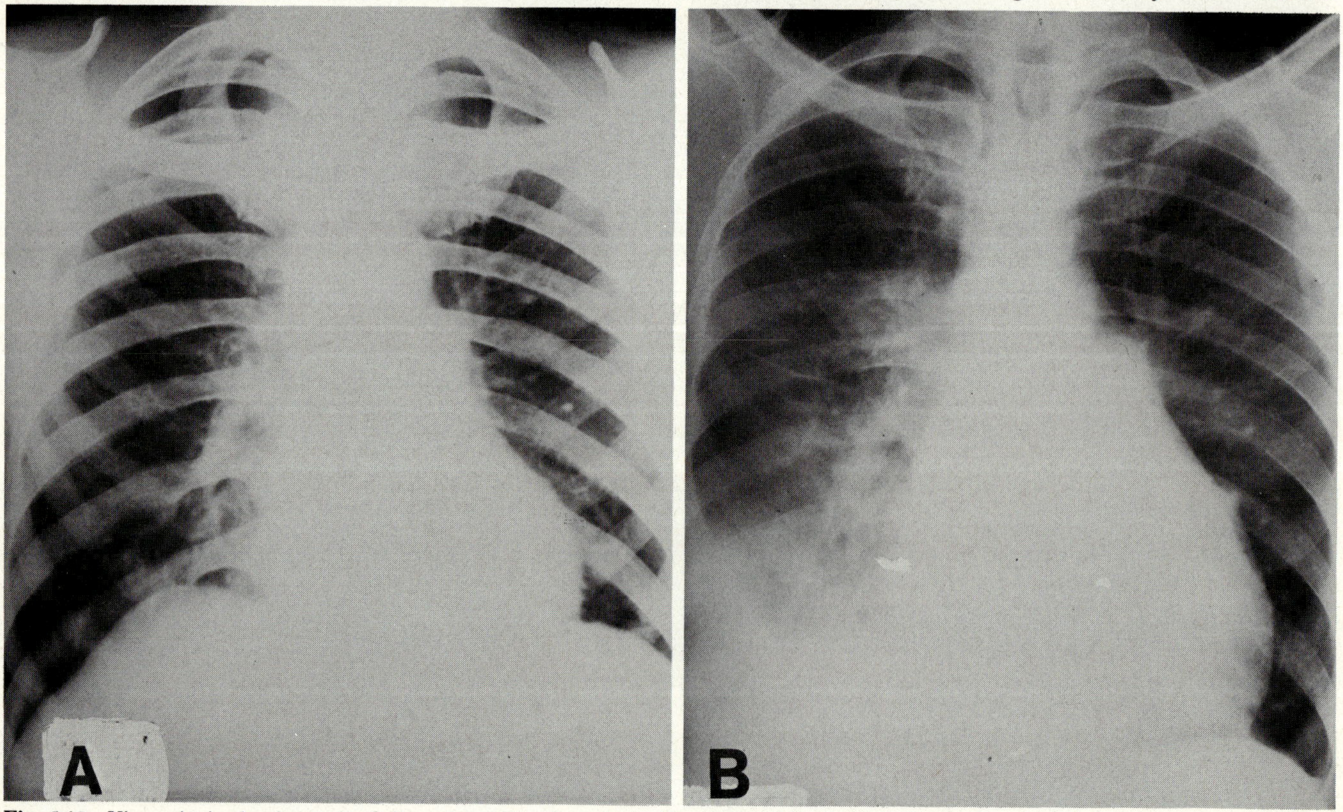

Fig. 5.10 Views obtained at intervals of six years to show the non-specific nature of the cardiac enlargement. In **A** the heart is big with left ventricular prominence. In **B** there is further enlargement and signs of biventricular failure.

vascularity to redistribution of flow, pulmonary oedema and septal lines. Generally only signs of early pulmonary venous distension are apparent. Pleural effusions are sometimes seen (Fig. 5.10).

In most respects the radiological picture of an enlarged heart altering in size and with lung evidence of left-sided failure depending on the degree of decompensation is similar to hypertensive and ischaemic heart failure, so that diagnosis can be difficult.

Left ventricular angiography indicates a poor stroke volume. The dilated chamber has a large end systolic volume and shows little change in size before and after contraction (Fig. 5.11). Apical thinning may be evident. If functional mitral incompetence is present a slightly enlarged left atrium is opacified. Injection of the right side of the heart may show concomitant right-sided dilatation (Antia *et al.*, 1969). The coronary circulation is normal or may appear to have a high flow.

It will be realised from this description that at the end of an angiographic study all the radiologist may be able to conclude is that the features are compatible with idiopathic cardiomegaly. Differentiation from hypertension can be difficult. A dilated aortic knuckle can be helpful (Ikeme *et al.*, 1976).

REFERENCES

Antia, A. V., Cockshott, W. P. & Thorpe, G. J. (1969) Idiopathic cardiomegaly in Nigerian children, *British Heart Journal*, **31**, 178–183.

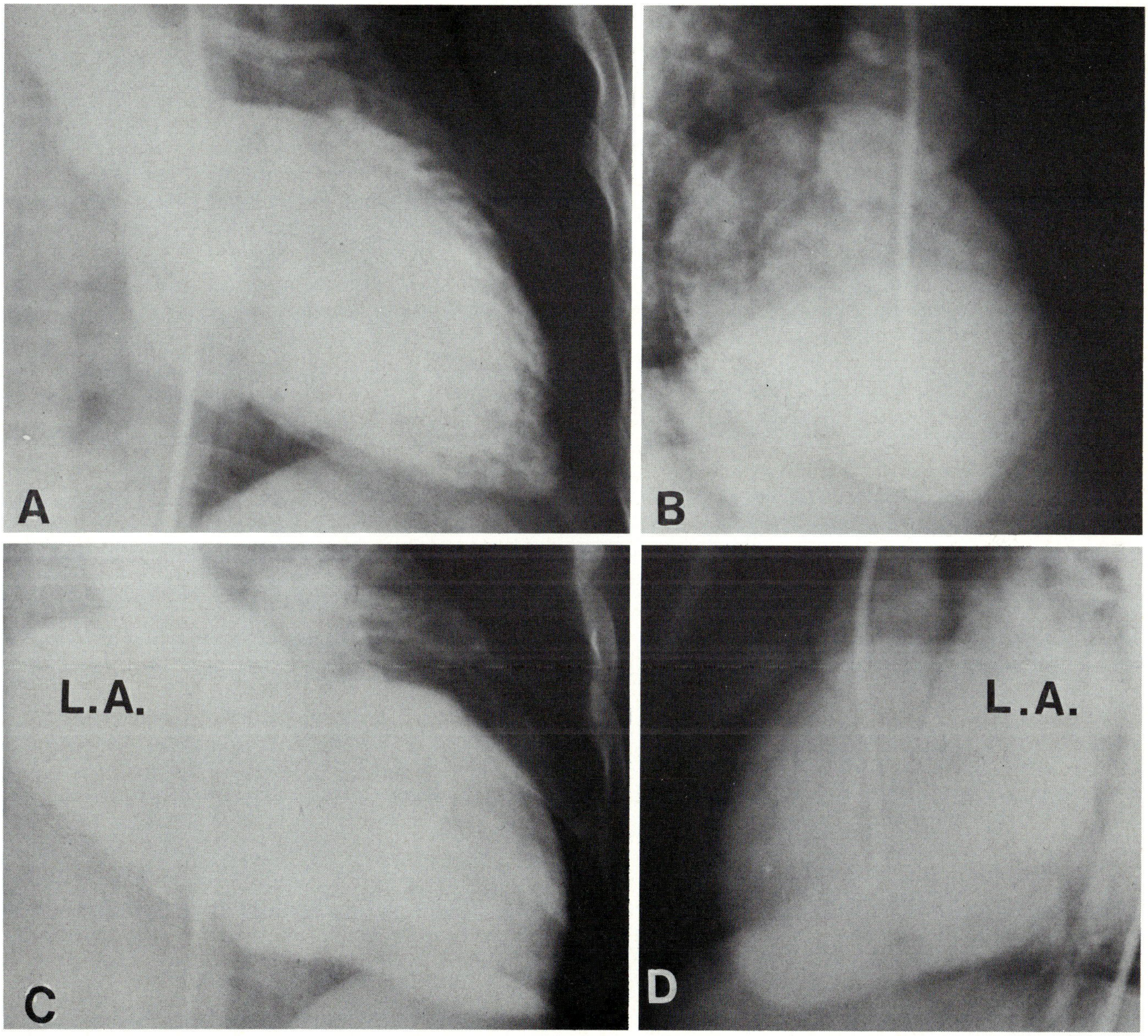

Fig. 5.11 Left ventricular angiogram **A** and **B** frontal and lateral views in systole and **C, D** similar later phase projections in another case. The enlarged dilated cavity with large end systole volume due to poor contractions is evident in **A, B**. There was no evidence of mitral incompetence. In **C, D** the left atrium L.A. is opacified due to valve dysfunction.

Brockington, I. F. & Bohrer, S. P. (1970) Enlargement of the aortic shadow in Nigerian heart muscle disease, *Acta Cardiologica*, **25**, 344–356.

*Cockshott, W. P., Thorpe, G. J. & Ikeme, A. C. (1967) Radiological aspects of heart muscle disease in Nigerian adults, *Circulation*, **36**, 460–467.

Falase, A. O. (1977) Cardiomegaly of unknown origin among Nigerian adults: role of hypertension in its aetiology, *British Heart Journal*, **39**, 671–679.

Ikeme, A. C. (1976) Idiopathic cardiomegaly in Africa, *Bulletin of the World Health Organisation*, **54**, 455–461.

Ikeme, A.C., Ogakwu, M. A. B. & Nwakanoki, F. A. (1976) The significance of the enlargement of the aortic shadow in adult Nigerians, *African Journal of Medical Sciences*, **5**, 195–199.

ENDOMYOCARDIAL FIBROSIS (E.M.F.)

This disease was initially described in West African troops during the second world war but became fully defined pathologically in Uganda and clinically in Nigeria some years later (Davies, 1948; Parry & Abrahams, 1965).

E.M.F. has been seen throughout equatorial Africa and the Sudan; in Brazil, Colombia and Venezuela; in New Guinea and in Sri Lanka and Southern India near Vellore and Kerala, and also in Indo China, Malaysia and Thailand. The condition can develop in all races and in individuals who may have spent only a short while in an 'endemic' part of the tropics (Brockington *et al.*, 1967). Loeffler's fibroplastic endocarditis, which has certain analogies, has been seen in temperate climates sporadically but this is not an identical disorder. Recently a condition with great pathologic similarity has developed in patients receiving adriamycin.

There are many aetiologic speculations arising from different centres where the disease occurs. Unfortunately none of these appears to be universally applicable. Epidemiological investigations suggest that an anomalous response to a streptococcus or a filaria may be important, but so far no accepted cause has been established.

The disorder can involve either ventricle or both at once. In a series of 102 patients from Ibadan there were 48 right-sided cases, 11 left-sided and 43 biventricular. The sex incidence is roughly 1 to 1 with about 80 per cent of those diagnosed being in the second or third decade of age (Cockshott *et al.*, 1967).

The hallmark of E.M.F. is the development of white fibrous tissue on the endocardial surface which slightly penetrates the myocardium. Typically the process starts near the apex and gradually extends superiorly along the surface of the inflow tract so that papillary muscle implication develops. Such extension tethers the leaflets of the mitral or tricuspid valve to the ventricular wall, rendering them incompetent. In right-sided E.M.F. the apex becomes obliterated, markedly reducing the ventricular volume inferiorly, whereas the distal outflow tract dilates and hypertrophies, seemingly to maintain the pulmonary flow. Owing to tricuspid incompetence the right atrium becomes aneurysmal (Fig. 5.12). In the pure left-sided disease mitral incompetence develops but the left atrium does not enlarge much. In the biventricular disease haemodynamically the right-sided restrictive changes lower the pulmonary lung flow so that the left side is in a sense protected from the effects of mitral insufficiency. Pericardial effusion is a frequent accompaniment of the right-sided form of the disease. Calcification beneath the plaques of thickened endocardium may develop in a proportion of patients. Mural thrombi sometimes form on the endocardial fibrotic areas so that from the left-sided condition systemic embolism is a danger and on the right, pulmonary embolism. The usual source of the latter is from clots forming in the stagnant area of the right auricular appendage. The coronary arteries are normal, apart from being displaced by the fibrotic distortion and chamber enlargement. Radiologically it is easiest to consider separately the pure right and left forms of the disease and the changes due to biventricular involvement.

Right-sided E.M.F. often produces characteristic physical findings of ascites, high central venous pressure with exaggerated tricuspid incompetence waves, and on palpation an active pulsating heave in the left parasternal area due to the hyperkinetic right ventricular outflow tract.

In chest radiographs the heart is always enlarged and at times the C.T. ratio is greater than 0·9 (Cockshott *et al.*, 1967). The globular shape suggests a pericardial collection, which is often present, or an aneurysmal right atrium, which is invariable (Fig. 5.12). There is probably little pericardial fluid if the outflow tract convexity can be distinguished. Cardiac calcification lying obliquely from the elevated R.V. apex to below the outflow tract may be seen in about 10 per cent of patients (Fig. 5.13). Because of the reduced cardiac output from loss of volume and contractibility of the right ventricle the lung fields show reduced vascularity. The superior vena cava and azygos vein are prominent.

Angiography confirms the diagnosis by demonstrating loss of the apex of the right ventricle and evidence that only the outflow tract of the R.V. is showing active contraction (Fig. 5.14). This process of ventricular obliteration can be shown to progress in serial studies (Fig. 5.15) (Cockshott, 1965). Clot may be seen in the auricular appendage. Because of this frequent occurrence care must be taken to avoid letting a catheter tip stray in this area and dislodge thrombi. The right ventricle and right atrium all usually show similar pressures and a 'dip and plateau' configuration. Angiography clearly shows whether there is a pericardial collection or merely a dilated right atrium (Fig. 5.12).

Left-sided E.M.F. is seen less frequently clinically than the right-sided disease—10 per cent as opposed to 47 per cent. The heart may be small or with a C.T. ratio up to 0·7. The heart may appear normal or show signs of right ventricular prominence consequent on the pulmonary hypertension arising from the mitral incompetence (Fig.

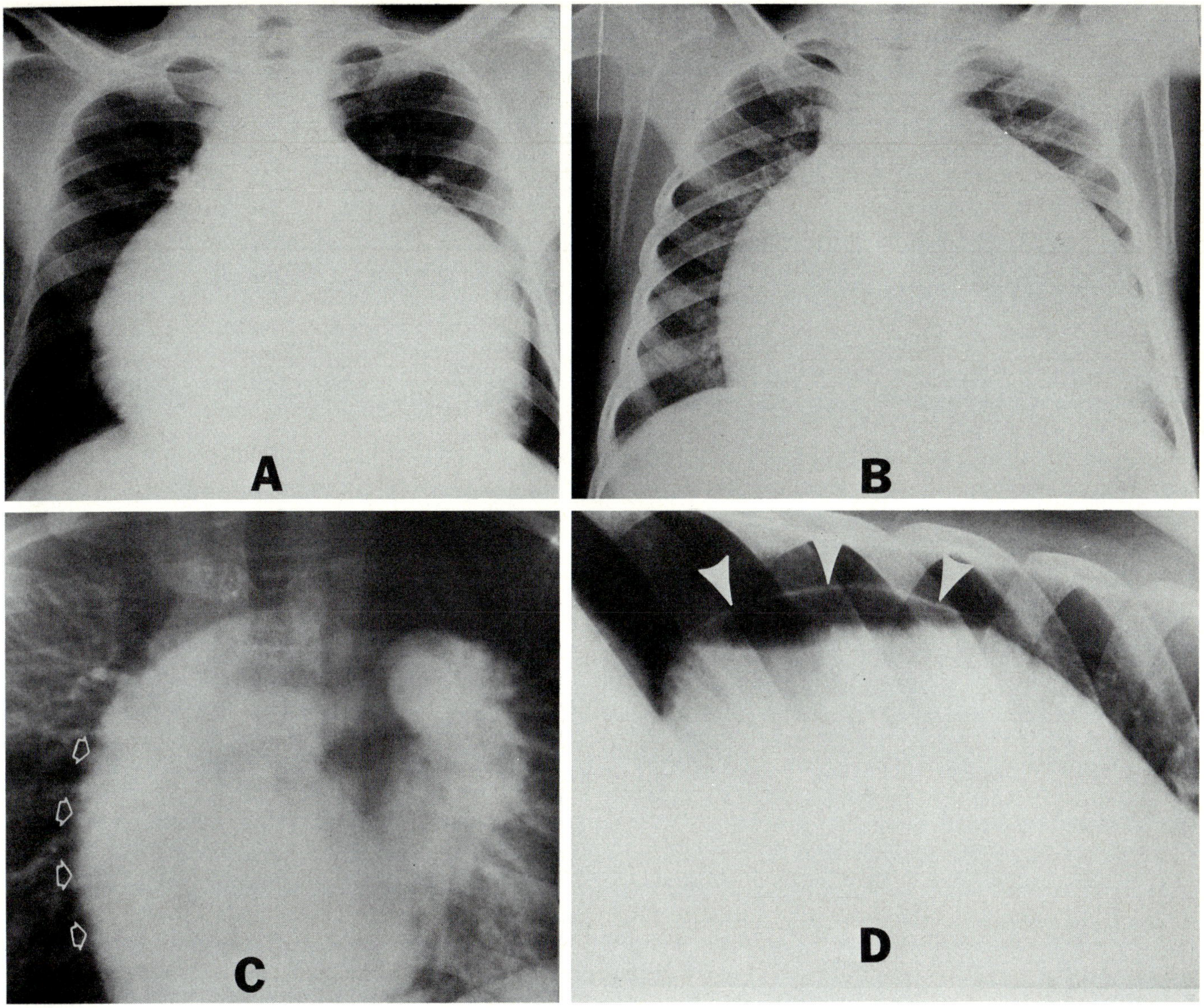

Fig. 5.12 **A & B** are anterior chest views of two patients with right-sided E.M.F. Both have similar greatly enlarged cardiac contours and oligaemic lung fields. An angiogram of **A** (**C**) clearly reveals that the heart enlargement is attributable to an enormous right atrium. The cardiac silhouette of **B** is revealed to be largely due to a large pericardial collection by the horizontal beam. (Courtesy of *British Journal of Radiology*.) Diagnostic pneumopericardium view **D.** Note that the thin pericardium, white solid arrows, is evident. In **C** the opacified atrium reaches the lateral cardiac border, proving the absence of pericardial fluid.

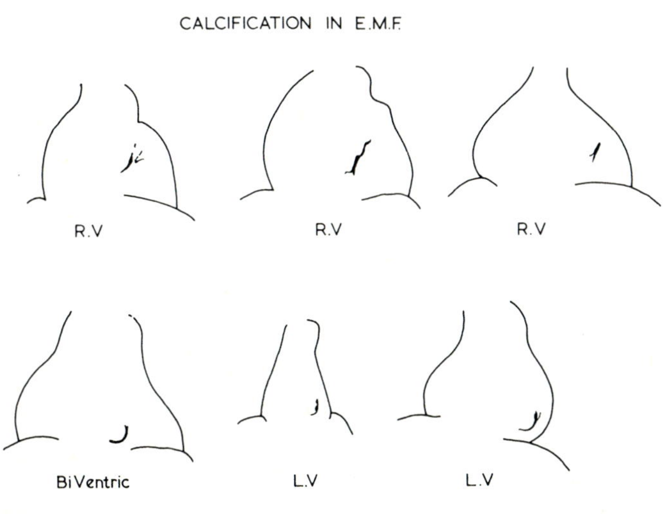

Fig. 5.13 Tracings of calcification in right ventricular, biventricular and left-sided E.M.F. The oblique linear deposition of calcium at the site of the obliterated apex in right E.M.F. is characteristic (top row). Calcification of left apex causes a curvilinear appearance (bottom row). (Courtesy of *British Journal of Radiology*.)

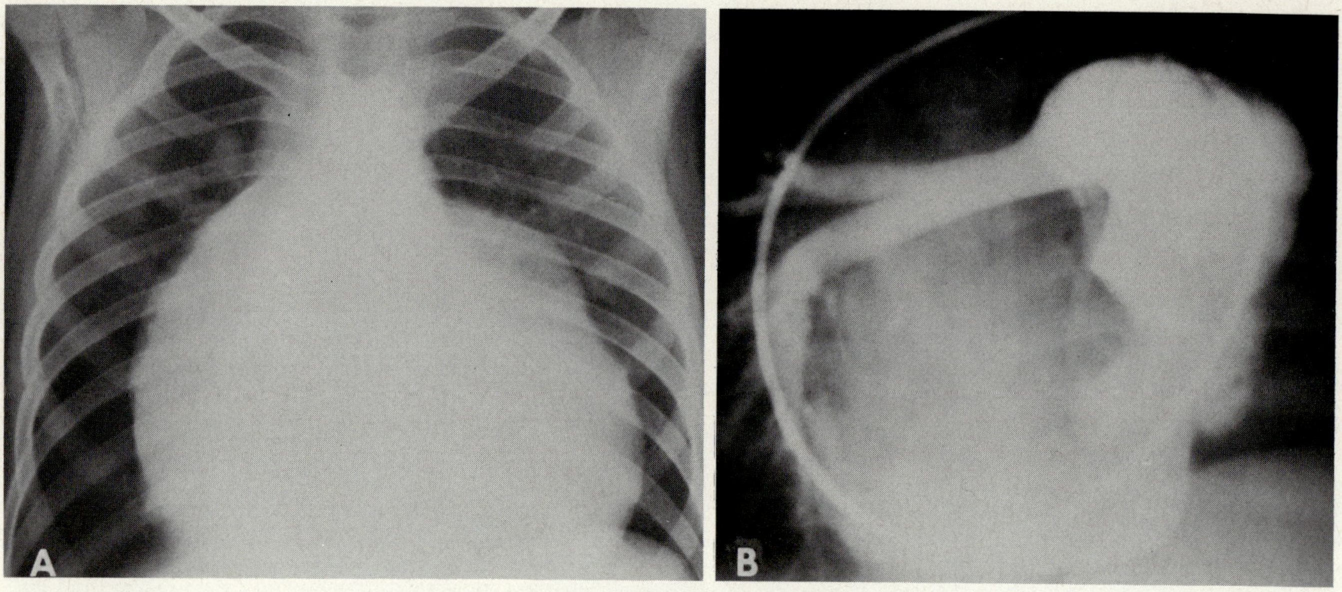

Fig. 5.14 Patient with right-sided E.M.F. **A.** In anterior view a bulge in the left side is due to prominence of the right ventricular outflow tract. Note the oligaemic lung fields in this low output state. **B.** The selective right ventricular angiogram confirms the dilated outflow tract and shows the obliterated ventricular apex, the reflux of contrast into large right atrium, and confirms the absence of pericardial collection.

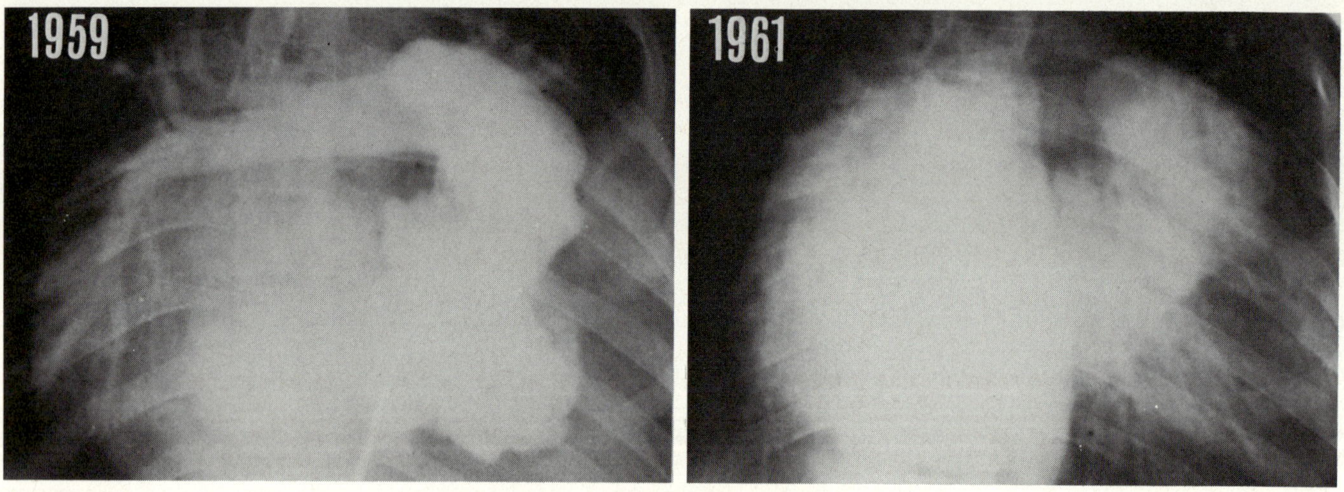

A B

Fig. 5.15 **A, B.** Right-sided angiocardiograms at two-year intervals in same patient to demonstrate progressive obliteration of the right ventricle. Note that in **B** the obliquity of the remaining right ventricle is identical in position to the line of calcification seen in right E.M.F. as shown in 5.13. (Courtesy of *British Journal of Radiology.*)

5.16). There may be curvilinear calcification at the apex of the ventricle (Fig. 5.13). There is no calcification around the mitral valve.

On angiography the left ventricle shows reduction in volume due to progressive obliteration of the apex, which gives rise to typical deformities (Fig. 5.17). The areas covered by endocardial plaques are akinetic or poorly contractile. Mitral incompetence is marked, with contrast reflux outlining a slightly or moderately enlarged atrial cavity which is actively contractile. Despite significant incompetence and a powerful muscular atrium with volume distension, there is incomplete atrial emptying—probably because the partially obliterated left ventricle cannot dilate to take the increased volume load (Fig. 5.18). With oblique projections one can show how the papillary muscles are incorporated with the ventricular wall. These patients do not have pericardial collections.

Biventricular E.M.F. is seen in about 41 per cent of cases and is more frequent in females. The heart is always enlarged, once again as in pure right-sided disease due to pericardial effusion, a dilated right atrium, or both. Pulmonary oligaemia is striking, but if the left side is severely involved there may be redistribution of flow to the upper lobe veins. Pleural collections occur at one stage or another in half the patients with biventricular disease. Since the right-sided involvement reduces the cardiac output the

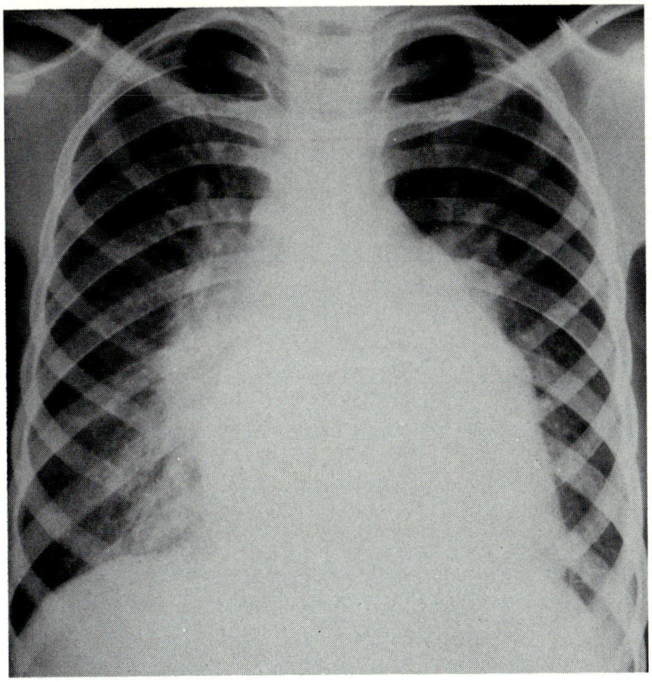

Fig. 5.16 Chest film of patient with left-sided E.M.F. Right-sided enlargement and pulmonary hypertension is evident. Here it is gross and the heart is larger in transverse diameter than at an earlier stage.

left side is protected from a full volume load, so that the left atrium is often small, as is the left ventricle and the aorta. However, the aorta often shows a bizarre displacement due to the right atrium. The right coronary artery also shows distortion, being elevated in an anterior arc by the right atrium (Fig. 5.19).

Do E.M.F. cases warrant angiography study? For purely diagnostic purposes the combination of clinical features and chest radiographs enable one usually to detect right-sided involvement. Constrictive pericarditis or tricuspid incompetence from other causes show enough differences that there should be no diagnostic confusion. Left-sided E.M.F. may be difficult to distinguish from rheumatic mitral disease unless there is left apical calcification. The relative small size of the left atrium may be a helpful point.

Recently successful open heart surgery with peeling off of the endocardial plaques combined with valve replacement has been carried out (Bertrand *et al.*, 1976; Bertrand *et al.*, 1977; Dubost *et al.*, 1977). As a prelude to such intervention angiography is needed to define the areas affected and to assess the secondary effects on the atria—as well as obtaining haemodynamic catheter data. The role of such therapy is for the present limited.

Ultimately angiography can be justified to establish the diagnosis when both clinical and simpler radiographic studies have failed to resolve a diagnostic problem. It would seem that in this disease echocardiography has an important diagnostic role in the future.

REFERENCES

Bertrand, E., Renambot, J., Chauvet, J., Assamoi, O. M. & Ekra, A. (1976) Le traitement chirurgical de la fibrose endomyocardique constrictive, *Cardiologie Tropicale*, **2,** 37–43.

Bertrand, E., Renambot, J., Metras, D., Chauvet, J. & Assamoi, M. O. (1977) Première évaluation à moyen terme du résultat du traitement chirurgical de la fibrose endomyocardique constrictive, *Cardiologie Tropicale*, **3,** 99–107.

Cockshott, W. P. (1965) Angiocardiography of endomyocardial fibrosis, *British Journal of Radiology*, **38,** 192–200.

Cockshott, W. P., Saric, S. & Ikeme, A. C. (1967) Radiological findings in endomyocardial fibrosis, *Circulation*, **35,** 913–922.

Davies, J. N. P. (1948) Endocardial fibrosis in Africans, *East Africa Medical Journal*, **25,** 10–16.

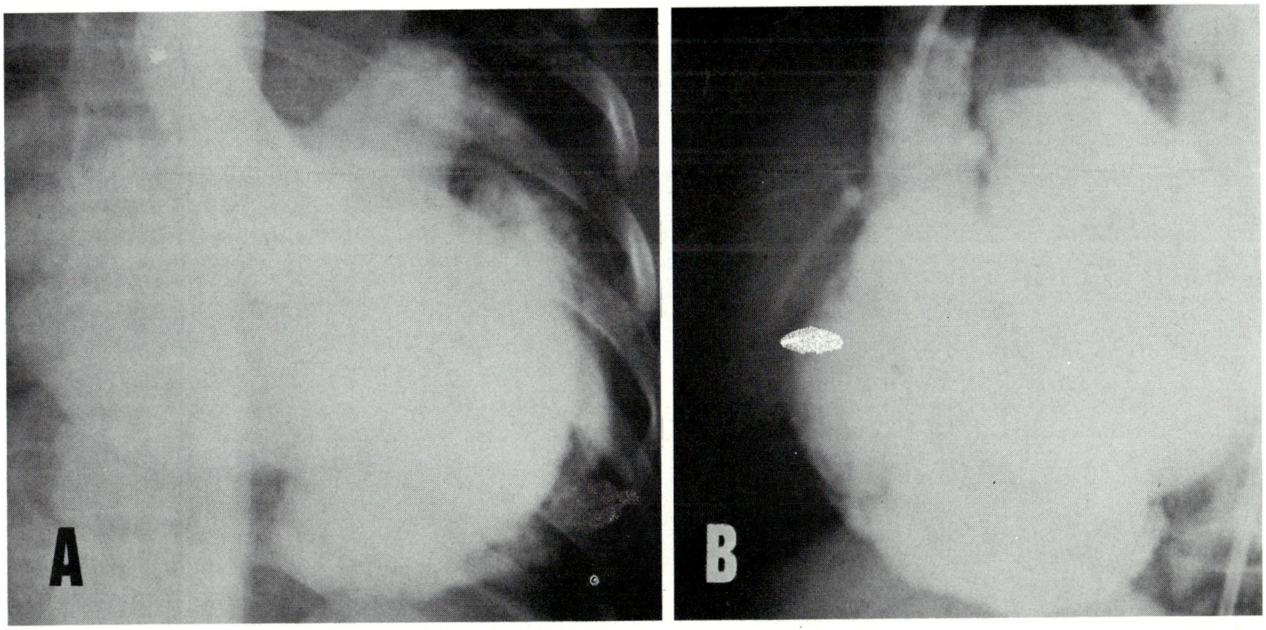

Fig. 5.17 Early left-sided E.M.F. frontal **A** and lateral **B** angiogram projections. The point of the apex has gone and was rigid with no change in shape with cardiac cycle. Marked mitral incompetence. (Courtesy of *British Journal of Radiology*.)

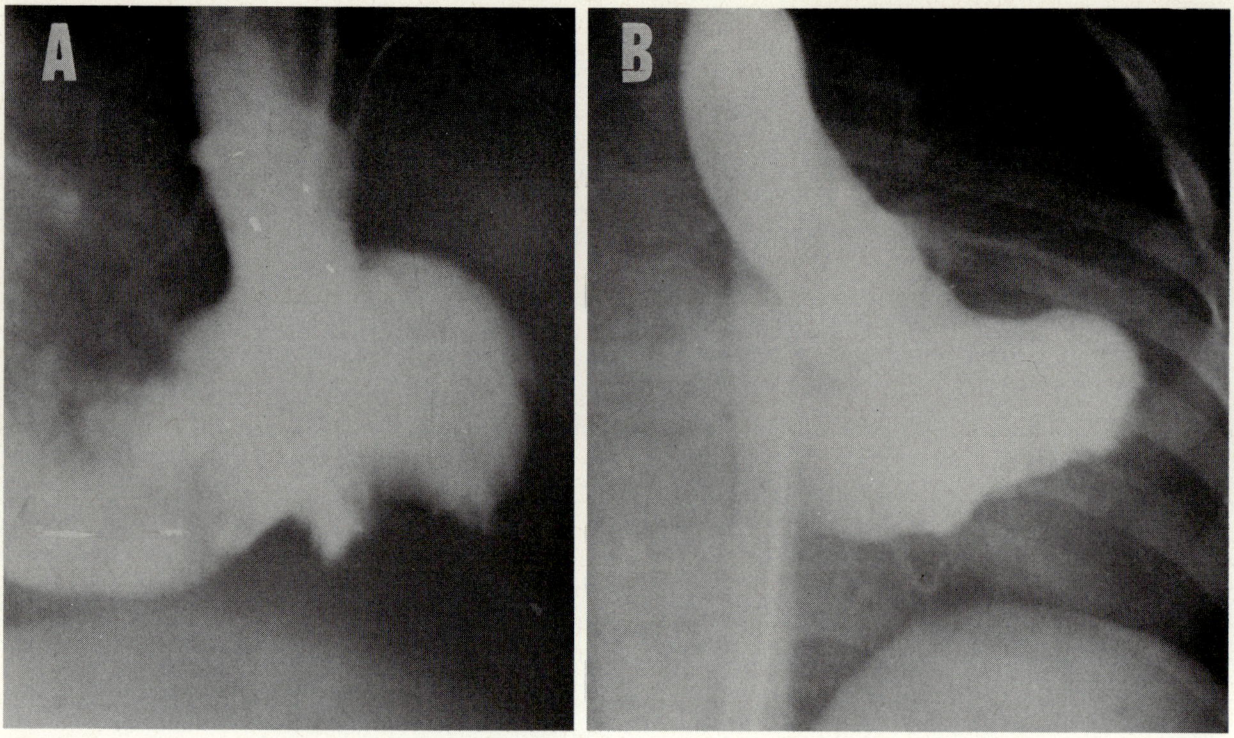

Fig. 5.18 A, B. More advanced obliteration of left ventricular cavity showing typical deformity of apex. The left atrium is small.

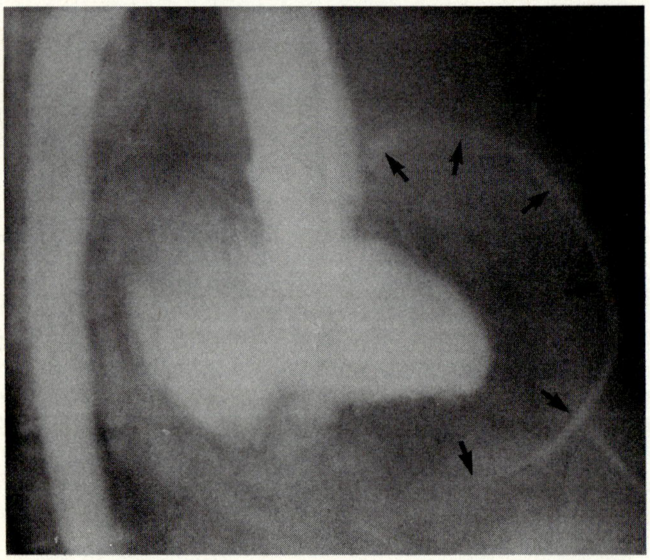

Fig. 5.19 Biventricular E.M.F. showing displacement of right coronary artery anteriorly by large right atrium.

Dubost, Ch., Maurice, P., Gerbaux, A., Rulliere, R., Bertrand, E., Barrillon, A., Vial, F., Prigent, C., Carpentier, A. & Soyer, R. (1977) L'endocardite fibreuse constrictive; traitement chirurgical, *Cardiologie Tropicale*, **3**, 17–20.

Parry, E. H. O. & Abrahams, D. G. (1965) The natural history of endomyocardial fibrosis, *Quarterly Journal of Medicine*, **34**, 383–408.

CHAGAS' CARDIOMYOPATHY

Chronic Chagas' heart disease is an enormous public health and human problem in much of Argentina, Brazil, Venezuela, Columbia, the countries of Central America and to a lesser extent southern Mexico. It has been estimated that at least seven million are afflicted. In some parts of this area 30 per cent of all autopsies reveal Chagasic heart disease. It is a major cause of sudden death from ventricular fibrillation.

The disease affects the lower socio-economic groups in rural areas, as their housing with cracks in the walls, thatched roofs and animals in the house provides an environment where the triatomid bugs flourish and can transmit the trypanasomes.

The responsible agent Trypanasoma cruzi multiplies and develops in the intestinal tract of species of Triatomidae. In the hind gut an infected bug excretes metacyclic trypanasomes with its faeces. Whilst taking a blood meal from man or an animal this insect defaecates on the skin. Because of the itch of the bite a scratch serves to inoculate the infected material into the bite wound. Circulating in the blood, the trypanasomes attach to cells to assume an intracellular leishmanial form that multiplies to later release further parasitising trypanasomes.

At the time of the initial bite an acute local reaction sets in with involvement of regional draining glands: the primary complex 'Chagoma'. During this phase there may be considerable systemic upset, fever, heart failure and central nervous system symptoms. There is a mortality of 5 to 10 per cent in the acute stage, but the main problems of the disease declare themselves slowly in the chronic phase that smoulders for many years, causing increasing symptoms. Then parasitaemia is difficult to detect except by Xeno diagnosis and intracellular parasitic forms are scanty. The patients' resistance develops and a serum gamma globulin factor reacts with certain tissues, including heart muscle, and more specifically autonomic cells in the heart and gastro-intestinal tract (dos Santos *et al.*, 1977). So it seems that auto-immune circulating antibodies create considerable destruction of the autonomic tissue of the body.

Chronic Chagasic heart disease may not clinically present for one to three or more decades after the initial insect inoculation. Thinning of the cardiac apex without necessarily significant cardiomegaly is an early gross abnormality. Whether this pathognomic change is due to relative ischaemia, unwinding of the bulbo spiralis fibres, or sympathetic overstimulation consequent on denervation, is not settled. The affected hearts are heavy, rounded with both hypertrophy and dilatation of the chambers. There is often bulging with some thinning of the right ventricular outflow tract. Intramural thrombus formation and embolic phenomena are frequent. Neuronal destruction of the S.A., A.V. nodes and bundles are the typical histological lesions (Koberle, 1973). It seems that the intracardiac neuronal destruction by an immunological process is the pathogenesis of the heart disease.

Patients at this stage frequently demonstrate conduction defects and arrhythmias which may lead to dizziness, loss of consciousness or death. However, most cases suffer from a biventricular heart failure, though right-sided congestive features usually dominate the clinical presentation. Consequently, since there is diminished right-sided output the lungs rarely develop pulmonary oedema even when the left ventricle is also gravely affected.

In the acute phase of Chagas' disease an enlarged dilated heart has been described radiologically, but there are few such descriptions (Laranja *et al.*, 1956; Anselmi *et al.*, 1967).

In the chronic stage the heart may be normal in size but slowly the left ventricle becomes more obvious in chest films, but eventually not only is there biventricular enlargement but also atrial dilatation (Fig. 5.20). The heart by then is globular and shows very small excursions on fluoroscopy. The lung vascular pattern is reduced and there is no redistribution of flow or pulmonary oedema. These oligaemic features reflect the low output state. Terminally small pleural effusions may be detected.

Angiography has established the presence of chamber dilatation, wall hypertrophy and thinning; the inefficient contractions causing a low ejection fraction; and sometimes, an apical aneurysm most obvious in diastole. Since these patients are in a precarious state of rhythm and little therapeutic advantage can follow angiography the indications for such studies are generally limited. At times in Chagas' heart disease there are anginal symptoms and electrocardiographic ischaemic changes, so that there may

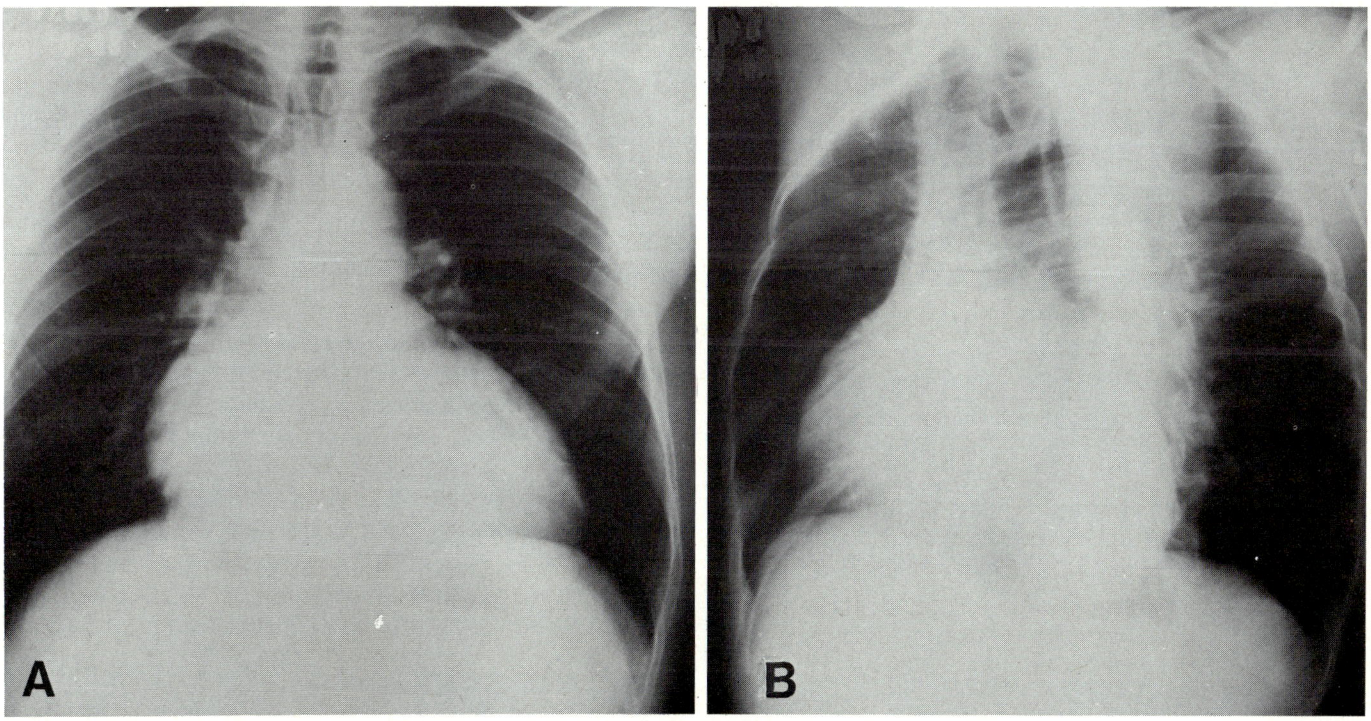

Fig. 5.20 A, B. Anterior A, and left anterior oblique position of chest of patient with Chagas' disease. There is generalised cardiomegaly with predominant left ventricular involvement. (Courtesy of Dr. Clovis Simao, Ribeirao-Preto.)

be confusion with atheromatous coronary artery disease. Since there is not a lot of overlap in the socio-economic status of these two disorders, consideration of a patient's economic circumstances may resolve the differential diagnostic problem and obviate the need for angiographic studies. The presence of mega-oesophagus is a useful additional diagnostic finding. Radiology is valuable in differentiating E.M.F. and Chagas' myocarditis in areas where both occur (Guimaraes *et al.*, 1977).

Myocardial scintigraphy by pyrophosphate with technetium tag can be positive in Chagas' heart disease and by so mimicking coronary infarction, results can be misleading (Lessem & Persson, 1977).

REFERENCES

Anselmi, A., Pisan, F., Suarez, J. A., Gurdiel, O. & Lapco, L. (1967) Cardiovascular radiology in acute and chronic Chagas' myocardiopathy, *American Heart Journal*, **73**, 626–639.

dos Santos, R., Furtado, Von G. C. C. & Rodrigues, W. (1977) In *Proceedings of the 13th Congress Brazilian Society of Tropical Medicine*—Abstract 62.

Guimaraes, A. C., de Abrev, W. N., Santos Filho, A., Vinhaes, L. S. A. & Souza, J. A. de A. (1977) Hemodynamics in chronic Chagas' myocarditis and its differential diagnosis with endomyocardial fibrosis, *Cardiologie Tropicale*, **3**, 87–95.

Koberle, F. (1973) *Tropical Pathology*, pp. 380–395. Heidelberg: Springer.

Laranja, F. S., Dias, E., Nobrega, G. & Miranda, A. (1956) Chagas' Disease. A clinical, epidemiologic and pathologic study, *Circulation*, **14**, 1035–1060.

Lessem, J. & Persson, B. (1977) Myocardial scintigraphy in Chagas' disease, *Lancet*, **2**, 310.

AFRICAN TRYPANOSOMIASIS—CARDIOMYOPATHY

Though cardiac manifestations of T. gambiense and T. rhodiense infections have for long been suspected, the existence of pathological lesions from trypanosomiasis is no longer in doubt (Poltera *et al.*, 1976). These authors, and others, have revealed the existence of a pancarditis. The myocardium shows a diffuse interstitial and perivascular inflammatory infiltrate, thickening of the endocardium, pericardium and valves, as well as scarring of the nodal and conducting tissues. The degree and intensity of involvement is less than in South American trypanosomiasis, but the lesions do have similarities, though apical aneurysms do not develop in the African form. Now that trypanosomiasis has been shown to exist in Asia it will be of interest to see if this form of cardiac pathology also is present there (Shrivasta & Shrivasta, 1974; Dissanaike *et al.*, 1974).

Patients with this complication of trypanosomiasis present in congestive failure. The diagnosis is difficult, not susceptible to proof in life. Rapid improvement in the clinical state and disappearance of conduction defects after specific therapy is suggestive, as are certain immunological and laboratory studies (Manson-Bahr & Charters, 1963; Bertrand *et al.*, 1973; Blackett & Ngu, 1976). The condition has been recorded in the Ivory Coast, Nigeria, Cameroons, Zaire, Uganda and Kenya.

Radiologically the hearts may be normal in size (45 per cent), enlarged (34 per cent), or even small (21 per cent) according to Bertrand (1973). Left ventricular angiography shows that the small hearts have a thick wall with normal diastolic filling. When large hearts have been present with evidence of right-sided failure a pericardial effusion may be associated (Manson-Bahr & Charters, 1963).

Thus the radiological features have no specificity and the diagnosis depends on isolation of trypanosomes from the blood and a therapeutic response to appropriate drugs.

REFERENCES

Bertrand, E., Serie, F., Rive, J., Compaore, P., Sentilkes, L., Bandin, L., Ekra. A. & Philippe, J. (1963) La symtomatologie cardiovasculaire dans la trypanosomiase humaine africaine à Trypanosoma gambiense, *Annales de l'Université d'Abidjan*, **7**, 84–86.

Blackett, K. & Ngu, J. L. (1976) Immunological studies in congestive cardiomyopathy in the Cameroons, *British Heart Journal*, **38**, 605–611.

Dissanaike, A. S., Ong, H. T. & Kan, S. P. (1974) Trypanosome infections in Arang Aslis (Aborigines) in West Malaysia, *Transactions of the Royal Society of Tropical Medicine and Hygiene*, **68**, 494–495.

Manson-Bahr, P. E. C. & Charters, A. D. (1963) Myocarditis in African trypanosomiasis, *Transactions of the Royal Society of Tropical Medicine and Hygiene*, **57**, 119–121.

*Poltera, A. A., Cox, J. N. & Dwor, R. (1976) Pancarditis affecting the conducting system and all valves in human African trypanosomiasis, *British Heart Journal*, **38**, 827–837.

Shrivistava, K. K. & Shrivistava, G. P. (1974) Two cases of Trypanasoma species infection of man in India, *Transactions of the Royal Society of Tropical Medicine and Hygiene*, **68**, 3–4.

PULMONARY HYPERTENSION IN THE TROPICS

In tropical areas such common 'Western' causes of pulmonary hypertension as chronic venous embolism, industrial pollution mediated chronic lung disease, congenital high flow state in the lung vascular bed, assume proportionately less significance. Other aetiological possibilities need to be considered such as: living at a high altitude, sickle cell anaemia, packed pulmonary emboli from malignant trophoblastic disease, embolism of parasitic elements as in schistosomiasis, cardiac hydatids and bancroftian filariasis, domestic air pollution and destructive lung diseases. In India up to 30 per cent of cardiac cases have cor pulmonale and the incidence in the New Guinea highlands is also high (Woolcock & Blackburn, 1967).

REFERENCE

Woolcock, A. J. & Blackburn, C. R. B. (1967) Chronic lung disease in the territory of Papua and New Guinea; an epidemiological study, *Australasian Annals of Medicine*, **16**, 11–19.

ALTITUDE PULMONARY HYPERTENSION

Those born and living at high altitudes, as in the Andes and the Himalayas, develop adaptive changes for acclimatisation which involve the cardiorespiratory system and give rise to radiological changes. After birth infants fail to develop hypertrophy of the left ventricle so that the neo-natal right ventricular dominance remains. This is due to persistence of the foetal type of muscularised pulmonary arterioles that does not proceed to the normal involution with age typical of those living at lower heights.

The elevation of resistance in the pulmonary circuit results in far more cases of ductus arteriosus. Thus in Peru those living at 3500 to 5000 metres have 18 to 30 times greater incidence of P.D.A. than those living on the coast. At 5000 metres the incidence is 30 times greater than in coastal dwellers (W.H.O., 1965). Despite elevated pulmonary arterial pressure, functional relief usually follows closure of the shunt. Cardiomegaly may be difficult to assess by cardiothoracic ratio since those living at high levels develop lungs of greater volume and greater thoracic transverse diameters. Discussion of high altitude sickness and pulmonary oedema lies outside the scope of this discussion.

A condition termed Ayerza's disease—'cardiacos negros'—in which cor pulmonale with cyanosis developed in gold miners working in Brazilian valleys at 4250 metres altitude was probably due to the combined effects of high altitude and silicosis rather than, as once thought, to bilharzial cor pulmonale (Tidy, 1949).

REFERENCES

Tidy, H. (1949) Ayerza's disease, silicosis and pulmonary bilharziasis, *British Medical Journal*, **1**, 977–978.

World Health Organisation (1965). Washington: Pan American Health Organisation Report R.E.S./40 Annex W.H.O., 27–38.

PULMONARY HYPERTENSION—DOMESTIC AIR POLLUTION

A form of pulmonary hypertension from emphysema is seen in young women of rural areas in northern and central India but not in the south (Padmavati, 1974). The condition is believed to be related to the practice of burning cow dung cakes as fuel and the inhalation of the smoke. In the southern part of the subcontinent there is no cold winter. In the northern parts the house is closed up for warmth and the inadequate ventilation permits high levels of smoke fumes to develop.

The smoking of wrapped tobacco leaves, especially if they have been 'cured' with mineral oils (black fat tobacco), can lead to pulmonary fibrosis and eventual pulmonary hypertension and cor pulmonale (Miller *et al.*, 1971). Blackfat tobacco contains lipids that volatilise and are inhaled to condense in the lungs, and thus sets up pulmonary fibrosis. This is a problem in both sexes in Guyana, Panama, Belize, Honduras, Surinam and elsewhere in the Caribbean.

The radiological changes precede the development of symptoms. There are widely scattered ill-defined nodular densities throughout the lung fields (Fig. 5.21). Right ventricular cardiomegaly and prominence of the main pulmonary artery and hilar vessels develop later.

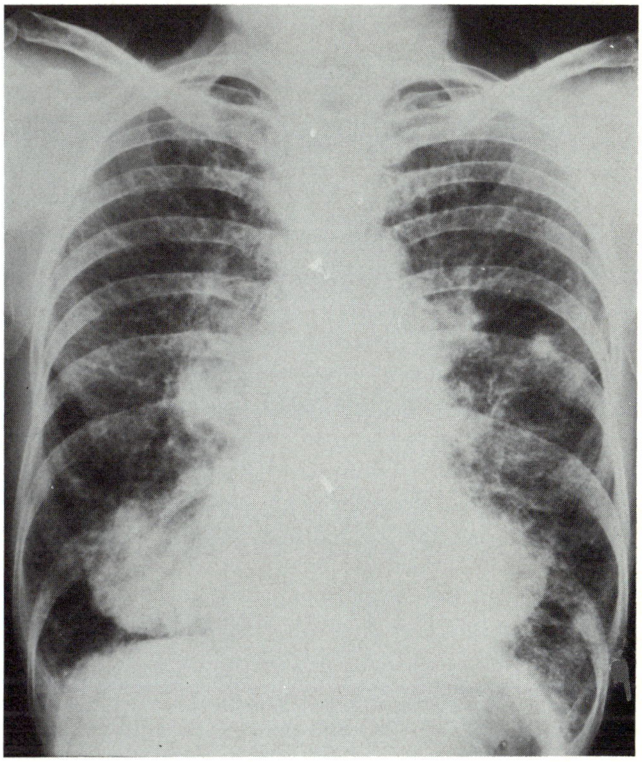

Fig. 5.21 Blackfat tobacco disease with lipid pneumonia, diffuse pulmonary fibrosis and evidence of pulmonary hypertension. (Courtesy of Dr. George G. Miller, Port of Spain, Trinidad.)

REFERENCES

Miller, G. J., Ashcroft, M. T., Bednell, H. M. S. G., Wagner, J. C. & Pepys, J. (1971) The lipoid pneumonia of blackfat tobacco smokers in Guyana, *Quarterly Journal of Medicine*, N.S. **40**, 457–470.

Padmavati, S. (1973) In *Cardio Vascular Disease in the Tropics*, pp. 291–296. London: British Medical Association.

SCHISTOSOMAL PULMONARY HYPERTENSION

The pulmonary vascular tree is vulnerable to damage from embolised ova, and less often worms, in bilharzia. The ova of paired flukes of S. haematobium lying in the perivesical, pelvic and prostatic plexuses may pass to the right side of the heart by anastamoses with the paravertebral venous system, whereas in S. mansoni and S. japonicum infections of the intestinal portal veins, entry into the vena cava and lungs must await the development of hepatic periportal fibrosis, portal hypertension and collaterals to bypass the obstructed liver vascular bed.

Live worms in the pulmonary vessels are relatively infrequent and benign, except in the case of S. japonicum infestations. By local ovideposition they can produce confluent focal granulomata that do not functionally reduce the pulmonary bed. However, should a worm die, a pronounced granulomatous reaction is set up which eventually scars and may show calcification histologically.

The eggs on the other hand are much more dangerous, not only because of their greater numbers but primarily because the contained miracidium exudes antigenic material when alive and releases even more reactive material with circulating antibodies after death and disintegration (Andrade, 1964).

Ova impact in the pulmonary arterioles and because of their mechanical and antigenic presence cause an acute necrotising arteriolitis. The ova tend to migrate out of the lumen to the perivascular tissues, focally destroying the vessel wall and resulting in perivascular fibrosis around the eggs. This process obstructs the arteriole, which may thrombose for a segment only to recanalise at a later date through fine channels, producing the so-called angiomatoid vessels. Since adjacent veins are also at times implicated, arteriovenous communications can develop through the angiomatoids dilating their lumen, which becomes nodular or cavernous. As the vascular bed is reduced the pulmonary pressure rises, and secondarily the lung arterial vessels develop medial hypertrophy and even atheroma, producing a self-perpetuating cycle. The right side of the heart hypertrophies in response to the imposed pressure load. If there are sufficient angiomatoid arteriovenous shunts peripheral arterial desaturation may ensue with cyanosis. Since there is extensive tissue reaction in the fibrous skeleton of the lung the bronchial arteries hypertrophy, due to increased flow. Because of the generalised lung vascular disintegration, anastamotic communications of oxygenated blood can develop from the bronchial systemic vessels to the pulmonary vasculature.

Histologically about a third of patients with S. mansoni infection and half of those with S. haematobium have specific lung lesions, but radiological changes are less frequent. These focal lesions are usually too small to be seen directly though small fine nodules have been attributed to their presence. One of the early signs is some redistribution of arterial flow with relative prominence of the upper lobe arteries but not of the veins. As the embolising process extends and the precapillary pressure rises, the hilar vessels become prominent, the pulmonary outflow tract enlarges and there may be some early right ventricular enlargement. This is progressive, so that the right heart is prominently enlarged in the radiograph with obvious hila, that may reach aneurysmal proportions, so that the poorly perfused peripheral lung fields stand out in contrast (Erfan & Deeb, 1949; Shafei, 1974; Bertram *et al.*, 1976) (Fig. 5.22).

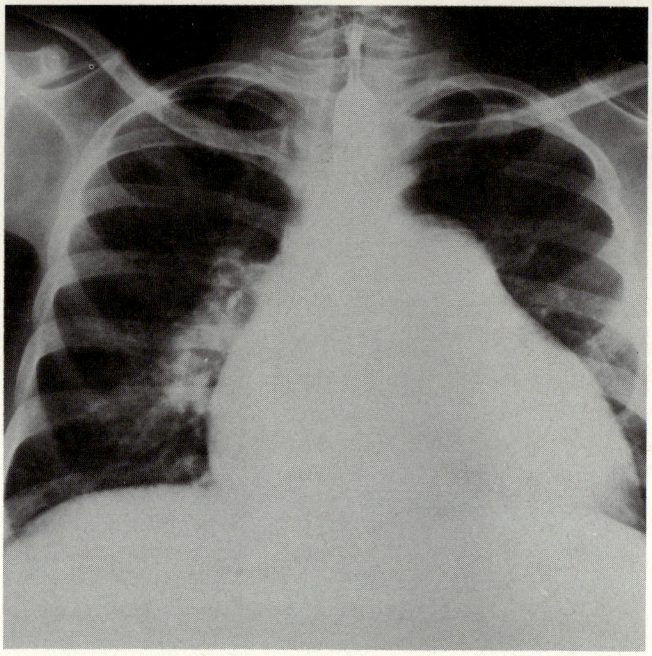

Fig. 5.22 Anterior chest film showing bulging main pulmonary artery and hila in patient with severe schistosomal pulmonary hypertension. The peripheral lung fields are oligaemic.

Pulmonary angiography serves little purpose and is hazardous in the face of severe pulmonary hypertension. When carried out at autopsy or in life it demonstrates the classic 'pruned winter tree' with loss of arborisation at about the fourth branching arterioles. Angiomatoid communication may be opacified in late films producing a nodular appearance; however, such shunts are more safely detected, as well as quantified, by isotopic means.

REFERENCES

Andrade, A. Z. (1964) Immunopathology of Manson's schistosomiasis, *Revista de Instituto de Medecina Tropical, Sao Paulo*, **6**, 181–187.

*Andrade, Z. A. & Andrade, S. G. (1970) Pathogenesis of schistosomal pulmonary arteritis, *American Journal of Tropical Medicine and Hygiene*, **19**, 305–310.

Bertrand, Ed., Dalger, Renambot, J. & Attia, Y. (1976) L'hypertension arterielle pulmonaire dans la bilharziose, *Afrique Médecine*, **15**, 537–544.

Erfan, H. & Deeb, A. A. (1949) The radiological features of chronic pulmonary schistosomiasis, *British Journal of Radiology*, **22**, 638–642.

Shafei, A. Z. (1976) Cardiovascular pulmonary schistosomiasis, *Tropical Cardiology*, **2**, 129–133.

'FILARIAL' PULMONARY HYPERTENSION

In Ceylon pulmonary hypertension is frequent, being about 15 times as common as in Britain (Obeyesereke, 1973). It develops mainly in the teens and early adult life with a female preponderance. Most patients have a chronic form of the disease with very high vascular pulmonary resistance, low cardiac outputs and severe pulmonary hypertension (120–200 mmHg). The capillary wedge pressure is normal but the right atrial pressure is elevated and the foramen ovale is patent in most cases. The latter leads to cyanosis from shunting but also serves to protect the right ventricle. When the foramen ovale remains closed a rapidly progressive fatal right-sided failure develops (Obeyesereke, 1973).

Epidemiological, haematological, histological and immunological studies suggest that filariasis is responsible (Obeyesereke & De Soysa, 1970). It is not clear whether the hypertension is a consequence of an antigenic response to microfilariae or results from their embolisation, but there does appear to be a causal relationship.

The radiological features conform to those expected from pulmonary hypertension: enlargement of the right ventricle and the right atrium, prominence of pulmonary artery and the hilar branches with translucency of the inadequately perfused lung fields. The pulmonary veins are small due to the small flow in these patients, with low output failure.

Cardiac catheterisation is dangerous in those with greatly elevated pressures.

The presence of eosinophilia, positive filarial skin test, and residence in an endemic filarial area support the diagnosis of this entity. Circulating microfilariae are not often found. This filarial aetiology of pulmonary hypertension is doubted by some workers.

REFERENCES

Obeyesereke, I. (1973) In *Cardiovascular Disease in the Tropics*, pp. 306–313. London: British Medical Association.

Obeyesereke, I. & De Soysa, N. (1970) 'Primary' pulmonary hypertension, eosinophilia and filariasis in Ceylon, *British Heart Journal*, **32**, 524–532.

PULMONARY HYPERTENSION FROM TROPHOBLASTIC TUMOURS

In much of South East Asia, the Philippines and most of Africa, where malignant trophoblastic disease is common, a severe form of dyspnoea, with pulmonary hypertension and cor pulmonale, develops acutely or in a slower fashion from tumour embolisation. This invasive fragile tumour has a propensity for venous spread and the dissemination of emboli to the lungs. Uterine curettage is a recognised cause of tumour embolism. The onset of dyspnoea is sudden and may be accompanied by cyanosis. In a series of 92 patients with malignant trophoblastic disease embolism was seen 15 times (Hendrickse *et al.*, 1965). Segmental pulmonary infarction often followed but was not a necessary consequence. Multiple small pulmonary emboli can cause significant obstruction to the pulmonary vascular bed but this can disappear with resolution of deposits and chemotherapy (Hendrickse *et al.*, 1965).

Radiologically the pulmonary hypertension usually gives rise to the traditional prominence of hilar vessels etc., but in acute packed pulmonary emboli these adaptive changes may not have time to develop. The progression of symptoms is often disproportionate to the meagre radiological changes, as these are partly masked by a concomitant high output state due to anaemia. Diagnostic difficulties are increased if a source of malignant trophoblastic disease is not suspected in the pelvis. Evidence of infarction, metastases, and pleural effusions can be of assistance (Evans *et al.*, 1965).

REFERENCES

Evans, K. T., Cockshott, W. P. & Hendrickse, J. P. de V. (1965) Pulmonary changes in malignant trophoblastic disease, *British Journal of Radiology*, **38**, 161–171.

Hendrickse, J. P. de V., Willis, A. J. P. & Evans, K. T. (1965) Acute dyspnoea with trophoblastic tumours, *Journal of Obstetrics and Gynaecology of the British Commonwealth*, **72**, 376–383.

PYOGENIC PULMONARY HYPERTENSION

Pulmonary hypertension has been recorded as a complication of Far Eastern pyogenic cholangitis due to showers of micro-emboli from the liver reaching the lungs (Lai *et al.*, 1968).

REFERENCE

Lai, K. S., MacFadzean, A. J. S. & Yeung, R. J. T. (1968) Microembolic pulmonary hypertension in pyogenic cholangitis, *British Medical Journal*, **1**, 22.

PULMONARY EMBOLISM

The incidence of venous thrombotic disease in a community generally matches that of other thrombotic disorders such as coronary thrombosis, atheroma and phlegmasia alba dolens. Where these are frequent pulmonary embolism and lung infarction constitute a significant cause of hospital morbidity and mortality. Americans and Caucasians living in Africa show an observed frequency of eight times that of Africans, matched by age and sex, for these disorders (Fisher & Nixon, 1952). Autopsy series confirm that pulmonary embolism does not occur to the same extent in Africa as in Europe and North America, though a threefold increase has been observed over a period of 21 years (Drury & Mylius, 1973). Out of 2800 autopsies in Ibadan 4·4 per cent showed evidence of pulmonary embolism, but of these 21 per cent were tumour emboli due to chorion carcinoma (Williams, 1974). Sickling is another factor that can cause lung infarcts by either segmental thrombosis or from fat and marrow emboli during a bone crisis.

In a study from Singapore Hwang (1968) found in 36 176 autopsies an incidence of 0·08 per cent of fatal pulmonary embolism overall, and 0·016 per cent in those over the age of 20. Fatal thrombo-embolism was more frequent in females and Indians were more prone than Chinese. He quotes a review of 52 861 major surgical cases operated on in Singapore with only five fatal pulmonary emboli, a rate of 0·009 per cent. This indicates an incidence over one hundred times less than some European series.

REFERENCES

Drury, R. A. B. & Mylius, E. A. (1973) The changing pattern of pulmonary embolism in Ugandan Africans, *African Journal of Medical Sciences*, **43**, 369–381.

Fisher, A. C. & Nixon, G. P. (1952) A comparison of the post-operative incidence of post-operative thromboembolism in African and European patients, *East African Medical Journal*, **29**, 186–188.

Hwang, W. S. (1968) The rarity of pulmonary thromboembolism in Asians, *Singapore Medical Journal*, **9**, 276–279.

Williams, A. O. (1974) In *Cardiovascular Disease in the Tropics*, pp. 314–322. London: British Medical Association.

CARDIAC HYDATID DISEASE

The endemic areas and biology of hydatid disease have been discussed in detail in the section on the liver.

Contributions to our knowledge of cardiac hydatids in recent years have come particularly from Francophone North Africa and France, where considerable experience has accumulated on the clinical features and the surgical management (Delahaye & Laaban, 1973).

It will be remembered that after entering the vascular bed most hexacanth embryos are arrested by the liver sinusoids or the lung capillaries, so that systemic dissemination occurs in only about 15 per cent of infections though a proportion as high as 25 per cent is reported from Baghdad (Al-Jeboori, 1976).

With vascular dissemination the heart is involved through the coronary vascular bed, so that because of its larger size the left ventricle is most often implicated. In a recent review of cardiac hydatids the left ventricle was involved in 60 per cent of cases; the right ventricle in 11 per cent; the atria each had a 6 per cent incidence; the remaining sites were pericardial, interventricular septum and pulmonary artery (Ben-Ismail *et al.*, 1975). The heart only is involved in 65 to 80 per cent of cases, with the remainder having other visceral foci in addition. In the heart the lesions are generally solitary, but multiple cardiac sites can be involved (Metras, 1976). A cyst can also spread by local vesicular extension to give rise to lesions in continuity. This process is responsible for some of the complications, notably extension from myocardium with rupture into the pericardial sac or into a cardiac chamber. The latter process of subendocardial extension develops most often from right atrial or right ventricular subendocardial lesions, since the myocardium is thin and cannot accommodate the extending cyst or cysts. Intracardiac rupture can be slow and result in embolism of cysts, causing pulmonary infarction, or with multiple emboli can lead to a very severe pulmonary hypertension. A rupture can also have immediate catastrophic effects from the immunological insult of release of hydatid contents into the circulation. In the rare left-sided intracardiac rupture the disturbances will depend on the site of lodgment of the intravascular cysts. Pericardial rupture is about a third as frequent as intracardiac.

Fortunately many of the cysts are asymptomatic. In endemic areas many cases were formerly undiagnosed as they were symptomless, but have been detected recently as a result of routine miniature mass radiography which has caused an apparent eight-fold rise in its prevalence (Ben-Ismail *et al.*, 1975).

A change in the contours of the cardiac silhouette is the most frequent radiological feature. There is a rounded elliptical bulge usually arising from the myocardium of the left ventricle. If calcification is present, usually ring calcification of the wall of the cyst, the appearance is characteristic and only has to be distinguished from calcified left ventricular annular aneurysm. Since in most areas of Black Africa where these are common there is no hydatid disease, differentiation thus is not difficult, as a rule.

A mass arising from the pulmonary artery can be difficult to recognise without angiography. This shows the mass to be avascular and the lumen may be seen to be compromised. At catheterisation a gradient can be detected (Ben-Ismail *et al.*, 1975; Metras, 1976).

Angiography should always be done, as beside the obvious focus other lesions not deforming the contours can be detected. This is of importance when planning open heart surgery, so that all lesions are removed.

Coronary angiography has been used by several workers to show the extent of the deposits. The vessels are stretched around the cyst and the affected area is seen not to be perfused.

The electrocardiographic changes are variable, depending on the location of the lesions. The complement fixation test is positive in about 25 per cent of cases.

Since cardiac hydatid disease can have such serious complications and surgery is proving successful, cases should have the benefits of adequate angiographic study to determine the full extent of the disease.

REFERENCES

Al-Jeboori, T. (1976) Hydatid disease: a study of the records of the Medical City Hospital, *Journal of the Faculty of Medicine, Baghdad*, **18**, 65–75.

Ben-Ismail, M., Fourati, M., Bousnina, A. & Lacronique, J. (1975) Le Kyste hydatique du cœur, *Tropical Cardiology*, **1**, 187–199.

Delahaye, R. P. & Laaban, J. (1973) *Radiologie Tropicale et Parasitaire*, pp. 201–204. Neuchatel: Delachaux & Niestle, S.A.

Metras, D. (1976) Le Kyste hydatique du cœur. *Tropical Cardiology*, **2**, 197–198.

CARDIAC BURKITT'S LYMPHOMA

Thirty-two per cent of patients dying from Burkitt's lymphoma have cardiac deposits. Obviously the incidence of such cardiac malignancy is lower at the time of presentation than at the terminal phase of the neoplasia. At autopsy tumour deposits may be found to infiltrate the pericardium, obliterate the pericardial cavity to encase the heart, or may form discrete nodular foci in the myocardium (Lothe & Somers, 1960).

In nine cases of cardiac involvement enlarged mediastinal glands were present in every instance. In a survey of chest radiographs obtained from 69 consecutive cases of Burkitt's, mediastinal enlargement or frank adenopathy

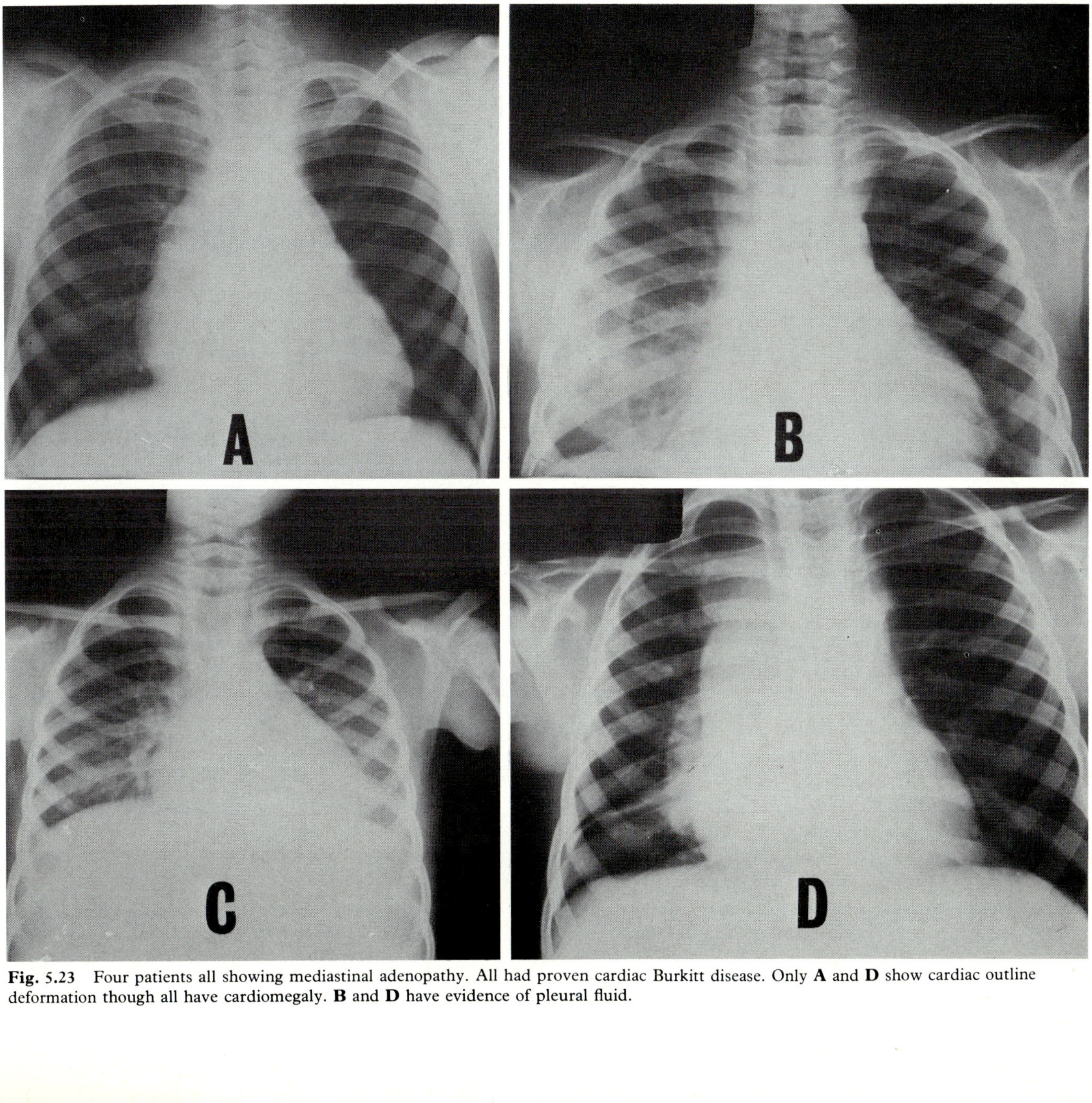

Fig. 5.23 Four patients all showing mediastinal adenopathy. All had proven cardiac Burkitt disease. Only **A** and **D** show cardiac outline deformation though all have cardiomegaly. **B** and **D** have evidence of pleural fluid.

was detected in eleven (Cockshott, 1964). Subsequently the nine autopsied cases had heart and mediastinal involvement. Thus it is probably valid to assume the presence of cardiac deposits when there is radiographic mediastinal enlargement (Fig. 5.23).

In addition to the mediastinal changes cardiomegaly and pleural effusions were both twice demonstrated in this series. Five examples of pleural effusions were seen but there was no evidence of any pulmonary involvement. The rarity of this radiological feature is in accord with the infrequency of lung involvement at necropsy.

REFERENCES

Cockshott, W. P. (1964) In *Symposium Lymphoreticular Tumours in Africa*, pp. 151–162. Basle: S. Karger.

Lothe, F. & Somers, K. (1960) Secondary tumors of the heart and pericardium in Uganda Africans, *Archives of Pathology*, **69**, 158–167.

PERICARDIAL DISEASES

Pericardial effusions can form in a considerable variety of conditions. In some tropical areas there are specific causes with a high prevalence, such as purulent pericarditis, tuberculosis and amoebic pericarditis (Assomoi *et al.*, 1975). In addition pericardial fluid collections may accompany right-sided endomyocardial fibrosis, rheumatic heart disease and possibly African trypanosomal heart disease (Manson-Bahr & Charters, 1963).

The clinical and radiological diagnosis of both acute and chronic pericardial disease can be very difficult, particularly as ultrasound facilities are not commonly available in non-industrialised countries.

A valuable, but rarely available help, is the presence of serial films documenting a rapid change of cardiac silhouette, particularly if accompanied by oligaemic lung fields due to scanty vasculature from the low cardiac output. Pneumonic consolidation may be an indicator towards pyogenic pericarditis. Since a large globular cardiac silhouette with oligaemic lung fields due to low cardiac output characterises some cardiopathies, particularly right-sided E.M.F., these radiographic features are not specific.

Fluoroscopy can be disappointing, as in cardiomyopathies the cardiac excursions can be of low amplitude and the bulging right atrium may change shape with position in a similar manner to pericardial fluid. To compound the problem in inflammatory collections the epicardial fat becomes oedematous and no longer radiologically evident as a translucent line in the A.V. groove during lateral fluoroscopy. Furthermore in many patients epicardial fat is scanty, so that this usually reliable sign of pericardial fluid has limited value.

When there is doubt it may be important to resolve the problem as to what should be done. Opacification of the right atrium by an intravenous bolus of iodinated contrast, or passage of an opaque catheter into the right atrium, can be useful procedures to determine whether the introduced material extends to the right lateral cardiac border. But often the time and the facilities do not permit such studies.

Pericardial tapping is of value in obtaining the specific diagnosis and therapeutically is a valid diagnostic technique. After the tap the injection of a small amount of air (20 ml) and the taking of a view of the right atrium with a horizontal beam with the patient lying on the left side

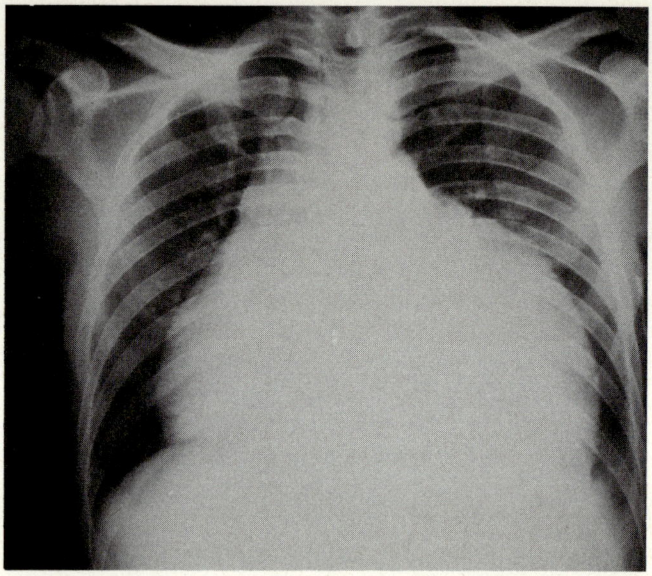

Fig. 5.24 Gross cardiac contour enlargement following rupture of a left lobe of liver, amoebic abscess and development of amoebic pericarditis.

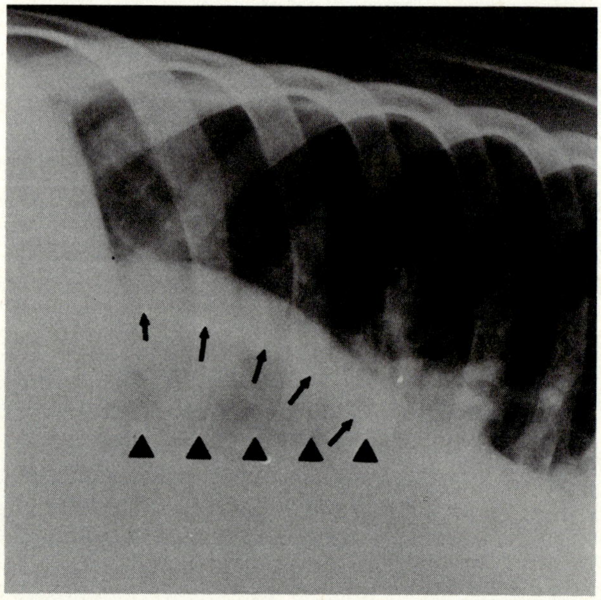

Fig. 5.25 Diagnostic pneumopericardium. Film taken with horizontal beam demonstrates fluid level and the thickened pericardial wall—arrows indicate medial aspect of thickened pericardium, black triangles the fluid level.

(left lateral decubitus) will demonstrate whether the pericardium is thickened or not (Fig. 5.12).

Purulent pericarditis, particularly staphylococcal, is not rare in West or East Africa. Amoebic pericarditis is classically due to rupture of a left hepatic lobe abscess but can occur in right-sided disease (Fig. 5.24). Later constriction is frequent in amoebic pericarditis (Faerber *et al.*, 1974).

Tuberculous pericarditis often shows a thick pericardial wall (Fig. 5.25). Later pericardial calcification is common, but is not specific to tuberculosis. In a significant proportion of patients with pericardial thickening or calcification the aetiology may never be clearly established.

Tropical splenic abscesses—often initially sterile infarcts of the spleen in sickle cell haemoglobinopathy—may rupture into the pericardium to produce a striking pneumopericardium (Fig. 3.63).

REFERENCES

Assamoi, O. D., Thomas, J. J., LeBras, M. & Bertrand, E. (1975) Les pericardites purulentes à Abidjan, *Tropical Cardiology*, **1**, 15–26.

Faerber, E. N., Segal, F. & Sischy, N. L. (1974) Amoebic pericarditis, *British Journal of Radiology*, 47, 816–818.

Manson-Bahr, P. E. C. & Charters, A. D. (1963) Myocarditis in African trypanosomiasis, *Transactions of the Royal Society of Tropical Medicine & Hygiene*, 57, 119–121.

AORTIC PAN ARTERITIS TAKAYASHU'S DISEASE, MIDDLE AORTIC SYNDROME, AORTIC ARCH SYNDROME

Though atheroma exists throughout the tropical world, it is commonly less advanced than in Europe or North America in all age groups. Throughout much of the tropical world a segmental inflammatory aortitis is far more frequent than in temperate and cold climates, and assumes greater importance. Unlike degenerative vascular disease, this is a disorder of the young and predominantly of females. The various clinical syndromes that ensue are determined by the anatomical localisation and the stage of the disease.

Originally this disease was described in Japan and became known as Takayashu or pulseless disease. The disease affected young women by obliterating one or more of the brachiocephalic vessels and their main branches. In the last three decades an extensive literature indicates that the original concept was too restrictive, since the thoracic and abdominal aorta and the iliac vessels and their primary branches can also be affected. At least 80 per cent of patients are female. The condition can begin in the first decade but onset is most frequent between the ages of 15 to 25.

Many reports come from under-doctored areas, so it is probable that the real prevalence is higher than the published figures would indicate.

In the East the condition is reported from Japan, China, Malaysia, Indonesia, the Philippines, and India (Danaraj & Wong, 1959; Inada *et al.*, 1962; Sen *et al.*, 1963). Reports have come from many parts of Africa; South Africa, Central Africa and all of West Africa, North Africa and to a lesser extent East Africa (Collomb, 1961; Abrahams & Cockshott, 1962; Joffe, 1965; Ben Naceur *et al.*, 1971). The disease exists in North, Central and South America (Lupi-Herrera, 1977). In Europe reports have been widely scattered (Gillanders & Strachan, 1965; Boely, 1969). Eskimo have been recorded with the disease (Steiness, 1965).

We have seen cases in Brazil, the West Indies, Ethiopia, Kuwait, Yemen, Singapore and Hong Kong, in addition to the areas already mentioned.

The multiracial prevalence and the global distribution make it difficult to conceive of any unifying genetic or environmental causative factor. The disease is inflammatory and not due to syphilis. In many reported cases from the tropics patients have shown evidence of tuberculosis, but this appears to be a casual rather than a causal association. Tuberculous arteritis is a well-defined entity that differs in several respects from primary arteritis. Yaws and syphilis have been aetiologically excluded. It is also probably distinct from temporal and giant cell arteritis, which mainly affects medium-sized vessels. An auto-immune disturbance has been suggested, particularly as circulating anti-aorta antibodies are present. High levels of IgG, IgM and IgA are also reported. North African cases have shown abnormally high rickettsial titres in about 90 per cent of their patients. However, the significance of this is uncertain (Comte *et al.*, 1960; Delande, 1963). Nematodes have also been suggested as causal agents (Munoz & Correa, 1970). Thus though a lot of data has accumulated in the last 120 years since the disease was first described, the cause remains speculative.

The pathologist rarely sees the early acute phase of the disease, though through angiography the radiologist may do so. The early change is in the adventitia, which becomes inflamed with round cell infiltration and an occlusive endarteritis of the vasa vasorum. This then results in a destructive process in which the media and elastic tissue are disturbed so that localised blow-out outpouchings or fusiform dilatations develop. The intima becomes thickened, and damaged so that mural thrombus formation takes place or obliterative thrombosis. The cicatrisation repair process may be followed by calcification in the vessel wall, readily evident in radiographs.

The clinical disturbances depend on the severity of the process, the anatomic location and the collateral circulation. The diagram indicates the main clinical locations and the resulting symptoms (Fig. 5.26). Patients initially show systemic disturbances and possibly fever. Absent pulses and vascular bruits are usual. Systemic hypertension from renal artery involvement and pulmonary hypertension from pulmonary arterial disease may cause heart failure.

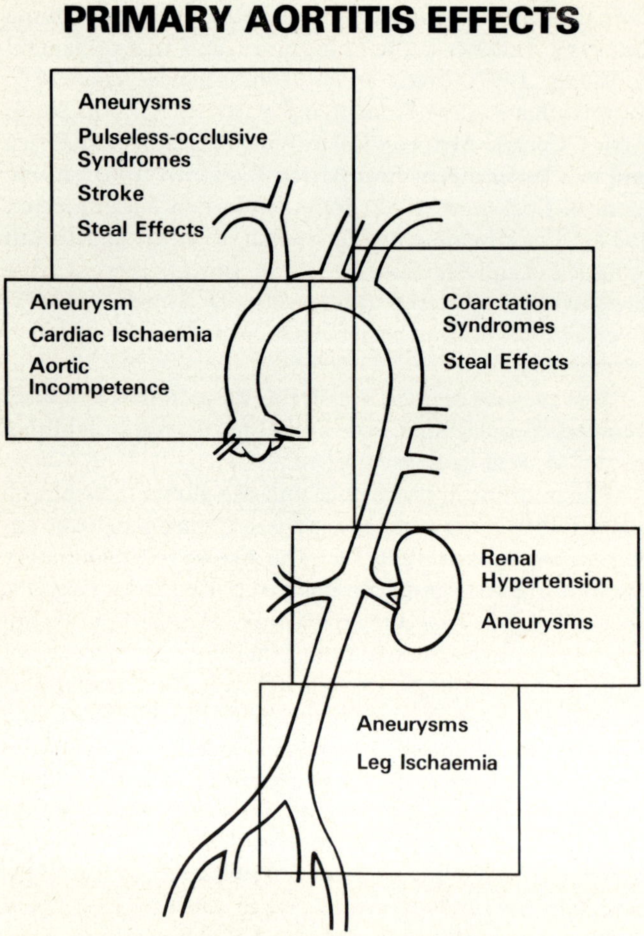

Fig. 5.26 Diagrammatic representation of syndromes due to lesions of primary aortitis according to anatomic sites of involvement.

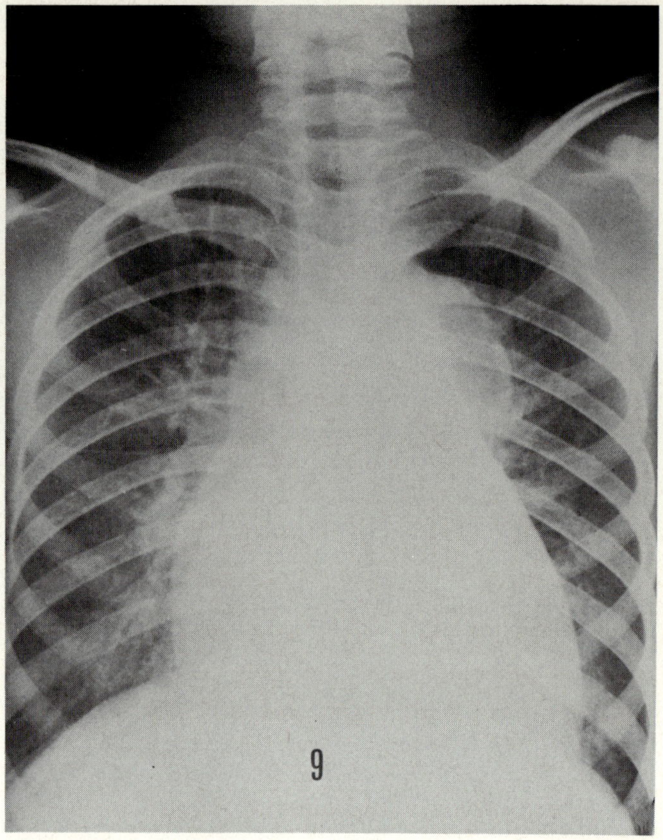

Fig. 5.27 Nine-year-old Nigerian girl showing cardiomegaly and gross widening of ascending arch and descending aorta. Hypertension and absence of left arm pulse were present.

Neurological symptoms result from cephalic vessel disease or implication of the spinal vessels at their origin.

Plain chest films may show in the acute phase a widened irregular aortic outline in the arch or descending portion (Fig. 5.27). In the chronic stage the aortic arch and even ascending aorta can be grossly dilated with intramural calcification (Fig. 5.28). Sometimes a degree of aortic valve incompetence may develop. About half the cases show cardiac enlargement, which is due to left ventricular hypertrophy in the majority. If pulmonary hypertension is present the right ventricle can be enlarged. In the lung fields there may be obvious segmental, patchy oligaemia. Pulmonary arterial disease can be functionally confirmed by lung scans and precisely delineated by angiography. In addition rib notching from collaterals is present in about 5 per cent of cases. Evidence of old or active tuberculosis should be sought.

Angiography may be difficult, particularly in children in the acute phase, as multiple pulses may be deficient. Since multiple segments are generally involved the whole of the aorta needs to be studied. Pulmonary angiography is rarely indicated. Since there is no specific therapy angiography is not necessary in every case. However, it is useful to explain hypertension, arm claudication, cerebral ischaemic attacks or strokes, and some instances of heart failure in children and young adults, particularly in females.

The ascending aorta and arch are implicated in about a quarter of patients and the descending aorta in two-thirds (Lupi-Herrera, 1977). The subclavian artery is the most frequent focus, being involved in over 80 per cent, followed by the renal vessels in about 60 per cent of cases (Lupi-Herrera, 1977). In the angiogram the process is often shown to be multifocal with perhaps subclavian or brachiocephalic or vertebral thrombosis and aneurysm formation or narrowing at the level of the renal vessels (Figs. 5.29 and 5.30). Steal syndromes and collaterals may be shown in late films. Often the disease shows exacerbation with new areas of occlusion or stenosis developing.

The frequency of hypertension in this disease, particularly in the young, needs emphasising. The series of Golding *et al.* (1977) contains 14 hypertensive children in a series of 18 with the disorder, and highlights this particular aspect.

The intravenous pyelogram when abnormal may show diminution in the size of one or both kidneys. Classical delay in the appearance of contrast and later increase in density of the collecting system may be present in predominantly unilateral disease.

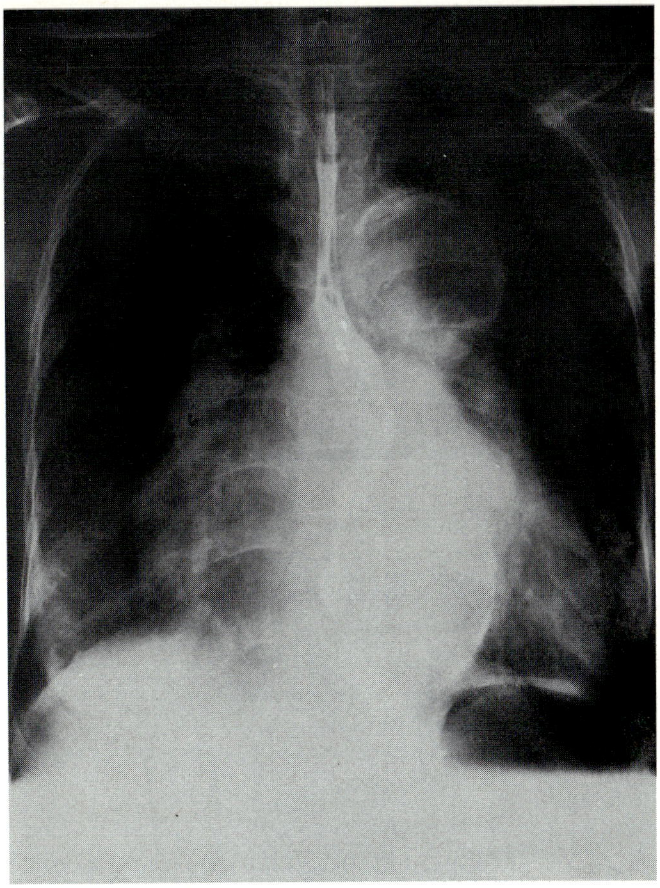

Fig. 5.28 Penetrated film with barium in oesophagus of an adult Nigerian female. Note greatly dilated aorta outlined by calcification in wall and by deviation of eosophagus. 'Healed' stage of primary aortitis.

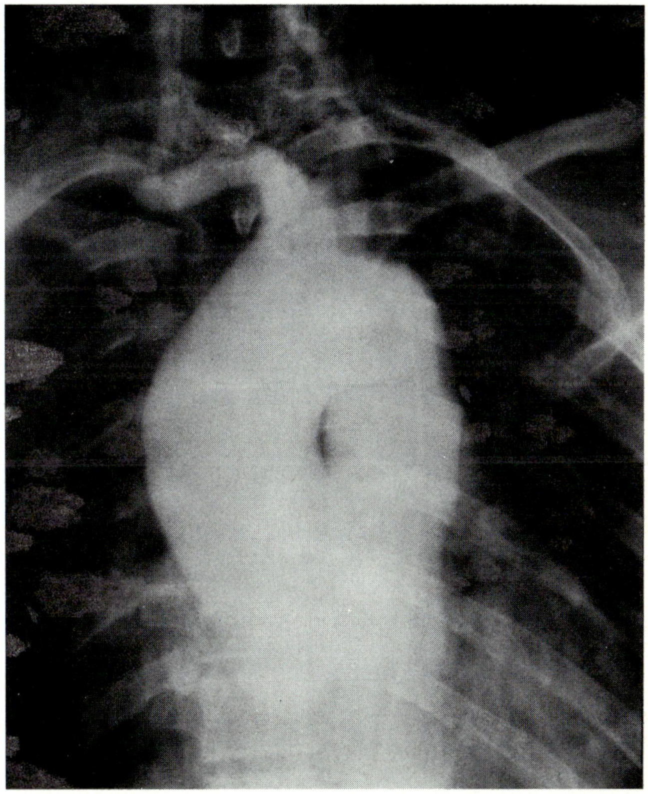

Fig. 5.29 'Pulseless syndrome' in 18-year-old female with absence of left subclavian artery and right carotid artery. Aorta is diffusely dilated and shows some luminal irregularity in descending portion. (Courtesy of Prof. Brian Cremin, Cape Town.)

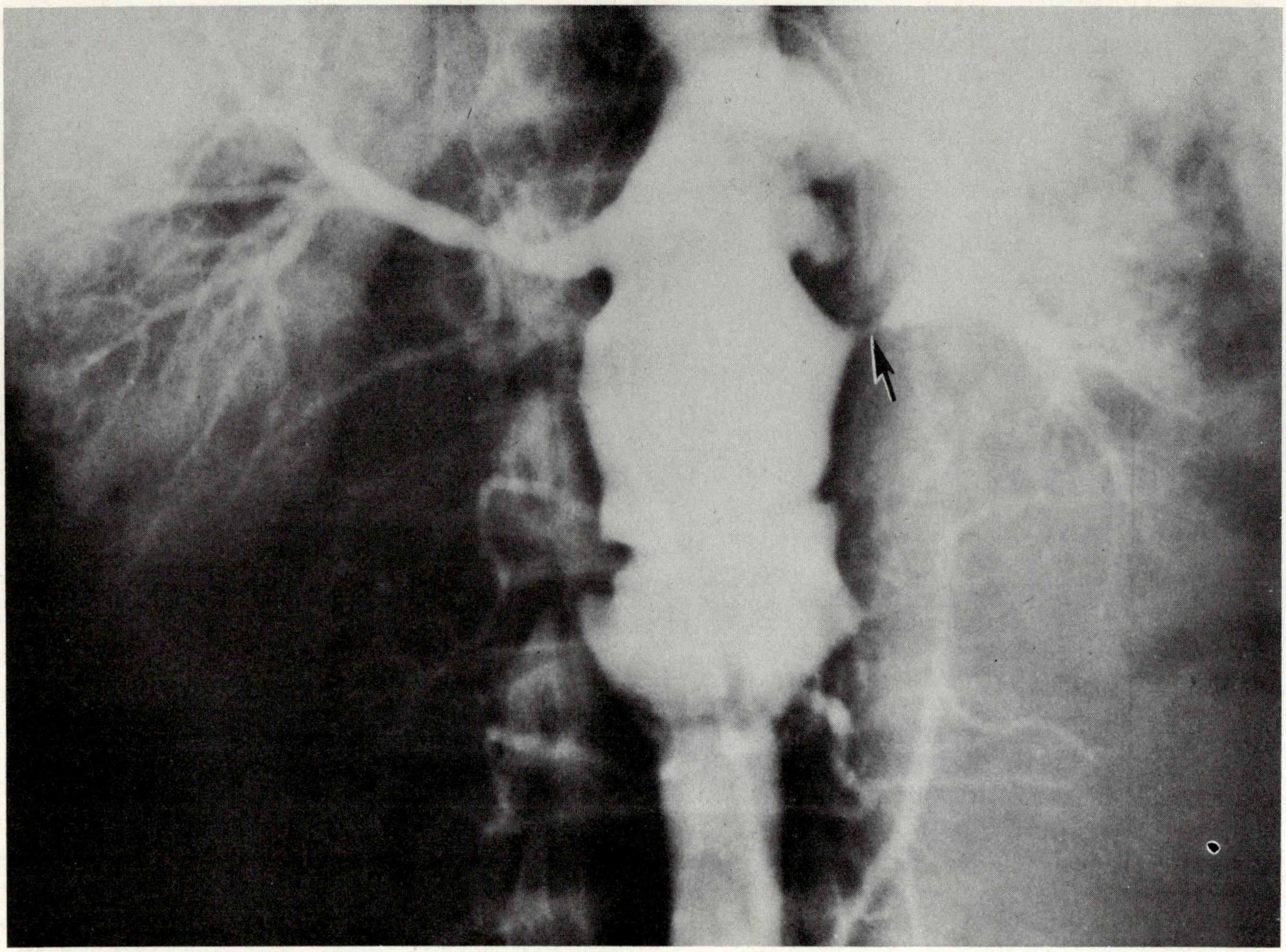

Fig. 5.30 Nigerian male youth who had an inominate aneurysm and severe hypertension. The upper abdominal aorta is diffusely involved with bizarre aneurysmal formation. Both renal arteries are implicated. There is severe stenosis of the left renal artery (arrow).

If drug treatment of hypertension fails, nephrectomy may help in unilateral disease. Bypass surgery is seldom done, as there is usually loss of patency from progression of the disease. The nature of the stenosing aortitis described by Gajaraj and colleagues (1977) is uncertain, because peri-aortic lymphadenitis was a prominent feature and was considered to be the cause of extrinsic pressure. There was no proof that tuberculosis was to blame and the process differs from tuberculous aortitis. Eleven cases of this disorder were seen in two years in Madras. Removal of chronically inflamed lymph nodes and perivascular scar tissue appears to provide relief.

REFERENCES

Abrahams, D. G. & Cockshott, W. P. (1962) Multiple non-luetic aneurysms in young Nigerians, *British Heart Journal*, **24,** 83–91.

Ben Naceur, M., Houissa, D., Maamouri, T., Hafsia, M. & Dite, B. (1972) Les Artériopathies tronculaire non athéroscléreuses, *Archives Maladie du Cœur*, **5,** 607–622.

Boely, C. (1969) Syndrome de Takayashu ou la maladie des gens sans pouls, *Presse Médicale*, **67,** 287–298.

Collomb, M., Philippe, Y. & Dumas (1961) Maladie de l'arc aortique, *Bulletin Médicine d'Afrique Noire*, **6,** 331–336.

Comte, H., Martin, L. A. & Quradou, J. A. (1960) A propos de 42 cas d'artérite dite juvenile, *Archives Institut Pasteur du Maroc*, **6,** 85–102.

Danaraj, T. J. & Wong, H. O. (1959) Primary arteritis of abdominal aorta in children causing bilateral stenosis of renal arteries and hypertension, *Circulation*, **20,** 856–863.

Delande, G. (1973) Sur le rôle des Rickettsioses atypique ou méconnues dans la pathologie vasculaire, *Semaine des hôpitaux de Paris*, 39–40.

Gajaraj, A., Victor, S. Aswathaman, A. S. & Ahmed, Q. (1977) Obscure stenosing aortitis and arteritis associated with perivascular lymphadenitis, *Clinical Radiology*, **28,** 555–559.

Gillanders, L. A. & Strachan, R. W. (1965) The role of radiology in the diagnosis of Takayasu's arteriopathy, *Clinical Radiology*, **16,** 119–129.

Golding, R. L., Perri, G. & Cremin, B. J. (1977) The arteriographic manifestations of Takayasu's arteritis in children, *Paediatric Radiology*, **5,** 224–230.

Inada, K., Shimuzu, M., Kobayashi, I. & Kawamoto, S. (1962) Pulseless disease and atypical coarction of the aorta, *Archives of Surgery*, **84,** 306–311.

Joffe, N. (1965) Aortitis of obscure origin in the African, *Clinical Radiology*, **16,** 130–140.

Lupi-Herrera, L., Sanchez-Torres, G., Marcushamer, J., Misperita, J., Horwitz, S. & Vela, J. E. (1977) Takayasu's arteritis. Clinical study of 107 cases, *American Heart Journal*, **93,** 94–103.

Munoz, N. & Correa, P. (1970) Arteritis of the aorta and its major branches, *American Heart Journal*, **80,** 319–328.

Rose, A. G. & Forman, R. (1976) Idiopathic aortitis with calcification of ascending aorta and aortic and mitral valve, *British Heart Journal*, **38**, 650–652.
Sen, P. K., Kinare, S. G., Engineer, S. D. & Parulkar, G. B. (1963) The middle aortic syndrome, *British Heart Journal*, **25**, 610–618.
Steiness, I. (1965) Hypertension due to renal artery obstruction in Eskimo girl, *British Heart Journal*, **2**, 1291.

TUBERCULOUS AORTITIS AND ANEURYSMS

Tuberculous aortitis can develop by two routes: haematogenous and by contiguity from caseating lymph nodes. Whichever way the organism reaches the aorta a focal granuloma is set up in the wall, which becomes weakened and may begin to bulge. When the process reaches the intima and ulcerates into the lumen the affected area is subject to systemic pressure, and in over half the cases a false aneurysm develops with a fibrous and granulomatous wall. Dissection and rupture are less frequent outcomes (Meehan *et al.*, 1957; German & Green, 1956). The condition is a well-defined entity (Neumann, 1952).

The aortic arch is sometimes involved, but the descending portion is the site of predilection in the thorax, probably because of the close relationship to the left hilar glands. Abdominal aneurysm also may develop. The inferior vena cava can become involved by continuity.

The condition may be suspected in a chest film if comparison with previous studies indicates a changed contour appearance of the aorta, which may be noted in the anterior or left oblique position. Needless to say it may be difficult to exclude primary aortic arteritis, particularly as most cases occur in the same young age group and evidence of pulmonary tuberculosis may be evident in both. Confusion with a developing mediastinal mass with the appearances of bronchial carcinoma has occurred (Myers, 1965).

Lesions of the abdominal aorta pose even greater diagnostic problems unless an older patient has displacement of calcified atheromatous plaques. A clinical suspicion of the presence of a tuberculous aneurysm may be entertained if the patient is of an age where degenerative disease is unlikely and he also has fever and other systemic disturbances.

Angiography has assumed importance in some centres as a prelude to surgery now that resection is possible (Kline & Durant, 1951). The position and extent of the aneurysm can usually be well demonstrated (Fig. 5.31) (Scully & McNeely, 1975).

REFERENCES

German, J. L. & Green, C. L. (1956) Fatal rupture of a tuberculous aortic aneurysm: a case report, *Annals of Internal Medicine*, **45**, 698–702.
Kline, J. L. & Durant, J. (1961) Surgical resection of a tuberculous aneurysm of the ascending aorta, *New England Journal of Medicine*, **265**, 1185–1187.
Meehan, J. J., Pastor, B. H. & Torre, A. V. (1957) Dissecting aneurysm of the aorta secondary to tuberculous aortitis, *Circulation*, **16**, 615–620.
Myers, L. F. (1965) Tuberculous aneurysm of the aorta simulating bronchogenic carcinoma, *South African Medical Journal*, **39**, 403–404.
Neumann, M. E. (1952) Tuberculous lesions of the circulatory system, *American Journal of Pathology*, **28**, 919–929.
Penn, I. (1962) Tuberculous aneurysm of the abdominal aorta, *British Journal of Surgery*, **50**, 288–290.
Scully, R. E. & McNeely, B. U. (1975) Case records of the Massachusetts General Hospital, *New England Journal of Medicine*, **292**, 579–586.

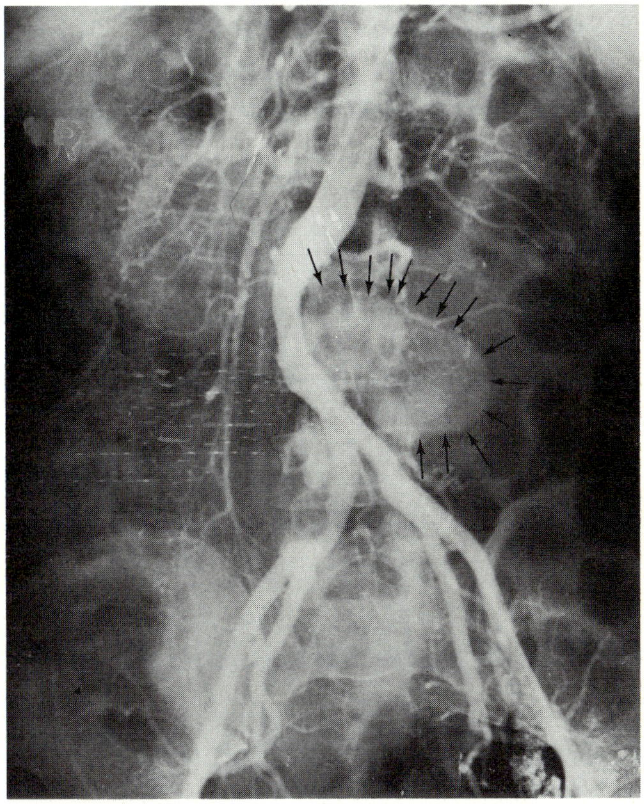

Fig. 5.31 Aortic displacement by tuberculous aortic aneurysm (arrowed). There is also some disruption of the right common iliac artery. (Courtesy of Prof. T. Kolawole, Ibadan.)

IDIOPATHIC PERIPHERAL GANGRENE

Reports from Rhodesia, Zambia, Nigeria, Kenya, Rwanda and Uganda describe patients who have acutely developed symmetric gangrene of the lower limbs, less often the upper and sometimes all four limbs. Males are more affected than females. Paediatric cases are common, but in one series the peak incidence was in the third and fourth decades (Steiner & Hutt, 1972).

Clinically the main pulses are normal and in those with only part of the fingers or toes affected digital vessel pulsation is detectable. A spontaneous line of separation forms between necrotic and healthy tissue. The level may be merely the tip of digits, all the fingers or toes, or sometimes amputation above the wrist and ankles.

Depression of plasma fibrinolytic activity due to increased levels of fibrinolytic inhibitors was noted in three young Kenyans by Turpie *et al.* (1967). Effects of cold agglutinins or drugs such as ergot have been excluded as aetiologic factors. Steiner and Hutt (1972) have shown histologically in their 14 cases mucoid swelling of all three layers of the implicated vessels, intimal hyperplasia and depositis of mucopolysaccharides in the intima and media. The process starts in the feeding artery or arterioles, with veins also being involved in a similar process which indicates a systemic disturbance.

Arteriography shows normal major vessels and muscular branches above the area of gangrene and as expected no distal perfusion or run-off.

There is an endemic ischaemic condition in Taiwan affecting the feet and progressing to gangrene. Though these individuals may have atherosclerosis the entity has been related to chronic arsenic intoxication from the water supply (Yeh & How, 1963).

REFERENCES

Steiner, I. O. & Hutt, M. S. R. (1972) Vascular changes in the idopathic peripheral gangrene of the tropics, *Tropical and Geographic Medicine*, **24**, 219–225.

Turpie, A. G. G., Forbes, C. D. & McNicol, G. P. (1967) Idiopathic gangrene in African children, *British Medical Journal*, **2**, 646–648.

Yeh, S. & How, S. W. (1963) A pathological study of the blackfoot disease in Taiwan, *Reports Institute of Pathology, National Taiwan University*, **14**, 25.

THROMBO-ANGIITIS OBLITERANS (T.A.O.) (BUERGER'S DISEASE)

Joginder Singh

Leo Buerger in 1908 suggested the name thrombo-angiitis obliterans for a peripheral arterial disease he had observed, but gave due credit to earlier workers who had described this disease under other names. Buerger extensively studied this disorder (1908, 1924) that has since become a distinct clinical entity by which he has been eponymously commemorated. This chronic occlusive disease of the peripheral arteries is for some unknown reason rare in the West today but is prevalent in Japan, Korea, India and South East Asia (Lambeth *et al.*, 1970). It was initially considered that the disease had a predilection for Jews of deprived economic circumstances who had migrated to the United States. Time has shown that Buerger's disease is not restricted to Jews, as it has been described in many ethnic groups throughout the world (Noble, 1931; Ishikawa *et al.*, 1962). Since the disease has become infrequent in the West some have questioned its existence. Wessler and his colleagues (1960) attempted to show that the pathologic changes in Buerger's disease were indistinguishable from those produced by atherosclerosis, embolism or thrombosis. However, strong evidence in support of it being a separate entity has come from workers who have studied the distinguishing clinical, early histopathological and arteriographic changes (McKusick *et al.*, 1962). The aetiologic and pathogenetic mechanism are still not well understood. This peripheral vascular disease often occurs in a setting where atherosclerotic disease and thrombo-embolic disease are infrequent (Horwitz, 1961).

Symptoms from peripheral limb ischemia affecting predominantly the feet, and in some cases the hands, is the usual presentation. In the foot the digits affected are mainly the big, second and the little toes, whereas in the hand the index and the middle fingers are most commonly affected. It is a disease found primarily in young male cigarette smokers between the ages of 20 to 45 years with a mean age of onset of 32 years. Women and non-smokers are rarely affected, though sporadic cases have been reported. No association with diabetes mellitus, hypercholesterolaemia or heart disease has been detected. Whatever is the underlying cause of this disease, prolonged smoking is an inevitable association. Failure to improve under treatment has been noted in patients who have continued to smoke, whereas prompt improvement is noticed in those who have abstained from smoking. Remissions and relapses are related to smoking, which can lead to amputation.

Peripheral arteriography establishes the presence of this disease. The arterial pattern is characteristic and has only to be differentiated from atherosclerosis in some cases. No calcium is visualised in the vessel walls on plain radiographs and the lumen is smooth and regular. Occlusion of the arteries is abrupt; the most common site in the lower extremities is the femoropopliteal segment at or above the adductor canal or in the popliteal fossa. Collateral vessels producing a tree root or a spider leg configuration together with several 'corkscrew' vessels form a very characteristic pattern. The anterior tibial artery is commonly affected and becomes occluded and narrowed close to its origin (Fig. 5.32).

In the upper extremities the most common site of occlusion is in the digital vessels. Occlusive changes in the radial and the ulnar arteries are next in frequency. It is interesting to note that the interosseus artery is rarely involved. Collateral vessels are not as abundant as with the lower extremities.

In Malaysia Buerger's disease is prevalent among rubber tappers, farmers, gardeners, fishermen, truck and taxi drivers. Similar observations were recorded by Noble in Siam in 1931. The tasks of these outdoor workers involve considerable stretching of the leg muscles over long hours. The popliteal artery after leaving the adductor canal enters a fibrous tunnel derived from the fascia on the deep surface of the gastrocnemius, and it is also overlapped by

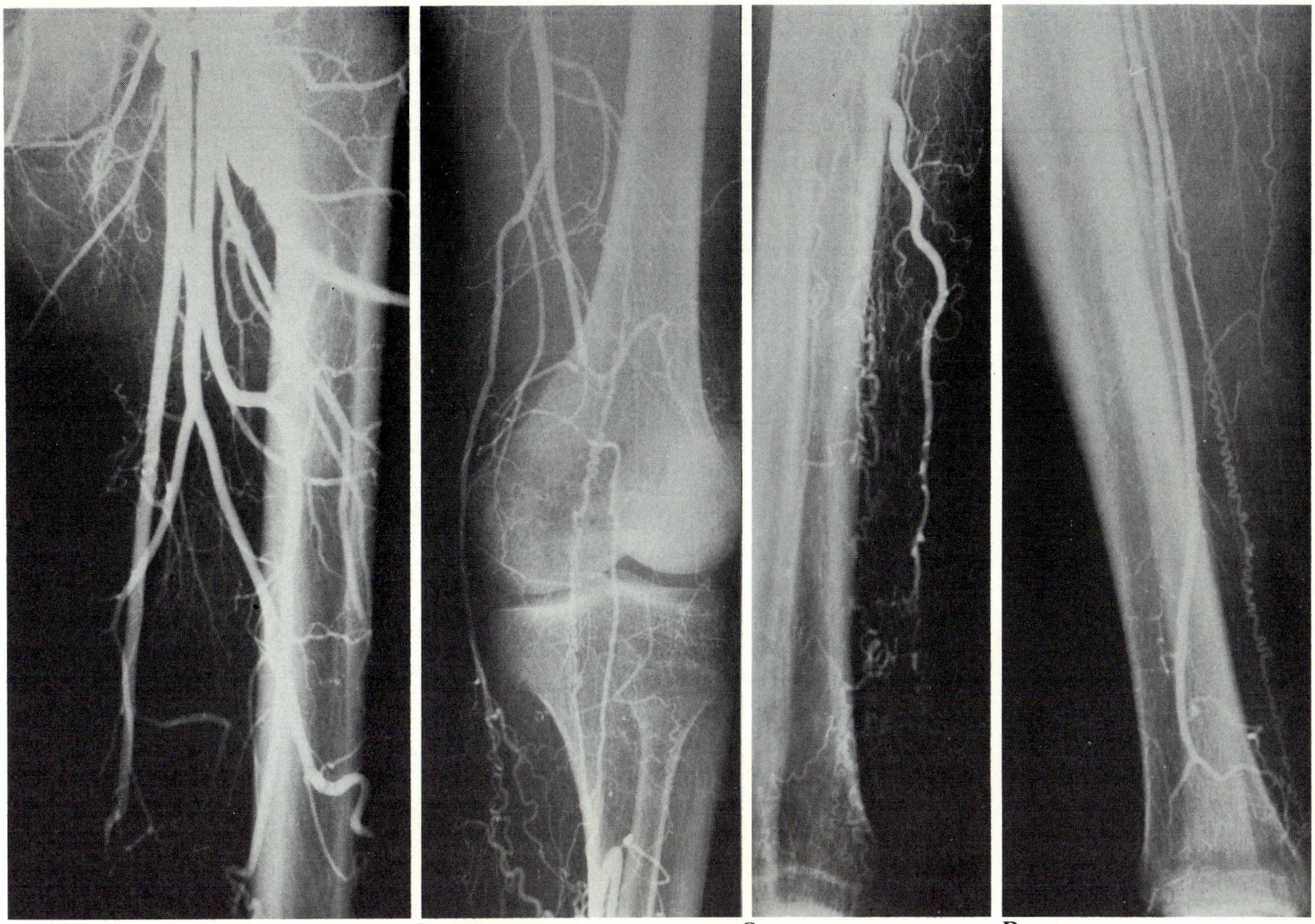

A B C D

Fig. 5.32 A–D. Femoral arteriograms in two Malaysian patients showing absence of luminal irregularities in Buerger's disease and the corkscrew collaterals providing 'run-off' distal to blocks.

the heads of the gastrocnemius muscle. In maximal plantar flexion or passive overstretching by dorsiflexion of the foot the popliteal artery has a tendency to be compressed and the peripheral pulses diminish. Perhaps it is the prolonged trapping of the popliteal artery by overstretched muscles of these active outdoor workers that provides continual trauma to the artery leading to thrombus formation. Tobacco smoking produces the vasoconstriction and thus stasis of blood could occur. These factors may explain why the femoropopliteal region of the artery is so commonly involved, and explain the rarity of interosseous artery involvement, since in its location in the forearm it is spared from the squeezing action of muscles. In atherosclerotic disease of the peripheral arteries the femoropopliteal segment is also a common site of occlusion.

The histologic features reveal organised recanalised thrombi with preservation of the architecture of the vessel walls. There also appears to be fusion between arteries and veins and at times envelopment of nerves with fibrous tissue.

Treatment is still unsatisfactory. Amputations and sympathectomies are still the commonest forms of surgery offered. Initial results in some patients are encouraging. Direct arterial surgery has been attempted in selected cases. Irrespective of the procedure used the long-term patency of the graft has been unsatisfactory, though initially there is often relief of symptoms. Perhaps direct arterial surgery has a role in delaying and limiting the severity of amputations. Serial arteriograms over a number of years in asymptomatic patients reveal little change in patients who have abstained from tobacco. It appears therefore that in a number of patients with Buerger's disease once the acute period of symptoms is arrested the condition does not progress as long as there is no smoking.

REFERENCES

Buerger, L. (1908) Thrombo-angiitis obliterans. Study of vascular lesions leading to presenile spontaneous gangrene, *American Journal Medical Sciences*, **136**, 567–580.

Buerger, L. (1924) *The Circulatory Disturbances of the Extremities: Including Gangrene, Vasomotor and Trophic Disorders*. p. 277. Philadelphia: W. B. Saunders Co.

Horwitz, O. (1961) Buerger's disease retrieved, *Annals of Internal Medicine*, **55**, 341–344.

Ishikawa, K., Kawase, S. & Mishima, Y. (1962) Occlusive arterial disease in extremities with special reference to Buerger's disease, *Angiology*, **13**, 398–411.

Lambeth, J. T. & Yong, Ñ. K. (1970) Arteriographic findings in thrombo-angiitis obliterans, *American Journal of Roentgenology*, **109**, 553–562.

McKusick, V. A., Harris, W. S., Ottesen, O. E., Goodman, R. M., Shelley, W. M. & Bloodwell, R. D. (1962) Buerger's disease: a distinct clinical and pathologic entity, *Journal of the American Medical Association*, **181**, 5–12.

Noble, T. P. (1931) Thromboangiitis obliterans in Siam, *Lancet*, **1**, 288.

Wessler, S., Ming, S. C., Gurewich, V. & Freiman, D. G. (1960) A critical evaluation of thrombo-angiitis obliterans: the case against Buerger's disease, *New England Journal of Medicine*, **262**, 1149–1160.

DEEP VENOUS THROMBOSIS AND VARICOSE VEINS

A low incidence of deep venous thrombosis has been noted clinically and at autopsy in many tropical areas, though expatriates dwelling there and affluent members of society do not usually share in these benefits (Fisher & Nixon, 1952; Drury & Mylius, 1952; Mathews, 1974; Burkitt *et al.*, 1977). In Thailand in a study of post-partum women the rate of D.V.T. was 17 per 100 000 compared with figures of 134 per 100 000 in the U.S.A. (Chumnijarakij, 1974). Figures for the low incidence of pulmonary embolism have already been cited earlier in this chapter.

Further evidence of the low frequency of venous thrombotic processes is afforded by a study of pelvic phleboliths. Radiologists have noted a low incidence of these in radiographs in much of Africa, the Persian Gulf, Polynesia, South East Asia and New Guinea compared with experience in Western Europe, North America and New Zealand. In the tropical areas mentioned phleboliths are rare, often single with the incidence slowly increasing with age. By contrast in the more affluent societies phleboliths are multiple and exist in almost half the adult population (Burkitt *et al.*, 1977). Adult blacks in the U.S.A. have a higher incidence than U.S. whites in two surveys, whereas in South Africa the Bantu population have a low incidence but there is a high incidence in whites. These points emphasise the presence of an unidentified environmental factor rather than a genetic determination for D.V.T.

Similar considerations appear to apply to varicose veins. In Europe certainly a proportion of patients develop varicose veins consequent on D.V.T.—particularly parous women. This is of course not the only factor. Alexander, in a series of papers, has commented on the epidemiology of this condition (Alexander, 1972a, b, c). He concludes that in Europe, based on French and English data, varicose veins exist in between 10 per cent to 20 per cent in a community overall, with a range of about 1 per cent at the age of 20 and between 40 per cent to 70 per cent by the age of 50 years, depending on sex and perhaps locality. On the other hand, he shows how in Egypt there was a 6 per cent incidence in women between the ages of 15 to 74 years; in Hong Kong 0·8 per cent in 1112 females of mean age 27 years; in Zululand 0·003 per cent in 115 000 hospital patients; 0·01 per cent in Senegalese; and no detectable incidence in Papua New Guinea Highlanders and Australian aborigines (Alexander, 1972a). In 18-year-old military recruits the incidence was six times higher in Germany than in Japan.

Alexander has also noted that in some areas in the tropics there is a higher male than female incidence of varicose veins. This is particularly noted in those of lean build and active occupation involving much walking or climbing. All these factors underline again the need to isolate the responsible aetiological factors in the development of varicose veins. An interesting thesis on the role of sitting has been put forward (Alexander, 1972c).

REFERENCES

Alexander, C. J. (1972a). The epidemiology of varicose veins, *Medical Journal of Australia*, **1**, 215–218.

Alexander, C. J. (1972b) The theoretical basis of varicose vein formation, *Medical Journal of Australia*, **1**, 258–261.

Alexander, C. J. (1972c) Chair sitting and varicose veins, *Lancet*, **1**, 822–824.

Burkitt, D., Latto, C., Janvrin, S. B. & Mayou, B. (1977) Pelvic phleboliths, epidemiology and postulated etiology, *New England Journal of Medicine*, **296**, 1387–1389.

Chumnijarakij, T. (1974) Incidence of post partum deep vein thrombosis in the tropics, *British Medical Journal*, **1**, 245–246.

Drury, R. A. B. & Mylius, E. A. (1973) The changing pattern of pulmonary embolism in Uganda Africans, *African Journal of Medical Sciences*, **43**, 369–381.

Fisher, A. C. & Nixon, G. P. (1952) A comparison of the post-operative incidence of post-operative thromboembolism in African and European patients, *East African Medical Journal*, **29**, 186–188.

Mathews, C. L. (1974) Cardiovascular disease in Lae—a five year review, *Papua and New Guinea Medical Journal*, **17**, 251–262.

6. Genito-urinary System

RENAL OUTLINES

Apart from schistosomiasis there are few conditions of the G.U. tract seen in the tropics that are not universal in distribution. Nevertheless there are some general remarks that are perhaps helpful.

In plain films of the abdomen the renal outlines are not distinguishable in some communities due to the paucity of perirenal fat deposits. This makes it difficult to determine the size and shape of the kidneys before injection of contrast provides nephrographic positive density. The low perirenal fat is related to diet and economic circumstance and not to a racial difference in size of fat depots. Probably the fat has never been laid down, since it has been noted that in adults who have lost considerable weight the renal fat depots persist longer than fat tissue in other sites.

We know of no work from the tropics establishing renal size standards for age, height or weight.

In the previous section on cardiovascular diseases the infrequency of pelvic phleboliths quantitatively and by specific age groupings has been commented on in the discussion on deep venous thrombosis (Burkitt *et al.*, 1977).

Intravenous pyelography appears to be associated with fewer reactions to contrast media in many tropical areas. Though the evidence is largely anecdotal, the experience from large hospital departments confirms the low incidence of urticarial and allergic manifestations. There is evidence that malnutrition affects cell-mediated immunity and depression of the immediate hypersensitivity response (Abbasy *et al.*, 1974; Neumann *et al.*, 1975). However, the relative anergy observed in contrast studies is unlikely to be explained only on the basis of malnutrition.

The incidence of renal tuberculosis is remarkably low in some parts of Africa. In Ibadan no case of renal tuberculosis was seen in a Nigerian in 10 years, yet numerous cases of tuberculosis at other sites were seen daily. Autopsy figures confirm the radiological experience. The American black is certainly not immune to renal tuberculosis. This variant in disease distribution remains a mystery. Renal tuberculosis is not rare in most of the tropics. Even when renal is infrequent tuberculosis of the female genital tract is not uncommon.

REFERENCES

Abbassy, A. S., Badr, El-Din, N. K., Hassam, A. I., Aref, G. H., Hammad, S. A., El-Araby, I. I., Badr, El-Din, A. A., Soliman, M. H. & Hussein, M. (1974) Cell mediated immunity and allergy in protein energy malnutrition, *Journal of Tropical Medicine and Hygiene*, 77, 13–21.

Burkitt, D., Latto, C., Janvrin, S. B. & Mayou, B. (1977) Pelvic phleboliths, epidemiology and postulated etiology, *New England Journal of Medicine*, **296,** 1387–1389.

Neumann, C. G., Lawlor, G. J. & Stiehm, E. R. (1975) Immunoligic responses in malnourished children, *American Journal of Clinical Nutrition*, **28,** 89–104.

URINARY CALCULI

The incidence of calculi, their location in the urinary tract and their composition show considerable variations in different parts of the world. Andersen (1969) considers that diet is of considerable importance in the vesical calculi of developing areas and in the upper urinary tract stones of industrialised communities. Vesical calculi tend to disappear from endemic areas with increasing standards of living and nutrition but to increase in the upper urinary tract. Genetic or racial factors are also probably involved, since there is such a wide difference in incidence between Bantus (0·0014 per cent) and Caucasians (0·12 per cent) in Africa. Renal calculi are frequent in Asia, whereas in Nigeria idiopathic renal calculi are rare but in Kenya they are not exceptional.

Vesical calculi

Vesical calculi, though once common in Europe, have virtually vanished in this century (Andersen, 1969). An improved diet is often invoked in explanation, since prevalence diminishes as protein content of the diet increases. Practising vegetarian Hindus have a higher rate of vesical calculi than their meat-consuming Moslem colleagues in the same community (Popelier & Gatera, 1976). An additional factor may be deficiency of fat-soluble vitamin A, as there is an association between vesical calculi and xerophthalmia due to lack of vitamin A. It is postulated that the deficiency leads to keratosis of the transitional epithelium of the urinary tract and desquamated portions form stone nuclei. This does not explain why the stones are nearly always solitary and occur almost only in boys. Of course the anatomical arrangements of the female urinary tract may allow the passage of stones before they enlarge. McLaren (1963) provides a good review of the nutritional aspects.

Vesical calculi in boys is prevalent in the Yemen, southwest Arabia, the Near East, areas abutting on the Sahara, Central Africa, Rwanda, Tanzania, the Congo delta, the Philippines, Northern India, Thailand, Indonesia and Vietnam. The size of the problem can be inferred from one hospital in Thailand where one-quarter of paediatric admissions were due to vesical calculi. 1780 stones were removed in two years (Andersen, 1969).

Radiologically such stones are usually solitary, oval in shape and show concentric rings of varying density (Fig. 6.1). Bladder wall calcification from bilharziasis may coexist, but such an association is probably fortuitous in endemic zones. Analyses of these vesical calculi show differences in various areas. Thus in the Yemen phosphate stones predominate, in Madagascar and India calcium oxalate, in Turkey and the Philippines ammonium urate and calcium oxalate, and in Rwanda calcium oxalate with a high trace content of rubidium (Popelier & Gatera, 1976).

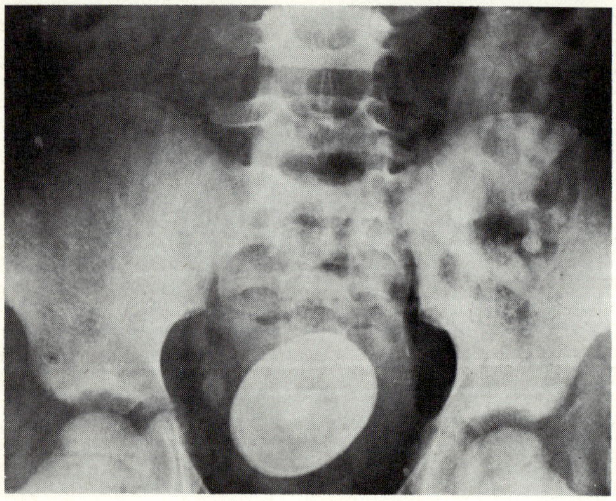

Fig. 6.1 Large vesical calculus in young boy.

In most parts of the world vesical calculi result from enlargement of a stone coming from the upper urinary tract but, as has already been emphasised, such a source would be unlikely in most Africans. A further feature suggesting a dietary or other environmental factor rather than a genetic cause is the patchy distribution of vesical calculi. They are rare in Uganda, the Ivory Coast and those areas of Nigeria lying south of the Savannah but not in the Sahel belt, Central Africa or the Congo mouth. Similarly vesical calculi occur in Northern India and not the South.

REFERENCES

Andersen, D. A. (1969) Historical and geographical differences in the pattern of incidence of urinary stones considered in relation to possible aetiological factors, *Proceedings of the Renal Stone Research Symposium*. Ed. Hodgkinson, A. pp. 2–31. London: A. Churchill.

McLaren, D. S. (1963) Nutritional factors in urinary lithiasis, *East African Medical Journal*, **40**, 178–185.

Popelier, G. & Gatera, G. (1976) La lithiase vesicale endemique chez les enfants du Rwanda, *Annales de la Société de Médecine Tropicale*, **56**, 25–35.

Wise, R. & Karle, A. (1961) Urinary calcium and serum levels in Africans and Indians, *South African Medical Journal*, **35**, 47–50.

URINARY SCHISTOSOMIASIS

It is estimated that schistosomiasis now affects approximately 200 000 000 people throughout the world. The complicated life cycle of this trematode worm that is parasitic in the circulatory system of man is described in chapter 3 in the section on 'Intestinal Schistosomiasis'. Of the three main species that affect man not all affect the urinary tract. Schistosoma haematobium infection is the form that does involve the urinary tract. It occurs in various parts of East, West, North and Central Africa, in various parts of the Middle East, and in Mauritius and Madagascar. On the African continent it occurs in many areas where Schistosoma mansoni infection is also endemic, and so mixed infections are not uncommon.

In S. haematobium infections the adult worms live in the veins of the pelvic plexus, from where eggs are passed mainly in the urine after traversing the blood vessels. This accounts for much of the haematuria. Eggs in the bladder and ureteric walls produce a cellular reaction, and this, together with the ulceration that results from the rupture of the blood vessels, is followed by fibrosis. Though eggs continue to be formed, many remain lodged in the fibrous tissue of the bladder and ureteric walls, where they eventually become necrotic. Bladder-wall fibrosis may lead to hydro-ureter with or without hydronephrosis. It has been shown that the prevalence of obstructive uropathy is related to the infection intensity (von Lichtenberg *et al.*, 1971; Smith *et al.*, 1977b). Ureteral dilatation, according to these authors, appears to result from functional inco-ordination and aperistalsis. Stenosis of the ureteral orifices at the trigone may also cause stasis and dilatation. Chronic schistosomal ulceration of the bladder has also been shown to develop at sites of very heavy egg burdens (Smith *et al.*, 1977a). In early infections the acute cellular response leads to oedematous inflammatory masses that mechanically can produce a reversible obstructive process (Lucas *et al.*, 1969).

There is a well-established causal relationship between the incidence of carcinoma of the bladder and long-standing schistosomiasis. This, however, is not seen everywhere but occurs predominantly in Egypt and Central Africa.

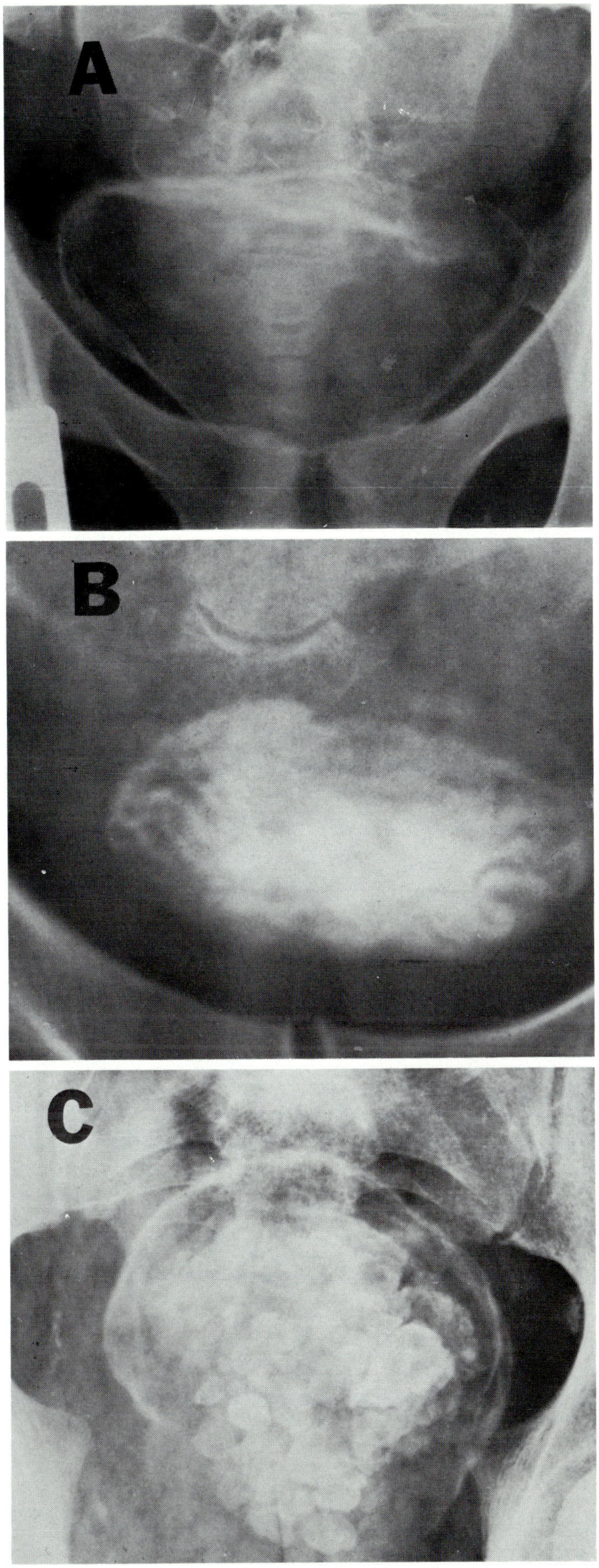

Fig. 6.2 **A.** Distended bladder with calcification visible where the x-ray beam traverses the bladder wall tangentially. **B.** Contracted bladder with dense calcification. Bladder folds can be seen. **C.** Densely calcified bladder with calcified nodular masses and encrustations.

Some workers in other parts of Africa (Attah & Nkposong, 1976) have discounted this relationship. Such differences may be explained by differences in the relative intensity of infections.

The radiological features that may be noted in this condition are as follows:

1. Calcification may be seen in the bladder wall or in other parts of the urinary tract as a late feature. Entombed ova remaining lodged in the fibrous tissue in the bladder wall or wall of the ureter eventually become necrotic and calcify. At first this is seen as a thin intermittent line of calcification in the bladder wall when seen tangentially, but subsequently it shows as a pencil line of calcification round the entire bladder, sometimes becoming very dense (Fig. 6.2). It can extend to outline the lower ureters, or even the lower half of a ureter or, rarely, the entire ureter (Fig. 6.3). If the ureter calcifies it is usually seen to be dilated. Other parts of the genito-urinary tract may be calcareous, such as the seminal vesicles or even the posterior urethra. Sometimes clusters of ova have been encased in mounds of granulation tissue or polyps and when they

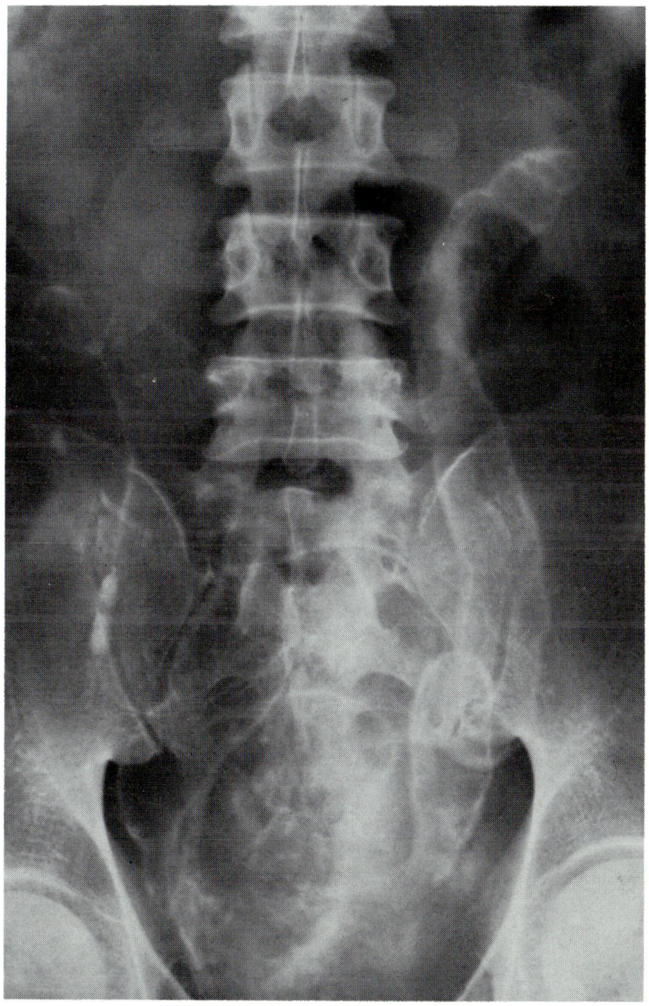

Fig. 6.3 Extensive bilateral ureteric calcification. The left ureter is greatly dilated.

calcify they show as nodules or undulations in the bladder wall. The persistence of such polyps has been shown (Smith *et al.*, 1977b) to follow heavy antecedent infection. Calcification in the bladder wall does not affect function of the muscle coat, as the bladder can be observed to distend and contract with filling and emptying (Middlemiss, 1967).

2. At excretion urography, ureteric narrowing, hydro-ureter, hydronephrosis, non-functioning kidney, or filling defects in the lower ureter and/or bladder may be demonstrated. The ureteric and renal changes may be unilateral or bilateral. If ureteric narrowing is demonstrated it is usually at the extreme distal end. It may show merely as the ureter tapering to a point. It is not known how much of this radiological feature is due to fibrotic stenosis or to reactive oedema and swelling of the ureteric mucosa. Occasionally filling defects are shown in the ureter. Quite often hydro-ureter is noted. In gross cases the ureter may be enormously dilated, and affected throughout its length (Figs. 6.4 and 6.5).

Similarly, a back pressure kidney may be demonstrated. This may vary from loss of cupping of calyces to gross calyceal dilatation, with delay in excretion of contrast medium. Finally, in these cases the function of the kidney may be so disturbed that little information about its structural state is obtained from the examination, and radiologically the organ is a non-functioning kidney. Such effects on the upper urinary tract may occur in young persons, changes having been observed from the age of six years upwards. They are more common in boys than in girls. Umerah (1977) has observed the ureteric appearances under fluoroscopic control and noted the ureters to be aperistaltic. He has also shown 'cobra-head' deformities of the lower ureters and ureteroceles. Al-Ghorab and colleagues (1966) have described ureteric reflux at ascending cystography in 44 per cent of patients with schistosomiasis haematobium.

3. In both East and West Africa, bladder lesions have been described at excretion urography, particularly in children, which are often symptomless (Lucas *et al.*, 1966; el Badawi, 1966; Bohrer *et al.*, 1971) (Fig. 6.6). These lesions, which are often multiple, appear as mound filling defects 1–3 cm in diameter, protruding into the bladder cavity. Similar mounds, smaller in size, have also been noted in the lower third of the ureter as already described (Fig. 6.7). The term 'granuloma' has been applied to these lesions, but it is possible that they are more in the nature of reactive oedema. They have been observed

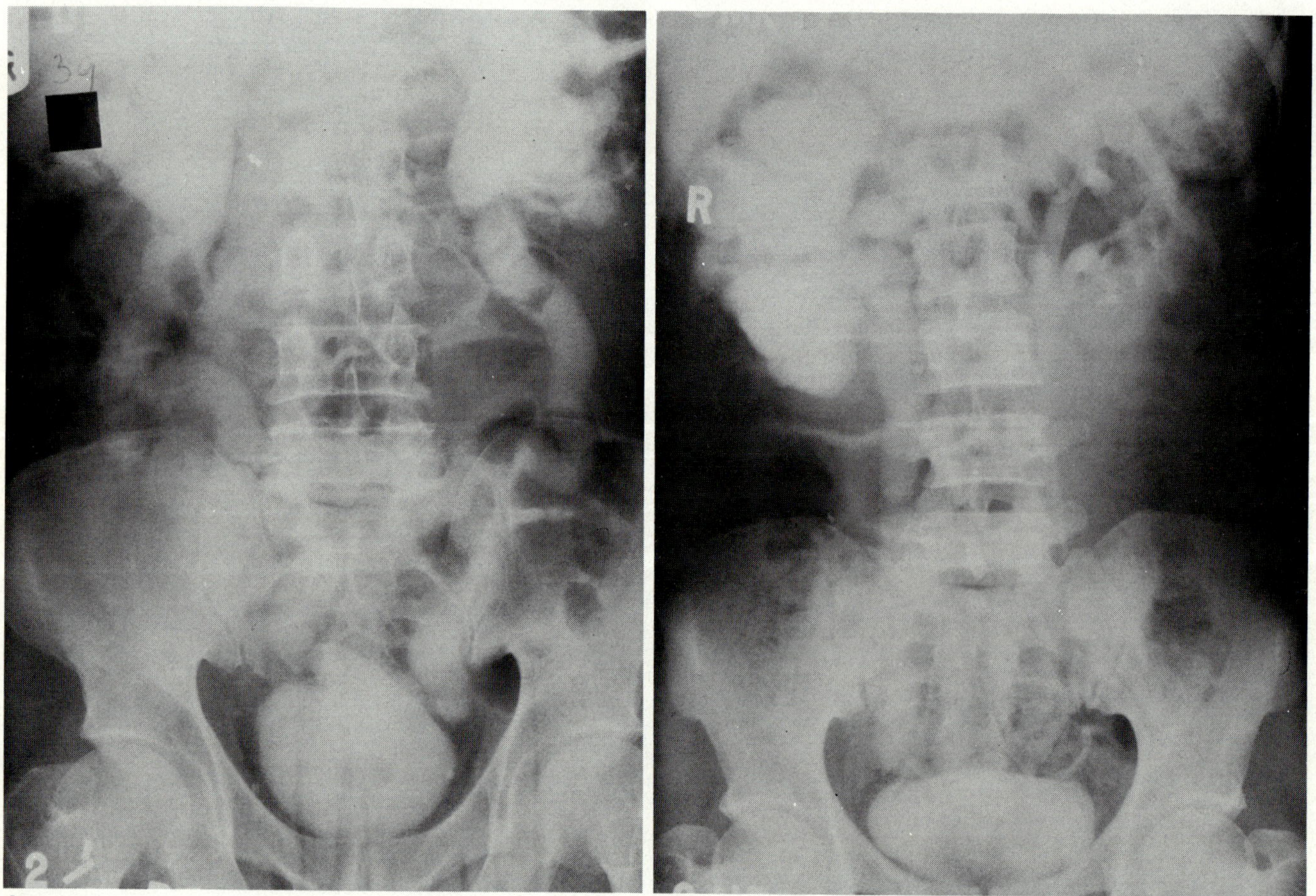

A B

Fig. 6.4 A, B. Patients with unilateral and bilateral back pressure kidneys due to schistosomiasis. The ureters are greatly distended and hydronephrotic.

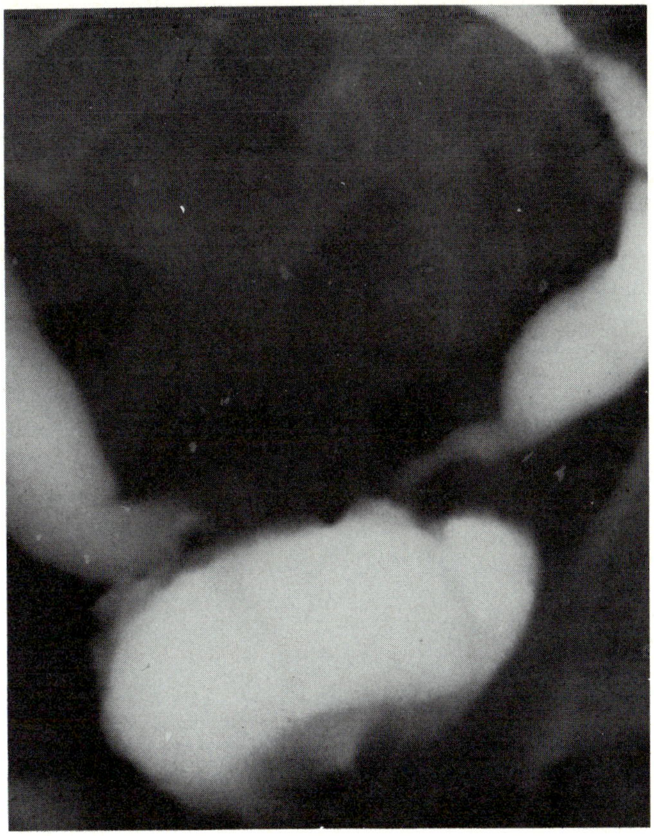

Fig. 6.5 Obstructive uropathy due to bilateral stenoses of lower ureters.

radiologically to resolve under specific therapy (Lucas *et al.*, 1969).

4. In adults, carcinoma of the bladder may be observed radiologically. At the same time carcinoma, either as a small mound or as malignant change in a long-standing ulcerative lesion, may not be noted at routine excretion urography.

5. Double contrast cystography has been employed in Egypt and elsewhere for showing schistosomal ulcers and neoplastic changes (Sinna, 1963). These features are relatively late events.

6. Studies with I^{131} Hippuran have shown renographic abnormalities which persist after a waterload and are more common in infected children than in normal controls. The renogram alterations are reversible following specific chemotherapy. The authors (Oyediran *et al.*, 1975) suggest that this may be a useful method for the assessment and follow-up of patients with visceral schistosomiasis.

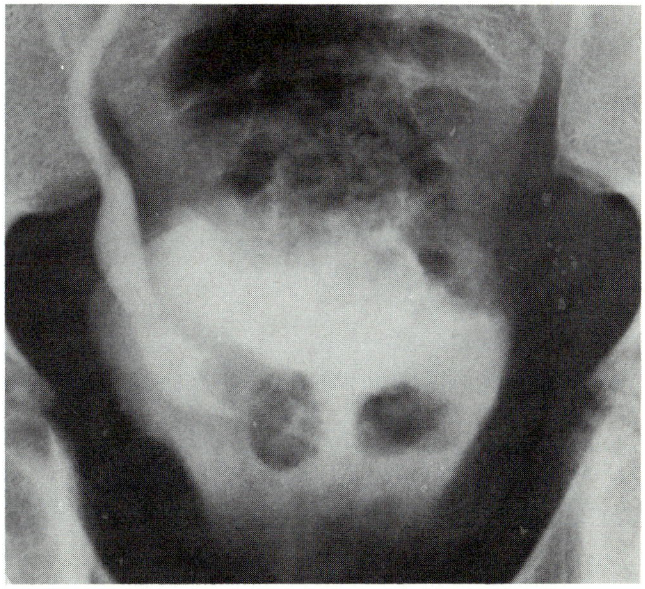

Fig. 6.7 A further example of mechanical obstruction to a ureter by vesical nodules related to the intramural course of the ureter.

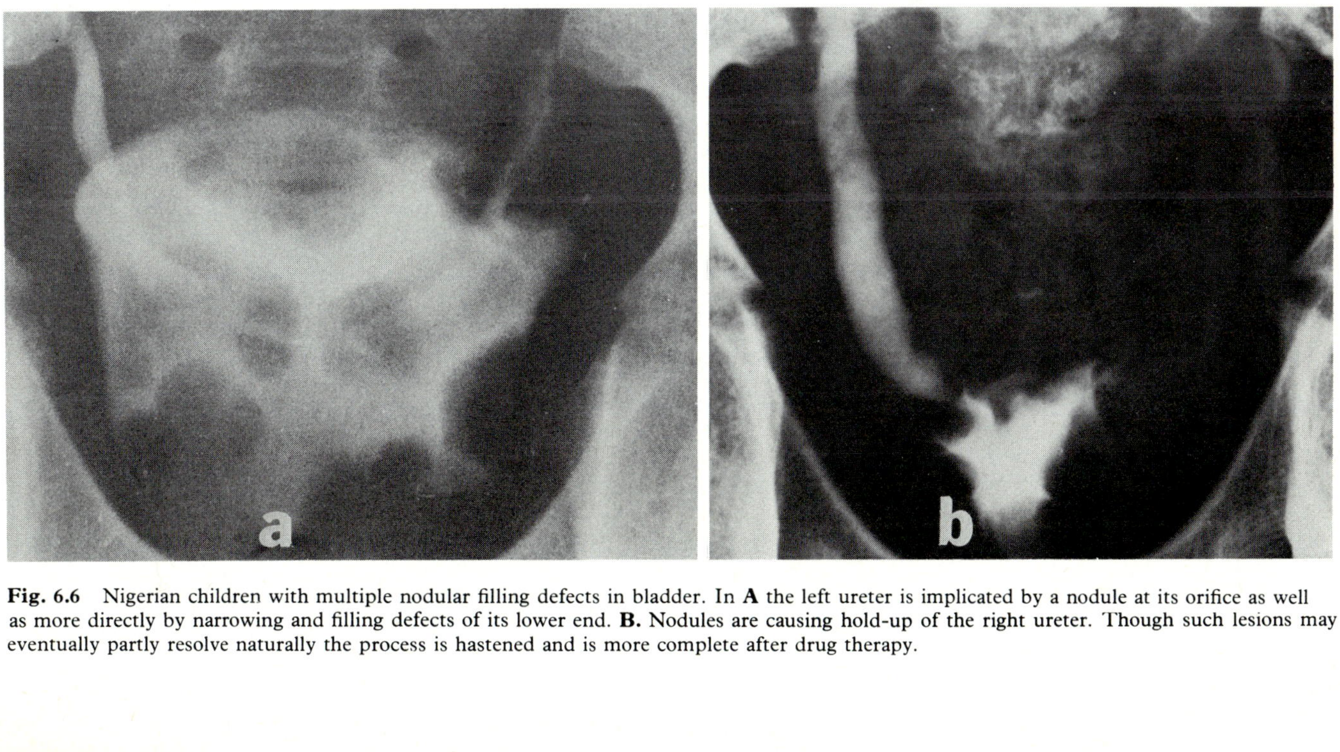

Fig. 6.6 Nigerian children with multiple nodular filling defects in bladder. In **A** the left ureter is implicated by a nodule at its orifice as well as more directly by narrowing and filling defects of its lower end. **B.** Nodules are causing hold-up of the right ureter. Though such lesions may eventually partly resolve naturally the process is hastened and is more complete after drug therapy.

REFERENCES

Al-Ghorab, M. M., el-Badawi, A. A. & Effat, H. (1966) Vesico-ureteric reflux in urinary bilharziasis—a clinico-radiological study, *Clinical Radiology*, **17**, 41–47.

Attah, E. B. & Nkposong, E. O. (1976) Schistosomiasis and carcinoma of the bladder, *Tropical and Geographical Medicine*, **28**, 268–272.

Bohrer, S. P., Lucas, A. O. & Cockshott, W. P. (1971) Roentgenographic features of schistosomiasis in children, *Zeitschrift für Tropenmedizin und Parasitologie*, **22**, 177–188.

Edington, G. M. (1967) Schistosomiasis in Ibadan. In *Bilharziasis*. Ed. Mostofi, F. K. Heidelberg: Springer-Verlag.

el Badawi, A. A. (1966) Bilharzial polypi of the urinary bladder, *British Journal of Urology*, **38**, 24–35.

Forsyth, D. M. & MacDonald, G. (1965) Urologic complications of endemic schistosomiasis in school children, *Transactions of the Royal Society of Tropical Medicine and Hygiene*, **59**, 171–178.

Gelfand, M. (1966) Filling defects of the bladder on intravenous pyelography in children passing schistosome ova in urine, *Journal of Tropical Medicine and Hygiene*, **69**, 4–6.

Girges, M. R. (1966) The syndrome of bladder-neck obstruction and ureteric fibrosis in Schistosoma haematobium infection, *Journal of Tropical Medicine and Hygiene*, **69**, 187–188.

Lucas, A. O., Adeniyi-Jones, C. C., Cockshott, W. P. & Gilles, H. M. (1966) Radiological changes after medical treatment of vesical schistosomiasis, *Lancet*, **1**, 631–633.

Lucas, A. O., Akpom, C. A., Cockshott, W. P. & Bohrer, S. P. (1969) Reversibility of the urological lesions of schistosomiasis in children after specific therapy, *Annals of New York Academy of Science*, **160**, 629–644.

Middlemiss, J. H. (1967) Radiological pathology and methods of investigation in schistosomiasis. In *Bilharziasis*. Ed. Mostofi, F. K. pp. 197–211. Heidelberg: Springer-Verlag.

Ovediran, A. B. O. O., Abayomi, I. O., Akinkugbe, O. O. Bohrer, S. P. & Lucas, A. O. (1975) Renographic studies in vesical schistosomiasis in children, *American Journal of Tropical Medicine and Hygiene*, **24**, 274–279.

Sinna, A. M. A. A. (1963) *Bilharziasis*. M.D. Thesis, Cairo University.

Smith, J. H., Torky, A. H., Kelada, A. S. & Farid, Z. (1977) Schistosomal polyposis of the urinary bladder, *American Journal of Tropical Medicine and Hygiene*, **26**, 85–88.

Smith, J. H., Kelada, A. S. & Khalil, A. (1977a) Schistosomal ulceration of the urinary bladder, *American Journal of Tropical Medicine and Hygiene*, **26**, 89–95.

Smith, J. H., Kelada, A. S., Khalil, A. & Torky, A. H. (1977b) Surgical pathology of schistosomal obstructive uropathy, *American Journal of Tropical Medicine and Hygiene*, **26**, 96–108.

von Lichtenberg, F., Edington, G., Nurabuebo, I., Taylor, J. R. & Smith, J. H. (1971) Pathologic effects of schistomiasis in Ibadan, *American Journal of Tropical Medicine and Hygiene*, **20**, 244–254.

Umerah, B. C. (1977) The less familiar manifestations of schistosomiasis of the urinary tract, *British Journal of Radiology*, **50**, 105–109.

FILARIAL CHYLURIA

Chyluria due to filariasis is caused by Wuchereria bancrofti and not Brugia malayi. Consequently it may develop in those who have lived in the endemic zones of Africa, parts of Central and South America and the Caribbean, Polynesia and south-west Pacific, southern Burma, Thailand, Assam, Malaysia, Indonesia and the islands in the East China sea.

Proof of a filarial aetiology in an individual case may be difficult to establish, since circulating microfilariae are rarely found and their presence in urine is even less frequent. Evidence of residence in an endemic area and absence of other forms of retroperitoneal lymphatic obstruction such as tuberculosis, haematomas, and chronic abscesses is strong circumstantial evidence of a filarial origin.

Clinical onset is often sudden and may be initially accompanied by slight haematuria. Chyluria is often intermittent, but episodes may continue for long periods and eventually periods of remission may cease.

The intravenous urogram may be abnormal. In under 10 per cent of cases paracalyceal lymphatics fill with contrast (Ko Ko *et al.*, 1975).

With retrograde pyelography pyelolymphatic backflow is visible in half the cases (Koehler *et al.*, 1968; Ko Ko *et al.*, 1975). The flow in opacified communicating lymphatics may be great enough to show the cisterna chyli.

Lymphangiography has become the standard way of demonstrating the abnormal lymphatic communications. Japanese radiologists working in islands near Okinawa, and Burmese radiologists have classified and illustrated the lymphangiographic features of filarial chyluria (Akisada & Tani, 1970; Ko Ko *et al.*, 1975). These workers and others have clearly shown that the chyluria is not due to an obstructive process of the thoracic duct as had once been postulated. It is due to an obliterative process of para-aortic glands and lymphatics, so that abnormal varicose pathways develop. A leash of dilated lymphatics

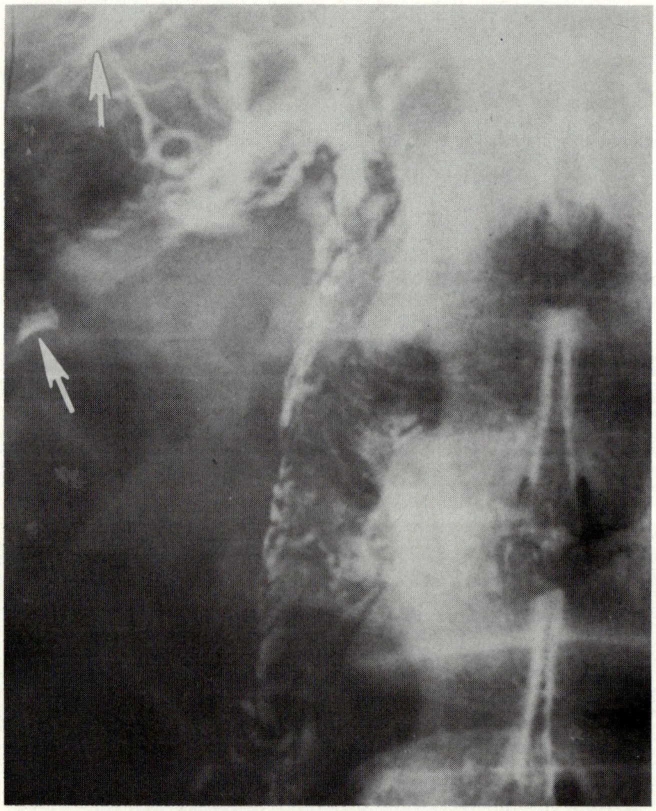

Fig. 6.8 Lymphangiogram in patient with filarial chyluria revealing dilated varicose lymphatics around the ureter and renal hilum. Contrast has reached the collecting system and calyces as shown by arrows (Courtesy of Dr. Robert Tuttle, Hamilton, Ontario.)

forms around the renal pedicle and a plexus of lymphatic vessels arborises around the collecting system of the kidney (Fig. 6.8). Contrast passes through one or more lymphatico-pelvic fistulae to partly outline calyces, renal pelvis, ureter and sometimes bladder. The pelvic lymphatics are often dilated, varicose and redundant.

Chyluria is a renal symptom due to abnormalities of abdominal lymph glands with dilatation of obstructed pathways and collaterals developing fistulous communications with the kidneys.

REFERENCES

Akisada, M. & Tani, S. (1970) Lymphangioadenopathy of filariasis. *Transactions of the Royal Society of Tropical Medicine and Hygiene*, **64,** 885–894.

Koehler, P. R., Chiang, T-C., Lin, C-T., Chen, K-C. & Chen, K-Y. (1968) Lymphography in chyluria, *American Journal of Roentgenology*, **102,** 455–465.

Ko Ko, U., Aye, T. T. & Aung, S. T. T. (1975) Chyluria, *Clinical Radiology*, **26,** 237–242.

RENAL HYDATID DISEASE

Oncospheres that manage to pass through the liver and pulmonary vascular filter beds lodge systemically. The kidneys with their rich blood supply are the site for about 4 per cent of all hydatid cysts. Most such cysts are for a long time clinically silent, but their presence may be declared as a result of the discovery of a mass or because of renal colic from rupture of a cyst and discharge of some contents into the urinary collecting system (Fig. 6.9).

Radiologically the existence of a cyst can be suspected from curvilinear calcification in the ectocyst wall, but of course there are other causes of calcification in the margin of a renal mass (Figs. 6.10 and 6.11). Calcification is a late stage.

Initially a renal hydatid causes a mass. Pyelography discloses no constant appearance. Calyces may be deformed

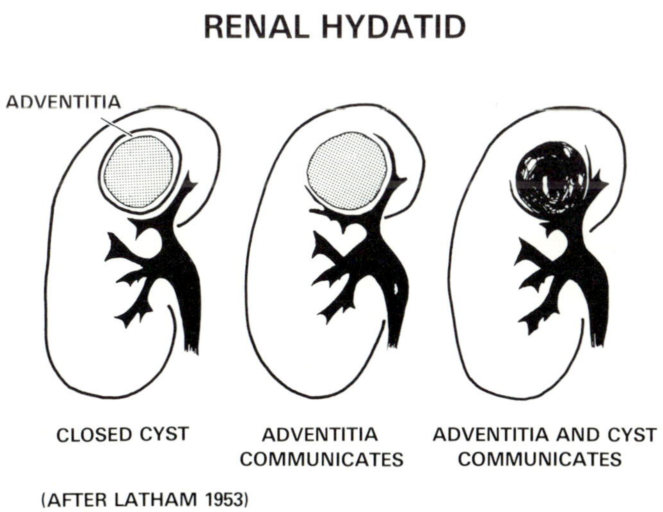

Fig. 6.9 Diagram to indicate pyelographic features of renal hydatid disease. A closed cyst displaces calyces; if ectocyst communicates with collecting system contrast enters the space between host and cyst; finally the cyst may communicate and fill with contrast and contain filling defects due to daughter cysts.

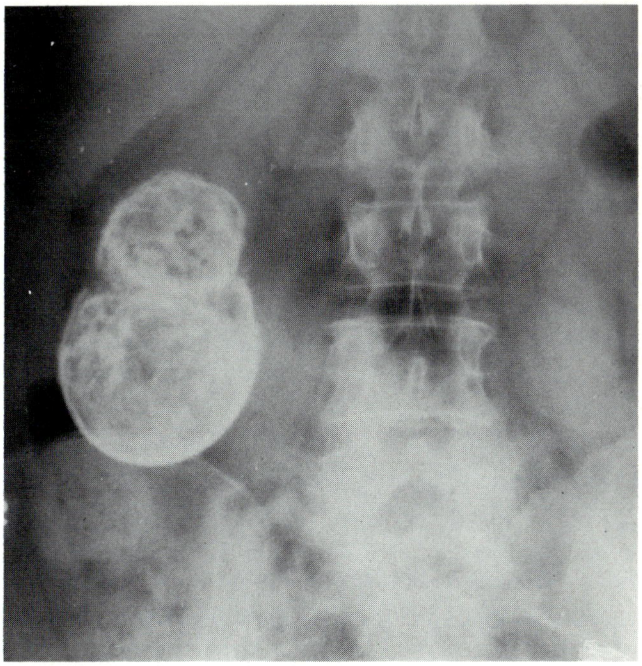

Fig. 6.10 Two densely calcified renal hydatid cysts.

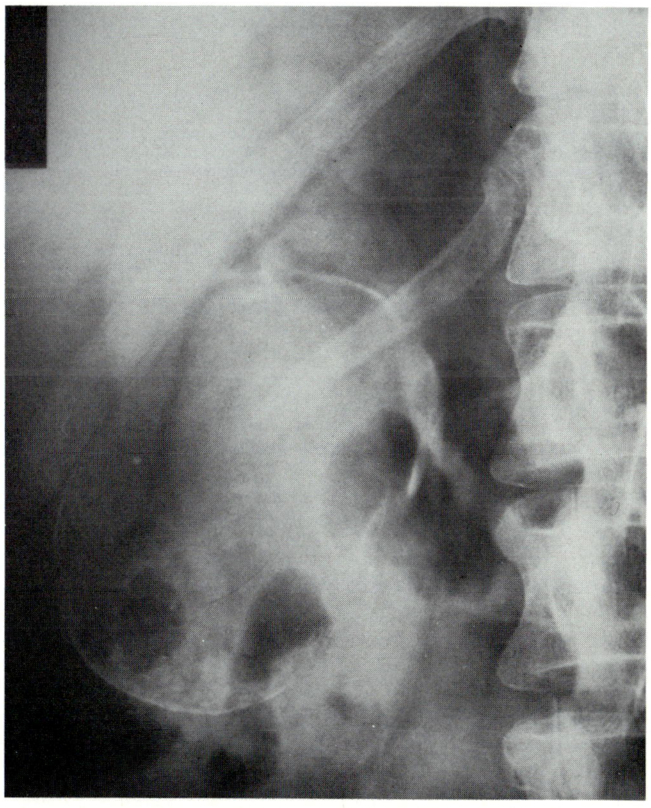

Fig. 6.11 Large renal hydatid with marginal calcification.

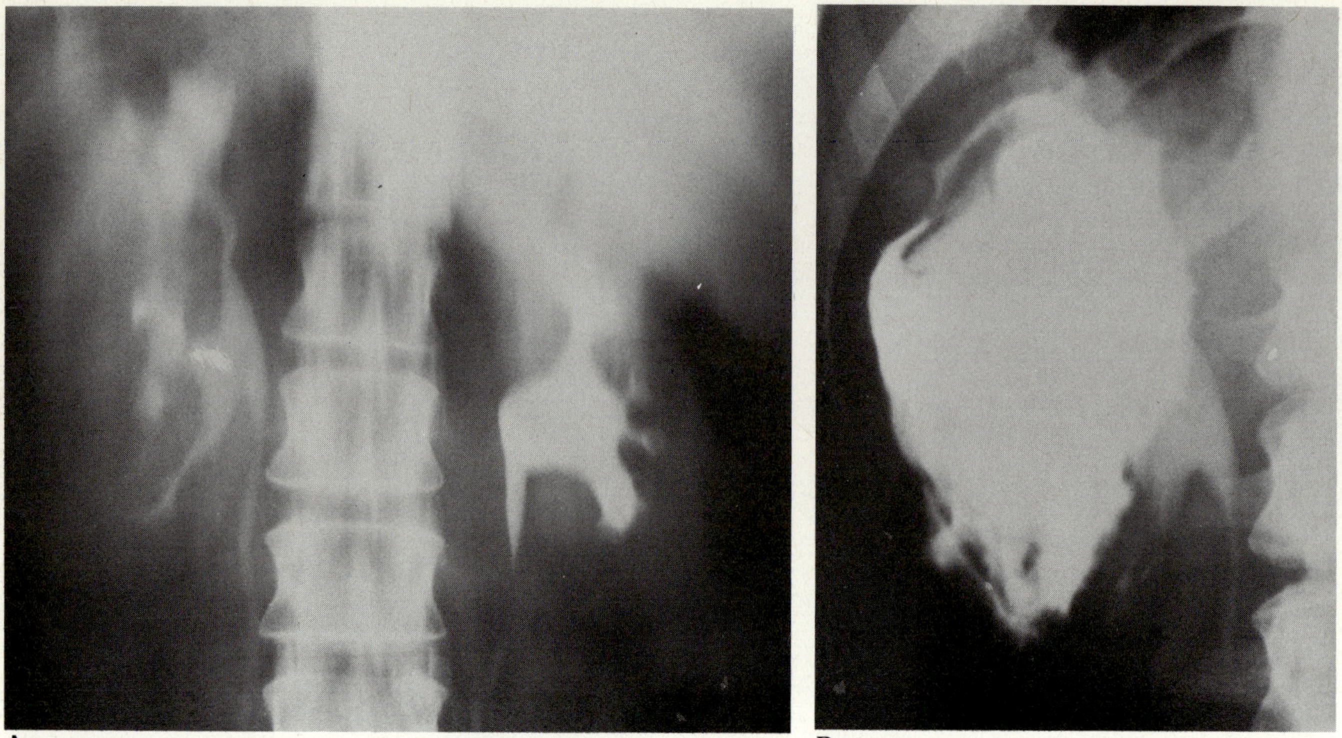

A B

Fig. 6.12 A, B. Enlarged right kidney with stretched calyces at excretion urography. Renal cyst puncture. Filling defects caused by daughter hydatid cysts. (Courtesy of Dr. J. Roylance, Bristol.)

and stretched and contrast may penetrate into or around cysts if there is communication with the drainage system. Angiography and isotope studies indicate that the mass is avascular. Ultrasonic and computerised tomography have shown that the cysts contain fluid and may be multilocular. Cysts have been inadvertently punctured for diagnosis when their true nature has not been known (Roylance *et al.*, 1973) (Fig. 6.12).

REFERENCES

Latham, W. J. (1953) Hydatid disease, *Journal of the Faculty of Radiologists*, **5**, 83–95.

Roylance, J., Rhys Davies, E. & Alexander, W. D. (1973) Translumbar puncture of a renal hydatid cyst, *British Journal of Radiology*, **49**, 960–963.

PAPILLARY NECROSIS

The conventional aetiologies considered for papillary necrosis are associations with phenacetin and aspirin abuse, diabetes and urinary tract infections.

It was noted during the second world war that nephrectomy for severe unilateral haematuria was occasionally carried out on negro soldiers and that the kidneys grossly were often unremarkable but histology showed the presence of sickled red cells. Subsequently severe haematuria has been noted in homozygotes as well as the AS, SC, and S thalassaemia heterozygotes. It is now recognised that papillary necrosis is present in many of these kidneys, though at the onset of haematuria the lesions may be minute. The combination of low oxygen tension, acidity and hyperosmolarity all make the peripapillary region vulnerable to sickling damage. We and others have seen papillary necrosis, usually multiple (Fig. 6.13), in all the sickle variants (Hurrow *et al.*, 1963). Jamaican investigators in a study of 181 sickle homozygotes found papillary

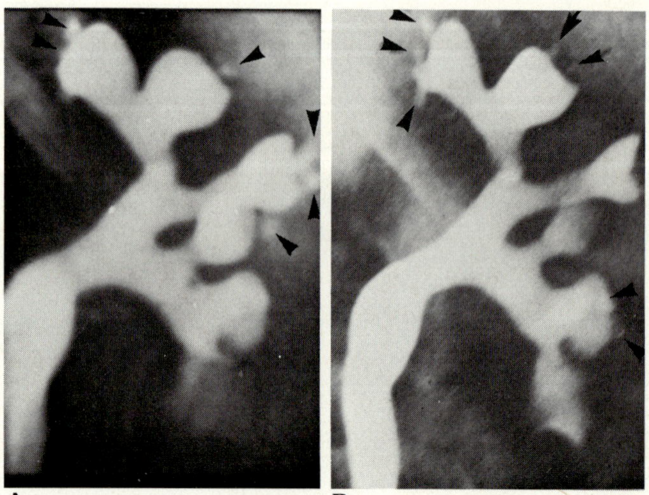

A B

Fig. 6.13 A, B. Examples of papillary necrosis demonstrated at pyelography in patients with A.S. haemaglobin genotype. Arrows indicate extension of contrast into damaged papillae.

necrosis in 41. This could be bilateral and was most frequent on the right side (McCall *et al.*, 1978). Function did not seem to be impaired by the presence of the lesions (Pandya *et al.*, 1976).

Papillary necrosis has been attributed to Dapsone (Dihydroxy phenyl sulfone) (Hoffbrand, 1978). Since this drug is widely employed in leprosy therapy and nocardial mycetoma, at times iatrogenic papillary necrosis may be encountered.

REFERENCES

Hoffbrand, B. I. (1978) Dapsone and renal papillary necrosis, *British Medical Journal*, **1**, 9.

Hurrow, B. R., Sloane, I. A. & Liebman (1963) Roentgenologic demonstration of renal papillary necrosis in sickle cell trait, *New England Journal of Medicine*, **268**, 969–976.

McCall, I. W., Moule, N., Desai, P. & Serjeant, G. R. (1978) Urographic findings in homozygous sickle disease, *Radiology*, **126**, 99–104.

Pandya, K. K., Koshy, M., Brown, N. & Presman, D. (1976) Renal papillary necrosis in sickle cell haemoglobinopathies, *Journal of Urology*, **115**, 497–501.

URETHRAL FISTULAE AND STRICTURES

In some tropical areas one may still encounter severe urethral strictures and urethral fistulae of a type that have vanished in well-doctored communities since the advent of antibiotics. Patients with these urethral tragedies are generally middle-aged or older and represent the natural history of untreated gonococcal urethritis.

Patients may be referred for retrograde urethrography when bouginage is difficult or to display the anatomy of fistulae. Strictures may be single or multiple, short or long (Fig. 6.14). The presence of prostatic and peri-urethral inflammatory spaces or of fistulae is readily demonstrated (Braband, 1964).

Urethrography is not without hazards in patients with an infected urethra, particularly if this is carried out shortly after bouginage. The injection of contrast may have to be forceful to proceed beyond a stricture and in a traumatised urethra contrast can readily extravasate, carrying with it infected material. This can cause septicaemia or even endotoxin shock with chills, dyspnoea and collapse. Bleeding per urethra is almost invariable after extravasation. When this is seen antibiotics should be given and the patient kept under observation.

REFERENCE

Braband, H. (1964) Zur Rontgendiagnostik urethraler strikturen und Fisteln, *Der Urologe*, **3**, 343–346.

OBSTETRICS

The use of radiology in obstetrics is diminishing greatly in response to concerns about radiation hazards coupled with the increased availability of ultrasound equipment. Many tropical areas do not possess ultrasound equipment nor do they have the facilities to maintain this complex equipment. In addition, ultrasound does not provide similar information to radiology. There is no doubt that it is ideal for locating the placenta and valuable to monitor the rate of growth. To convert dimensions to maturation can be difficult in the tropics, as most published charts are based on well-nourished Caucasian communities. Such data may err if applied without correction to other communities of different genetic and dietary background. In Africa babies are small for dates compared with European standards but yet are mature if assessed by psychomotor parameters and, to a lesser extent, by skeletal maturation.

These comments are made to emphasise the need to relate assessments of age and maturity to a local context. Generally used standards should only be a guide and clinicians should be made aware of the wide range of standard deviations.

Where there is no ultrasound facility radiological information may be sought for determining whether there is multiparity; the presence of fetal abnormality; maturation of fetus; maternal disproportion; and the placental site.

The first two requests present no great difficulty.

Maturation is best assessed by development of local standards, but standard tables provide a guide with plus or minus one and a half weeks being applied as the standard deviation (Russell, 1973). Assessment by fetal head size is more subject to error radiographically. It should be recollected that slight movement can readily blur a small ossific nucleus and render it invisible. The date of the appearance of fetal fat has not to our knowledge been studied in many communities. Whether the dietary state of the mother affects this is also unknown.

Disproportion standards invariably vary with race due to variations in size and degree of pelvic funnelling. Thus obstructed labour is infrequent in the Chinese of Hong Kong and Singapore in comparison with their sisters in West Africa. A comparative study between Welsh Caucasians and Nigerian negroes documents such racial pelvic differences (Kolawole *et al.*, 1978). African women have a greater sacral inclination, shorter A.P. brim measurements and generally smaller pelvic dimensions, despite being taller than the Caucasians.

A tragic sequel of obstructed labour is the development of vesico-vaginal fistulae. This is discussed later.

Multiparity is more frequent in some parts of the world. Thus in parts of West Africa twins occur about four times

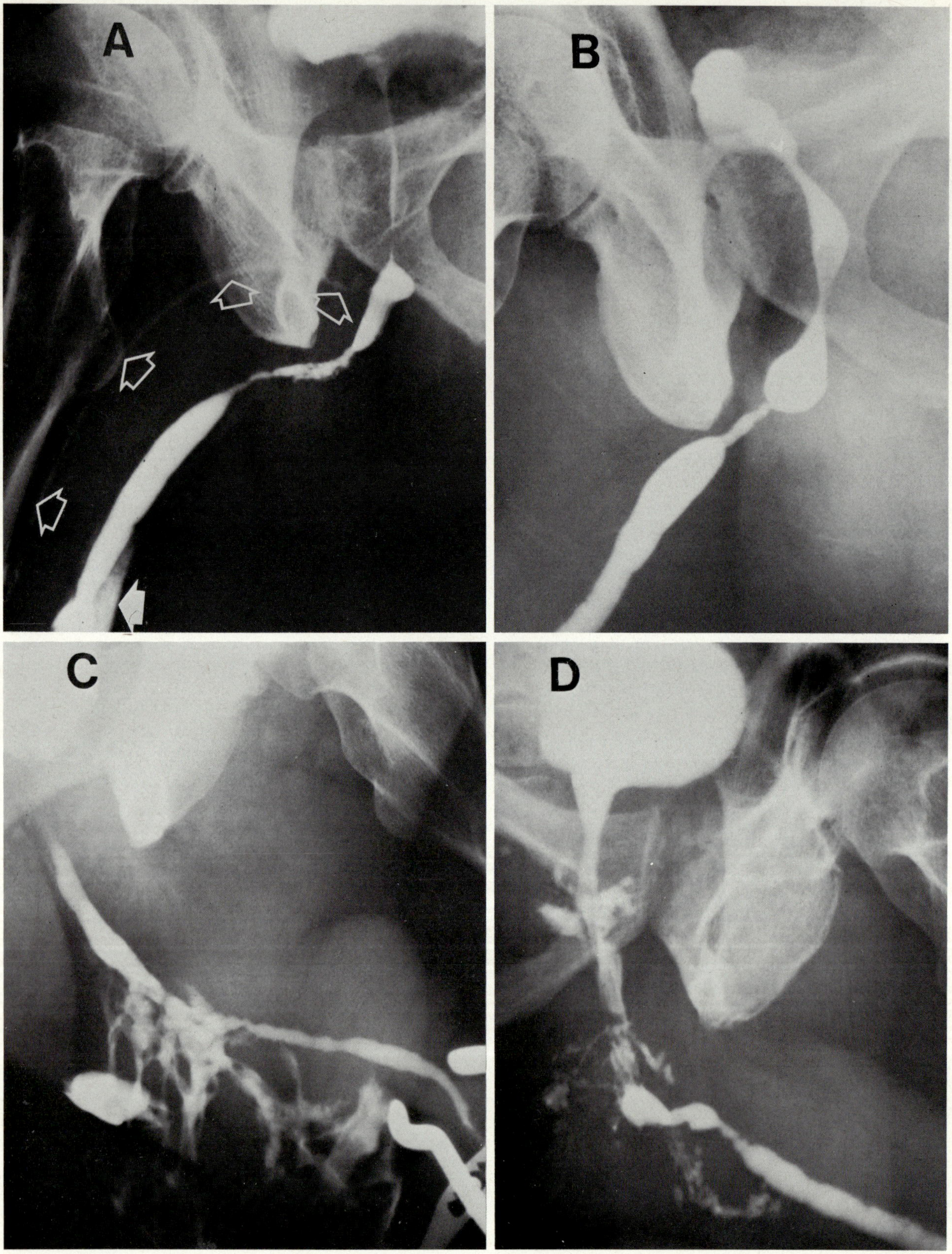

Fig. 6.14 Composite view of gonococcal urethral strictures demonstrated by retrograms. **A.** Posterior urethral stricture with anterior contrast extravasation (solid arrow) and faint draining contrast in dorsal vein (open arrow). **B.** Short stricture, **C, D** are complicated strictures with multiple fistulae—a watering can scrotum.

more frequently than in Europe. Conjoined twins are in consequence more frequent.

REFERENCES
Kolawole, T. M., Adamu, S. P. & Evans, K. T. (1978) Comparative pelvic measurements in Nigerian and Welsh women, *Clinical Radiology*, **29**, 85–90.
Russell, J. G. B. (1973) *Radiology in Obstetrics and Antenatal Paediatrics.* London: Butterworth.

ADVANCED EXTRA-UTERINE GESTATION

In under-doctored areas where there is a high prevalence of inflammatory pelvic disease ectopic gestations have a high incidence. If, for various circumstances, a ruptured tubal gestation maintains a placental blood supply the foetus will continue to develop. This combination of circumstances is not restricted to the tropics but can occur in deprived inner city areas in North America.

Patients may present because they have 'gone beyond their date' and not delivered or the diagnosis may be suspected on clinical grounds. Radiological confirmation is generally not difficult. Often the fetus is lying high with a bizarre lie that is sometimes transverse (Fig. 6.15). Close inspection may show that some fetal part lies closely applied to the maternal properitoneal translucent fat line—often in the flank. The best way to elicit this very reliable radiographic sign is to palpate the maternal abdominal wall to detect the most superficial hard foetal part. The patient is then rotated so that this portion of the abdomen is 'skylined' tangentially and a film obtained at about 60 kV. This technique will show such close approximation of maternal and foetal parts that there is no room for the 1 to 1·5 cm needed for the uterine wall (Fig. 6.16) (Cockshott & Lawson, 1972).

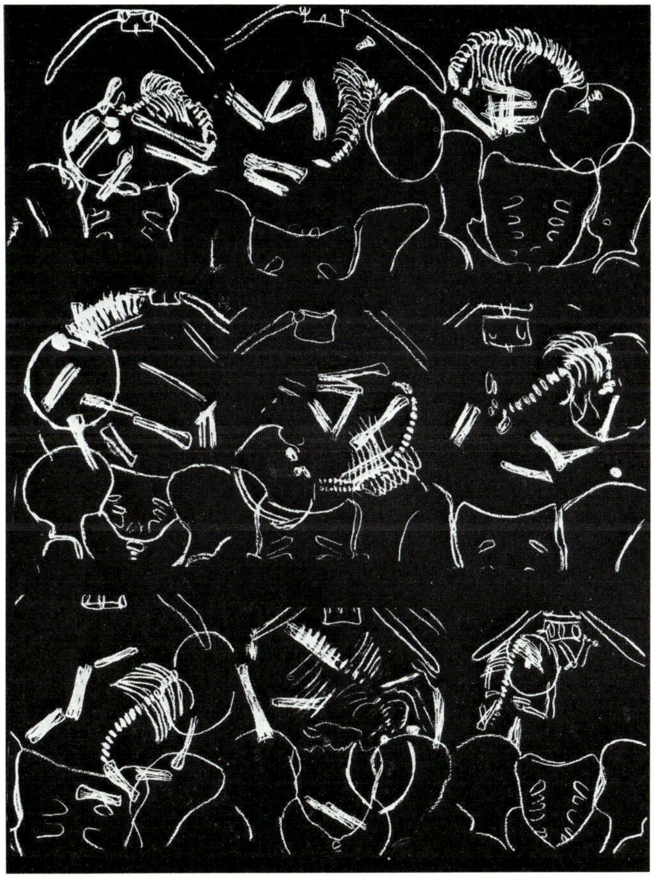

Fig. 6.15 Composite tracing of nine abdominal radiographs of mothers with extra-uterine gestation. The lies are bizarre and with transverse elements. (With acknowledgement to *Radiology*.)

Extra-uterine gestation sacs may become filled with excess fluid (hydramnios) or may become infected with the development of a pyogaseous abscess and abdominal ileus.

Confirmation of the diagnosis by hysterography is not indicated, since this is inadvisable in an intra-uterine gestation and unnecessary if one is confident of the diagnosis of an extra-uterine pregnancy.

Angiography has an occasional role in showing whether the placenta is still being perfused and in revealing the site of the placenta and its main feeding vessel (Cockshott & Lawson, 1972) (Fig. 6.17).

REFERENCE
Cockshott, W. P. & Lawson, J. (1972) Radiology of advanced abdominal pregnancy, *Radiology*, **103**, 21–29.

VESICO-VAGINAL FISTULAE

Vesico-vaginal fistulae (VVF) as a result of tissue necrosis following obstructed labour is a tragic problem in Africa, Arabia, India and New Guinea, and to a much lesser extent in some parts of the Far East.

Renal back pressure changes of varying degrees occur in a significant number, but this morphological alteration generally has little effect on function. Urography should be delayed at least three months post-partum to allow resolution of the obstetric dilatations of the urinary tract. The purpose of the study is not diagnosis, as this is only too evident to the patient and visible to the clinician, but rather to obtain a base line for the future and to provide information on the course of the ureters (Lawson & Stewart, 1967) (Fig. 6.18).

In initial films post-partal changes in the symphysis pubis will be evident. Most of such changes are non-specific and follow normal pregnancy. However, severe changes varying from frank osteitis to bony obliteration of the symphysis suggest considerable tissue necrosis and

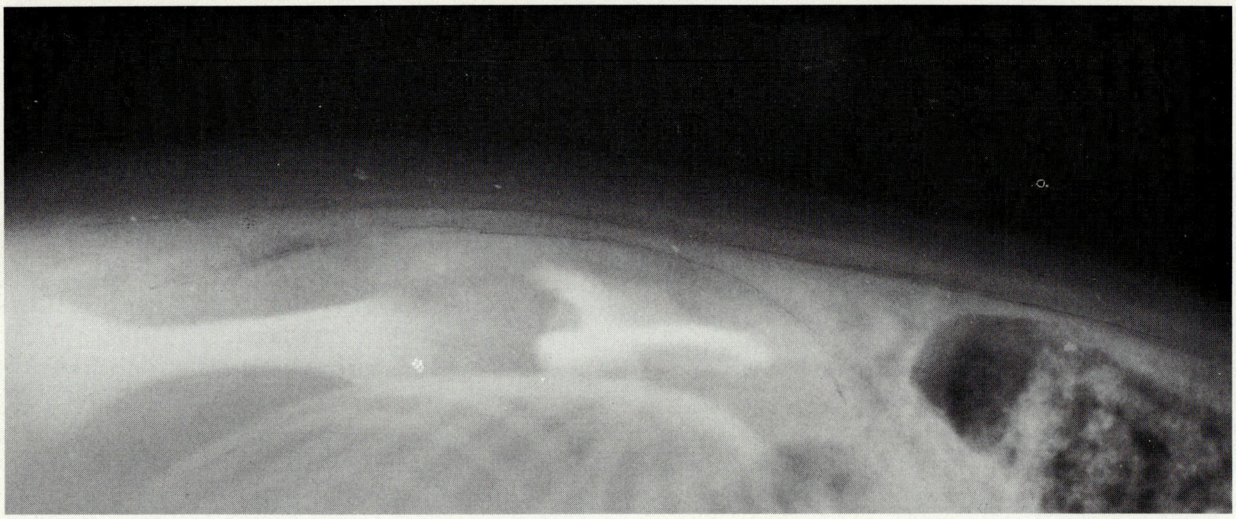

Fig. 6.16 Tangential abdominal view to show approximation of fetal fat and maternal peritoneal fat in an extra-uterine gestation.

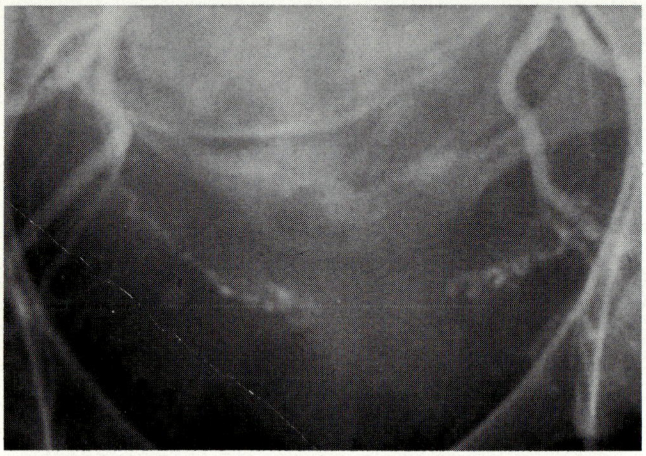

Fig. 6.17 Angiogram reveals small uterine vessels close together in advanced extra-uterine gestation.

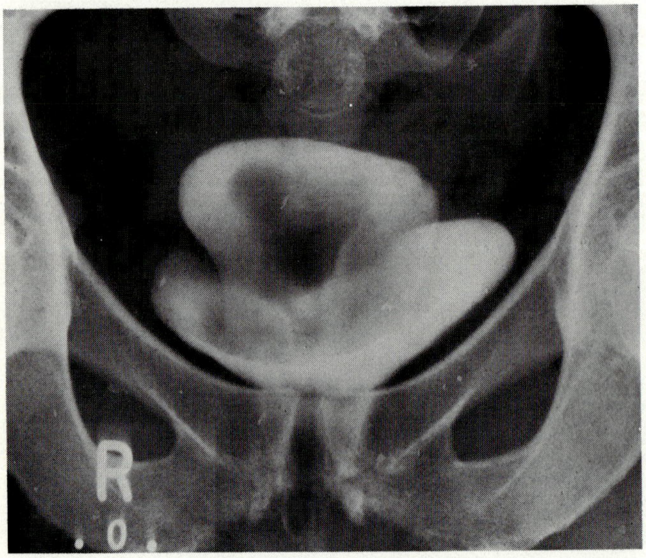

Fig. 6.18 Intravenous urogram in a woman with a V.V.F. Due to supine position contrast pours into the vagina, producing a central opacity superimposed on the bladder outline.

the presence of a low bladder-neck fistula with bone forming its anterior wall (Cockshott, 1973). In the plain film gas may be seen in the bladder and, less often, vesical calculi. Medial deviation of the ureters by scar tissue formation may be marked (Lagundoye *et al.*, 1976). Hydroureter and back pressure kidney changes of varying degree are frequent (Lagundoye *et al.*, 1976).

REFERENCES

Cockshott, W. P. (1973) Pubic changes associated with obstetric vesico-vaginal fistulae. *Clinical Radiology*, **24,** 241–247.

Lagundoye, S. B., Bell, D., Gill, G. & Ogunbode, O. (1976) Urinary tract changes in obstetric vesico-vaginal fistulae: a report of 216 cases studied by intravenous urography, *Clinical Radiology*, **27,** 531–539.

Lawson, J. B. & Stewart, D. B. (1967) *Obstetrics and Gynaecology in the Tropics.* London: Ballantyne.

MALIGNANT TROPHOBLASTIC DISEASE

In parts of the Far East (the Philippines, Malaysia, Hong Kong, Singapore), in New Guinea, West Africa, Mexico and the West Indies hydatidiform mole and chorion carcinoma are more prevalent than in Europe or North America. In the latter the incidence of hydatidiform mole is about one in 2500 pregnancies, whereas in Singapore it is one in 823 (Teoh *et al.*, 1971) and in Kuala Lumpur one in 302 pregnancies (Ang *et al.*, 1975). Similarly the rate of chorion carcinoma is greatly elevated, being as high as 17·4 per 100 000 in the Philippines (Baltazar, 1976). Thus in several tropical areas malignant trophoblastic disease (M.T.D.) is a serious problem. Since the results of chemotherapy of this disease are so encouraging early diagnosis is important. In the section on the chest we have already mentioned that certain lung changes in a woman

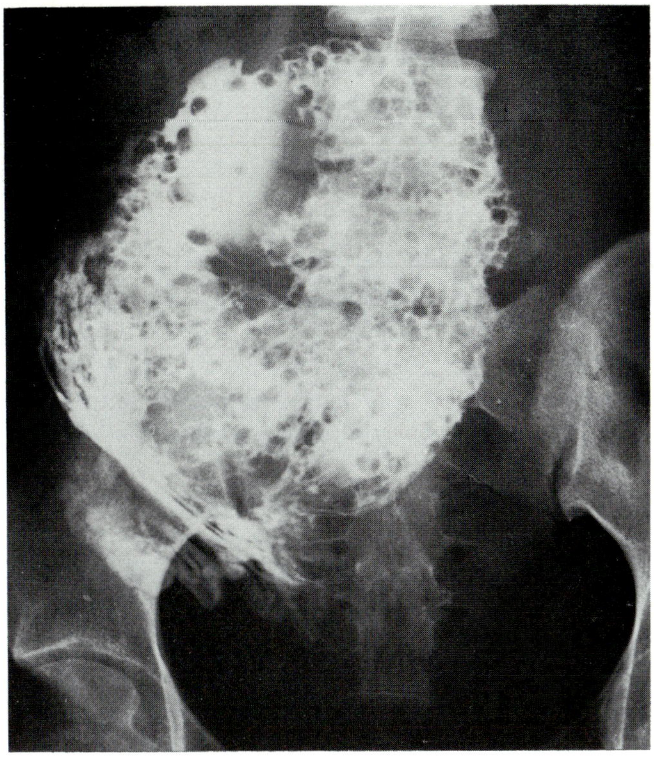

Fig. 6.19 Injection into uterine cavity in a patient with hydatidiform mole displays multiple filling defects due to vesicles. Contrast drains rapidly via uterine and ovarian veins. (Courtesy of Prof. Ang, Kuala Lumpur.)

of reproductive years may provide the first diagnostic indication of the presence of M.T.D.

The most benign form, hydatidiform mole, is generally not too difficult to suspect clinically, as too rapid growth of the uterus, bleeding, the passage of molar tissue etc. will alert the clinician. Confirmation by examination of molar tissue, ultrasound examination of the uterus, absence of fetal parts in a radiograph (exceptionally a normal and a molar pregnancy may coexist) and a positive pregnancy test with H.C.G. at a high titre generally make any further radiographic contrast study unnecessary, since histological material will be available after uterine evacuation. In cases of uncertainty amniography, or perhaps more correctly visualisation of the intervillous spaces, can be useful. This is most readily accomplished by direct injection of contrast by a percutaneous puncture into the uterine mass with the display of numerous filling defect due to hydropic vesicles (Fig. 6.19). The intervillous space drains by uterine and ovarian veins which are also often evident (Ang *et al.*, 1975). This form of study does not indicate whether there is any invasive area of chorio-adenoma destruens or chorion carcinoma. Furthermore if the os is patent and has been discharging such injection is contra-indicated because of the danger of the spread of sepsis. A further hazard is the possibility of inducing embolisation of trophoblastic tissue to the lung via the pelvic veins (Hendrickse *et al.*, 1965).

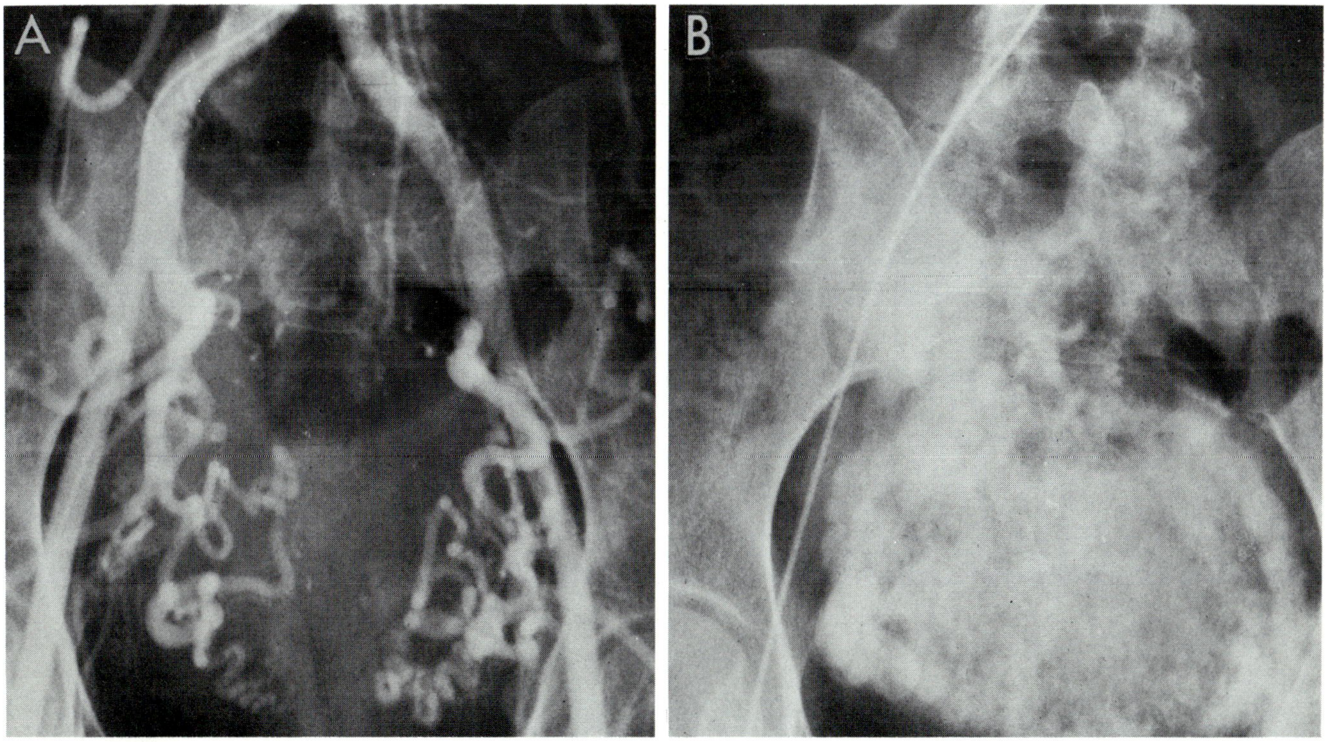

Fig. 6.20 A, B. Aortogram in chorion cancer showing dilated uterine and ovarian vessels and a large hypervascular uterine mass with early venous drainage.

Though angiography shows characteristic features in hydatidiform mole (Borell & Fernstrom, 1961; Cockshott *et al.*, 1964) we do not believe it is generally necessary in the typical clinical case at this stage but should be reserved for patients with a continuing high H.C.G. level, recurrent vaginal bleeding, or in individuals with high H.C.G. lung disease and an uncertain state in the pelvis.

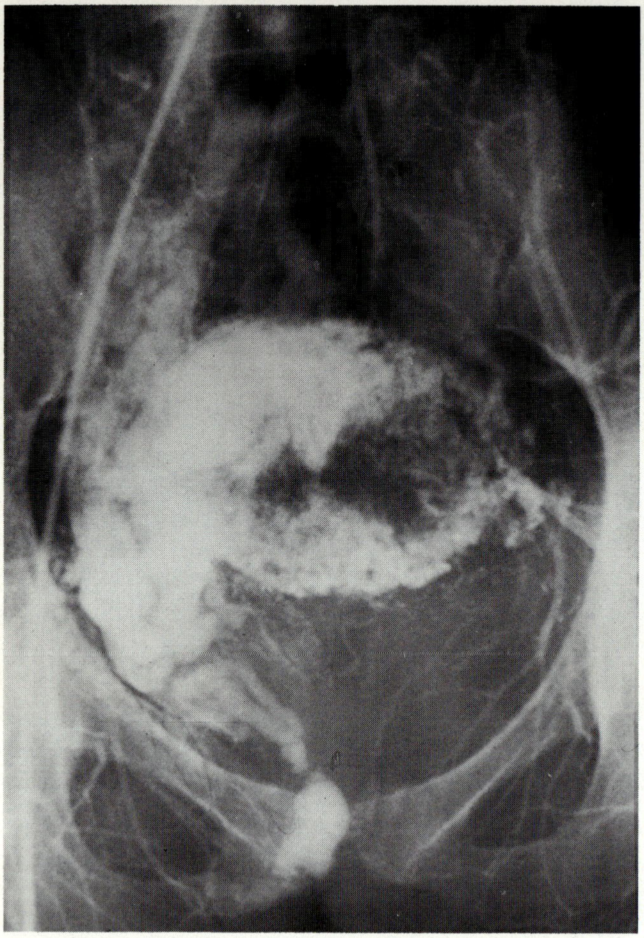

Fig. 6.21 Angiogram revealing a right-sided uterine mass with venous shunting and a hypervascular retropubic deposit.

Though arteriography does not necessarily define the degree of malignancy a focal vascular lesion is suspect, especially if associated with shunting (Fig. 6.20). Lesions not communicating with the endometrium lying in the myometrium, parametrium or retropubic area will be displayed (Fig. 6.21). Thus at times angiography can reveal lesions out of the reach of an exploring curette. Furthermore it is probably a safer procedure than curettage. Lastly, it can suggest the site of the most malignant area for a curettage to obtain appropriate tissue (Hendrickse *et al.*, 1964).

In some patients after chemotherapy a persistent vascular pelvic souffle may indicate the presence of an arteriovenous fistula through the site of a former M.T.D. deposit. This should not be confused arteriographically with active disease, since the features differ (Cockshott & Hendrickse, 1967).

In conclusion, a clinical and immunological diagnosis of hydatidiform mole is usually possible. Malignant trophoblastic disease can be more perplexing and then angiography may occasionally assist in diagnosis and management.

REFERENCES

Ang, A. H., Chan, W. F. & Ng, K. K. (1975) Amniography in the early diagnosis of hydatidiform mole, *British Journal of Radiology*, **48**, 979–981.

Baltzar, J. C. (1976) Epidemiological features of choriocarcinoma, *Bulletin World Health Organisation*, **54**, 523–532.

Borell, V. & Fernstrom, I. (1961) Hydatidiform mole diagnosed by pelvic angiography, *Acta Radiologica*, **56**, 113–118.

Cockshott, W. P., Evans, K. T. & Hendrickse, J. P. de V. (1964) Arteriography of trophoblastic tumours, *Clinical Radiology*, **15**, 1–8.

Cockshott, W. P. & Hendrickse, J. P. de V. (1967) Persistent arteriovenous fistulae following chemotherapy of malignant trophoblastic disease, *Radiology*, **88**, 329–333.

Hendrickse, J. P. de V., Cockshott, W. P., Barton, C. J. & Evans, K. T. (1964) Pelvic angiography in diagnosis of malignant trophoblastic disease, *New England Journal of Medicine*, **271**, 859–866.

Hendrickse, J. P. de V., Willis, A. J. & Evans, K. T. (1965) Acute dyspnoea with trophoblastic tumours, *Journal of Obstetrics and Gynaecology of the British Commonwealth*, **72**, 376–383.

Teoh, E. S., Dawood, M. Y. & Ratnam, S. S. (1971) Epidemiology of hydatidiform mole in Singapore, *American Journal of Obstetrics and Gynaecology*, **33**, 352–356.

7. Central Nervous System

PINEAL CALCIFICATION

Calcification of the pineal gland is a useful fixed point from which displacements of intra-cerebral contents may be gauged. In temperate countries when dealing with Caucasians the pineal can be radiographically located in approximately 46 per cent between the ages of 13 to 40 and in 69 per cent of individuals over the age of 40 (Adeloye & Felson, 1974). Figures for other parts of the world are considerably less in adults: 2 per cent in Uganda, 5 per cent in Nigeria, 9·9 per cent in Japanese, 14 per cent in Iranians, 15·6 per cent in Fijians and up to 24 per cent in Indians (Murphy, 1968; Daramola & Olowu, 1972; McKay, 1973). Adeloye & Felson confirmed the racial difference in incidence between U.S. whites and U.S. blacks, but in America the black subjects had a higher rate of pineal calcification than in a similar series from Africa. They attribute this to racial admixture in the new world.

In autopsy series where excised pineals have been directly radiographed calcification is much more obvious, since within the head adjacent tissues of closely related density cause considerable scattering and loss of contrast, causing problems in the perception of calcification. In Uganda at autopsy it has been shown that 43 per cent of pineals are calcified by the age of 10, so that it is the degree of calcification that differs in different societies (Poltera & Mugondi, 1976).

REFERENCES

Adeloye, A. & Felson, B. (1974) Incidence of normal pineal gland calcification in skull roentgenograms of black and white Americans, *American Journal of Roentgenology*, **122**, 503–507.

Daramola, G. F. & Olowu, A. O. (1972) Physiological and radiological implications of low incidence pineal calcification in Nigeria, *Neuroendocrinology*, **9**, 41–57.

McKay, R. T. (1973) Pineal calcification in Indians and Fijians, *Transactions of the Royal Society of Tropical Medicine and Hygiene*, **67**, 214–216.

Murphy, N. B. (1968) Carotid angiography in Uganda. Review of 100 consecutive cases, *East African Medical Journal*, **45**, 47–60.

Poltera, A. A. & Mugondi, S. G. (1976) The degree of calcification and the weight of pineal glands in Ugandan Africans, *African Journal of Medical Sciences*, **5**, 169–174.

CEREBRAL PARASITISM

Echinococcus granulosus

The brain is infected either during the early dissemination by oncospheres that have evaded the hepatic and pulmonary filtration to reach systemic vessels, or by rupture of a lung hydatid cyst into a pulmonary vein. Perhaps 3 per cent of cases of hydatid develop cerebral or spinal cord complications.

Because of the vascular route of infection most lesions are found in the territory of the middle cerebral arteries.

The cysts grow slowly and can reach considerable dimensions, extending from the cortex to the lateral ventricles. Becaue of their mass the skull will show the usual radiographic features of accommodation to a slowly expanding process which raises the intracranial pressure. Over the convexity of the lesion there may be calvarial erosion (Danziger & Bloch, 1975). Cyst calcification may be seen which can be curvilinear in part of the wall or more amorphous in part of a dead cyst. When the latter is seen the cyst is usually larger than the calcification indicates. Most lesions are in the parietal lobe and are clearly revealed in angiograms as avascular masses displacing vessels (Fig. 7.1).

Pneumo-encephalography is dangerous because of the elevated pressure and ventriculography, unless one is confident of the position of the cyst, is potentially even more hazardous, as the cyst may be punctured.

The ideal technique of investigation is computerised axial tomography but this is not readily available in most areas.

Coenurosis

Various species of multiceps are dog tapeworms that are found in areas associated with sheep raising. The brain of sheep is the normal site of development of the cystic stage. The cysts are single and have no daughter cysts, though numerous scolices can present as nodules within the cyst. The cysts may be rounded or nodular and racemose, so that their size can vary from 1 cm up to several centimetres. They may locate in man in relation to the ventricles, or in the meninges.

The effects of the cysts depends on their location. If

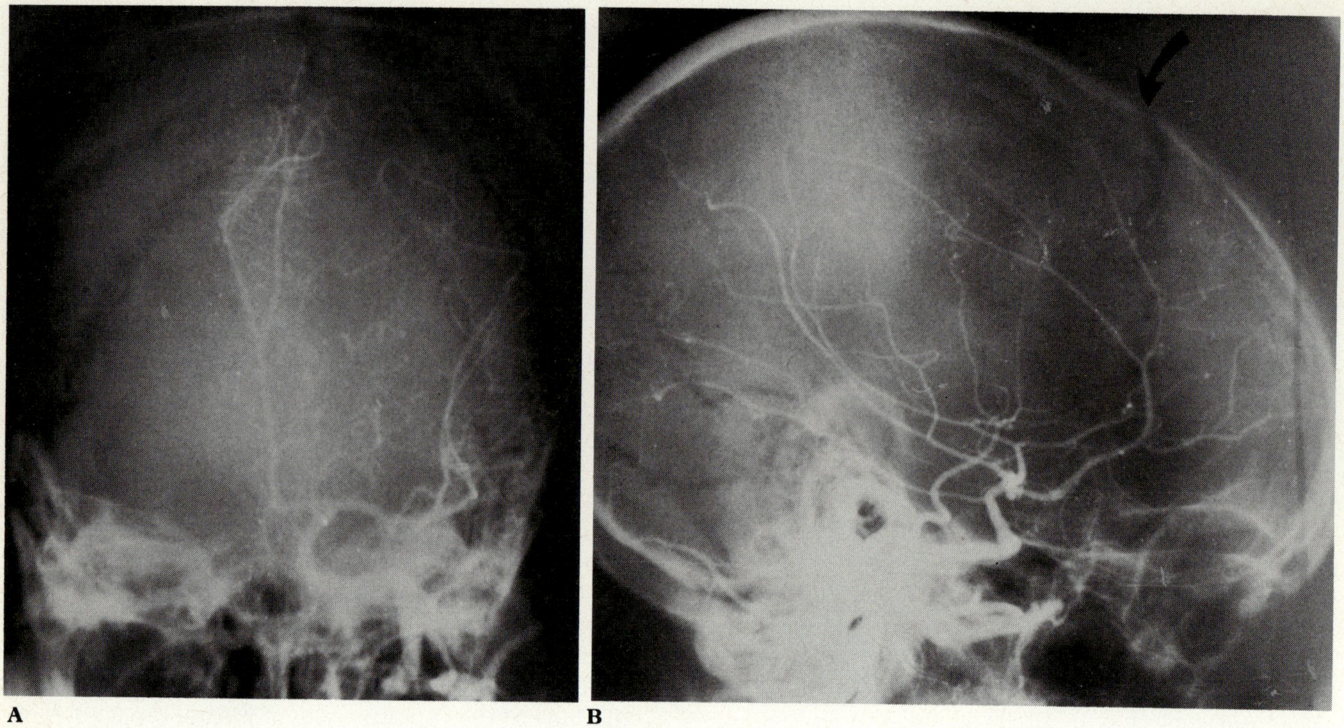

A B

Fig. 7.1 A, B. Frontal and lateral projections left carotid angiogram. Large avascular left-sided parietal mass displacing and stretching vessels. The large intracerebral hydatid has caused separation of the coronal suture (arrow). (Courtesy of Prof. L. Whittaker, Nairobi.)

they obstruct cerebrospinal fluid pathways obstructive hydrocephalus develops. With meningeal implication a cystic arachnoiditis can form which can cause direct pressure symptoms or obstruction of foraminae. Pneumoencephalography is the procedure of choice to detect these cysts.

When man is accidentally infected by certain Multiceps multiceps species they develop in the nervous tissue and the eye as a site of predilection. Such cases are recorded from Europe, Central America and Mexico and Brazil and South Africa. The majority of African cases develop cysts as subcutaneous granulomata (Templeton, 1971; Wilson *et al.*, 1972). This may be because the species is Multiceps brauni, which may not have the same neurotropic behaviour as in Brazilian and European multiceps.

REFERENCES

Danziger, J. & Bloch, S. (1975) Tapeworm cyst infestations of the brain, *Clinical Radiology*, **26**, 141–148.

Templeton, A. C. (1968) Human coenorus infection. A report of 14 cases from Uganda, *Transactions of the Royal Society of Tropical Medicine and Hygiene*, **62**, 251–255.

Wilson, V. C. L. C. (1972) Human coenurosis in Ghana, *Transactions of the Royal Society of Tropical Medicine and Hygiene*, **66**, 611–623.

Paragonimiasis

Brain involvement represents the most frequent of the extrapulmonary manifestations of paragonimiasis and has been estimated to occur in approximately a quarter of those affected by the disease in the Far East by P. westermani (Galatius-Jensen & Uhm, 1965). By contrast to date there have been no proven reports of this complication developing in the West African foci of paragonomiasis where P. africanus and P. uterobilateralis are the endemic pathogens. It is still too early to say whether this difference between Asia and Africa will be maintained, as Nwokolo in Nigeria (1977) has seen patients with paragonomiasis develop epilepsy.

According to Chung (1971) cerebral involvement is more frequent in males and children. The first symptoms develop three to ten months following lung symptoms.

The mode of invasion is controversial. (For details of the life cycle see pulmonary section pages.) Doubtless on occasions eggs may directly embolise from the lung foci to the brain, but this does not explain the more usual presence of intracranial flukes. Two main routes are believed to be used on the basis of animal experiments and human experience (Yokogawa, 1921). Aberrant young flukes migrate through the soft tissues of the neck along neurovascular bundles and enter the cranium via the jugular and other foraminae. In other instances the flukes enter into the venous system in the neck and enter the large sinuses—transverse and sagittal—and then pass through a side branch into the cerebral tissue. Whatever path is actually traversed, once in the brain the fluke appears to destroy by colliquative necrosis an area of the brain in its vicinity. This may be mechanically by venous infarction. The parasite eventually dies and little trace of it may be evident later except for ova that persist in the wall of the cystic cavity that has formed. The cyst-wall may show foreign body reaction and eventually calcifies. Such cysts may be multilocular or multiple and show a significant preponderance for the occipital, posterior parietal and posterior temporal zones and considerably less frequent involvement of the anterior parietal and temporal zones or frontal lobes or infratentorially. The right side is more involved than the left. Foci of arachnoiditis and dural adhesions are frequent. Spinal manifestations, usually epidural, are infrequent.

The symptoms obviously vary depending on the location of the cysts. A fit, rather than headache, is the usual presenting symptom. Pressure effects leading to hemiplegia, aphasia, visual disturbances, homonymous hemianopia are common. Meningitic features may be evident.

Several excellent clinical reviews of the radiologic appearances in cerebral paragonimiasis have come from South Korea (Kim & Bahk, 1964; Galatius-Jensen & Uhm, 1965; Oh, 1968).

Plain skull radiography will show an abnormality in over two-thirds of those affected. The features can be non-specific evidence of raised intracranial pressure evident in over a third, or intracranial calcification seen in about half of the patients.

Calcification is uncommon in Chinese and Japanese reports, though in Korea figures of 57 per cent (Oh, 1968) and 43 per cent (Galatius-Jensen & Uhm, 1965) have been recorded. The cause of the difference in incidence in various parts of the Far East is not known. The frequency and intensity of calcification certainly rises steadily with the duration of symptoms. It does not occur under a year and by three years over two-thirds of patients will have evidence of cranial calcification.

The varying forms of calcification have been classified into four types by Oh (1968). Punctate and curvilinear lines that can simulate that seen in gliomata; round nodular spotty deposits 5 to 7 mm in size with ill-defined borders; solitary well-defined rounded calcification 1 to 2 cm; and characteristic clusters of round well-defined dense calcification in walls of cysts (Fig. 7.2). It is likely that the patterns of calcification would ultimately become dense, well-defined 'cystic' type ultimately and that the more faintly opacified lesions are earlier phases in the dystrophic calcification process.

Calcification is supratentorial and mainly seen in the posterior half of the cerebral hemispheres. It is usually unilateral.

Pneumo-encephalography has been used to locate the space-occupying lesions. Authors remark that it may prove difficult to visualise the subarachnoid spaces due to the chronic arachnoiditis that results from the meningitis of the acute phase of cerebral invasion. In addition there may be blocks at interventricular foraminae. Cortical atrophy, ventricular dilatation and displacements are frequent. Filling into the ventricular system may also be seen.

Cerebral angiography provides further evidence of focal mass lesions and ventricular enlargement. Abnormal vessels, or capillary staining are not features of this parasitic process (Fig. 7.3).

The investigation of cases suspected of having intracranial involvement must be matched to the clinical and plain film findings. It is obvious that when available C.A.T. scanning provides the ideal non-invasive diagnostic tool. When calcification is present in a patchy 'early'

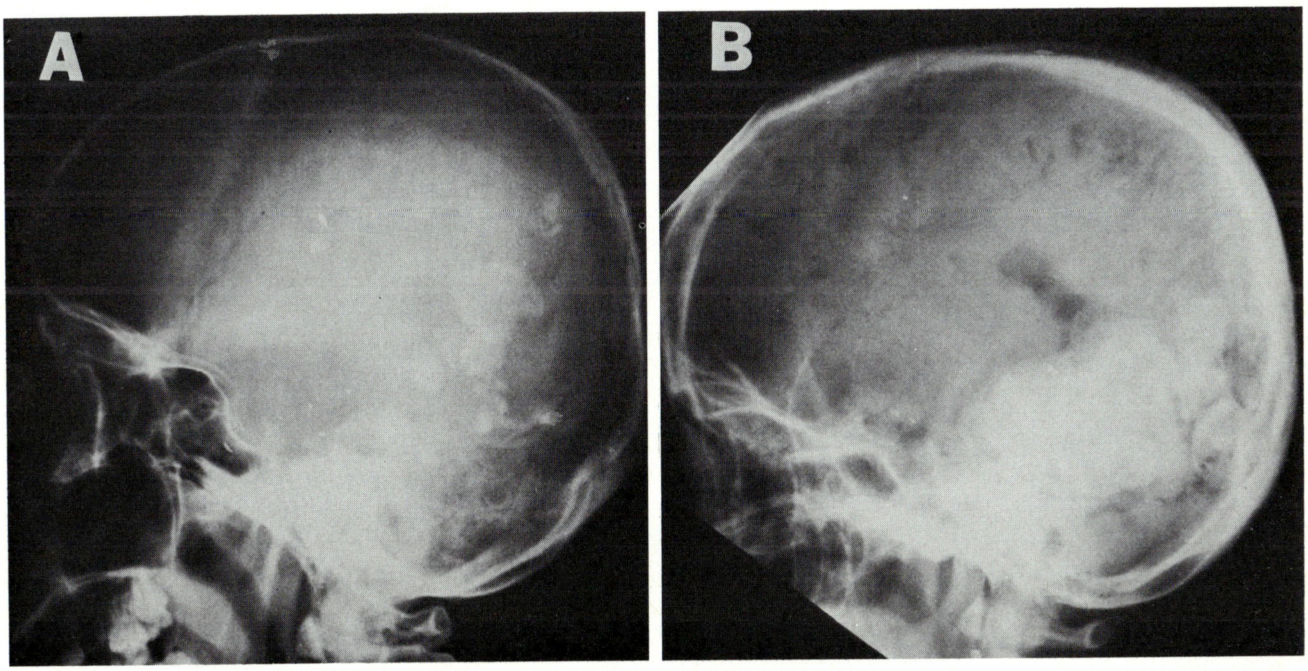

Fig. 7.2 **A.** Lateral skull with multiple calcified foci in tempero-occipital area. **B.** Pneumo-encephalogram with displacement of temporal and occipital horns by calcified paragonimus cysts. (Courtesy of Prof. Yong Whee Bahk, Seoul, Korea.)

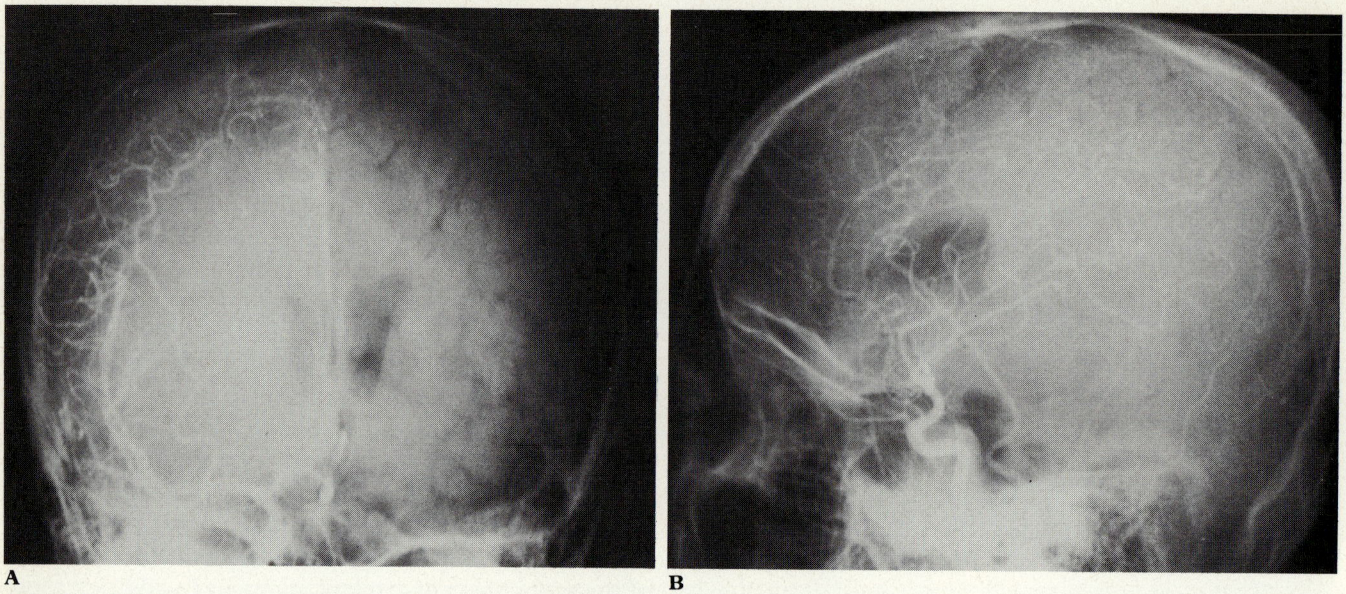

Fig. 7.3 A, B. Frontal and lateral views of right carotid angiogram and pneumo-encephalogram in patient with thalamic paragonimus cysts which are displacing the third and lateral ventricles to the left side and shifting the middle cerebral artery superiorly and forwards. (Courtesy of Prof. Yong Whee Bahk, Seoul, Korea.)

stage, differentiation from tuberculomata and tumours may be difficult. Pneumo-encephalography defines the extent of the parasitic involvement but may not be advisable if there is raised intracranial pressure. In such circumstances angiography can provide essential information for localisation rather than indicating a specific diagnosis. For that studies of the sputum and the chest radiographs are essential.

REFERENCES

Chung, C. H. (1971) Human paragonimiasis, *Pathology of Protozoal and Helminthic Diseases*, Marcial-Rojas, R. A. pp. 504–535. Baltimore: Williams & Wilkins.

Galatius-Jensen, F. & Uhm, I. K. (1965) Radiological aspects of cerebral paragonimiasis, *British Journal of Radiology*, **38**, 494–502.

Kim, E. O. & Bahk, Y. W. (1964) Intracranial calcifications in cerebral paragonimiasis, *British Journal of Radiology*, **37**, 670–673.

Nwokolo, C. (1977) Personal communication.

Oh, S. J. (1968) Roentgen findings in cerebral paragonimiasis, *Radiology*, **90**, 292–299.

Yokogawa, S. & Suyemori, S. (1921) An experimental study of the intracranial parasitism of the human lung fluke Paragonimus westermani, *American Journal of Hygiene*, **1**, 63–78.

CEREBRAL CYSTICERCOSIS

When man accidentally acquires the larval stage of Taenia solium, the pork tapeworm, by ingesting ova from proglottids, he becomes the intermediate host. The ova on reaching the stomach liberate oncospheres which penetrate the gut wall and attain the circulation. These settle mainly in muscle, the brain and cerebrospinal fluid pathways.

The relative proportion deposited in muscle and the nervous system is uncertain. When they are dead and calcified the muscular foci are readily apparent to radiologists, whereas the intracranial forms have been more difficult to display until the advent of computerised scanning. At autopsy the intracranial foci are more obvious to the pathologist than those located in muscle. Other viscera can be involved but this is unusual.

The infective vesicle Cysticercus cellulosae is usually about half by one centimetre and consists of a liquid-filled bladder containing an invaginated scolex with 22 or more hooklets. The scolax may degenerate and a larger form C. racemosus may form that can be several centimetres in size. These are generally found in areas of little resistance to expansion, as in the cerebrospinal fluid pathways.

The disease is particularly frequent in Mexico, Central and South America, Eastern Europe, Spain and Portugal, India and the Lebanon.

The radiological features depend on the sites involved and the stage of the disease.

Plain skull films rarely show sutural separation or evidence of raised intracranial pressure. For these changes to occur a lesion must be intraventricular to obstruct the cerebrospinal fluid pathways or cause obstructive arachnoiditis. Calcification in the cyst is a well-known radiographic sign but can only develop after the death of the larva and may take up to ten years to develop. Calcification is said to appear first in the scolex which is about 1 mm in size and difficult to detect. Later the cyst-wall is involved so that the focus of calcification is about 1 cm in size. Usually the lesions are multiple (Santin & Vargas, 1966; Soto Ramos & Palomino, 1967).

Many cysticerci are closely related to the ventricles and cerebrospinal fluid pathways and so can be shown by air

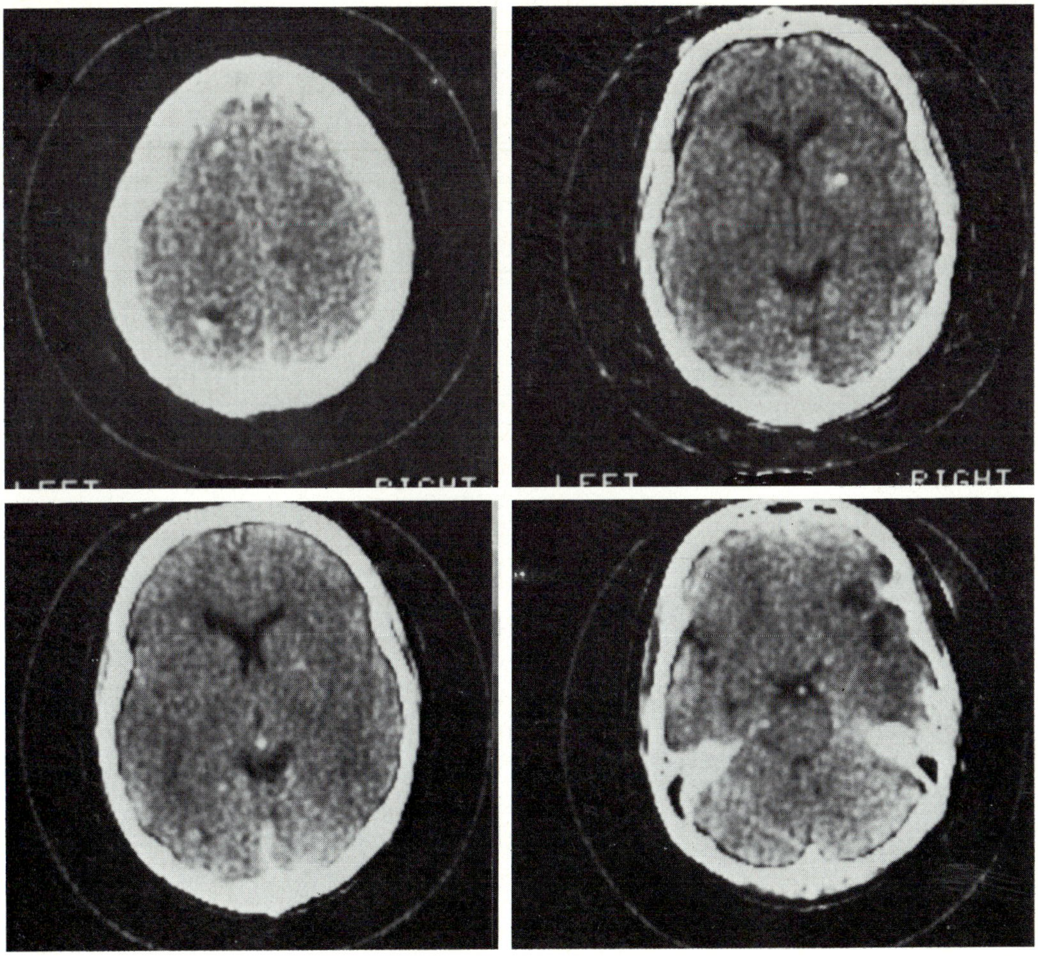

Fig. 7.4 Thirty-seven-year-old Guatemalan who had headache and grand mal for seven years. In his thigh calcification were evident in the musculature. The scan reveals a few calcified foci and a number of water density cysts. (Courtesy of Dr. Marjorie Le May, Boston.)

studies. Ventricles may be enlarged if obstructed or may show spherical filling defects protruding from the brain tissue (Santin & Vargas, 1966; Balaparameswararao & Dinakar, 1970; Danziger & Bloch, 1975). Basal changes of adhesive arachnoiditis are difficult to demonstrate.

Angiography provides little guidance, since the cysts are small and can be multiple.

When a computerised tomographic scanner is available it provides the best display of the lesions, as the cysts are clearly evident as rounded lesions containing water density and calcific foci are clearly revealed (Fig. 7.4) (Carbajal *et al.*, 1977).

Spinal deposit can be shown by myelography. Examination of cerebrospinal fluid can be of diagnostic assistance. These may be a high protein, pleocytosis, eosinophilia and a positive complement fixation test.

In suspected patients a radiograph of the thigh musculature is worthwhile. Calcification develops in muscle cysticerci before those in the brain.

REFERENCES

Balaparameswararao, M. S. & Dinaker, I. (1970) Ventriculographic features of cerebral cysticercosis, *British Journal of Radiology*, **43,** 267–268.

Carbajal, J. R., Palacios, E., Azar-Kia, B. & Churchill, R. (1977) Radiology of cysticercosis of the central nervous system including computed tomography, *Radiology*, **125,** 127–131.

Danziger, J. & Bloch, S. (1975) Tapeworm cyst infestation of the brain, *Clinical Radiology*, **26,** 141–148.

Santín, G. & Vargas, J. (1966) Roentgen study of cysticercosis of central nervous system, *Radiology*, **86,** 520–528.

Soto Ramos, B. & Palomino, L. (1967) Aspects radiologiques de la cysticercose cérébrale, *Annales de Radiologie*, **11,** 31–42.

TUBERCULOMA

At the beginning of this century a tuberculoma was the most common brain tumour reported in the English literature. Now they have virtually disappeared from Europe and North America but are still encountered in tropical Africa, India and Latin America (Asenjo *et al.*, 1951; Ramamarthi & Varadarajan, 1961; Higazi, 1963). In a

1968 Indian survey tuberculomas comprised 20 per cent of intracranial space occupying lesions overall and 47 per cent of those occurring in patients under the age of 15 (Sinh *et al.*, 1968).

These figures highlight that over 90 per cent of tuberculomas present in children. The mass may declare its presence early, if subcortical and causing fits, but usually it is not clinically apparent until there is evidence of raised intracranial pressure as well as, possibly, some localising signs. Though said to be more frequent in the posterior fossa in children they can be anywhere intracranially, and consequently cause no specific grouping of signs to suggest the diagnosis. Over 80 per cent of lesions are solitary in the brain, but careful search may indicate tuberculous foci elsewhere in the body, such as bone or lung etc.

Radiologically the classical features of raised intracranial pressure with suture diastasis is frequent. Calcification is noted in about 5 per cent of cases. It may be faint specks, amorphous nodules, curvilinear or a mixture of these. Calcification depends on duration of the caseous process and degree of glial reaction. The opacified area is the tip of the iceberg, so that one can be sure that the mass is larger than the visible portion.

Ventriculography may show displacements of dilatation of the ventricles according to the location of the masses. 'Young' lesions can be vascular enough to give a blush due to the hyperaemic brain surrounding a tuberculoma (Berlin, 1963). As the process matures it is avascular and its site can only be inferred by vessel displacement.

C.A.T. scanning is obviously the optimal study for this condition (Price & Danziger, 1978).

With specific antituberculous therapy the dreaded surgical complication of T.B. meningitis can be controlled so that the surgical prognosis is good.

Following tuberculous meningitis from whatever cause, calcification of the meninges around the base and the chiasmatic and ambient cysterns can develop as soon as 18 months, and in nearly all cases by the end of three years after treatment (Lorber, 1958).

REFERENCES

Asenjo, A., Valladares, H. & Fierro, J. (1951) Tuberculomas of brain—report of one hundred and fifty-nine cases, *Archives Neurology and Psychiatry*, **65**, 146–160.

Berlin, L. (1963) Tuberculoma of the brain, *American Journal of Roentgenology*, **90**, 1185–1192.

Higazi, I. (1963) Tuberculoma of brain, *Journal of Neurosurgery*, **20**, 378–386.

Lorber, J. (1958) Intracranial calcification following tuberculous meningitis in children, *Acta Radiologica*, **50**, 204–210.

Price, H. I. & Danziger, A. (1978) Computed tomography in cranial tuberculosis, *American Journal of Roentgenology*, **130**, 769–771.

Ramamarthi, B & Varadarajan, M. G. (1961) Diagnosis of tuberculoma of the brain, clinical and radiological correlation, *Journal of Neurosurgery*, **18**, 1–7.

Sinh, G., Pandya, S. K. & Dastur, D. K. (1968) Pathogenesis of unusual intracranial tuberculomas and tuberculous space occupying lesions, *Journal of Neurosurgery*, **29**, 149–159.

CEREBRAL AFRICAN TRYPANOSOMIASIS

On the basis of a pneumo-encephalographic study of 20 patients with trypanosomiasis with cerebral symptoms, Collomb and his co-workers (1956) documented that ventricular enlargement was consistently present. This involved a generalised dilatation of the lateral ventricles; with rounding of the third ventricle in the anterior posterior films; occasional dilatation of the aqueduct; basal cystern enlargement; and inconstant widened sulci over the cerebral hemispheres. These changes were related by the authors to the demyelinating process mediated by immunologic factors that caused a generalised atrophic loss of volume which at times could also implicate the brain stem.

In Chagas' disease sometimes the prefrontal gyri are atrophied and there is reduction in nerve cells, so that similar changes may be present though we have not seen these demonstrated.

REFERENCE

Gallais, P., Collomb, H., Miletto, G., Dutertre, J. & Berard-Badier (1956) L'Apport de la pneumo-encéphalographie dans l'interpretation et le classement de l'encéphalite de la trypanosomiase humaine africaine, *Medicine Tropicale*, **16**, 6–46.

INFLAMMATORY PARAPLEGIA

Tuberculosis

Tuberculosis is still the dominant aetiology of paraplegia in the young of many developing countries. Paraplegia may develop during the active phase of bone infection or be tardy in onset as a consequence of the long-standing angular deformity.

In the active phase the paraplegia is spastic in nature, but should it later convert into a flaccid form, the prospects of neurologic recovery are poor.

The classical radiologic features of Pott's disease are well known. The vertebral body destruction with erosive loss of the intervertebral disc and extension to the next body; the development of paraspinal abscesses; the collapse of vertebral bodies and wedge angular deformities require no emphasis (Konstam & Blesovsky, 1962). However, about 2 per cent of patients have anomalous presentations that are not as well recognised.

Sometimes there is destruction of a vertebral pedicle, unilaterally or bilaterally, at a single level, or extending over several segments. Extension into the posterior aspect of a vertebral body or the head of a rib are common (Fig. 2.10). The disc normally remains preserved. This combination of changes is at first suggestive of metastases, apart from the presence of paravertebral abscesses. Dimorphic yeasts can give a similar picture. As surgery and chemotherapy have much to offer to these patients who are paraplegics or have nerve deficits, prompt diagnosis is important (Bell & Cockshott, 1971).

The second unusual tuberculous variety is uniform collapse of a body with maintenance of intact discs above and below to produce a Calve-like vertebra plana of the type that is normally associated with histiocytosis. However, the sclerosis that is often present and the older age of occurrence may be useful differentiating points (Figs. 2.7 and 2.11).

Thirdly there may be involvement of the other posterior appendages of the vertebra: lamina, transverse processes and the spinous process. Once again yeast infections can simulate this (Fig. 2.12).

REFERENCE
Bell, D. & Cockshott, W. P. (1971) Tuberculosis of the vertebral pedicles, *Radiology*, **99,** 43–48.

YEAST VERTEBRAL GRANULOMATA

Yeast vertebral granulomata have been discussed in detail in the osseous section of this book. Foci of infection are found in red marrow, and as the spine is the largest depot of this tissue in adults, vertebrae are frequently implicated. Bodies, appendages or the pedicles may be the first site of involvement (Fig. 7.5). Extradural extension of a fungal granuloma may lead to neurologic disturbances (in 10 per cent of cases of Histoplasma duboisii infections) or collapse and deformity can cause pressure effects on the cord (Cockshott & Lucas, 1964). The fungal granuloma do not appear to be proteolytic and the intervertebral discs remain preserved until late in contrast to vertebral tuberculosis.

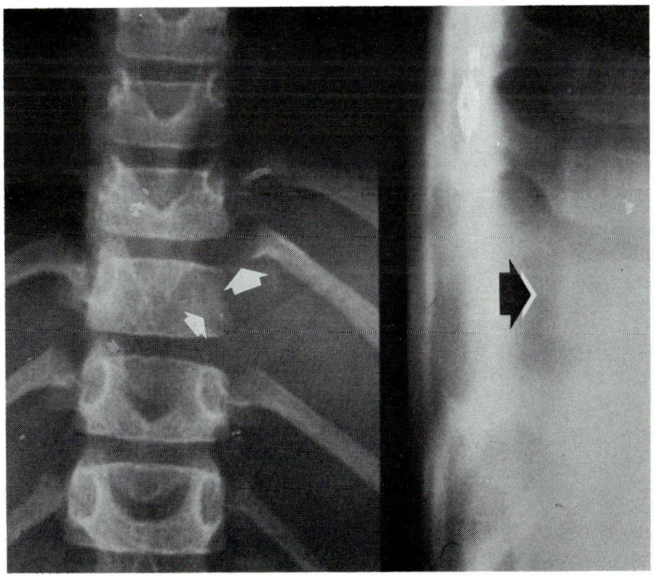

Fig. 7.5 There is loss of the left pedicle of D10 (small white arrow) and destruction of the transverse process of D10. This has resulted in upwards subluxation of the left 10th rib (large white arrow). In the tomogram the black arrow indicates the focal pedicular destruction by H. duboisii granuloma.

Extradural mycetoma has been recorded (Lytton & Hamilton, 1975).

REFERENCES
Cockshott, W. P. & Lucas, A. D. (1964) Radiological findings in Histoplasma duboisii infections, *British Journal of Radiology*, **37,** 653–660.
Lytton, D. G. & Hamilton, D. R. (1975) Mycetoma in Papua New Guinea with special reference to a case of extradural mycetoma, *Papua New Guinea Medical Journal*, **18,** 61–65.

BRUCELLOSIS MYELOPATHY

Brucellosis myelopathy is said to occur in about 2 per cent of those with bone brucellosis (Ganado & Craig, 1958). This has been described in the section on the skeleton earlier in the book. Cord compressive symptoms are usually due to extradural extension of bony foci, though primary brucellar meningitis has been reported. Spine tomography and myelography are indicated when the diagnosis is suspected.

REFERENCE
Ganado, W. & Craig, A. J. (1958) Brucellosis myelopathy, *Journal of Bone and Joint Surgery*, **40A,** 1380–1387.

PARAPLEGIA AND CEREBRAL SCHISTOSOMIASIS

Nervous tissue can be implicated in Bilharzia by embolisation of ova via collaterals to the paravertebral plexus of Batson and its intracranial connections; by embolisation from aberrant trematodes in the pulmonary vascular bed; or migrating schistosomes in venous pathways close to the spine, producing localised ova deposition. Frequently focal collections of eggs with tuberculoid granulomas are noted histologically in the paraspinal lesions, suggesting that the latter mode is responsible for most dural and extradural masses. Some authors believe that in addition to mechanical factors, the presence of circulating immune complexes may be important in the development of myelitis (Cohen *et al.*, 1977).

S. japonicum is the chief offender for cerebral lesions, possibly because the smaller ova embolise more readily.

This is further borne out by the greater number of cerebral cases. This in a series of 97 patients with nervous involvement 60 were due to S. japonicum with 58 involving the brain and only 2 the cord, whereas of the 11 S. haematobium, in 8 the cord was affected, and 7 of the 26 S. mansoni patients had implication of the cord (Marcial-Rojas, 1971).

Sometimes a focal deposition of eggs may cause symptoms suggestive of a brain tumour.

Radiology is of more specific value in the study of cord compression syndromes. Myelography can disclose an intramedullary expanding process, a subdural or epidural mass, or a complete block (Hutton & Holland, 1960; Odeku *et al.*, 1968; Lechtenberg & Vayda, 1977). Complete transverse myelitis is not rare. The development of sensory paraparesis and sphincter disturbance can be rapid.

REFERENCES

Cohen, J., Capildeo, R., Clifford-Rose, F. & Pallis, G. (1977) Schistosomal myelopathy, *British Medical Journal*, **1**, 1258.

Hutton, P. W. & Holland, J. T. (1960) Schistosomiasis of the spinal cord, *British Medical Journal*, **2**, 1931–1933.

Lechtenberg, R. & Vayda, G. A. (1977) Schistosomiasis of the spinal cord, *Neurology*, **27**, 55–59.

Marcial-Rojas, R. A. (1971) *Pathology of Protozoal and Helminthic Diseases*. p. 404. Baltimore: Williams & Wilkins.

Odeku, E. L., Lucas, A. O. & Richards, D. R. (1968) Intramedullary spinal cord schistosomiasis, *Journal of Neurosurgery*, **29**, 418–423.

GUINEA WORM PARAPLEGIA

Migration of female guinea worms to aberrant sites when the intensity of infection is high is well known. Location in the extradural vertebral tissues results in cord pressure. If infection develops the abscess that forms can lead to vascular effects that may in addition produce an ischaemic focal myelitis. Accordingly early diagnosis is imperative if there is to be relief of neurologic deficits.

Myelography will show the presence of an extradural space-occupying mass that initially deviates the flow of contrast media and at a later stage results in a total block (Reddy & Valli, 1967; Mitra & Haddock, 1970). Since the radiological features are not in themselves specific the only pre-operative indications of the nature of the aetiology would be evidence of a recent 'crop' of emerging guinea worms and perhaps the presence of eosinophilia.

REFERENCES

Mitra, A. K. & Haddock, D. R. W. (1970) Paraplegia due to guinea worm infection, *Transactions of the Royal Society of Tropical Medicine and Hygiene*, **64**, 102–106.

Reddy, C. R. R. M. & Valli, V. V. (1967) Extradural guinea worm abscess, *American Journal of Tropical Medicine and Hygiene*, **16**, 23–25.

GNATHOSTOMIASIS

Gnathostomiasis due to Gnathostoma spinigerum, is acquired by eating raw fish in endemic areas in Thailand, Indonesia and some other parts of South East Asia. The parasites may burrow in the nervous system in the course of their migration. If the spinal cord is implicated by haemorrhagic tunnels paraplegia may develop (Sorasuchart *et al.*, 1968). These intramedullary lesions are not expansile and it is doubtful if there would be any significant changes on myelography. With the cerebral forms the mortality is high. Eosinophilia of the cerebrospinal fluid may help in the diagnosis.

This condition should not be confused with the syndrome of eosinophilic meningitis that has a somewhat similar geographic distribution, though more extensive, as Hawaii, Tahiti, Okinawa and New Caledonia are also implicated. The causative agent Angiostrongylus cantonensis is a lung parasite of the rat. Man becomes infected by eating contaminated raw snails.

REFERENCE

Sorasuchart, A., Khunadorn, N. & Edmeads, J. (1968) Parasitic diseases of the nervous system in Thailand, *Canadian Medical Association Journal*, **98**, 859–867.

SPINAL HYDATID DISEASE

Spinal hydatid disease can be due to extension of a bony focus that extradurally compresses the cord, but meningeal cysts, which can be multiple, can cause paraplegia in the absence of vertebral foci.

HAEMATOPOIESIS PARAPLEGIA

The formation of thoracic extramedullary blood-forming masses in chronic haemolytic anaemias, such as spherocytosis, or in failures of haemoglobin synthesis, as in Thalassaemia, has at times resulted in extradural cord compression (Sorsdahl *et al.*, 1964). A multilobulated paravertebral mass is evident in the chest film. No bone erosion can be detected, by myelography reveals contiguous extradural masses. Needle biopsy is the preferred means of confirming the diagnosis.

REFERENCE

Sorsdahl, O. S., Taylor, P. E. & Noyes, W. D. (1964) Cord compression by extramedullary hematopoiesis, *Journal of the American Medical Association*, **189**, 343–347.

BURKITT'S PARAPLEGIA

In those parts of the world where Burkitt's tumour is prevalent spinal and dural deposits causing paraplegia are not rare. This complication developed in 18 per cent of children with Burkitt's in Ibadan (Cockshott & Evans, 1963). Only Pott's disease was a more frequent cause of childhood paraplegia. Other types of lymphoma in children cause paraplegia infrequently. Thus at the Mayo clinic there was only a single example of lymphoma out of 56 spinal tumours in children seen in the space of 25 years (Dodge *et al.*, 1956).

Children usually present with an initial flaccid paraplegia rather than the spastic form of Pott's disease. The sensory changes vary from paraesthesia to complete loss of sensation.

In the investigation of a patient where the paraplegia may be due to a lymphoma deposit, views of the jaws and any other part of the body where there may be a focal destructive osseous lesion can be helpful. This is of particular value when the plain films of the spine do not disclose any abnormality. A paravertebral mass can, however, be detected in 61 per cent of patients. It is usually noted on both sides of the vertebral column and can extend in length from 2 to 6 vertebral segments. The visible extravertebral soft tissue masses do not necessarily correspond to the level of cord involvement, which can be at multiple levels.

Vertebral bone destruction is present in 39 per cent of paraplegics. Compression of a vertebral body and erosion of a pedicle were most frequent. The intervertebral disc space remains intact (Fig. 7.6).

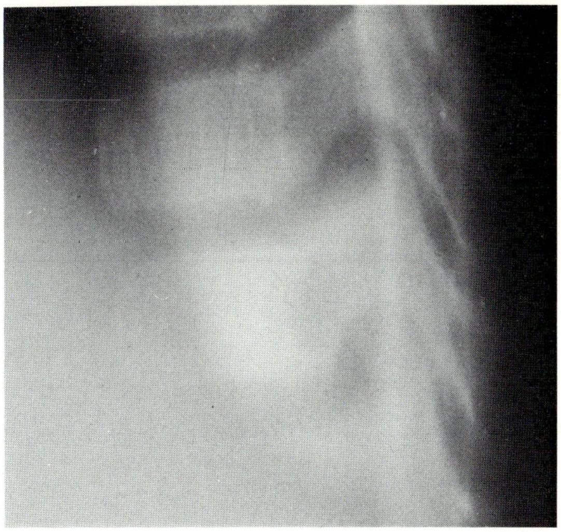

Fig. 7.6 Tomogram showing localised destruction of posterior part of D11 in a six-year-old boy with Burkitt's lymphoma. (Courtesy of *British Journal of Radiology*.)

Myelography defines the exact site affected by extradural compression. If more than one level appears to be involved both cysternal and lumbar puncture may prove necessary to obtain precise morphologic information. However, as surgery offers little hope of improvement once flaccid changes are present there is little purpose in subjecting a patient to a full work-up. With chemotherapy there is no need for such precise localisation, but myelography can be useful to monitor progress so that it is unnecessary to remove the oily contrast medium.

REFERENCE
Cockshott, W. P. & Evans, K. T. (1963) Childhood paraplegia in lymphosarcoma (Burkitt's tumour), *British Journal of Radiology*, **36**, 914–920.

Index

Italicized entries denote species

Abscess
amoebic of liver, 130–132
amoebic of lung, 167–168
guinea worm, 5, 13
pyomyositis, 12, 13
splenic, 146–148
Adenopathy
abdominal tuberculosis, 105, 107
inguinal tuberculosis, 15
Kaposi sarcoma, 17
leptospirosis, 156, 157
lymphogranuloma venereum, 117, 118
plague, 155, 156
pulmonary tuberculosis, 161
Ainhum, 69
Altitude
chest configuration, 191
Alveolar hydatid, *see* liver hydatid
Ameloblastoma, 82
Amoebiasis
colonic, 113–117
liver, 130–132
lung, 167, 168
pericardium, 168
pleura, 167
Amoeboma, 114, 116
Anaemia
cardiac effects, *see* Haemoglobinopathy, 175–177
Aneurysms
left ventricular, 178–180
primary arteritis, 197–200
tuberculous, 201
Angiostrongylus cantonensis, 226
Angiostrongylus costaricensis, 112
Anisakiasis
bowel, 94
stomach, 92–94 *see* Helminthoma
Ankylostoma duodenale, *see* Hookworm
Annular subvalvar left ventricular aneurysm, 178, 180
Aortic dilatation
aortic pan arteritis, 197–201
hypertension, 177
Aortic pan arteritis
aneurysm, 197–200
calcification, 197, 199
hypertension, 198
Armiliffer species, 10
Arthritis
guinea worm, 6
rheumatoid, 86
septic, 85
tropical polyarthropathy, 87
Ascariasis, 97, 98
biliary tree, 136, 137
intestinal, 97, 98
obstructive, 98
pulmonary larval, 150–152

Aspergillosis
osteomyelitis, 60, 61
paranasal, 60

Basidiobolus species, 14
Bile ducts
ascariasis, 136
calculi, 130
carcinoma, 139
cholangitis, Far Eastern, 142
clonorchiasis, 137, 138
fascioliasis, 139, 140
hydatid, 133, 134
opisthorchiasis, 137–139
Bilharzia, *see* Schistosomiasis
Black fat pneumonia, 170, 171, 191
Bladder
calculi, 205–206
carcinoma, 206, 209
fistulae (VVF), 215–216
schistosomiasis, 206–210
Blastomyces dermatitidis, 51
Blount's disease, 71
Bone infections
Allescheria boydii, 56–59
aspergillus osteitis, 60
aspergillus paranasal, 60
Blastomyces, 51, 55
brucellosis, 36–38
Coccidioides immitis, 51
Cryptococcus neoformans, 52
donovanosis, 40
granuloma inguinale, 40
Histoplasma capsulatum, 51
Histoplasma duboisii, 52–54
hydatid disease, 66, 67
Klebsiella, 39–40
Lagochilascaris, 65
leprosy, 46–50
Leptosphaeria senegalensis, 56–59
Madurella species, 56–59
melioidosis, 38, 39
mycetoma, 56–59
nocardia, 56–59
osteomyelitis, 27
osteomyelitis variolosa, 64, 65
paragonimiasis, 65
Phialaphora species, 56–59
rhinoscleroma, 62, 63
salmonella, 41, 42, 76, 172
schistosomal, 65, 66
smallpox, 64, 65
sporotrichosis, 58
Streptomyces species, 56–59
treponematosis, 42–46
tropical ulcers, 34–46
tuberculosis, 27–34
vaccinial osteomyelitis, 63
yaws, 42–46

Brucellosis
of bone, 36–38
myelopathy, 38, 225
Brugia malayi see Filariasis
Buerger's disease, 202–204
Burkitt's lymphoma
bone, 81, 82
cardiac, 195, 196
gastro-intestinal, 127–128
mediastinal, 195, 196
paraplegia, 227
ribs, 173, 174
vertebral, 227
Buruli ulcer, 14, 15

Calcification
amoebic abscess, 132
aneurysms, 197, 199, 201
Armilifer infections, 10
cysticercosis, 9, 222, 223
endomyocardial fibrosis, 185
guinea worm, 5
helminthoma, 112
hydatid, 166, 211, 219
injection site, 1
kikuyu bursa, 2, 3
left ventricular aneurysm, 180
leprosy, in nerve, 48
loaisis, 6
myositis ossificans, 3
oesophagostomum, 112, 113
onchocerciasis, 7
pancreatic lithiasis, 144
paragonomiasis, 221
pericardial, 196, 197
phleboliths, 204, 205
pineal, 219
porocephalosis, 10, 11
primary arteritis, 197–199
sarcocystis, 7
schistosomiasis, 206, 207
sparganosis, 8
tuberculous, 162, 224
tumoral calcinosis, 1–3
Calculi
biliary, 130
enteroliths, 107, 108
pancreatic, 144
urinary, 205, 206
vesical, 205, 206
Cancrum oris, 88
Capillariasis
C. aerophila, 152
C. philippinensis, 101
Cardiomegaly
African trypanosomiasis, 190
anaemia, 175, 176
Burkitt's lymphoma, 195–196
Chagas' disease, 188–190

Cardiomegaly—cont.
endomyocardial fibrosis, 184
idiopathic, 182
L.V. aneurysm, 178–181
sickle cell anaemia, 177
Carpal fusions, 70
Caustic stricture, 89, 90
Chagas' disease
cardiomyopathy, 188–190
megacolon, 118, 119
mega-eosophagus, 88, 89
sigmoid volvulus, 119, 122, 123
Chlamydia trachomatis,
Cholangitis
ascariasis, 136, 137
clonorchiasis, 137–139
Far Eastern, 142
opisthorchiasis, 137–139
Chyluria, filarial, 210, 211
Clonorchiasis, 137–139
Coccidioides immitis, 51
Coenurosis, 219, 220
Colitis
amoebic, 113–117
angiostrongylus costaricensis, 112
Crohn's, 120
dysenteric, 120, 121
fungal, 119
Gastrodiscoides species, 113
helminthoma, 112, 113
lymphogranuloma, 117, 118
non-specific, 120
schistosomal, 110, 111
strongyloidal, 95, 96
trichuris, 119, 120
tuberculous, 105–110
ulcerative, 120
Colon
carcinoma, 128
diverticula, 126
Congenital dislocation of hip, 70, 71
Contracaecum osculatum, 112
Cryptococcus neoformans, 52
Cysticercosis
cerebral, 222, 223
muscle, 9
spinal, 226

Dirofilaria immitis
coin lesion, 169
embolic, 169
pulmonary eosinophilia, 149
Disaccharide malabsorption, 126
Diverticular disease (colon), 126
Donovanosis, 40
Dracunculosis, *see* Guinea worm
Drechslera hawaiensis, 61
Duodenum
hookworm, 94
strongyloidiasis, 95, 97
tuberculosis, 105, 110
ulcer, 91–92
ulcer biliary fistula, 91

Echinococcus granulosus, *see* Hydatid disease
Echinococcus multilocularis, *see* Hydatid disease
Echinostoma ilocanum, 113
Endomycardial fibrosis, 184–188
Entomopthora coronata, 61, 62
Eosinophilia, *see* Pulmonary eosinophilia
Eosinophilic meningitis, 226
Extra-uterine gestation, 215, 216

Fascioliasis, 139, 140
Fasciolopsis, 112
Filariasis
calcification in, 6–7
chyluria, 210, 211
loa loa, 6, 7
lymphoedema, 16, 17
onchocerciasis, 7
pulmonary eosinophilia, 149, 150
pulmonary hypertension, 193
pulmonary infarction, 169
Fluorosis, 24–26

Gallbladder calculi, 130
Gangosa, *see* Yaws
Gangrene, symmetrical, 201, 202
Gastric outlet obstruction
carcinoma, 127
corrosive antritis, 89, 90
peptic ulcer, 91, 92
tuberculosis, 105–110
Gastric ulcer, 91, 92
Gastrodiscoides hominis, 113
Giardiasis, 98–100
Gnathostoma spinigerum
paraplegia, 226
pulmonary eosinophilia, 153
Goundou, *see* Yaws
Granuloma inguinale, 40
Guinea worm,
abscess, 12, 13
arthritis, 85
calcification, 5, 6
paraplegia, 226

Haemoglobinopathy, 73–79
haemoglobin C, 76
haemoglobin E, 79
sickle cell disease, 74–76
sickle thalassaemia, 79
thalassaemia, 77
Heart calcification
aneurysms, 178–80
endomyocardial fibrosis, 184–188
hydatids, 194–195
tuberculosis, 196
Helminthoma, 112, 113
angiostrongyliasis, 112
anisakiasis, 92, 94
Contracaecum osculatum, 112
hookworm, 94
Spirurida physalopteridae, 112
Hepatoma, 84, 142–143
Hernia, obstruction, 122
Heterophyes heterophyes, 113
Histoplasma capsulatum, 51
Histoplasma duboisii, 52
bone, 52–54
colon, 119
paraplegia, 225
subcutaneous, 14
Hookworm
cardiac effects, 176–177
small bowel, 94
Hydatid disease
bone, 66, 67
cardiac, 194, 195
cerebral, 219, 220
hepatic, 133–136
pulmonary, 165–166
renal, 211, 212
spinal, 226

Hydrocephalus
African trypanosomiasis, 224
cysticercosis, 223
hydatid, 219
paragonomiasis, 220, 221
Hypertension, 177, 198

Idiopathic cardiomegaly, 182–184
Idiopathic tropical sprue, 125, 126
Inermicapsifer madagascarensis, 103
Injection calcification, 1
Intestinal obstruction, 122–124
ascariasis, 98
herniae, 122
intussusception, 122
sigmoid volvulus, 122
typhoid, 103–105

Kaposi sarcoma, 17–21, 128
Kwashiorkor, 23, 175

Lagochilascaris minor, 66
Leprosy, 46, 50
Leptospirosis, 156–158
Lymphangiography
abdominal tuberculosis, 105, 107
chyluria, 210, 211
filariasis, 16–17
inguinal, 15
Kaposi sarcoma, 18
leptospirosis, 157
lymphoedema, 16
lymphogranuloma venereum, 117, 118
Lymphoedema, 15–17
filarial, 16–17
tuberculosis, 15
Lymphogranuloma venereum, 117, 118
Lymphoma
Burkitt's, 81, 82, 173, 195, 196, 227
Mediterranean, 129
Lymphostatic verrucosis, 15

Madura foot, 56–59
Madurella grisea, 59
Madurella mycetomi, 59
Malabsorption pattern
capillariasis, 101
disaccharide deficiency, 126
fasciolopsis, 112
giardiasis, 98–100
intestinal Burkitt, 127, 128
intestinal tuberculosis, 105–110
Mediterranean lymphoma, 129
sprue, 125, 126
strongyloidiasis, 95, 96
Malaria shock lung, 169
Malignant trophoblastic disease, 171, 216–218
pulmonary hypertension, 193
Malnutrition
chest wall, 154, 175
giardiasis, 99
growth, 22, 23
heart size, 175
maturation, 22
Mastoid
Lagochilascaris species, 66
Paragonimus species, 65
Poikilorchis congolensis, 66
tuberculosis, 31
Measles pneumonia, 154, 155
Mediterranean lymphoma, 129
Megacolon, 119
Mega-oesophagus, 88, 89

Melioidosis
bone, 38, 39
pulmonary, 158–159
Metagonimus yokogawai, 113
Mossy Foot, 16
Mucocele, 72
Multiceps multiceps, 220
Mycetoma, 56–59, 225
Mycobacteria ulcerans, 14, 15
Myositis ossificans, 3–5, 26
sleeping sickness, 5
tetanus, 3, 4, 5, 68

Nasal dentition, 72
Necator americanus, *see* Hookworm
Nocardiosis
mycetoma, 56–59
pulmonary, 159, 160

Oesophagostomum apiostomum, 13, 112
Oesophagus
carcinoma, 127
Chagas' disease, 88
corrosive stricture, 89, 90
Onchocerciasis, 7
Opisthorchiasis
cholangiocarcinoma, 139
cholangitis, 137–139
Osteomyelitis, *see* Bone infection
Osteomyelitis variolosa, 64, 65

Pancreatic lithiasis, 144
Papillary necrosis, 212, 213
Paracoccidioides brasiliensis, 51, 55
Paragonomiasis
cerebral, 220–222
mastoid, 65
pulmonary, 162–165
Paraplegia
brucellar, 38, 225
Burkitt, 227
fluorosis, 26
fungal, 225
gnathostomiasis, 226
guinea worm, 226
haematopoiesis, 226
schistosomal, 225
tuberculosis, 224
Peptic ulceration, 90–92
Perforation, intestinal
amoebiasis, 115
ascariasis, 97
helminthoma, 113
typhoid, 104
Pericardial disease, 196
African trypanosomiasis, 190
amoebic, 168
endomyocardial fibrosis, 184–187
purulent, 196
splenic abscess, 197
tuberculous, 196
Phialaphora jeanselmei, 59
Phlebitis,
deep venous, 204
tropical, 15, 16
Phleboliths, 204, 205
Phycomycosis, 14
Pineal calcification, 219
Plague, 154–156
Pneumomediastinum, 154, 155
Pneumothorax,
Poikilorchis congolensis, 65
Polyps, intestinal, 110, 111
Porocephalosis, 10

Portal hypertension, 140, 141
Primary arteritis, *see* Aortic pan arteritis
Pseudomonas pseudomallei, 158, 159
Pubis, post-partal, 72
Pulmonary amoebiasis, 167
Pulmonary embolism, 193, 194, 204
cardiac hydatids, 167, 194, 195
dirofilarial, 169
filarial, 169
schistosomal, 191, 192
tumour, 193
venous, 193, 194
Pulmonary eosinophilia, 149–153
ascariasis, 149–152
capillariasis, 152
filarial, 149, 150
gnathostomiasis, 153
schistosomal, 149
strongyloides, 153
Pulmonary fibrosis, 170, 171, 191
Pulmonary hypertension, 190–195
altitude, 191
black fat, 191
filarial, 193
hydatid, 194, 195
pyogenic cholangitis, 193
schistosomal, 191, 192
sickle cell, 177
smoke pollution, 191
trophoblastic tumour, 193
Pyomyositis, 12, 13

Rallietina celebensis, 103
Rhinoentomopthoromycosis, 61, 62
Rhinophycomycosis, 61, 62
Rhinoscleroma, 62, 63
Ribs
histoplasmosis, 52, 54
infarcts, 172, 173
lymphoma, 173, 174
melioidosis, 38
salmonella, 172
tuberculosis, 173
Rickets, 24, 25

Salmonella, 41, 76, 172
Sarcocystis, 7
Schistosomiasis
calcification, 207
carcinoma, 206, 209
cerebral, 225, 226
intestinal, 110, 111
paraplegia, 226
portal hypertension, 141
pulmonary hypertension, 191, 192
urinary, 206–210
Septic arthritis, 85
Sickle disease
bone infarcts, 73–74
heart, 177
kidney, 212
rib involvement, 172, 173
salmonella infection, 41, 172
spleen, 145–148
spondylitis, 41, 42
Sigmoid volvulus
Chagas' disease, 119
Sinuses
aspergillosis, 60
Burkitt's lymphoma, 81, 82
ectopic dentition, 72
mucocele, 72
rhinophycomycosis, 61, 62

Sparganosis
calcification, 8, 9
helminthoma, 112, 113
Spirurida physalopteridae, 112
Spleen
abscess, 146–148
calcification, 146
size, 145
tropical splenomegaly, 148
Sporotrichosis, 59
Sprue, 125, 126
Stomach
anisakiasis, 92–94
lymphoma, 127
Streptomyces species, 59
Stricture, colon
amoebic, 113–117
helminthoma, 112, 113
Kaposi, 128
lymphogranuloma, 117, 118
schistosomal, 110
tuberculous, 108, 109
Stricture, oesophagus
corrosive, 89, 90
malignant, 127
Stricture urethra, 213, 214
Strongyloides stercoralis
intestinal, 95–97
pulmonary, 153

Taenia saginata, 101, 102
Taenia solium, *see also* Cysticercosis, 103
Takayashu arteritis, 197–200
Tapeworms, 101–103
Tetanus,
fractures, 67–69
myositis ossificans, 3, 4
Tibia vara, 71
Treponematoses, 42–46
Trichuris trichiuria, 119, 120
Tropical
enteropathy, 125, 126
eosinophilia, 149–153
phlebitis, 15, 16, 204
polyarthropathy, 87
splenomegaly, 148
sprue, 125, 126
ulcer, 34–36
Trypanosome cruzii, *see* Chagas' disease
Trypanosomiasis, African
cardiomyopathy, 190
cerebral, 224
myositis ossificans, 3
Tuberculosis
aortitis, 201
cerebral, 223, 224
duodenal, 105–110
gastric, 105–110
ileo-caecal, 105–110
left bronchus, 161
lymphoedema, 15
mesenteric, 105, 107
osseous, 27–34
paraplegia, 224, 225
pericardial, 196
pulmonary, 160–162
renal, 205
spine, 27–34
Tumoral calcinosis, 1–3
Typhoid, 103–105, 130

Umbilical sepsis, 140
Urethral stricture, 213

Vaccinial osteomyelitis, 63
Varicose veins, 204
Venous thrombosis, 204
Vesical calculi, 205–206
Vesicovaginal fistulae, 215–216
Volvulus, sigmoid, 119, 122, 123
  small bowel, 124

Whipworm, 119, 120
Wuchereria bancrofti, 7

Yaws, 42–46
Yersinia enterocolitis, 94, 121
Yersinia pestis, 154–156